Tumors of the Peripheral Nervous System

AFIP Atlas
of
Tumor Pathology

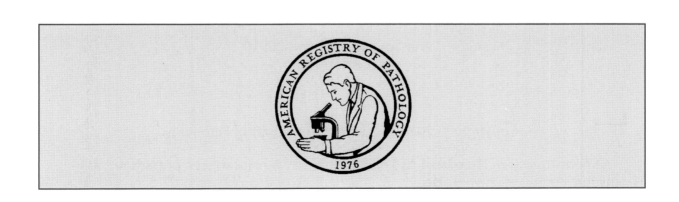

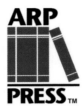

ARP PRESS

Silver Spring, Maryland

Editorial Director: Mirlinda Q. Caton
Production Editor: Dian S. Thomas
Editorial Assistant: Magdalena C. Silva
Editorial Assistant: Alana N. Black
Copyeditor: Audrey Kahn

Available from the American Registry of Pathology
Silver Spring, Maryland 20910
www.arppress.org
ISBN 1-933477-30-X
978-1-933477-30-5

AFIP ATLAS OF TUMOR PATHOLOGY

Fourth Series
Fascicle 19

TUMORS OF THE PERIPHERAL NERVOUS SYSTEM

by

Cristina R. Antonescu, MD
Attending Pathologist
Director of Bone and Soft Tissue Pathology
Memorial Sloan-Kettering Cancer Center
New York, New York

Bernd W. Scheithauer, MD
Consultant in Pathology
Mayo Clinic
Professor of Pathology
Mayo Graduate School of Medicine
Rochester, Minnesota

James M. Woodruff, MD
Attending Pathologist
Memorial Sloan-Kettering Cancer Center
Associate Professor of Pathology
Cornell University Medical College
New York, New York

Published by the
American Registry of Pathology
Silver Spring, Maryland
2013

AFIP ATLAS OF TUMOR PATHOLOGY

EDITORS' NOTE

The Atlas of Tumor Pathology has a long and distinguished history. It was first conceived at a cancer research meeting held in St. Louis in September 1947 as an attempt to standardize the nomenclature of neoplastic diseases. The first series was sponsored by the National Academy of Sciences-National Research Council. The organization of this formidable effort was entrusted to the Subcommittee on Oncology of the Committee on Pathology, and Dr. Arthur Purdy Stout was the first editor-in-chief. Many of the illustrations were provided by the Medical Illustration Service of the Armed Forces Institute of Pathology (AFIP), the type was set by the Government Printing Office, and the final printing was done at the Armed Forces Institute of Pathology (hence the colloquial appellation "AFIP Fascicles"). The American Registry of Pathology (ARP) purchased the Fascicles from the Government Printing Office and sold them virtually at cost. Over a period of 20 years, approximately 15,000 copies each of nearly 40 Fascicles were produced. The worldwide impact of these publications over the years has largely surpassed the original goal. They quickly became among the most influential publications on tumor pathology, primarily because of their overall high quality, but also because their low cost made them easily accessible the world over to pathologists and other students of oncology.

Upon completion of the first series, the National Academy of Sciences-National Research Council handed further pursuit of the project over to the newly created Universities Associated for Research and Education in Pathology (UAREP). A second series was started, generously supported by grants from the AFIP, the National Cancer Institute, and the American Cancer Society. Dr. Harlan I. Firminger became the editor-in-chief and was succeeded by Dr. William H. Hartmann. The second series' Fascicles were produced as bound volumes instead of loose leaflets. They featured a more comprehensive coverage of the subjects, to the extent that the Fascicles could no longer be regarded as "atlases" but rather as monographs describing and illustrating in detail the tumors and tumor-like conditions of the various organs and systems.

Once the second series was completed, with a success that matched that of the first, ARP, UAREP, and AFIP decided to embark on a third series. Dr. Juan Rosai was appointed as editor-in-chief, and Dr. Leslie Sobin became associate editor. A distinguished Editorial Advisory Board was also convened, and these outstanding pathologists and educators played a major role in the success of this series, the first publication of which appeared in 1991 and the last (number 32) in 2003.

The same organizational framework applies to the current fourth series, but with UAREP and AFIP no longer functioning, ARP is now the responsible organization. New features include a hardbound cover and illustrations almost exclusively in color. There is also an increased emphasis on the cytopathologic (intraoperative, exfoliative, or fine needle aspiration) and molecular features that are important in diagnosis and prognosis. What does not change from the three previous series, however, is the goal of providing the practicing pathologist with thorough, concise, and up-to-date information on the nomenclature and classification; epidemiologic, clinical, and pathogenetic features; and, most importantly, guidance in the diagnosis of the tumors and tumorlike lesions of all major organ systems and body sites.

As in the third series, a continuous attempt is made to correlate, whenever possible, the nomenclature used in the Fascicles with that proposed by the World Health Organization's Classification of Tumors, as well as to ensure a consistency of style. Close cooperation between the various authors and their respective liaisons from the Editorial Board will continue to be emphasized in order to minimize unnecessary repetition and discrepancies in the text and illustrations.

Particular thanks are due to the members of the Editorial Advisory Board, the reviewers (at least two for each Fascicle), the editorial and production staff, and the individual Fascicle authors for their ongoing efforts to ensure that this series is a worthy successor to the previous three.

Steven G. Silverberg, MD
Ronald A. DeLellis, MD
William A. Gardner, MD
Leslie H. Sobin, MD

PREFACE

This monograph describes the spectrum of neoplasms, hamartomas, hyperplasias, reactive lesions, and inflammatory pseudotumors arising from or associated with peripheral nerves. Included are lesions affecting spinal nerves and extradural portions of cranial nerves. Specifically excluded from this discussion are lesions of the optic nerve, a central nervous system structure.

Peripheral nerve tumors are generally classified as soft tissue tumors, but they differ significantly from most neoplasms in this category. Notable differences include the frequent association of nerve sheath tumors with genetic disorders and the origin of a majority of malignant nerve sheath tumors from neurofibroma, a benign precursor lesion. Furthermore, tumors of peripheral nerves are histologically diverse and arise in a complex tissue with distinctive anatomic compartments. Nerves consist not simply of axons but of specialized ensheathments and compartments. These include: 1) Schwann cells that enwrap axons and form the boundary for the inner limits of the endoneurium; 2) the endoneurium, which consists of capillaries, fibroblasts, macrophages, and mast cells; 3) a specialized barrier layer, the perineurium, that forms the outer limit of the endoneurium; and 4) the epineurium, an external layer of fibroadipose tissue. Vascular elements are present in all three layers. Hamartomas, hyperplasias, reactive lesions including true neuromas and inflammatory pseudotumors, as well as neurofibromas typically involve several if not all these components of peripheral nerve. Although, theoretically, neoplasms may arise from Schwann cells, perineurial cells, fibroblasts, and other cells comprising the nerve sheaths, most peripheral nerve neoplasms are in fact derived from Schwann cells. The latter are neuroectodermal cells of neural crest origin, ones unique to peripheral nerves. The histologic diversity so characteristic of peripheral nerve tumors is, in large part, attributable to the metaplastic repertoire of neoplastic Schwann cells which produce not only a variety of collagens and melanin, but display a remarkable capacity for divergent differentiation toward rhabdomyoblasts, chondroblasts, and epithelial cells of varying type. Also, unique to peripheral nerves are perineurial cells, tumors of which are rare. Whereas vascular and adipose tumors of peripheral nerves have been reported, ones presumably derived from fibroblasts are not well defined.

The authors believe that this volume will be a useful reference for pathologists, residents, and students for many years.

Cristina R. Antonescu, MD
Bernd W. Scheithauer, MD
James M. Woodruff, MD

ACKNOWLEDGMENTS

On September 19, 2011, Dr. Bernd Scheithauer passed away prematurely at age 65. His departure is a tremendous loss for our entire pathology community and huge circle of personal friends. He touched many lives with his boundless generosity and willingness to teach anyone who wanted to learn. He enthusiastically delivered all of his contributions to this Fascicle, but was not able to see it in its final version. We dedicate this latest Fascicle tour de force to his career and his remarkable professional accomplishments. He will be truly missed, and his legacy will live on in our hearts forever.

The authors are also grateful to the following physicians for their discussions and for providing invaluable illustrations: Thomas Seemayer, Omaha, NE; Christopher Fletcher, Boston, MA; John Fetsch, Washington, DC; and Ioannis Koutlas, Minneapolis, MN. We would also like to thank our dedicated assistants, Denise Chase, Mayo Clinic, and Milagros Soto, Memorial Sloan-Kettering Cancer Center, for their relentless assistance with secretarial and editorial help.

Cristina R. Antonescu, MD
James M. Woodruff, MD

Permission to use copyrighted illustrations has been granted by:

American Medical Association
    JAMA 1962;180:522. For figures 3-31 and 3-32.
    JAMA 1997;278:52. For tables 15-2 and 15-3.

Elsevier
    South Med J 1975;68:89. For figure 3-15.

Lippincott
    Am J Surg Pathol 1995;19:1326. For figure 11-10.
    Am J Surg Pathol 1996;20;1214. For figure 4-2A.
    Neurosurgery 1994;35:128-29. For figures 6-5 and 6-8.
    Neurosurgery 2010;67:1135, 1139-41. For figures 11-3 right, and 11-4 through 11-7.

Mayo Foundation
    Atlas of Neuropathology. New York: Gower; 1988. For figures 3-4, 3-24, 8-5, 15-8C, 15-21C and D, 15-24, 15-25 above, 15-26 above, 15-28, 15-29A, and 15-30.

Springer
    Die Krankhaften Geschwülste: Dreissig Vorlesungen, gehalten während des Wintersemesters 1862-1863 an der Universität zu Berlin. Berlin: Verlag von August Hirschwald; 1863:II. For figure 15-1.

Wiley
    Cancer 2000:89:1580-82. For figures 12-46A and B.
    J Peripher Nerv Syst 2010;15:218. For figure 4-1.

CONTENTS

1. Peripheral Nerve Tumors: Overview 1
   Historical Background 2
      Early Key Investigators 2
   Specimen Presentation, Handling, and Assessment 6
2. The Normal Peripheral Nervous System 11
   Development 11
   Gross Anatomy 11
   Microanatomy 14
      Peripheral Nerves 14
      Sensory and Autonomic Ganglia 20
      Interstitial Cells of Cajal 25
      Specialized Nerve Endings 26
   Immunohistochemistry 28
   Ultrastructure 30
3. Reactive Lesions 33
   Traumatic Neuroma 33
   Localized Interdigital Neuritis 41
   Pacinian Neuroma 45
   Oral Pseudoperineurioma 49
   Intraneural Injury Neuroma 51
   Epithelial Sheath Neuroma 52
   Ganglion Cyst of Nerve 53
   Endometriosis of Sciatic Nerve 58
   Heterotopic Ossification of Nerve (Neuritis Ossificans) 60
4. Inflammatory and Infectious Lesions Simulating Tumors of Nerve 67
   Inflammatory Pseudotumor of Nerve 67
   Sarcoidosis of Peripheral Nerve 71
   Mycobacterial Pseudotumor 73
   Leprous Neuropathy 75
5. Hyperplastic Lesions 81
   Palisaded Encapsulated Neuroma 81
   Multiple Endocrine Neoplasia 2B-Associated Mucosal Neuroma, Mucosal
      Neuromatosis, and Intestinal Ganglioneuromatosis 87
   MEN 2B-Unassociated Neuroma, Ganglioneuroma/Ganglioneuromatosis, and
      Localized Hypertrophic Neuropathy 95

Neuroma 95

Mucosal Ganglioneuroma and Ganglioneuromatosis 98

Localized Hypertrophic Neuropathy 101

6. Lipomatosis and Neuromuscular Choristoma of Nerve 111

Lipomatosis of Nerve 111

Neuromuscular Choristoma 117

7. Schwannoma 129

Conventional Schwannoma 129

Cellular Schwannoma 165

Plexiform Schwannoma 178

Congenital and Childhood Plexiform (Multinodular) Cellular Schwannoma 184

Melanotic Schwannoma 187

8. Neurofibroma 211

General Features 211

Genetics 212

Clinicopathologic and Anatomic Variants 212

Microscopic Findings 228

Diagnostically Confusing Microscopic Findings 233

Immunohistochemical Findings 244

Ultrastructural Findings 244

DNA Flow Cytometry 245

Histologic Atypia and Malignant Change 245

Tumor of Proposed Neurofibromatous Nature but Unconfirmed 253

Differential Diagnosis 253

Treatment and Prognosis 259

9. Perineurial Cell Tumors 265

Perineurioma 265

Intraneural Perineurioma 266

Soft Tissue Perineurioma 274

Intestinal Perineurioma 286

Hybrid Benign Peripheral Nerve Sheath Tumors 289

Hybrid Schwannoma/Perineurioma 289

Hybrid Reticular (Retiform) Schwannoma/Perineurioma 289

Significance of Hybrid Benign PNSTs with Intimately Admixed Phenotypically
Different Tumor Cell Types 289

Differential Diagnosis 292

10. Miscellaneous Benign Neurogenic Tumors 297

Nerve Sheath Myxoma 297

Benign Granular Cell Tumor 305

Ganglioneuroma 319

11. Benign and Malignant Non-Neurogenic Tumors 347

    Benign Non-Neurogenic Tumors 347

        Lipoma 347

        Paraganglioma 347

        Angiomas of Nerve 350

        Glomus Tumor Variants 351

        Hemangioblastoma 356

        Meningioma 361

        Cutaneous Meningioma 366

        Adrenal Adenoma 366

    Malignant Non-Neurogenic Tumors 366

        Synovial Sarcoma 366

        Angiosarcoma 372

        Hemangiopericytoma 372

        Primary Non-Hodgkin Lymphoma 372

        Amyloidoma of Nerve 373

12. Malignant Tumors of the Peripheral Nerves 381

    Conventional Malignant Peripheral Nerve Sheath Tumors 381

    Perineurial Cell MPNST 414

    Variants of Schwann Cell-Derived MPNST 416

    Epithelioid MPNST 416

        Deep Epithelioid MPNST 416

        Superficial Epithelioid MPNST 423

        Conventional Schwannoma with Epithelioid Malignancy 423

        Neurofibroma with Malignant Epithelioid Cell Differentiation 427

    MPNST with Divergent Differentiation 429

        MPNST with Divergent Mesenchymal Differentiation 431

        PNST with Divergent Epithelial Differentiation 438

    MPNST Arising in Peripheral Neuroblastic Tumors 450

        MPNST Presenting in Ganglioneuroma or Ganglioneuroblastoma 450

        MPNST Arising in Pheochromocytoma 455

    Primitive Neuroectodermal Tumor of Peripheral Nerve 457

    Malignant Granular Cell Tumor 458

13. Tumors of the Neural Transmitting Mesenchymal Cell Component of the

    Peripheral Nervous System 475

    Gastrointestinal Stromal Tumor 475

14. Secondary Neoplasia 491

    Metastases and Direct Extension of Neoplasms to Nerve 491

        Carcinoma 491

        Sarcoma 494

        Neurotropic Melanoma 495

        Lymphoma-Leukemia 502

        Miscellaneous Involvement 503

    Metastases to Nerve Sheath Tumor 503

15. Neurofibromatosis 1 and 2, and Schwannomatosis 507

    Neurofibromatosis 1 507

    Neurofibromatosis 2 521

    Schwannomatosis 535

    Index 545

1 PERIPHERAL NERVE TUMORS: OVERVIEW

This monograph describes the neoplasms, hamartomas, hyperplasias, reactive lesions, and inflammatory pseudotumors arising from or associated with peripheral nerves. Discussed are lesions affecting spinal nerves (intradural and extradural nerve roots and ganglia), peripheral nerves, specialized sensorimotor endings of peripheral nerves, and cranial nerves. Also included are autonomic nerves, their paravertebral and visceral ganglia, and associated neurotransmitter cells of Cajal. Specifically excluded from consideration are lesions of the optic nerve, a central nervous system structure, as well as nontumefactive disorders affecting nerve. Nonneural tumors affecting the substance of nerves, such as metastatic carcinoma, rare examples of melanoma, lymphoma, and direct extensions from surrounding soft tissue neoplasms are also discussed.

Peripheral nerve tumors (PNTs), which account for the large majority of tumors of the peripheral nervous system, are generally classified as soft tissue tumors but differ significantly from other neoplasms in this category. Notable differences include their frequent association with genetic disorders, particularly neurofibromatosis type 1, and the origin of a majority of malignant PNT from a benign precursor lesion, the neurofibroma. PNTs arise from complex tissue with distinctive anatomic compartments. Nerves consist not simply of axons but of specialized ensheathments and compartments. These include: 1) Schwann cells, which ensheath axons to form "nerve fibers"; 2) accompanying endoneurium consisting of capillaries, fibroblasts, macrophages, and mast cells; 3) perineurium, a specialized barrier layer located at the outer limit of the endoneurium and contributing to a "blood-nerve" barrier; and 4) epineurium, an external layer of fibroadipose tissue. Vascular elements are present in all three layers. Hamartomas, hyperplasias, reactive lesions including true neuromas and inflammatory pseudotumors, and neurofibromas involve several if not all these components simultaneously. Non-neural tumors, with the exception of carcinoma, neurotropic melanoma, and lymphoma, are commonly extrinsic to nerve fascicles and their perineurium, and do not exhibit the endoneurial pattern of spread so characteristic of many primary PNTs.

Primary tumors of peripheral nerve originate from cells of the nerve sheath. Although, in theory, peripheral nerve sheath tumors (PNSTs) may arise from Schwann cells, perineurial cells, fibroblasts, and other cells comprising the nerve sheath, most are derived from Schwann cells. This cell is neuroectodermal in nature, originates in the neural crest, and is unique to peripheral nerve. One characteristic of PNTs is their histologic diversity, a feature in large part attributable to the metaplastic repertoire of neoplastic Schwann cells, which may produce not only a variety of collagens and melanin, but display a remarkable capacity for divergent differentiation toward rhabdomyoblasts, chondroblasts, and various epithelial cell types. Also unique to peripheral nerves are perineurial cells, the tumors of which are uncommon but increasingly encountered. Whereas vascular tumors of the peripheral nerves have been reported, fibroblast-derived neoplasms are not well defined.

The process of diagnosis and classification of tumors of the peripheral nervous system requires correlation with clinical and surgical data, as well as considerable attention to the histologic features. In many instances, an immunohistochemical evaluation is also necessary. Although some authors have concluded that electron microscopy is no longer of diagnostic value, it has played a crucial role in the classification of PNTs and remains useful in recognizing: 1) advanced schwannian differentiation in cellular schwannoma, a lesion that must be distinguished from rare diffusely S-100 protein–positive malignant peripheral nerve sheath tumors (MPNSTs), which often demonstrate only minor degrees of Schwann cell differentiation; 2) the fully one third of MPNSTs that lack light microscopic or immuno-histochemical evidence of nerve sheath differentiation; and 3) occasional perineurial tumors not expressing epithelial membrane antigen immunoreactivity. Most recently, molecular genetics has come to play a role in identifying malignant change in neurofibroma and in distinguishing MPNSTs from other soft tissue tumors, particularly synovial sarcoma.

HISTORICAL BACKGROUND

Due to the lessons learned from the application of electron microscopy and immunohisto-chemistry, we now have unequivocal evidence that the Schwann cell plays the major role in the formation of peripheral nerve neoplasms. An appropriate classification system for PNTs, however, has generated much controversy over the years. Ideal classifications are based on the cell type or composition of a tumor since tumor differentiation reflects its "cell of origin." Since the mid-19th century, this concept and the controversy surrounding it, propelled by differing views as to the histologic make-up of PNTs, initially involved European pathologists. After World War I, North American views were expressed. Opposing views pitted investigators favoring a Schwann cell origin against those favoring a mesenchymal or fibroblastic derivation. In the absence of general agreement, recourse was also made to a classification based on less specific noncell-oriented criteria. Perineurial cell tumors, both intraneural and extraneural, went unrecognized until recent years when modern methods quickly resolved their nature.

More recently, it has been shown that neural innervation of the gastrointestinal musculature is augmented and aided by the activity of a plexus of cells referred to as interstitial cells of Cajal (ICC) (1). Linked to both enteric nerves and to smooth muscle cells, the plexus is a network of electrically coupled cells functioning as a syncytium (2). ICCs express ionic conductances facilitating the generation and propagation of slow wave, rhythmic activity in gastrointestinal smooth muscles and, in addition, transduce neural inputs (1). Rather than originating from the neural crest, developmental studies have provided convincing evidence of a mesenchy-

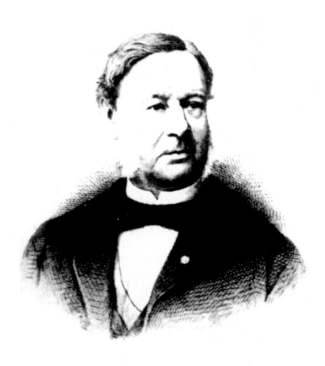

Figure 1-1

THEODOR SCHWANN

mal origin and smooth muscle differentiation (1). ICCs are thought to give rise to the gastrointestinal stromal tumor (GIST) (3,4), a neoplasm that unlike peripheral nerve sheath tumor arises from an electrical impulse-generating cell.

Early Key Investigators

Theodor Schwann (1810-1882). Born in Neuss, Germany, and medically trained in Bonn, Schwann (fig. 1-1) was the first student of the celebrated microscopist, Johannes Mueller of Berlin, to achieve prominence. He became known for his 1839 joint observation with Matthias Schleiden that cells are the fundamental particles of both plants and animals (5). Key among his many observations was a description of the cellular envelope intimately surrounding peripheral nerve axons, a structure that bears his name.

Rudolf Virchow (1821-1902). Berlin based and also a one-time Mueller student who emphasized the importance of microscopy in medicine, Virchow (fig. 1-2) became the most influential pathologist and physician of the 19th century. Guided by observations made earlier by Robert

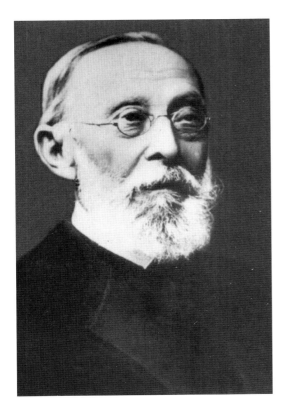

Figure 1-2

RUDOLF VIRCHOW

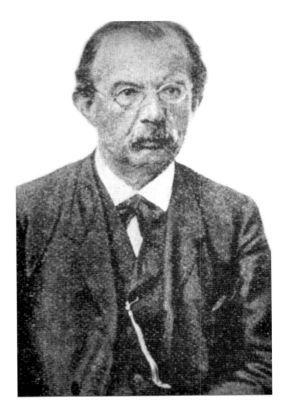

Figure 1-3

FREDERICK VON RECKLINGHAUSEN

Remak that cells originated from other cells by cell division (6,7), and through the application of his own concept of the cellular basis of disease (8), Virchow instituted a revolution in medical investigation. This wide-ranging study included peripheral nerve neoplasms which, in keeping with his view regarding soft tissue tumors (9), he concluded were fibroblastic in nature (10). He coined the term neurofibroma.

Frederick von Recklinghausen (1833-1910). Von Recklinghausen (fig. 1-3) completes the triad of German pioneers in peripheral nerve investigation. As Virchow's favorite disciple, he undertook his 1886 detailed re-examination of patients with multiple peripheral nerve tumors and associated cutaneous pigmented macules (11). The topic had been reported upon by Virchow some 30 years earlier (10). Von Recklinghausen's work established the disorder as a distinctive syndrome and his name became synonymous with it. This work further promoted the term neurofibroma.

Jose Verocay (1876-1927). A Uruguayan physician of Austrian and Italian ancestry, Verocay (fig. 1-4) received a general education in Italy and medical education, including pathology training, in Prague. During the first decade of the 20th century he described in detail a type of peripheral nerve tumor he regarded as Schwann cell in nature (12). This coincided with findings first reported as early as 1878 and credited to French investigators (13) that peripheral nerve neoplasms were unlikely mesenchymal in nature given their frequent nerve association and cellular fasciculation. Verocay called attention to the presence of distinct bodies with palisaded cells, structures now referred to as "Verocay bodies." Verocay's tumor, with its palisaded cell bodies and related processes, was so convincingly indicative of a peripheral nerve tumor distinct from neurofibroma that his report had a significant impact on work in this area. The designation of "neurinoma" which Verocay selected for this tumor was likely based on his

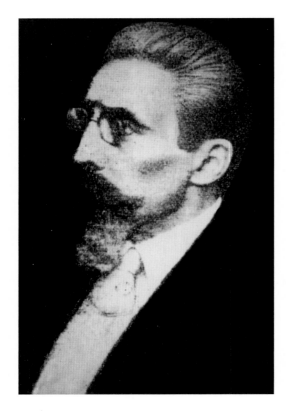

Figure 1-4

JOSE VEROCAY

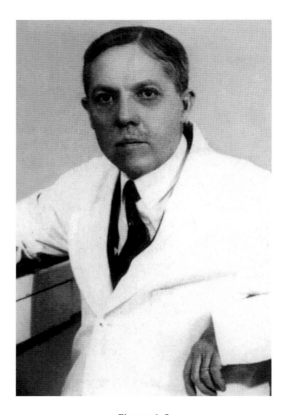

Figure 1-5

PIERRE MASSON

conclusion that the neoplastic Schwann cells contained portions of nerve fibers, an observation in keeping with Schwann's view that the cells he had described encasing axons actually participated in their formation.

Pierre Masson (1880-1959). From Dijon, France, and schooled in biological research before obtaining a medical degree, Masson (fig. 1-5) was an extraordinarily insightful anatomic pathologist. He came to occupy academic Chairs in the field at Strasbourg and later at the University of Montreal in Canada (14). In the latter capacity, assumed in 1927, he acted as a conduit for infusion of French concepts in pathology into North America. A major interest in neuroectodermal neoplasms included the peripheral nerve tumors. Among these was neurinoma, which he concluded was Schwann cell in nature, given the apparent syncytial structure of the neoplastic cells (15). Unconvinced that Schwann cells form axons, he set aside the term "neurinoma" for the cell composition-based designation of "schwannoglioma." Masson

considered neurofibroma and MPNST to also be Schwann cell neoplasms. Schwann cells are neural crest derived (16), and since the neural crest gives rise to the musculature in the head and neck regions, his concept that the majority of nerve sheath neoplasms are Schwann cell derived provided him an explanation for his discovery of examples of MPNST with rhabdomyosarcomatous differentiation (15,17).

Arthur Purdy Stout (1885-1967). A key figure in the development of surgical pathology as a specialty, and one of its foremost experts (18), Stout (fig. 1-6), New York City born, was medically trained and pursued a career at Columbia University. His interests were diverse but none captured his attention more than the pathology of the peripheral nervous system. In 1935, a time when the mesenchymal theory of the origin of peripheral nerve tumors prevailed among American neuropathologists (19), Stout published two important papers, both regarding his own and previously reported cases, dealing with Verocay's neurinoma (20) and MPNST (21).

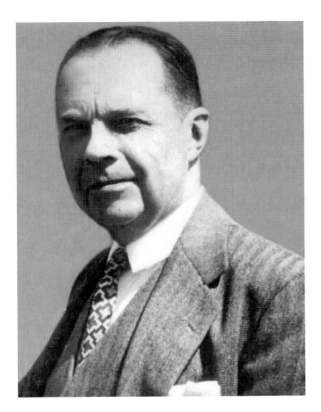

Figure 1-6

ARTHUR PURDY STOUT

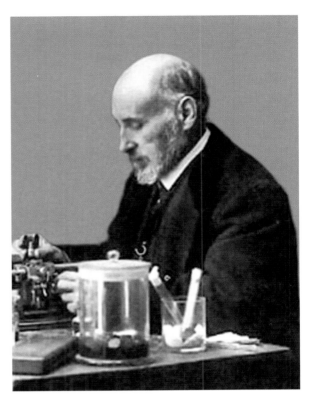

Figure 1-7

SANTIAGO RAMON Y CAJAL

With respect to neurinoma, Stout thought the term inappropriate because it literally means "nerve fiber tumor," which it is not, and suggested its replacement with the designation "neurilemoma," his own creation and meaning "nerve sheath tumor," which it is. The final determination of the tumor's originating cell he left to future studies. Regarding MPNST, he was convinced that in the past the designation had often been misapplied to spindle cell sarcomas of other derivation. To correct this, he recommended that specific criteria such as origin from a nerve, transformation from neurofibroma, or occurrence in a patient with von Recklinghausen neurofibromatosis be met before making the diagnosis. At this time he still accepted the view that MPNSTs were derived from mesoblastic endoneurium, only rare cases having a neuroectodermal origin (13). Because Stout correlated a defined histology with clinical findings and a routinely benign course, his paper on neurilemomas was a major contribution. Nonetheless, the terminology for

this tumor had a drawback. The benefit of a cell-based designation was lost even though 6 years later, on the basis of Murray's cell culture work (22), he adjusted his view to coincide with Masson. His landmark 1949 fascicle on tumors of the peripheral nervous system (23), which propounded the Schwann cell derivation of all major peripheral nervous system tumors, was instrumental in the general acceptance of that view. Unfortunately, Stout's characterization of neurilemoma as a consistently benign tumor was not understood by subsequent investigators providing the initial assessments of MPNST (24,25), who referred to the latter as "malignant neurilemoma," a misuse of the term that sowed confusion among later workers in the field.

Santiago Ramon y Cajal (1852-1934). Santiago Ramon y Cajal (fig. 1-7), Spain's most illustrious physician, was a founding father of modern neuroscience. His Nobel Prize was in recognition of a life of intense labor, exhaustively studying the microanatomy of the nervous system. Using the modifications of

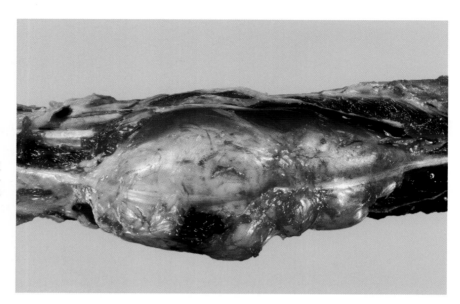

Figure 1-8

ELONGATED "FUSIFORM" SCLEROSING EPITHELIOID FIBROSARCOMA

Attachment to peripheral nerve led to a false initial assumption that this was a nerve sheath tumor.

Camillo Golgi's silver impregnation method and an artist's facility for fine drawing, he painstakingly recorded his findings. His anatomic studies of nervous tissue were conducted at a series of institutions, lastly at the University of Madrid. Here, he established the prestigious Laboratory of Investigative Biology, a mecca for future leaders in the field. Cajal's principal achievement was proving that individual nerve cells (neurons) are the basic units of the central nervous system, a novel concept that displaced the reticular theory. Cajal was also the first to describe cells interposed between nerve endings and smooth muscle cells of the gastrointestinal tract, cells now referred to as the interstitial cells of Cajal (ICC). His investigation of these cells, believed by him to be a type of primitive neuron, was solely confined to their description (1,26–28).

SPECIMEN PRESENTATION, HANDLING, AND ASSESSMENT

Specimen Types. Tissues to be evaluated in cases of PNT vary greatly in size, ranging from fine needle aspiration, to needle biopsy, to open biopsy or a resection specimen. The clinical presentation is usually of a soft tissue mass of uncertain type, or of a lesion clinically or operatively related to peripheral nerve.

Diagnostic Pitfalls Related to Presentation. Any suggestion or assurance of a tumor's origin in nerve must be weighed against imaging and operative findings regarding its location, gross features, and histology. When inconsistencies arise, the clinical reports and gross descriptions should be re-examined. An illustration of the problem, based on the experience of one of the authors, relates to an unusual elongated tumor that partially encircled an arm. Its configuration led to the conclusion of a peripheral nerve origin, but doubt was subsequently raised because most nerves of limbs are longitudinally, not horizontally, disposed. Histologic review showed features inconsistent with a peripheral nerve primary but, rather, compatible with a sweat gland adenoma. Another problematic case was a sclerosing epithelioid fibrosarcoma of the lower extremity that grew as an elongated mass in the calf where, along its length, it was attached to a nerve (fig. 1-8). An erroneous initial assumption that it represented a primary MPNST was made. Yet another example of striking mimicry of a peripheral nerve tumor was provided by an elongated, smooth muscle tumor arising within a limb and involving a neurovascular bundle. The correct diagnosis became apparent on microscopic examination with the finding of an origin in a vessel coursing through the tumor.

Histologically similar neoplasms may simulate a PNST. Two lesions in this category are synovial sarcoma of nerve and primitive neuroectodermal tumor (PNET) of soft tissue, which can masquerade as a primary nerve sheath tumor. Synovial

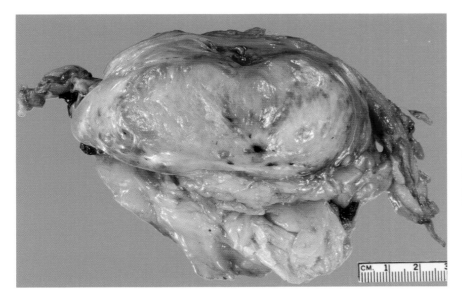

Figure 1-9

**AIR-INDUCED
TUMOR DISCOLORATION**

Gross photo of monophasic synovial sarcoma taken over 3 minutes after sectioning shows beginning pink artifactual discoloration of a usually gray soft tissue tumor.

sarcomas primary in nerve pose a particular diagnostic challenge (see chapter 12). Their identification is greatly aided by demonstrating the diagnostic translocation t(x;18). The nerve most frequently involved by PNET is the sciatic. Typically, the nerve, irregularly invaded by tumor, is partly or completely surrounded by a soft tissue PNET (see fig. 13-9). Distinguishing a primary soft tissue PNET secondarily involving nerve from a rare MPNST showing PNET differentiation rests upon demonstrating a malignant spindle cell tumor component in the latter.

Gross Features. Like other tumors of soft tissue, each of the principal forms of PNT exhibits a distinctive range of gross features. External features of importance in the assessment of PNTs but not evaluable in small specimens include: tumor boundary (circumscription with or without encapsulation versus invasion of adjacent normal tissues) and tumor shape after being freed from surrounding tissue (ovoid, flattened, elongate, cylindrical, fusiform, multinodular, or plexiform). On cut section, color is a key feature in the evaluation of all soft tissue tumors and the one requiring immediate assessment following tumor transection in order to avoid the common artifactual, pink discoloration that occurs after 3 minutes exposure to air (figs. 1-9, 1-10). Other key features include texture, uniformity, tissue homogeneity, and the presence and extent of necrosis.

Before dissection, external specimen examination includes: 1) recording gross features by color photography; 2) measuring in centimeters the specimen's three dimensions; 3) accurately describing gross features, particularly tumor configuration and the presence or absence of a nerve; and 4) if considering malignancy, coating the external surface of the specimen with India ink to permit accurate assessment of resection margins. Having completed these steps, assessment of the specimen interior begins with transection along its long axis by a sharp knife, if possible by a single passage. An exception is made when the tumor is long, cylindrical, and of generally uniform diameter, in which case multiple cross sections are more informative. Generous sections are then submitted for microscopy, at least one for every centimeter of maximal lesion diameter. These should be fully representative of the variations in tumor color and texture. Lastly, sections are taken of proximal, distal, and lateral margins of resection. Additionally, particularly when confronted with a tumor having unusual gross features, a sample in fixative should be set aside for electron microscopy. Although preservation in either glutaraldehyde or Trump fixative is optimal, formalin fixation suffices. In selected cases, setting aside fresh tissue in appropriate media, such as RPMI, facilitates cytogenetic and flow cytometric studies. In addition, a sample can be quick frozen in liquid nitrogen for molecular genetic studies.

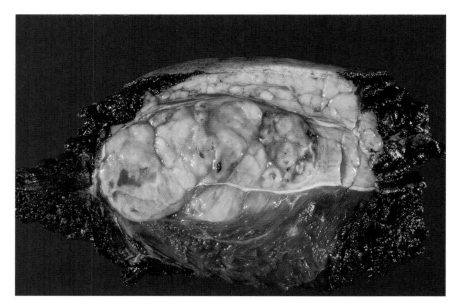

Figure 1-10

AIR-INDUCED TUMOR DISCOLORATION

Monophasic synovial sarcoma with complete pink discoloration following prolonged exposure to air.

REFERENCES

1. Sanders K, Ordog T, Koh S, Torihashi S, Ward S. Development and plasticity of interstitial cells of Cajal. Neurogastroenterol Motil 1999;11:311-338.
2. Kobilo T, Szurszewski J, Farrugia G, Hanani M. Coupling and innervation patterns of interstitial cells of Cajal in the deep muscular plexus of the guinea-pig. Neurogastroenterol Motil 2003;15:635-641.
3. Hirota S, Isozaki K, Moriyama Y, et al. Gain-of-function mutations of c-kit in human gastrointestinal stromal tumors. Science 1998;279:577-580.
4. Kindblom LG, Remotti HE, Aldenborg F, Meis-Kindblom JM. Gastrointestinal pacemaker cell tumor (GIPACT): gastrointestinal stromal tumors show phenotypic characteristics of the interstitial cells of Cajal. Am J Pathol 1998;152:1259-1269.
5. Schwann T. Microscopical researches into the accordance of the structure and growth of animals and plants. London: The Syndeham Society; 1847.
6. Remak R. Uber extracellulare Entstehung thierischer Zellen und über vermehrung derselben durch Teilung Arch Pathol Anat Phys Wiss Med 1852;49:57.

7. Virchow R. Handbuch der speziellen Pathologie and therapie. Erlangen: Enke; 1854.
8. Virchow R. In: Rather RL, ed. Disease, life, and man: selected essays by Rudolf Virchow. Stanford, CA: Stanford Univ. Press; 1958:71-101.
9. Fitzgerald P. From demons and evil spirits to cancer genes. Washington, DC: American Registry of Pathology, Armed Forces Institute of Pathology; 2000:67.
10. Virchow R. Die Krankhafte Geschwulste: Dreissig Vorlesungen, gehalted wahrend des Wintersemesters 1862-1863 an der Universität zu Berlin. Berlin: A Hirschwald; 1863:1.
11. von Recklinghausen F. "Uber die multiplen Fibromeder Haut und ihre Beziehung Zuden multiplen neuromen. Berlin: A. Hirschwald; 1882.
12. Verocay J. Zur Kenntnis der "Neurofibrome." Beitr Pathol Anat Allg Pathol 1910;48:1-69.
13. Woodruff JM. Arthur Purdy Stout and the evolution of modern concepts regarding peripheral nerve sheath tumors. Am J Surg Pathol 1986;10(Suppl 1):63-67.
14. Seemayer TA. A life and legacy of Professor Pierre Masson. Am J Surg Pathol 1983;7:179-183.

15. Masson P. Experimental and spontaneous schwannomas (peripheral gliomas). Part II. Spontaneous schwannomas. Am J Pathol 1932;8:389-416.

16. Harrison RG. Neuroblast versus sheath cell in the development of peripheral nerves. J Comp Neurol 1924;37:123-205.

17. Masson P, Martin JF. Rhabdomyomes des nerfs. Bull Assoc Fr Etud Cancer 1938;27:751-767.

18. Lattes R. Surgical pathology at the college of physicians and surgeons of Columbia University. In: Rosai R, ed. Guiding the surgeon's hand. The history of American surgical pathology. Washington, DC American Registry of Pathology, Armed Forces Institute of Pathology, 1997:41-60.

19. Penfield W. Tumors of the sheaths of the nervous system. In: Penfield W, ed. Cytology and cellular pathology of the nervous system, Vol 3. New York: P. Hoeber; 1932.

20. Stout AP. The peripheral manifestations of the specific nerve sheath tumor. Am J Cancer 1935;24:751-96.

21. Stout AP. The malignant tumors of the peripheral nerves. Am J Cancer 1935;25:1-36.

22. Murray MR, Stout AP, Bradley CF. Schwann cell versus fibroblast as the origin of the specific nerve sheath tumor. Observations upon normal nerve sheaths and neurilemomas in vitro. Am J Pathol 1940;16:41-60.

23. Stout AP. Tumors of the peripheral nervous system. Atlas of Tumor Pathology. 1st Series, Fascicle 6. Washington DC: Armed Forces Institute of Pathology; 1949.

24. D'Agostino AN, Soule EH, Miller RH. Primary malignant neoplasms of nerves (malignant neurilemomas) in patients without manifestations of multiple neurofibromatosis (von Recklinghausen's disease). Cancer 1963;16:1003-1014.

25. Vieta J, Pack GT. Malignant neurilemomas of peripheral nerves. Am J Surg 1951;82:416-431.

26. Cajal S. Sur les ganglions et plexus nerveux de l'intestin. CR Soc Biol (Paris) 1893;45:217-223.

27. Cajal S. Histologie du systeme nerveux de l'homme et des vertebres. Paris: Maloine; 1909: 891-942.

28. Courville CR. Santiago Ramon Y Cajal (1852-1934). In: Haymaker W, F Shiller F, eds. The founders of neurology. Springfield, Ill: Charles C Thomas; 1970:147-151.

2 THE NORMAL PERIPHERAL NERVOUS SYSTEM

DEVELOPMENT

In early embryogenesis, the midline dorsal ectoderm forms the neural plate, which, in turn, develops a longitudinal groove. The walls of the groove fold and fuse to form the neural tube. The lateral portions of the fold form the neural crest, which extends from the level of the diencephalon through the distal neuraxis. Neural crest derivatives include sensory and autonomic nerves as well as their respective ganglia, Schwann cells and their variant satellite cells, and melanocytes. Neural crest cells are not only pluripotential, but their differentiation is affected by their milieu and by interaction with surrounding cells. For instance, neurite outgrowth and its direction is, in part, genetically determined but is also influenced by Schwann cell growth factors, among which is nerve growth factor (NGF), a 14-kD polypeptide encoded on chromosome 22. Particularly during development, Schwann cells not only produce NGF but possess NGF receptors. By its chemotactic properties and action upon the cytoskeleton of receptor-bearing axons, NGF promotes growth cone mobility in growing axons. The latter, by way of receptors, also are affected by extracellular substances such as collagen, laminin, fibronectin, and entactin. Early neurotransmitter synthesis is also induced by NGF. Lastly, trophic substances produced by target organs also determine the direction of neurite growth.

With a few exceptions, neurons giving rise to sensory nerves lie within either cranial nerve sensory ganglia (I, II, III, V, VII, VIII, IX, X) or dorsal root ganglia. The cells of the latter are large and round, feature centrally situated nuclei, and are encircled by satellite cells, specialized but indistinguishable from Schwann cells. The initially single process of a sensory ganglion cell divides in a T-fashion, sending a proximal axon into the substance of the spinal cord (efferent fiber) and another distally within the sensory nerve (afferent fiber). In contrast, motor neurons lie within the central nervous system, either in motor nuclei (III, IV, V, VI, VII, IX, X, XI, XII) of the brain stem or in anterior horns of the spinal cord. They send a single efferent process distal within a motor nerve root. The central portions of sensory and motor axons are ensheathed by central myelin, the product of oligodendrocytes, while the distally directed processes of cranial and spinal sensory and motor axons are ensheathed by Schwann cell–derived peripheral myelin. Their tinctorial characteristics differ, even with Luxol-fast blue, a myelin stain.

Myelination of the peripheral nervous system precedes that of the central nervous system and is initiated by axon-Schwann cell contact. Functionally, segments of the myelin sheath, the product of individual Schwann cells, insulate and facilitate rapid saltatory conduction along the fiber. During development, Schwann cells follow elongating axons and form concentric sheaths around them. Myelination begins by the 18th week of gestation. Large axons tend to be myelinated to a greater extent than small axons. Only a few peripheral nerves and their fibers are myelinated, but all axons are encircled by Schwann cells, regardless of size. Although the term "nerve fiber" has been used to denote either the axon alone or the axon with its accompanying Schwann sheath, we favor the latter definition, since the axon and Schwann sheath function as a unit, both physiologically and in reaction to injury. In myelinated fibers, a single Schwann cell provides myelin for only a segment of a single axon. In unmyelinated nerves, a number of axons are ensheathed by a single Schwann cell.

GROSS ANATOMY

Anterior (motor) and posterior (sensory) spinal nerve roots exit the spinal cord separately, traverse the subarachnoid space, and coalesce just proximal to the dorsal root ganglia to form peripheral nerve trunks surrounded by a dural sleeve that continues into the intervertebral foramen (fig. 2-1). Proximally, cranial and spinal nerves are surrounded by a layer of arachnoid membrane (leptomeninges). Distally, the relationship of the latter to epiperineurium is unclear (fig. 2-2).

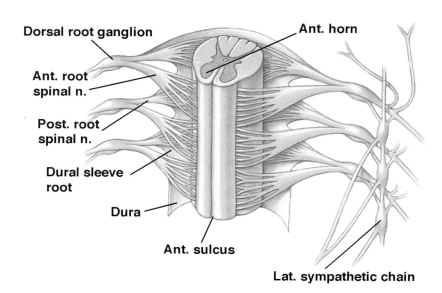

Figure 2-1

SCHEMATIC REPRESENTATION OF THE SENSORIMOTOR AND AUTONOMIC NERVES AND THEIR GANGLIA RELATIVE TO THE SPINAL CORD AND MENINGES

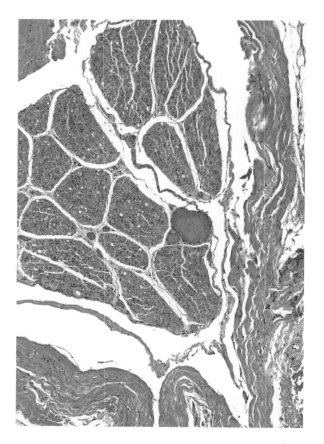
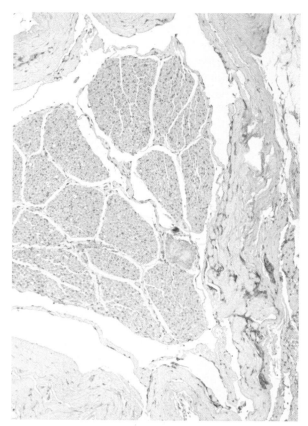

Figure 2-2

SPINAL NERVE TRUNK: RELATIONSHIP OF PERINEURIUM TO MENINGES

Left: The relationship of the meninges to the spinal nerve trunks is intimate.

Right: The delicate arachnoid membrane encircles and is partly in continuity with the epithelial membrane antigen-reactive perineurium surrounding nerve fascicles. Both are contained within the much thicker, collagen-rich dura.

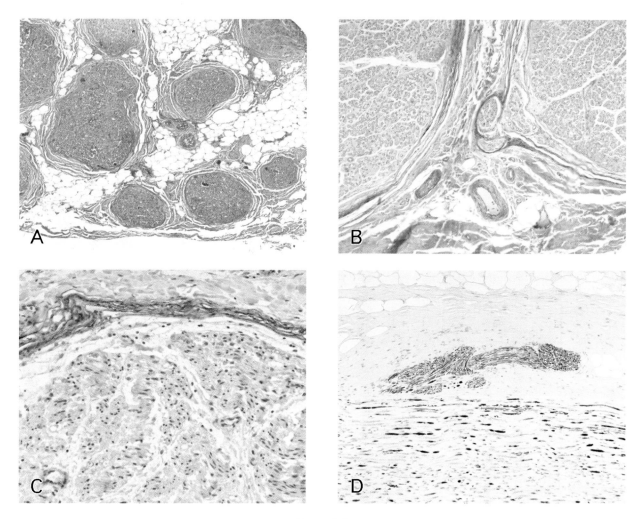

Figure 2-3

NORMAL NERVE IN CROSS SECTION

A: Nerve fascicles are embedded in fibrofatty epineurial tissue.

B: With the Luxol-fast blue–periodic acid–Schiff (LFB-PAS) stain, two nerve fascicles are seen, each surrounded by PAS-positive perineurium. The vasa nervorum is delineated. The endoneurium contains numerous nerve fibers, each surrounded by a blue cylinder of myelin.

C: Epithelial membrane antigen stains the perineurium.

D: On occasion, nerve fascicles branch, here shown with a neurofilament protein immunostain.

Having traversed the intervertebral foramen, each spinal nerve trunk divides into dorsal and ventral rami, the former supplying the posterior portion of the body and the latter the anterior portion and limbs. The brachial and lumbosacral plexuses are formed by fusion of ventral rami of adjacent spinal nerves. Thus, major peripheral nerves originating from a plexus actually contain nerve fibers from multiple spinal cord segments. Peripheral nerves progressively divide into smaller nerves as, grouped or single, their fascicles exit

from them. As a result, nerve fibers comprising a peripheral nerve fascicle do not necessarily remain with that parent fascicle. Instead, some fiber bundles extend from one fascicle to another ("bridging fascicles") (fig. 2-3).

All peripheral nerves are compound in nature, consisting of a variable admixture of motor, sensory, and autonomic nerve fibers. Motor nerve fibers terminate on somatic muscle end-plates. Sensory fibers terminate in specialized structures or transducers in skin, muscle,

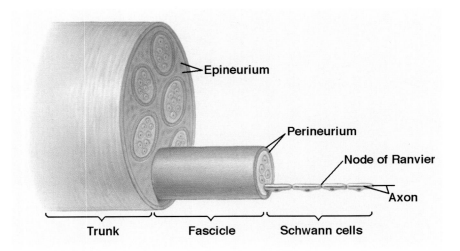

Figure 2-4

SCHEMATIC
REPRESENTATION OF
THE BASIC ARCHITECTURE
OF NORMAL NERVE

and other organs (see below). Unlike spinal nerves, cranial nerves originate from the brain at irregular intervals, having neither dorsal nor ventral roots. Instead, their efferent and afferent fibers exit and enter the brain at the same site.

Autonomic nerves of both parasympathetic and sympathetic type innervate viscera, blood vessels, and smooth muscle of the skin and eye. Parasympathetic preganglionic neurons are craniosacral in origin, their nerve fibers exiting the brain stem in cranial nerves 3, 7, 9, 10, and 11 as well as in sacral ventral roots 2 and 3 or 3 and 4. Parasympathetic ganglion cells are located near or within the structures they innervate. In contrast, sympathetic preganglionic fibers arise from the intermediolateral gray columns of the thoracolumbar spinal cord (T1-L2), exit via anterior nerve roots, are myelinated, and terminate in sympathetic ganglion cells in perivertebral or prevertebral locations.

For a more detailed discussion of the anatomic features of the peripheral nervous system, the reader is referred to an authoritative text (1).

MICROANATOMY

Peripheral Nerves

The basic anatomic features of peripheral nerves are schematically illustrated in figures 2-4 and 2-5. Normal peripheral nerves consist of shiny, white bundles or fascicles surrounded and separated by a highly variable amount of adipose stroma termed epineurium. This layer is grossly distinct from surrounding soft tissue

when adipose tissue is scant but not so evident when adipose tissue is ample. Epineurial tissue contains collagen types 1 and 3 as well as elastic fibers, the latter concentrated around the fascicles. Whereas large nerves, particularly of the lower extremities and nearby joints, feature ample epineurial adipose tissue as well as nutrient arteries, veins, and lymphatics, all of which follow the course of the nerve (fig. 2-3A,B), minute nerves consisting of but one or two fascicles often possess little epineurial tissue. Mast cells in small number are also present in epineurium.

A functionally specialized structure, the perineurium, is contiguous with the arachnoid membrane (figs. 2-2, 2-5). It ensheathes not only individual peripheral and autonomic nerve fascicles (figs. 2-3A–C, 2-6A,B), but their ganglia as well. Although perineurial and arachnoidal cells share some immunophenotypic features (positivity for vimentin, epithelial membrane antigen, Glut-1, Claudin-1), they differ at the ultrastructural level (see below), and the cytogenesis of perineurial cells, whether derived from Schwann, fibroblastic, or arachnoidal cells, remains unsettled (2). Thus, the terms "perineurial fibroblasts" and "perineurial epithelium" should be avoided.

Perineurium consists of layers of concentrically disposed, flattened, polygonal cells separated by thin layers of collagen, primarily type 4 (figs. 2-7, 2-8). The number of perineurial cells ensheathing any one fascicle varies in proportion to its size. Distal nerve twigs often possess only a single layer of perineurial cells, whereas large

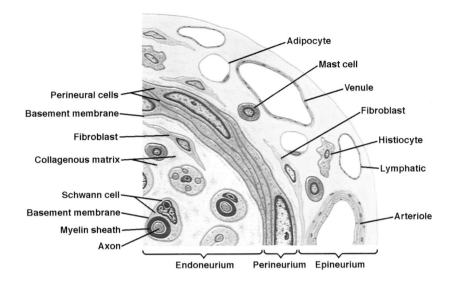

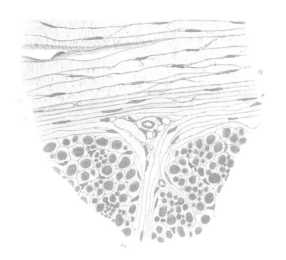

Figure 2-5

THE ESSENTIAL ELEMENTS OF EPINEURIUM, PERINEURIUM, AND ENDONEURIUM

Top: Diagrammatic representation.

Bottom: The intricate microanatomy of perineurium is illustrated in this line drawing by Key and Retzius in their classic monograph of 1876. Septa form between portions of the endoneurium.

fascicles possess ten or more. At the termination of sensory nerves, perineurium becomes incorporated into the architecture of specialized sensory structures (see below). In motor nerves, perineurium ends in a funnel-like aperture capping the motor end-plate. Perineurial cells function as a diffusion barrier. As such, in conjunction with the specialized vasculature of the peripheral nerve, they maintain the physiologic milieu of the endoneurium.

Contained within the encircling perineurium, the endoneurium is a compartment surrounding axons and their accompanying Schwann cells, and containing fibroblasts, macrophages, mast cells, and capillaries (figs. 2-4; 2-5, top; 2-6;

2-7). These cellular constituents are similar in spinal nerve roots and peripheral nerves. Approximately 20 to 30 percent of endoneurium consists of fluid and connective tissue matrix. Albumin is the major protein component of the fluid and its transfer through the blood-nerve barrier may be increased in pathologic conditions. The connective tissue matrix is composed of collagen fibrils, mainly of type 1, but also 2 and 3. Longitudinally oriented and in part closely ensheathing nerve fibers, the fibrils form what were once termed the sheaths of Plenk and Laidlaw, and of Key and Retzius. A distinct but inconspicuous feature of endoneurium is the finding of Renaut bodies, cylindrical

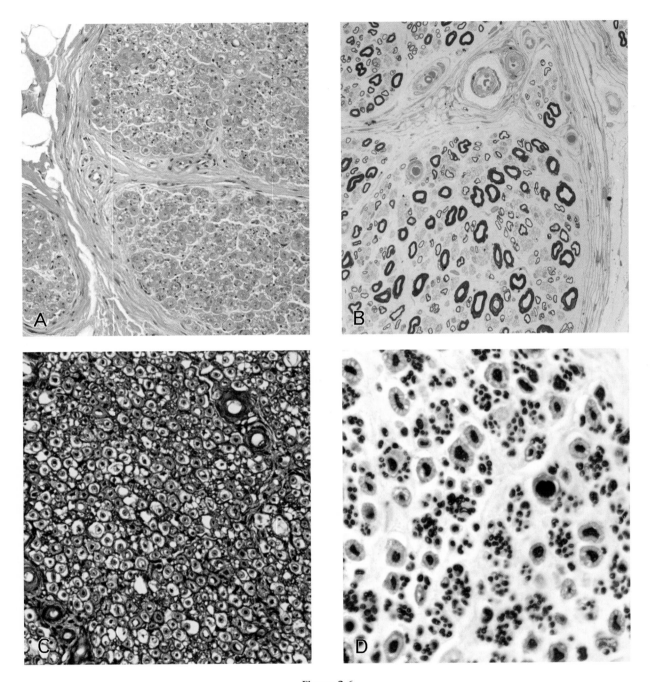

Figure 2-6

NORMAL NERVE IN CROSS SECTION

A: The H&E stain delineates a nerve fiber-filled fascicle surrounded by perineurium. Myelinated axons are numerous and mainly appear as dots, each surrounded by a cuff of myelin. Unmyelinated axons are minute and inapparent.

B: The toluidine blue-stained semi-thin section shows these microanatomic features in greater detail, particularly the direct relationship between the axon diameter and the thickness of the myelin sheaths. An arteriole is present within a perineurial septum.

C: A LFB-PAS-Bielschowsky stain shows prominent myelin in sensorimotor nerves compared to largely unmyelinated autonomic nerves (see fig. 2-17B).

D: A combination immunostain (PG 9.5) and LFB preparation underscores the considerable variation in axon and myelin sheath size. (B and D, courtesy of Dr. P.C. Johnson, Tucson, Arizona.)

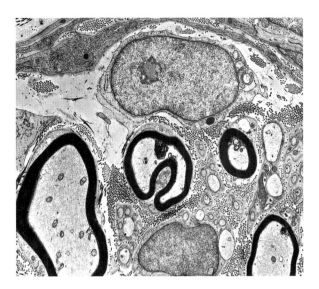

Figure 2-7

NORMAL CUTANEOUS NERVE

Myelinated and unmyelinated axons and endoneurial collagen fibrils are seen. A three-cell thick sheath of perineurial cells, the perineurium, is present at the top.

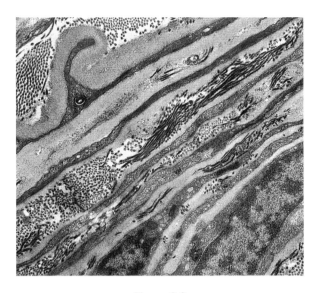

Figure 2-8

**SURAL NERVE
PERINEURIAL SHEATH**

Seven layers of perineurial cells are illustrated. The thin cytoplasmic processes of the perineurial cell contain prominent pinocytotic vesicles and are coated on both sides by a thick continuous basement membrane. Collagen fibrils are found in the intercellular matrix.

hyaline structures lying on the inner aspect of the perineurium. They are collagen rich and Alcian blue positive, as is the remainder of the endoneurium. The function of Renaut bodies is uncertain, but their increased number near normal joints as well as in the setting of compressive neuropathies suggests that they may have a mechanical role as cushions.

The vasa nervorum, the vascular supply of the peripheral nerves, is derived from regional arteries entering the epineurium. Here, they run longitudinally to form an anastomosing plexus (figs. 2-3A,B; 2-5; 2-6A,B). In order to gain access to the endoneurial space, arteriolar branches obliquely penetrate the perineurium, carrying with them a short sleeve of perineurium. Longitudinally oriented, the endoneurial capillary network is surrounded by pericytes. Its nonfenestrated endothelium is in part the basis of the "blood-nerve barrier," a structure lacking in dorsal root and autonomic ganglia. Unlike epineurium, endoneurium lacks lymphatics.

Whether engaged in myelin production or not, Schwann cells ensheath axons of all sizes (figs. 2-5; 2-6C,D). Distributed along the length of the axons, the cytoplasm of the myelin-forming Schwann cells is wrapped around

them in a spiral fashion. In myelinated nerves, single Schwann cells ensheath each segment of axon length. In unmyelinated fibers, portions of several axons are individually encased in a simple, cuff-like manner by a single Schwann cell. These relationships are schematically and ultrastructurally illustrated in figures 2-5, 2-7, 2-9, and 2-10. Although on transverse hematoxylin and eosin (H&E)-stained sections, large axons are recognized as eosinophilic dots at the center of myelin sheaths, the microanatomic relationship is more readily apparent with special stains (fig. 2-6). In longitudinal sections, Schwann cell nuclei appear elongated and serially arranged along the length of the axon (fig. 2-11A,B). The cytoplasm varies from pink to inconspicuous depending on whether the nerve is myelinated or not. Axons are difficult to visualize since, when longitudinally cut, they typically enter and exit the visual plane. On routine H&E-stained sections, only sizable myelinated axons are discernible. The visualization of axons is greatly enhanced, however, by silver impregnation methods (Bodian or Bielschowsky stain) and, of course, on immunostain for neurofilament protein

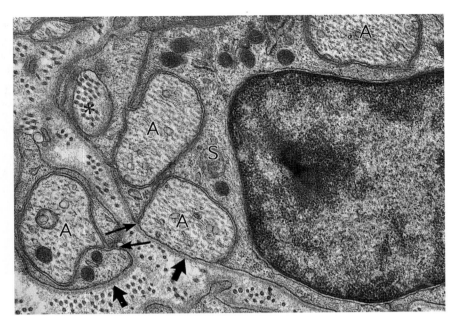

Figure 2-9

UNMYELINATED NERVE FIBERS

A biopsy of the sural nerve shows numerous unmyelinated axons (A) embedded within the surface of a single Schwann cell (S). The processes are entirely surrounded but no spiral of myelin is present. The Schwann cell nucleus is seen at the right. A continuous basement membrane surrounds the entire Schwann cell (arrows). A "collagen pocket" is also noted (asterisk). This characteristic grouped arrangement of axons is known as a Remak bundle. (Courtesy of Dr. G. Moretto, Verona, Italy.)

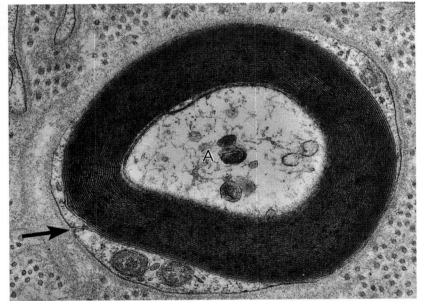

Figure 2-10

MYELINATED NERVE FIBER

The small myelinated fiber and its ensheathing Schwann cell are surrounded by a continuous basement membrane. The nucleus of the Schwann cell is not present at this level. The axon (A) contains neurofilaments, microtubules, and a few smooth endoplasmic reticulum profiles. The characteristic periodicity of the myelin sheath is apparent, with clearly visible major dense lines. Inner mesaxon formation is seen at the inner aspect of the myelin sheath in the adaxonal space. The external mesaxon is obliquely cut but can be clearly identified (arrow). The Schwann cell cytoplasm contains abundant rough endoplasmic reticulum, glycogen, and a small, spherical Elzholz body. (Courtesy of Dr. G. Moretto, Verona, Italy.)

(fig. 2-11D,E). Some structures, such as the nodes of Ranvier, points of abutment between adjacent Schwann sheaths, are most clearly seen in plastic-embedded, semi-thin sections (fig. 2-12). At the light microscopic level, the intimate relationship between the Schwann cells and the axons is best appreciated on teased fiber preparations. Histochemically, Schwann cells exhibit pericellular reticulin or periodic acid–Schiff (PAS) staining which corresponds to their surface basement membrane, a structure composed of laminin, fibronectin, entactin, heparin sulfate, and collagen, primarily of type 4.

Myelin is a complex substance consisting largely (75 percent) of lipids, particularly cholesterol, sphingomyelin, and galactolipids. Proteins comprise the remaining 25 percent. In the peripheral nervous system, the bulk of the protein consists of glycoprotein Po, a substance not found in central myelin. This appears to underlie the differing antigenicity and perhaps the tinctorial characteristics of central and

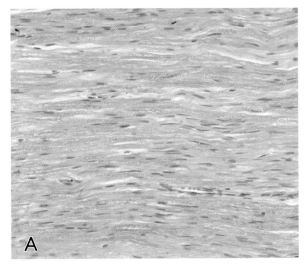

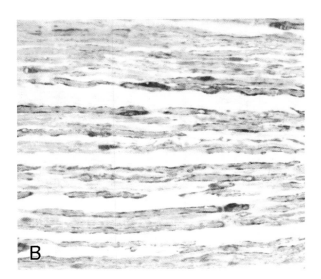

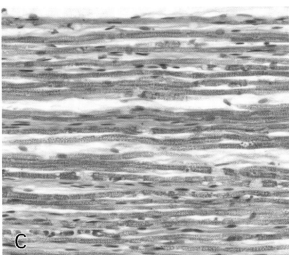

Figure 2-11

**NORMAL PERIPHERAL NERVE: LONGITUDINAL
SECTION OF A SINGLE NERVE FIBER**

A: With the H&E stain, axons are barely discernible as delicate gray threads obscured by myelin and Schwann cells.

B: Schwann cells, particularly their nuclei, are best seen with S-100 protein staining.

C: Myelin is most apparent with the LFB-PAS stain.

D: Axons are identified with silver stains, such as the Bielschowsky preparation.

E: Neurofilament protein immunostains more reliably demonstrate axons than do silver impregnations.

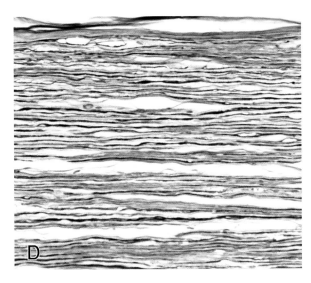

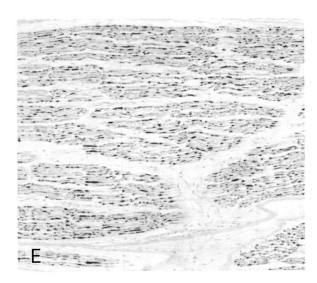

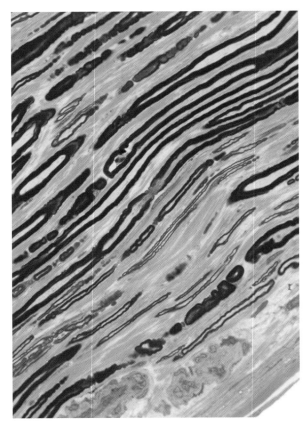

Figure 2-12

MYELINATED PERIPHERAL NERVE IN A SEMI-THIN, OSMIUM- AND EOSIN-STAINED SECTION

The node of Ranvier (center), the juncture of two myelin sheaths, is seen. (Courtesy of Dr. P.C. Johnson, Tucson, Arizona.)

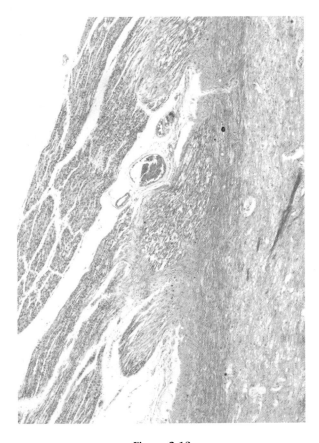

Figure 2-13

NORMAL SPINAL CORD AND NERVE ROOT IN LONGITUDINAL SECTION

This LFB-PAS stain shows the transition zone between the central and peripheral nervous systems. Central, oligodendrocyte-derived myelin of the spinal cord (right) is lighter stained than peripheral or Schwann cell myelin in nerve roots (left).

peripheral myelin (fig. 2-13). Myelin-associated glycoprotein (MAG) also plays an important role in myelination, being present in myelin-forming Schwann cells, but not in ones accompanying unmyelinated fibers.

In neurophysiologic terms, peripheral nerve fibers are classified by their diameters, a feature directly related to conduction velocity. Myelin facilitates conduction, thus myelinated fibers do so more rapidly than nonmyelinated fibers. In most peripheral nerves, the fibers are of both myelinated and unmyelinated type (figs. 2-5, 2-7, 2-9, 2-10). Their relative frequencies can only be assessed by counting them at the ultrastructural level. Although myelinated fibers are readily evident in epoxy-embedded, toluidine blue–stained sections

(fig. 2-6B), unmyelinated fibers are not. As previously noted, longitudinal sections of peripheral nerve are less informative than are cross sections. Transversely cut nerve demonstrates not only variations in fiber type but pathology, including axonal degeneration, demyelination, architectural features peculiar to reactive processes, and the localization of nerve-associated neoplasms such as intraneural perineurioma.

Sensory and Autonomic Ganglia

Despite significant differences in size, the general architectural features of dorsal root and autonomic ganglia are similar (fig. 2-14).

Sensory Ganglia. As stated above, nerve fibers giving rise to sensory nerves originate

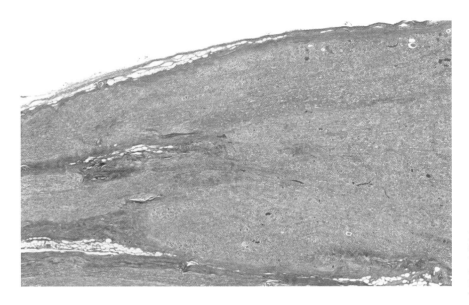

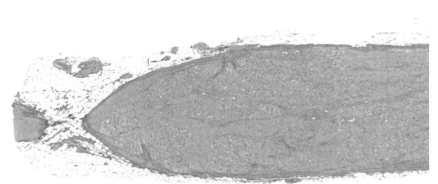

Figure 2-14

DORSAL ROOT AND SYMPATHETIC GANGLIA

Dorsal root (top) and sympathetic ganglia (bottom), at the same magnification and stained with Masson trichrome stain, differ markedly in size but exhibit basic architectural similarities. These include a delicate fibrous capsule, traversing bundles of afferent and efferent nerve fibers, and clustering of ganglion cells, a feature most apparent in dorsal root ganglia.

either in cranial nerve ganglia or in dorsal root ganglia. The latter, aside from differences in their size and content of cytoplasmic Nissl substance, show no significant differences in the appearance of their ganglion cells. All possess centrally situated round nuclei with open chromatin and prominent nucleoli. They are ensheathed by perineurial cells and dura. The dorsal root ganglia consist of clustered cell bodies separated by bundles of myelinated nerve fibers (fig. 2-15). The neurons or ganglion cells in dorsal root ganglia consist of small and large cells. These vary in neurotransmitter content and are functionally distinct.

In any case, individual ganglion cells are surrounded by specialized Schwann cells termed satellite or capsular cells. In dorsal root ganglia, these specialized cells totally surround ganglion

cells with delicate overlapping cytoplasmic processes, and are invested by basement membrane. Special histochemical and immunocytochemical preparations clearly distinguish satellite and nerve fiber–associated Schwann cells of ganglia from the ganglion cells and their processes (fig. 2-16). No synapses are present in dorsal root ganglia. Instead, the ganglion cells possess proximal and distal processes originating from the branching of a short, initially unipolar and highly coiled process termed the glomerular segment. In an ill-defined region of transition proximal to the ganglion, Schwann cells of the root are replaced by oligodendrocytes on centrally directed processes (fig. 2-13). The extent of this transition zone varies, and does not strictly correspond to the anatomic interference between nerve root and spinal cord surface.

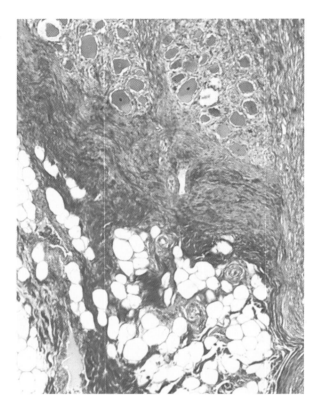 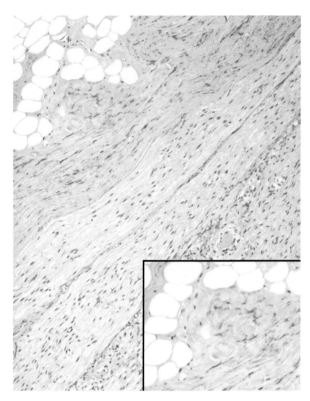

Figure 2-15

DORSAL (SENSORY) ROOT GANGLION

Left: With the trichrome stain, the ganglion is seen to be surrounded by a collagenous capsule.
Right: The connective tissue capsule surrounding the ganglion contains perineurial cells as evidenced by epithelial membrane antigen staining (inset).

Autonomic Ganglia. Ganglia occur in both the sympathetic and parasympathetic divisions of the autonomic nervous system. Sympathetic ganglia and dorsal root ganglia are structurally similar (figs. 2-16, 2-17). Both are invested by a fibrous capsule contiguous with epineurium. Their ganglion cells are surrounded by satellite or capsular cells; however, unlike in dorsal root ganglia, this investment of sympathetic ganglia is often incomplete. Autonomic ganglion cells are multipolar and receive synapses from preganglionic fibers, the majority of which are dendrites. As in dorsal root ganglia, autonomic ganglion cells are not uniform in size. Some are large and feature eccentric nuclei, vesicular chromatin, prominent nucleoli, and abundant Nissl substance. Their dense core granule-containing cells are adrenergic. There is often a second, minor population of smaller ganglion cells. The nuclei of smaller cells are ovoid or convoluted, contain more heterochro-

matin, and feature larger dense core granules, which are dopaminergic in nature.

Of parasympathetic ganglia, those arising in the gastrointestinal tract are the most relevant to surgical pathology. Lying within the wall of the gastrointestinal tract and connected with the vagus nerve and sacral outflow, such intramural ganglia occur in two locations, the submucosa (Meissner plexus) and between the layers of the muscularis propria (myenteric or Auerbach plexus). Their cells are surrounded by satellite cells, typically have eccentrically situated nuclei of vesicular type with prominent nucleoli, and possess many dendrites. Parasympathetic ganglia and nerves of the gastrointestinal tract are cholinergic. They contain not only acetylcholine but also a number of other peptides, particularly the gastrointestinal hormone vasoactive intestinal polypeptide. Their stimulation generally increases muscular

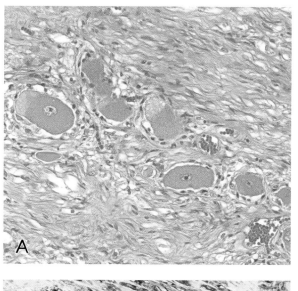

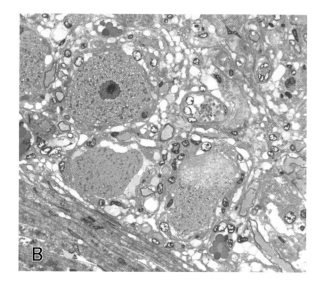

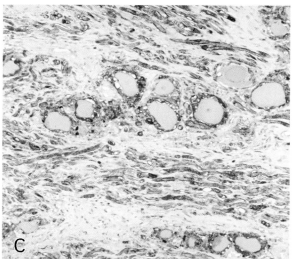

Figure 2-16

DORSAL (SENSORY) ROOT GANGLION

A: The clustered ganglion cells lie separated by bundles of their nerve fibers.

B,C: The ganglion cells with their centrally situated nuclei are surrounded by satellite cells best seen on toluidine blue–stained semi-thin sections (B) and with the S-100 protein immunostain (C).

D,E: Myelinated nerve fiber bundles traversing the ganglion are seen with the LFB-PAS-Bielschowsky stain (D) as well as with a neurofilament immunostain (E).

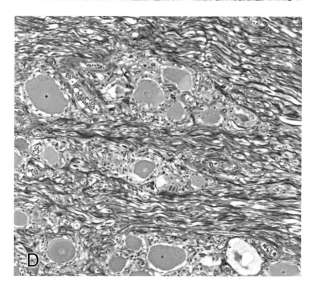

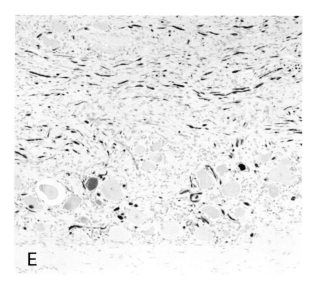

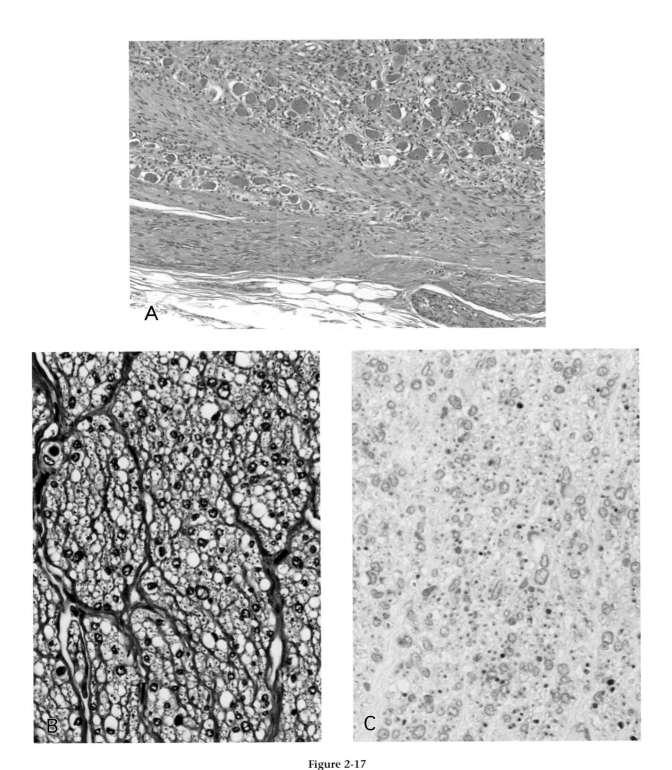

Figure 2-17

CERVICAL SYMPATHETIC GANGLION AND NERVE

Although these ganglia closely resemble dorsal root (sensory) ganglia (fig. 2-12), at least three differences are apparent. Sympathetic ganglia appear more cellular, and their neurons are both smaller and feature eccentric nuclei (A). With the LFB-PAS-Bielschowsky stains (B), sympathetic nerves are largely unmyelinated and contain minute axons. The small size of these axons is best seen with neurofilament protein immunostains (C).

Table 2-1

HISTOLOGIC TECHNIQUES FOR PERIPHERAL NERVES

Stains	Purpose
General Stains	
Hematoxylin and eosin	Detection of inflammation including vasculitis, fibrosis; myelin and axons
Reticulin	Basement membrane surrounding Schwann cells in normal nerve barely evident but are more readily demonstrated in nerve sheath tumors
Masson trichrome	Fibrosis; fibrinoid necrosis in vasculitis; myelin, red
Alcian blue	Glycosaminoglycans, blue
Toluidine blue	Mast cells, metachromatic; general stain for semi-thin resin sections
Stains for Myelin	
Luxol-fast blue	Myelin, blue; can be combined with silver stains for axon
Periodic acid–Schiff	Degenerating myelin and macrophages; perineurium
Osmium	Myelin, black
Congo red	Amyloid
Stains for Axons	
Bodian, Bielschowsky, or Palmgren (silver stains)	Axons, black
Stains for Immunochemistry	
S-100 protein	Schwann cells, normal and neoplastic
Leu-7 (CD57)	Schwann cells, normal and neoplastic
Glial fibrillary acidic protein	Some Schwann cells and Schwann cell tumors
Myelin basic protein	Myelin
Epithelial membrane antigen	Perineurial cells
Glut-1	Perineurial cells
Claudin-1	Perineurial cells
Synaptophysin	Axons, neurons
Neurofilament protein	Axons, neurons
Collagen 4, laminin	Basement membranes

activity, circulation, and secretion. These same activities are decreased by stimulation of sympathetic nerves, the ganglia of which lie outside the gut.

The principal histologic and immunohistochemical stains useful in the study of peripheral nerve pathology are summarized, as are their tissue specificities, in Table 2-1.

Interstitial Cells of Cajal

Described by Cajal in 1911 (3), and rightly identified as having the capacity to modify smooth muscle contraction, the interstitial cells of Cajal (ICCs) are modified smooth muscle cells situated between intramural neurons of the gastrointestinal tract and smooth muscle cells. By generating electrical slow waves, they underlie gastrointestinal motility and are termed "pacemaker cells" since they literally drive peristalsis (4). Patients with gastrointestinal motility disorders may have decreased numbers of such cells in their bowels (4–6).

Interstitial cells are identified throughout the gut, and are variously distributed in its layers (4). In the small and large bowel, these layers include the lamina propria, but their density is greatest around the myenteric plexus and at the submucosal border (4). In the myenteric plexus and muscularis propria, they are disposed in a reticular network, their elongated processes aligned with muscle cells.

Cytologically, ICC appears in routine H&E-stained specimens as a fusiform cell with an oval nucleus (fig. 2-18A). The same configuration is evident in silver impregnations where their processes are also evident. In optimally oriented sections, immunohistochemistry reveals two or more dendritic processes connecting ICCs to one another, to ganglion cells, or to adjacent smooth muscle cells. They exhibit reactivity for CD34 and CD117 (c-kit), a transmembrane protein kinase involved in the development of a variety of cell lineages, but are negative for S-100 protein (fig. 2-18B,C). Associated with nerve

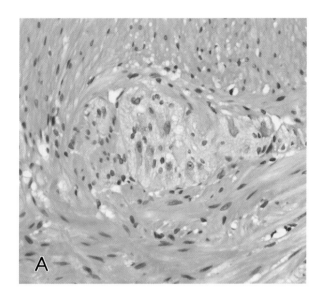

Figure 2-18

MYENTERIC PLEXUS OF COLON

The myenteric plexus consists of ganglia and nerves distributed as a circumferential layer between the inner and outer muscle coats (A). Cajal cells in the myenteric plexus of the colon are highlighted by immunostaining for CD34 (B) and CD117 (C).

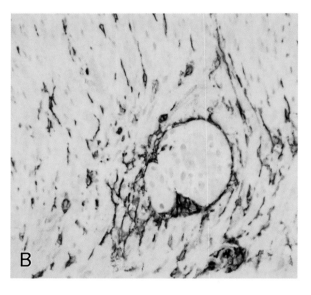

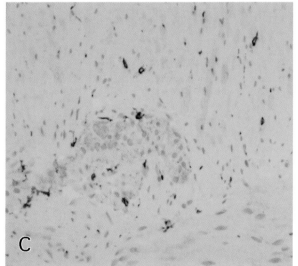

bundles and innervated by enteric neurons, they bear receptors for neurotransmitters, thus facilitating transmission. With respect to neoplasms of the peripheral nervous system, gastrointestinal stromal tumors show the phenotypic characteristics of ICC (see chapter 13) (7).

Specialized Nerve Endings

Non-neoplastic lesions may affect specialized nerve endings. Furthermore, a variety of peripheral nerve tumors mimic the cytoarchitecture of sensory endings. Thus, a brief discussion of these distinctive structures is in order (8–10).

Among nerve endings, the sensory ones are the most numerous transducers of stimulation.

The three main sensory subtypes are free nerve endings, expanded tip endings, and terminal corpuscles (encapsulated endings). Free nerve endings are unassociated with specialized receptor structures. Collectively, they subserve pain and touch. Their fibers usually measure less than 1 mm in diameter and they lose their Schwann sheaths near their terminations. Such receptors are most numerous in the dermis, epidermis, mucosa, cornea, about tendons, and within soft tissue. Free nerve endings of the epidermis are sometimes associated with modified, disc-shaped tactile cells of Merkel about which they form networks. Terminal corpuscles (encapsulated corpuscles) are among the most frequent

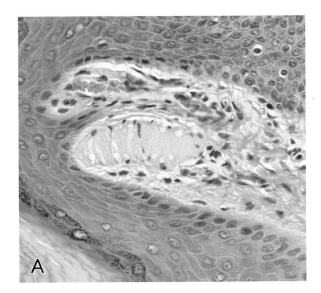

Figure 2-19

MEISSNER CORPUSCLES

These tactile bodies lie within the papillary dermis (A) and consist of stacked lamellae of S-100 protein–positive Schwann cells (B) between which are interposed neurofilament protein–positive axons (C).

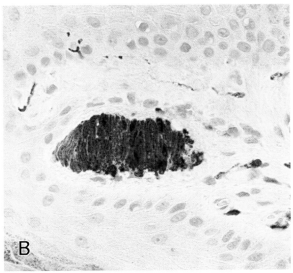

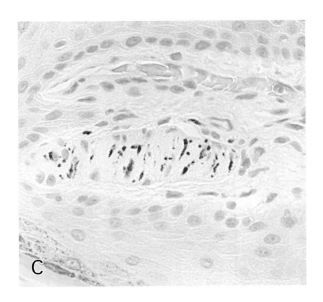

of sensory endings encountered in peripheral nerve pathology. They include Meissner and pacinian (Vater-Pacini) corpuscles as well as muscle and tendon spindles.

Meissner Corpuscles. These receptors sense low frequency vibrations and touch, and are most numerous in the glabrous skin of the fingertips, palms, and soles, as well as on sensitive mucosal surfaces. They measure 50 to 150 μm and thus are small in comparison to pacinian corpuscles. Meissner corpuscles are laminated structures (fig. 2-19) composed of flattened layers of Schwann cells oriented across the long axis of one or several of the myelinated nerve fibers that enter at one end of the corpuscle.

Once having lost their myelination, such fibers branch or spiral in a zigzag fashion, making contact with the specialized Schwann cells of the corpuscle. The latter are S-100 protein immunoreactive and, as expected, the axons are neurofilament protein-positive (fig. 2-19B, C). Normal Meissner corpuscles lack epithelial membrane antigen reactivity (10).

Pacinian (Vater-Pacini) Corpuscles. As the first receptors to be recognized, these structures have been particularly well studied (8). Fully differentiated in the 20-cm fetus and functional as pressure or tension receptors able to sense high frequency vibrations, stimulation of pacinian corpuscles may not produce subjective sensations. Numerically, they are most abundant in deep dermal tissue of the hands and feet, and a single finger contains up to 350 such corpuscles (8). Their association with arteriovenous anastomoses of the skin suggests that pacinian corpuscles also play a vasoregulatory role. Pacinian corpuscles also occur in the vicinity of joints, tendons, periosteum, and perimysium, as well as within mesentery and sensitive mucosal surfaces. In association with large vessels, they appear to act as pressor receptors. Single or occasionally paired pacinian corpuscles are connected to their parent nerve by a myelinated fiber. Less often, they are more intimately associated with the parent nerve, lying either within the epineurium or near the perineurium.

Pacinian corpuscles are the largest of sensory receptors, measuring up to 4 mm in adulthood. Their structure and function are the basis of a review (11). Distributed singly or in groups, oval or occasionally folded, these rice grain-like structures are surrounded by a collagenous capsule. They consist of an outer and inner bulb (fig. 2-20A, B), the outer composed of 20 to 60 onion-like lamellae of flattened perineurial cells with scant intervening collagen fibrils (fig. 2-20B,C). Each layer measures approximately 1 μm in thickness and is epithelial membrane antigen immunopositive (fig. 2-20D) (10). A sizable artery enters the mid-portion of the corpuscle, and its capillaries ramify within the interlamellar spaces. At the avascular center of the corpuscle lies the inner bulb. Within it is a large, neurofilament protein-positive nerve fiber (fig. 2-20E) which loses its myelin sheath, and becomes flattened, branched, and coiled.

Pacinian corpuscles grow by the addition of lamellae and by retrograde extension along their nerve. In the process, the myelinated nerve fibers come to lie more deeply within the corpuscle (fig. 2-20F). With age, corpuscles undergo regressive changes, including shrinkage, irregularity in configuration, and interlamellar as well as pericorpuscular fibrosis.

Muscle Spindles. These highly specialized receptors are involved in proprioception. They are present in all striated muscles, and are most numerous in muscles subserving delicate movements of the eye, hand, and neck. Muscle spindles consist of 3 to 20 modified striated muscle fibers ranging from 1 to 5 mm in length and up to 2 mm in diameter. Also termed intrafusal fibers, they are smaller than normal skeletal muscle fibers and include one or two long, thick fibers with central aggregated nuclei (nuclear bag fibers) and numerous short, thin fibers in which nuclei are arranged longitudinally (nuclear chain fibers). Both fibers exhibit cross striations. Myelinated motor and sensory nerve fibers enter the spindle to branch and spiral among the muscle fibers at its center. The nerves maintain tone within the spindle and sense its degree and rate of stretch. Analogous structures also occur in tendons (tendon spindles of Golgi). The reader is referred to authoritative texts for a more detailed discussion of the microanatomy of the muscle spindle (12,13).

IMMUNOHISTOCHEMISTRY

Familiarity with the immunoreactivities of nerve is essential in order to understand nerve sheath tumors. Schwann cells engaged in myelin formation as well as those accompanying nonmyelinated nerves are characterized by strong staining for vimentin and S-100 protein, an acidic protein of unknown function. Leu-7, an antibody directed against human killer T cells, also stains Schwann cells by recognizing a carbohydrate epitope on MAG (14). The latter plays a role in myelination, being present in the membranes of Schwann cells engaged in myelin formation but not in those accompanying nonmyelinated axons. Some Schwann cells stain for glial fibrillary acidic protein (GFAP), the principal component of glial fibrils in both astrocytes and ependymal cells (15). This antigen is present mainly in Schwann cells unengaged in myelin formation (16). As previously noted, the basement membrane surrounding Schwann cells contains laminin, fibronectin, entactin, and various collagens, mainly type 4. Reactivity for collagen 4 and laminin shows Schwann cell–associated basement membranes.

Perineurial cells also exhibit vimentin staining but unlike Schwann cells, lack immunoreactivity for S-100 protein, Leu-7, and GFAP (14,17). Perineurium and arachnoid membrane (17,18) share some similarities in that both are reactive for epithelial membrane antigen, a group of carbohydrate-rich, protein-poor, high molecular weight substances present in nearly all epithelia and in plasma cells. Nerve sheath fibroblasts are immunoreactive for vimentin alone.

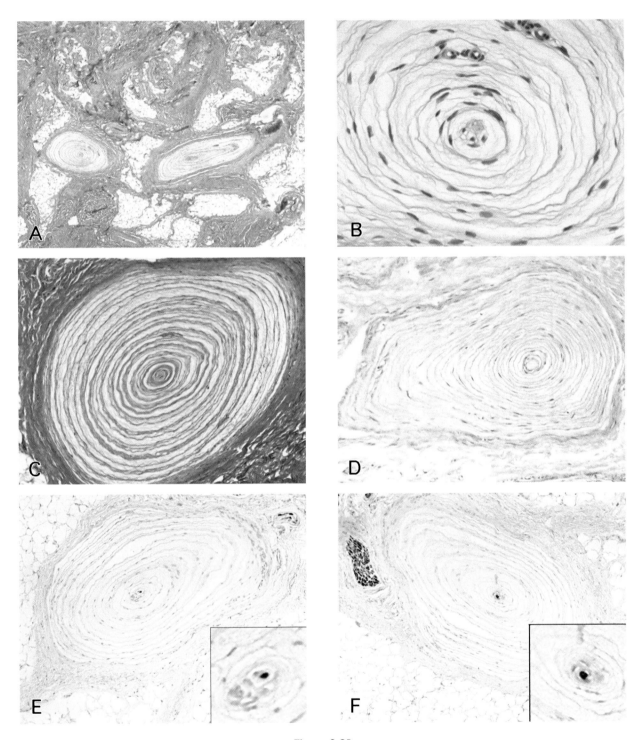

Figure 2-20

PACINIAN CORPUSCLES

These specialized receptors, here seen at the dermal-subcutaneous junction (A), consist of an outer core composed of spherical laminae of perineurial cells (B) with interposed delicate collagen (C, trichrome stain). The perineurial cells stain for epithelial membrane antigen (D). The delicate central nerve fiber (E and F, inset) and accompanying Schwann sheath that comprise the inner core are best seen with neurofilament protein (E) and S-100 protein (F) immunostains.

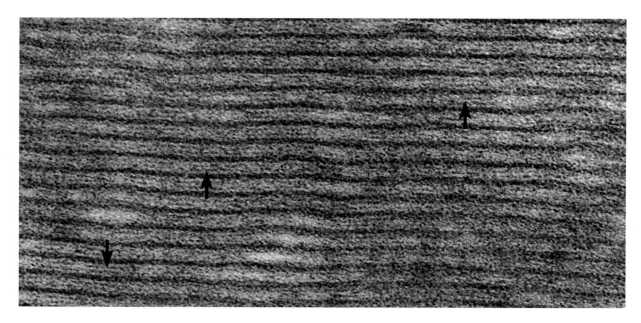

Figure 2-21

MYELIN SHEATH

Detail of the myelin sheath of a medium-sized myelinated nerve from the parotid gland. The myelin sheath consists of alternating major dense lines with a periodicity of approximately 12 nm and two intraperiod lines with a 2-nm intraperiod gap. The double intraperiod lines are seen in favorable planes of section (arrows).

ULTRASTRUCTURE

On transmission electron microscopy, the cellular composition and fine structural features of peripheral nerves are readily apparent (fig. 2-7). Unmyelinated axons in varying number are enclosed by the cytoplasm of a single Schwann cell (fig. 2-9). Regardless of size, axons are readily recognized by the presence of numerous, fairly evenly spaced microtubules having an average diameter of 25 nm in association with 10-nm neurofilaments. Occasional mitochondria and ribosomes also are found within the axoplasm.

Unlike nonmyelinated nerve fibers, myelinated examples appear as a single axon surrounded by a myelin sheath formed by concentric wrappings of the Schwann cell membrane (fig. 2-10). The space formed by the outer invaginating Schwann cell membranes is termed the external mesaxon (fig. 2-10), whereas the junction where the membranes separate to surround the axon is referred to as the inner mesaxon. Ultrastructural studies show that the myelin sheath is formed of uniform, multilayered, spiral wrappings of the Schwann cell membrane. At high magnification, these feature 3-nm thick major dense lines alternating with an intraperiod line doublet separated by a space known as the intraperiod gap (fig. 2-21) (19). The periodicity of the major dense lines is approximately 12 nm.

The outer Schwann cell membrane of both myelinated and nonmyelinated axons is separated from the endoneurial matrix by a continuous basement membrane (figs. 2-9, 2-10). The electron-lucent endoneurial matrix contains primarily collagen fibrils. The cellular constituents of endoneurium include endothelial cells and pericytes of small blood capillaries, fibroblasts rich in rough endoplasmic reticulum, mast cells, and macrophages.

The endoneurium is surrounded by the perineurial sheath (fig. 2-7). On cross section, the latter consists of multiple layers of elongated perineurial cells bound on their inner and outer aspects by a continuous, irregularly thick basement membrane and a scant matrix consisting mainly of collagen fibrils (fig. 2-8). Perineurial cells with their elongated, blunt-ended nuclei are characterized by long, thin, bipolar cytoplasmic processes, the cell membranes of which exhibit pinocytotic vesicles. These vesicles are also evident in the cytoplasm of perineurial cells (fig. 2-8). Organelles are sparse, although diffuse arrays of both actin microfilaments and vimentin intermediate filaments may be prominent. For a more detailed discussion of the fine structure of peripheral nerves, the reader is referred to several authoritative texts (13,19).

REFERENCES

1. Gardner E, Bunge RP. Gross anatomy of the peripheral nervous system. In: Dyck PJ, Thomas PK, eds. Peripheral neuropathy. 3rd ed. Philadelphia: W. B. Saunders, Co; 1993:8-27.

2. Erlandson RA. The enigmatic perineurial cell and its participation in tumors and in tumorlike entities. Ultrastruct Pathol 1991;15:335-351.

3. Cajal RR. Histologie du systéme nerveux de l'homme et des vértebrés, Vol. 2. Paris: Maloire; 1911:891-942.

4. Streutker CJ, Huizinga JD, Driman DK, Riddell RH. Interstitial cells of Cajal in health and disease. Part I: normal ICC structure and function with associated motility disorders. Histopathology 2007;50:176-189.

5. Rolle U, Piaseczna-Piotrowska A, Puri P. Interstitial cells of Cajal in the normal gut and in intestinal motility disorders of childhood. Pediatr Surg Int 2007;23:1139-1152.

6. Vanderwinden JM, Rumessen JJ. Interstitial cells of Cajal in human gut and gastrointestinal disease. Microsc Res Tech 1999;47:344-360.

7. Kindblom LG, Remotti HE, Aldenborg F, Meis-Kindblom JM. Gastrointestinal pacemaker cell tumor (GIPACT): gastrointestinal stromal tumors show phenotypic characteristics of the interstitial cells of Cajal. Am J Pathol 1998;152:1259-1269.

8. Cauna N, Mannan G. The structure of human digital pacinian corpuscles (corpus cula lamellosa) and its functional significance. J Anat 1958;92:1-20.

9. Malinovsky L. Sensory nerve formations in the skin and their classification. Microsc Res Tech 1996;34:283-301.

10. Vega JA, Haro JJ, Del Valle ME. Immunohistochemistry of human cutaneous Meissner and pacinian corpuscles. Microsc Res Tech 1996;34:351-361.

11. Bell J, Bolanowski S, Holmes MH. The structure and function of Pacinian corpuscles: a review. Prog Neurobiol 1994;42:79-128.

12. Poppele RE. The muscle spindle. In: Dyck PJ, Thomas PK, eds. Peripheral neuropathy. Philadelphia: W. B. Saunders; 1993:121-140.

13. Thomas PK, Berthold CH, Ochoa J. Microscopic anatomy of the peripheral nervous system. In: Dyck PJ, Thomas PK, eds. Peripheral neuropathy. Philadelphia: W. B. Saunders; 1993:28-92.

14. Perentes E, Rubinstein LJ. Recent applications of immunoperoxidase histochemistry in human neuro-oncology. An update. Arch Pathol Lab Med 1987;111:796-812.

15. Gould VE, Moll R, Moll I, Lee I, Schwechheimer K, Franke WW. The intermediate filament complement of the spectrum of nerve sheath neoplasms. Lab Invest 1986;55:463-474.

16. Gray MH, Rosenberg AE, Dickersin GR, Bhan AK. Glial fibrillary acidic protein and keratin expression by benign and malignant nerve sheath tumors. Hum Pathol 1989;20:1089-1096.

17. Perentes E, Nakagawa Y, Ross GW, Stanton C, Rubinstein LJ. Expression of epithelial membrane antigen in perineurial cells and their derivatives. An immunohistochemical study with multiple markers. Acta Neuropathol 1987;75:160-165.

18. Ariza A, Bilbao JM, Rosai J. Immunohistochemical detection of epithelial membrane antigen in normal perineurial cells and perineurioma. Am J Surg Pathol 1988;12:678-683.

19. Angevine JB. The nervous tissue. In: Bloom, Fawcett, eds. A textbook of histology. New York: Chapman & Hall; 1994:309-364.

3 REACTIVE LESIONS

TRAUMATIC NEUROMA

Definition. *Traumatic neuroma* is a non-neoplastic, disorganized proliferation of axons, Schwann cells, and perineurial cells, all in a fibrocollagenous stroma and forming a mass at the site of the partial or complete transection of a nerve. Traumatic neuroma is also known as *amputation neuroma*.

General Features. Although in physiologic terms, normal peripheral nerve is a site of intense activity, it is quiescent in terms of cell turnover, particularly with respect to Schwann cell proliferation. Injury is required to prompt proliferative changes in nerve, both in axons and sheath cells. The most commonly encountered example of a reparative proliferation is traumatic neuroma. It is the prototypic *true neuroma*, a reactive lesion composed of all the elements of normal nerve.

An understanding of traumatic neuroma requires familiarity with the events following an experimental nerve transection (1–3). Successful reinnervation of the distal stump of a fully transected nerve requires: 1) proximity of the injury to the end organ; 2) a close association of the severed proximal and distal nerve segments; and 3) no obstruction to the path of regenerating axons. With reference to the distal segment, complete degeneration of residual axons and myelin sheaths (wallerian degeneration) is required to prepare the nerve for ingrowth of new proximal neurites. The process is evident even at 24 hours, a time when fiber fragmentation is underway. Lysosomal enzymes alter the degenerating myelin, with resultant loss of birefringence and its characteristic tinctorial properties. During the process, normally Luxol-fast blue–positive myelin is transformed into periodic acid-Schiff (PAS)-, sudanophilic-, oil red O-, and Marchi-positive debris. By 4 weeks, Schwann cells and macrophages have removed most, if not all, axonal and myelin debris. In its place, cords or tubes of basement membrane-enshrouded Schwann cells, termed *bands of Büngner,* await the ingrowth of regenerating proximal axons. In the absence of distally traveling axons, the bands atrophy (4).

Alterations that occur proximally affect both the neuronal cell body and the axons. The cell body shows chromatolysis, a decrease in prominence of Nissl substance indicating intense synthetic activity. The proximal axon also undergoes dramatic changes. Between 1 and 3 weeks after transection, the proximal stump forms an organelle-rich, 50- to 100-µm diameter expansion. Neurites emerge from the expansion under the influence of nerve growth factor, a substance elaborated by surrounding Schwann cells, as well as trophic factors secreted by macrophages. Growing 1 to 2 mm per day, the new axons cross the trauma-induced gap, reach the distal nerve segment, and colonize the bands of Büngner. Fibers regenerate down the bands, mature, and, if possible, reconnect with their original or with a different, albeit meaningful, target. If misdirection occurs and connections cannot be established, the nerve fibers atrophy.

A traumatic neuroma results when effective regeneration is thwarted because the outgrowing axons are too removed from the distal stump or encounter scar tissue. In simplistic terms, the lesion represents a frustrated attempt at re-establishment of nerve continuity. It consists of massive, disorganized tangles of nerve fibers, some forming microfascicles, each a crude caricature of a nerve, replete with axons, Schwann sheaths, and a surrounding perineurium.

Clinical Features. Following nerve injury, either complete transection or crush (traumatic neuroma in continuity), the previously described degenerative and reparative changes follow. The growth of new axons from the proximal nerve stump begins even before the degeneration of distal axons is complete. The neuroma resulting from unsuccessful regeneration is a firm, often tender or painful nodule.

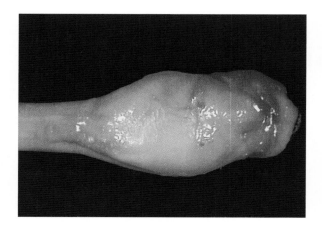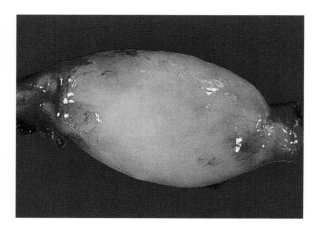

Figure 3-1

TRAUMATIC NEUROMA

Left: This intact lesion forms a localized bulbous expansion at the distal end of a once transected nerve.
Right: On cut section, neuromas appear as localized, gray-tan and translucent masses.

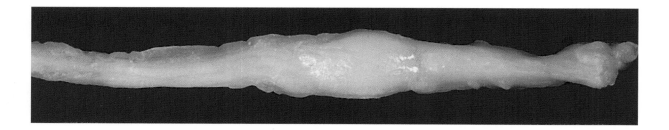

Figure 3-2

TRAUMATIC NEUROMA

Above: This example formed after trauma without complete division of the nerve. As a result, the nerve is still in continuity.

Right: Using the Bielschowsky stain, tangled, newly formed microfascicles are seen to comprise the bulk of the lesion. Large entering nerve fascicles are present on the right with only small fascicles within the lesion (left).

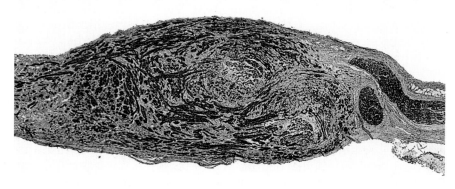

Most traumatic neuromas arise in the postsurgical setting, but in some instances, they follow insignificant injuries. A rare form occurs in utero after autoamputation of a supernumerary digit (5,6). The lesion(s) usually appear on the proximal, ulnar aspect of the hand. Visceral sites, particularly the gallbladder (7) and bile ducts (8,9), are also affected. Most, but not all (10), occur months to years after cholecystectomy or in association with lithiasis. Some examples are polypoid (11).

Gross Findings. Traumatic neuromas are somewhat circumscribed, gray-white, nodular masses that occur either at the proximal stump of a transected nerve (fig. 3-1) or along the course of an incompletely transected, crushed, or otherwise traumatized nerve (fig. 3-2). In the case of a nerve plexus, severe injury may result in the formation of multiple neuromas (fig. 3-3). Nearly all traumatic neuromas measure less than 5 cm in maximal dimension. On longitudinal section, the proximal portion of the nerve splays, disappearing into a firm, fibrous mass, features readily appreciated in whole mount sections (figs. 3-2, 3-4A,B).

Microscopic Findings. The essential features of traumatic neuroma are haphazard tangles of regenerated axons accompanied by ensheathing Schwann cells. The lesion is unencapsulated and consists of nerve fibers organized into microfascicles of varying size lying within fibrous tissue (figs. 3-2, 3-4C,D). The nerve fibers are far less myelinated than those of the parent nerve (fig. 3-5A). Microfascicles vary in size and appearance. When well formed and seen in cross section, they are surrounded by a uniform, albeit thin, perineurial membrane (fig. 3-5D). Occasionally, circumferential proliferation of nerve fibers surrounds residual or parent nerve fascicles (fig. 3-6). Within the newer fascicles, proliferating nerve fibers may lie embedded in a mucoid matrix (fig. 3-7A); in well-established neuromas, they often lie enmeshed in fibrocollagenous tissue (fig. 3-7B). Extension of neuroma into adipose tissue or even nearby skeletal muscle fibers is less often seen (fig. 3-7C,D). Chronic inflammation and focal foreign body reaction at the transection site is uncommon but may be seen at wound sites inadequately cleansed (fig. 3-8).

Immunohistochemical Findings. As expected, the immunoreactivities of normal nerve are represented in traumatic neuromas. Axons are positive for neurofilament protein (fig. 3-5B), Schwann cells react for S-100 protein (fig. 3-5C) or Leu-7, and perineurial cells surrounding microfascicles react for epithelial membrane antigen (EMA) (fig. 3-5D).

Ultrastructural Findings. In the early phases of nerve fiber regeneration, axons are often unmyelinated and surrounded only by the cytoplasm of Schwann cells (fig. 3-9). With time, limited myelin formation results from Schwann cells wrapping about axons while perineurial cells delimit microfascicles.

Differential Diagnosis. Since traumatic neuromas occur at almost any site, the differential diagnostic considerations are broad. Simulators include localized interdigital neuritis (Morton neuroma), palisaded encapsulated neuroma,

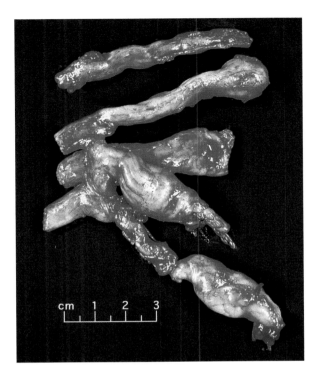

Figure 3-3

TRAUMATIC NEUROMA

In severe injuries, such as this example of avulsion of the brachial plexus, traumatic neuromas are multiple and involve several nerve trunks.

mucosal neuromatosis, schwannoma, and neurofibroma.

As a response to chronic nerve injury, localized interdigital neuritis (LIN) is etiologically related to traumatic neuroma in continuity. Given the stereotypic clinical setting and anatomic location of LIN, the two lesions are usually easily distinguished. With rare exception, LINs are limited to the feet of females. Both lesions, but mainly the latter, affect grossly recognizable nerves. Unlike traumatic neuroma, which is a proliferative, reparative lesion composed of microfascicles of axons with accompanying Schwann cells, LIN consists of a recognizable nerve with marked degenerative changes affecting epineurium, perineurium, and endoneurium. Schwann cell, myelin, and axonal loss characterize the lesion. What remains within the endoneurium are aligned, but very much diminished, axons and Schwann cells. Due to the preservation of gross architectural features, LIN

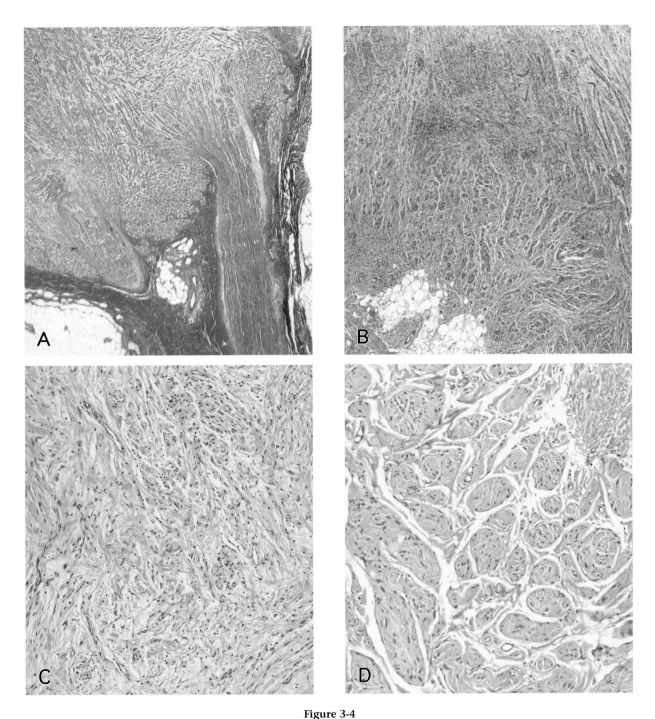

Figure 3-4

TRAUMATIC NEUROMA

A: A whole mount section of a globular example is associated with a small myelinated nerve (lower left). The transition of the nerve to neuroma is clearly seen. Despite apparent circumscription, these lesions lack a capsule. Instead, this trichrome preparation highlights associated perilesional fibrosis. (Fig. 3.402 from Okazaki H, Scheithauer BW. Atlas of neuropathology. New York: Gower; 1988:180. With permission from the Mayo Foundation.)

B: The neuroma (center and right) erupts from the parent nerve (left).

C,D: Varying in size from small and disorganized (C) to larger and better defined (D), newly formed microfascicles make up the substance of a traumatic neuroma.

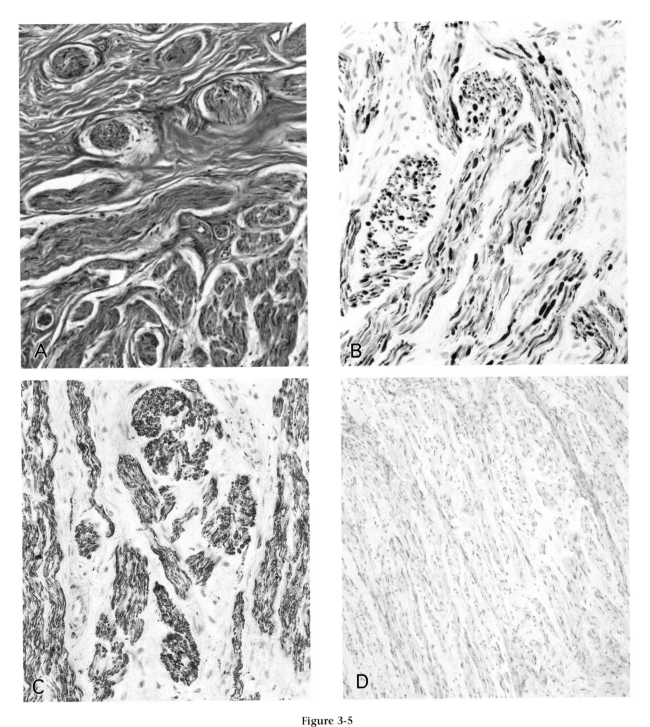

Figure 3-5

TRAUMATIC NEUROMA

A: Regenerating nerve fiber bundles (microfascicles) are arranged in uniform, tangled bundles, which with a Luxol-fast blue–periodic acid–Schiff (PAS) stain are seen to be composed of variably myelinated nerves.

B,C: A delicate collagenous stroma separates the fascicles. Immunostains for neurofilament protein and S-100 protein highlight the axons and Schwann sheaths, respectively.

D: A perineurial investment, best seen here with an epithelial membrane antigen (EMA) immunostain, surrounds the microfascicles.

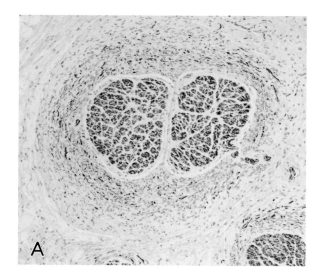

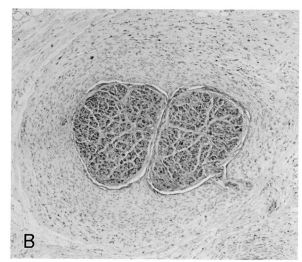

Figure 3-6

TRAUMATIC NEUROMA

Unusual findings are proliferation of axons (A), accompanying Schwann cells (B), and perineurial cells (C) in a circumferential pattern about the parent nerve fascicles (A: neurofilament protein; B: S-100 protein; C: EMA immunostains).

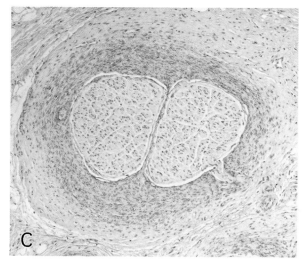

is more orderly than the random meandering of new microfascicles that characterizes traumatic neuroma. Lastly, LINs feature perineurial fibrosis and elastic tissue deposition as well as epineural vascular thrombosis and sclerosis.

A number of features aid in the distinction of palisaded encapsulated neuroma (PEN) from traumatic neuroma. Unlike the latter, PENs mainly affect females, are superficially situated, and usually lie within skin rather than in deep soft tissue. Traumatic neuromas are more often associated with a recognizable nerve and are usually microscopically less circumscribed than are PENs. Although both lesions consist of axons, Schwann cells, and perineurial cells, traumatic

neuroma represents a more orderly physiologic response, featuring axons uniformly ensheathed by Schwann cells as well as microfascicle formation, replete with perineurial ensheathment. In contrast, PEN consists mostly of Schwann cells; orderly ensheathment of axons and well-formed microfascicle formation are lacking. Instead, a delicate perineurium often surrounds all but the most superficial portions.

Also in the differential diagnosis of traumatic neuroma is mucosal neuroma. When multiple and consisting of well-formed nerves, as in multiple endocrine neoplasia (MEN) 2B, the distinction is easy. Solitary mucosal neuromas, however, such as those of the biliary system,

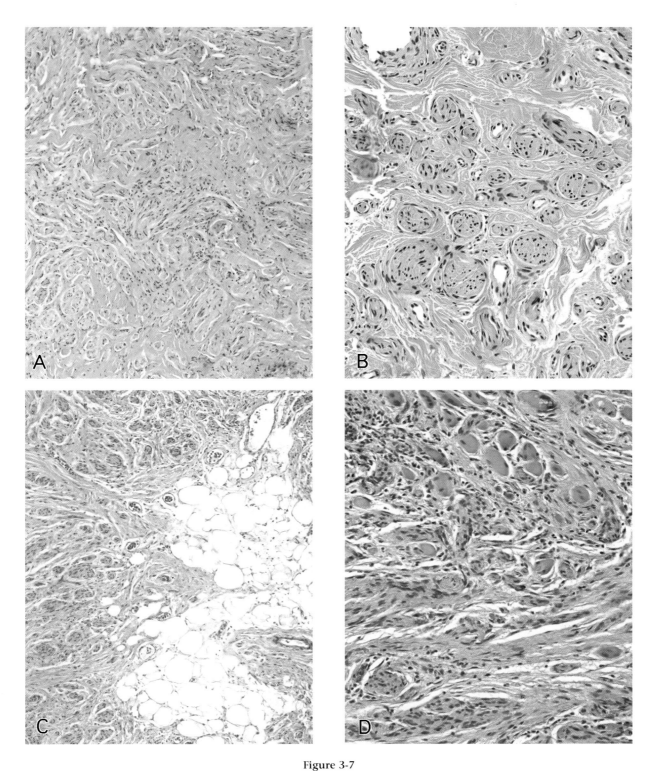

Figure 3-7

TRAUMATIC NEUROMA

The stroma of traumatic neuroma varies from partly mucinous (A) to dense fibrous connective tissue (B). Some lesions, due to their loose texture or to extension into surrounding fibroadipose tissue (C) or muscle (D), superficially resemble neurofibroma.

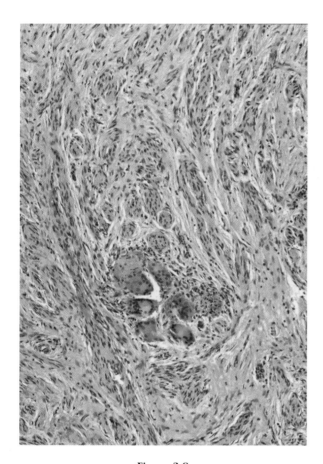

Figure 3-8

TRAUMATIC NEUROMA

Chronic inflammation and foreign body reaction related to the original trauma, although an uncommon finding, may be a hint to the diagnosis.

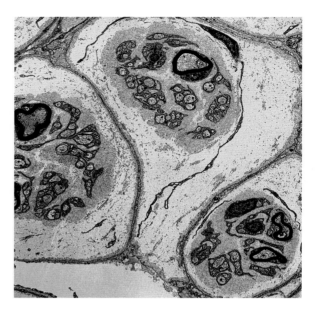

Figure 3-9

TRAUMATIC NEUROMA: ULTRASTRUCTURE

Resected 8 years after traumatic amputation of the lower leg, this stump neuroma arising from a small nerve shows three microfascicles, each composed largely of unmyelinated axons, surrounded by a delicate perineurium.

duodenum, and appendix, may closely resemble traumatic neuroma. In fact, we believe the two lesions may be etiologically related (see figs. 4-12, 4-13).

Particularly in cases in which biopsies are small and nonrepresentative, schwannoma enters into the differential diagnosis. Unlike traumatic neuromas, schwannomas are unassociated with antecedent trauma. Whereas traumatic neuromas are solid, gray-white, ill-defined, complex lesions composed of regenerating axons with accompanying Schwann and perineurial cells, schwannomas are encapsulated, often partially cystic, tan or yellow lesions, composed only of Schwann cells. The features typical of schwannoma, including Antoni A and B patterns as well as Verocay bodies, are not compo-

nents of traumatic neuroma. The maximal size of traumatic neuroma is approximately 5 cm, but schwannomas are often considerably larger. Schwannomas feature an entering and exiting nerve. Whereas Schwann cell-ensheathed axons are present throughout traumatic neuromas, in schwannomas the parent nerve is usually eccentric and essentially displaced by the proliferation. However, neurofilament protein stains may show axons in the subcapsular region and even some deeper in the schwannoma. Schwannomas exhibit S-100 protein reactivity but lack epithelial membrane staining in all but their capsules. Fibrosis, granulation tissue, and focal inflammation, common features of traumatic neuroma, are not seen in small schwannomas. At the ultrastructural level, axons are usually not encountered in schwannomas.

Soft tissues are a common site of neurofibromas. Both they and traumatic neuromas vary in gross appearance, from localized to ill-defined. Although soft tissue infiltration may be widespread in neurofibroma, it is limited in traumatic neuroma (fig. 3-7C,D). Due in large part to the presence of a mucopolysaccharide matrix, neurofibroma grossly appears less cellular than does traumatic neuroma. This matrix is often conspicuous within the "worm-like" branches of plexiform neurofibromas. As a result, neurofibromas differ in appearance from the far smaller, complex microfascicles of traumatic neuromas. Histochemical stains and immunostains show axons in traumatic neuroma to be spread out, whereas they are centrally situated in intraneural neurofibromas.

Treatment and Prognosis. The treatment of fully developed traumatic neuroma is simple excision. The proximal nerve stump is embedded into normal soft tissue. This is not only required for traumatic neuromas associated with pain or dysesthesia, but also distinguishes them from what grossly may appear as recurrent neoplasm in the setting of prior cancer surgery (12). Their formation may be avoided if, at the time of nerve injury, the ends of traumatized nerves are optimally approximated to facilitate orderly regeneration. Graft placement may be required when proximity cannot be achieved.

LOCALIZED INTERDIGITAL NEURITIS

Definition. *Localized interdigital neuritis* (LIN) is a non-neoplastic, localized, degenerative lesion that usually affects a plantar digital nerve and is characterized by axon and Schwann cell/myelin loss with accompanying fibrosis. Synonyms include *Morton neuroma, plantar neuroma, Morton toe,* and *Morton node.*

General Features. LIN is caused by chronic nerve trauma or ischemia resulting from vascular and perivascular fibrosis (13). The role of vascular injury is supported by the observation, in early cases, of fibrodegenerative alterations surrounding the neurovascular bundle (14).

Clinical and Radiologic Features. The clinicopathologic features of LIN, a common lesion, have been well studied (15). Although its precise incidence is unknown, it affects primarily, but not exclusively, the feet of adult females. The process is often unilateral. Fully 90 percent of patients present with paroxysmal pain beneath the metatarsal arch between the third and fourth toes. The second and third interspaces may also be affected. Point tenderness is noted on compression. Pain is often present for weeks to years and is typically exacerbated by exercise and relieved by rest. The condition is usually at-

tributed to the compressive effects of ill-fitting shoes. On occasion, a similar lesion affects the hands, usually of males with chronic, repetitive occupational trauma.

Gross Findings. LIN is a localized, fusiform, firm expansion, usually at the bifurcation of the fourth plantar digital nerve (fig. 3-10). In well-established cases, the nerve sheath is often adherent to the intermetatarsal bursa and the adjacent digital artery. Most lesions are small, less than 1 cm in size, and grossly resemble either traumatic neuroma in continuity or neurofibroma. On cut section, they appear gray-tan and fibrous.

Microscopic Findings. Despite obvious enlargement of the plantar digital nerve, LIN is primarily a degenerative rather than a proliferative process. All compartments of the nerve are involved. Only the basic architectural features are preserved. Epineurial tissue is often extensively fibrotic (fig. 3-11A,B). Vessels, including the digital artery, become hyalinized (fig. 3-11A) and frequently thrombosed. Perineurium, although showing mucinous degeneration in early cases, becomes thickened over time (fig. 3-11B), clearly evident with a trichrome stain (figs. 3-11C, 3-12). Laminated collagenous nodules, a nonspecific feature, may be seen within the endoneurium (fig. 3-11D). Stromal deposition of elastic tissue (elastofibrosis) is a late-stage feature (fig. 3-12C) (14).

Although special stains are generally not required to make the diagnosis, silver stains for axons as well as stains for myelin typically show a reduction of both (fig. 3-13). Loss of axons and Schwann sheaths is also evident with immunostains (fig. 3-14). In keeping with the chronic nature of the lesion, the changes are unaccompanied by obvious wallerian degeneration or Schwann cell hyperplasia. No significant inflammation is seen, although fibrin deposits are common and the nearby synovium, included in an occasional biopsy, may show mild nonspecific chronic inflammation.

Immunohistochemical Findings. Residual axons are seen with a neurofilament stain but are reduced in number. S-100 protein stains show a proportionate reduction in Schwann sheaths. EMA preparations highlight the abnormal architecture of the hyalinized perineurium.

Ultrastructural Findings. Aside from fibrosis of extraneural tissues, electron microscopy

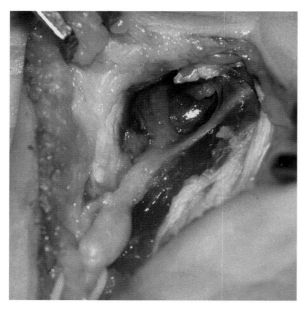 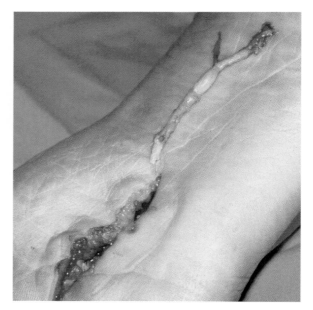

Figure 3-10

LOCALIZED INTERDIGITAL NEURITIS

Left: This sequence of intraoperative photographs shows the neuroma as a firm, gray, fusiform to somewhat nodular expansion of the digital plantar nerve.

Right: Still in situ, the size of the lesion (bottom) is contrasted with the normal-appearing remainder of the nerve (upper right).

reveals a variety of changes, including degenerative changes in nerve fibers, myelin loss, endoneurial vessel thickening due to multilayering of basement membrane, edema and sclerosis of endoneurium with collagen fibril deposition, and thickening of the perineurial sheath (16).

Differential Diagnosis. The clinicopathologic features of LIN are so characteristic that few lesions enter into the differential diagnosis. Unlike traumatic neuroma, a proliferative process, the nerve is intact and lacks the low-power, tangled, microfascicular architecture of that lesion. LIN is degenerative in nature: the axons are decreased in number and aligned rather than regenerating and haphazardly arranged.

Treatment and Prognosis. Although a change of footwear or steroid/anesthetic injection may alleviate symptoms (17), resection may be required. The failure rate of neurectomy is approximately 10 percent. This is due, in nearly all instances, to the formation of a traumatic neuroma, the subsequent resection of which is curative (18).

PACINIAN NEUROMA

Definition. *Pacinian neuroma*, a neuroma variant, results from hypertrophy or hyperplasia of pacinian corpuscles, with or without associated degenerative changes. It is also known as *pacinian corpuscle neuroma, pacinian corpuscle hyperplasia*, and *pacinioma*.

General Features. The basic anatomy and physiology of pacinian corpuscles as well as their immunohistochemical and ultrastructural features were described in chapter 2. Briefly, they are mechanoreceptors most numerous in the subcutaneous tissue of the hands and feet, but also occur in the walls of viscera, in mesentery, and within the adventitia of vessels. In the hands, the site most often affected by pacinian neuroma, corpuscles are preferentially situated in palmar fat beneath the level of the sweat glands, near the periosteum on the lateral aspects of the proximal and middle phalanges, between flexor tendons and periosteum, and at the bases of proximal phalanges (19). At surgery, their characteristic locations serve as anatomic landmarks for nerves.

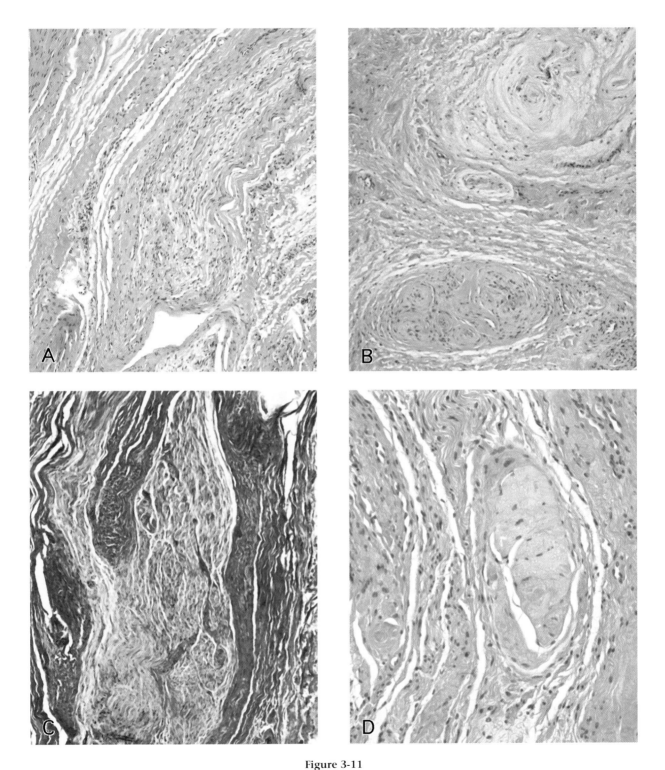

Figure 3-11

LOCALIZED INTERDIGITAL NEURITIS

A,B: At low magnification, the digital nerve, its perineurium and epineurium, as well as surrounding vasculature are fibrotic.
C: These changes are most conspicuous with a trichrome stain.
D: Intraneural collagenous nodules are also a feature of some examples.

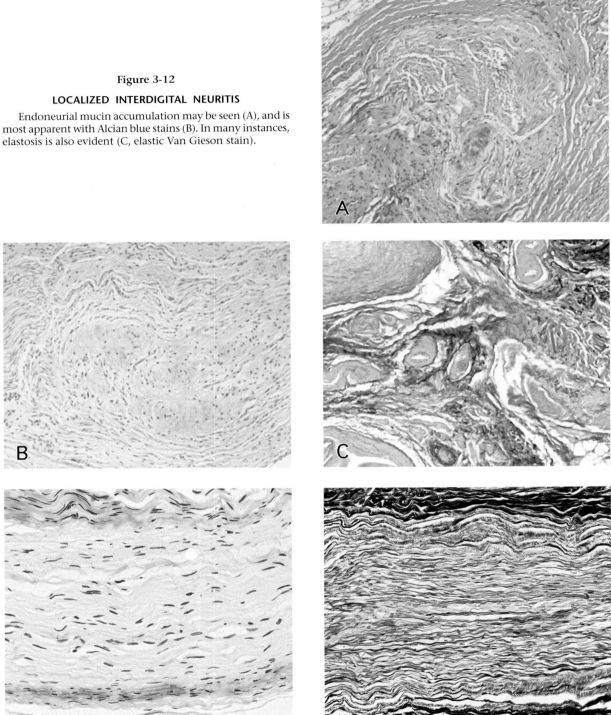

Figure 3-12

LOCALIZED INTERDIGITAL NEURITIS

Endoneurial mucin accumulation may be seen (A), and is most apparent with Alcian blue stains (B). In many instances, elastosis is also evident (C, elastic Van Gieson stain).

Figure 3-13

LOCALIZED INTERDIGITAL NEURITIS

A reduction in axons and myelin loss are apparent with silver impregnation for axons (left) and with myelin stains (right). (Left, Bielschowsky; right, Luxol-fast blue-PAS.)

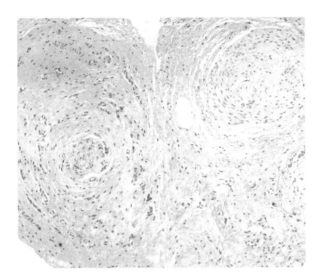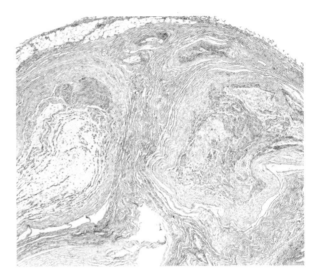

Figure 3-14

LOCALIZED INTERDIGITAL NEURITIS

The effects of degenerative changes upon the architecture of the digital nerve are best appreciated with neurofilament protein (left) and S-100 protein (right) immunostains which show nerve fibers and Schwann sheaths to be reduced in number, dispersed, and distorted.

Pacinian corpuscles undergo morphologic changes in response to trauma or physiologic stimuli. In both animals (20) and man (21), they are capable of regeneration from terminations of their nerves. Given the frequent association of pacinian neuroma with prior trauma and the near normal morphology of many examples, we view them not as neoplasms but as being akin to true neuroma (22). A diagnostic word of caution is in order: in view of the frequent operative finding of a sizable corpuscle(s) in the absence of an alternative explanation for symptoms, pacinian neuromas are no doubt overdiagnosed.

Clinical Features. Pacinian neuromas occur most frequently in the hands and enter into the differential diagnosis of digital pain. The English literature contains more than 20 reported cases affecting the hands (5,23–38). Pacinian neuromas affecting the feet may present with a compression syndrome resembling LIN (39,40). With the rare exception of two extremely long-standing and perhaps congenital examples (26,34), both bilateral and affecting the thumbs, most pacinian neuromas affect adults and occur in the fifth and sixth decades. Females are twice as often affected. Most lesions are associated with prior direct or nearby trauma, with

an interval to clinical presentation of weeks to years. Pacinian neuromas of the hands are all related to digital nerves. Nearly all affect fingers, mainly the index and middle, or rarely, the palm (27). Unusual patterns of involvement include multiple digits (26,29,34) and two nerves of the same digit (24,31,32,38). Erosion of adjacent bone is uncommon (29,33). Pain is present in nearly all cases, but sensory loss is uncommon. Asymptomatic lesions incidentally encountered at surgery are uncommon (29,83).

On rare occasion, pacinian neuromas occur within the abdomen, specifically in the pancreatic region (41), mesentery (42), and aortic adventitia (43). Most occur at a site of prior surgery. Pacinian neuromas have also been described in association with spinal dysraphism (44,45).

Gross Findings. Pacinian neuromas do not form a tumor-like mass. Whether hypertrophic or of relatively normal size, single or multiple, the corpuscles comprising the neuroma are pearl gray, often ovoid, rice-like nodules embedded in fibroareolar tissue. Their entering nerves may be prominent or numerous enough to make multiple corpuscles appear interconnected.

Pacinian neuromas vary considerably in terms of their surgical anatomy. Based on the

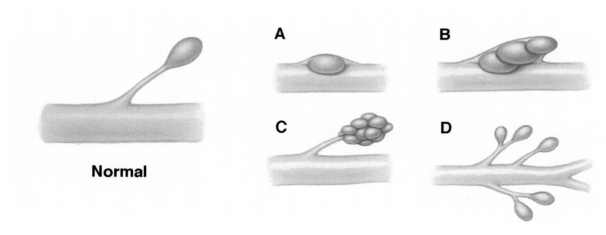

Figure 3-15

PACINIAN NEUROMA

Schematic representation of the most common growth patterns: type A, a single enlarged subepineural corpuscle; type B, enlarged corpuscles arranged in tandem beneath the epineurium; type C, a grape-like cluster of pacinian corpuscles of normal size attached to the digital nerve by a fine filament; and type D, multiple hyperplastic corpuscles arranged along the length of the affected nerve. (Modified from fig. 6, reference 35.)

number of constituent corpuscles, their spatial distribution, and their relation to the parent nerve, Rhode and Jennings (35) developed a simple four-tier classification for pacinian neuromas (fig. 3-15). The shortcoming of this scheme is that its application is predicated upon data obtained only by detailed or extensive dissection. Overall, most pacinian neuromas are of type B, whereas C and D type lesions are rare. Normal corpuscles as well as most hypertrophic and hyperplastic examples are attached to a digital nerve by a minute nerve fiber. Some type A examples are actually intraperineurial (23,24,28,35,38). Although not always apparent at surgery, nerve compression is thought to be the basis of symptoms. As a rule, no gross nerve injury is seen.

Microscopic Findings. Pacinian neuromas consist of enlarged or multiple pacinian corpuscles (fig. 3-16), some associated with fibrosis. When aggregated in a mass, their smooth-contoured profiles lie jumbled in fibroareolar tissue but not encompassed by a fibrous capsule. Corpuscles vary in shape (fig. 3-17, left) or appear to be "budding." Hypertrophic examples generally measure greater than 1.6 mm (29) and most feature more than 20 concentric lamellae (up to 60 in some cases). Degenerative changes are often seen and take the form of capsular and interlamellar collagen deposition (fig. 3-17, left) as

well as perineural and endoneurial fibrosis of the nerves entering the corpuscles (fig. 3-17, right). Capsular elastosis is an uncommon finding, even in neuromas of the feet, a site at which elastic fibers are a normal feature of corpuscle capsules (46). In some cases, fibrosis is marked (fig. 3-18, left) and the inner core lacks a nerve fiber (fig. 3-18, right).

Given the frequent association of pacinian neuromas with antecedent injury, it is not surprising that an occasional example is associated with a traumatic neuroma (26). Also, since normal pacinian corpuscles are associated with arteriovenous anastomoses, pacinian neuromas may occur in association with glomus tumors, either contiguous or spatially separate (30).

Immunohistochemical Findings. The immunoprofile of pacinian neuroma is that of normal pacinian corpuscles. The perineurial cell lamellae comprising the outer core are EMA positive, whereas the Schwann cells and axons within the inner core are reactive for S-100 protein and neurofilament protein, respectively (25,47,48).

Ultrastructural Findings. Electron microscopy has shown that the outer lamellae of normal pacinian corpuscles consist of long, thin perineurial cell processes with prominent pinocytotic vesicles (see chapter 2). Since these outer lamellae are immunoreactive for EMA (see below), and

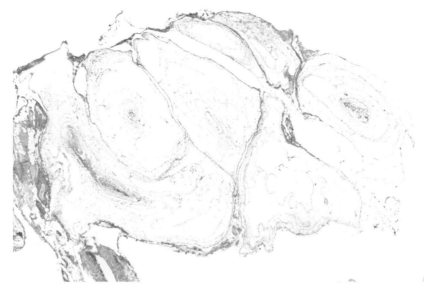

Figure 3-16

PACINIAN NEUROMA

The clustering of corpuscles (Rhode and Jennings pattern C), as in this example from the transverse mesocolon, represents a common form of pacinian neuroma.

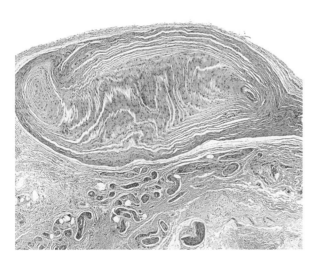 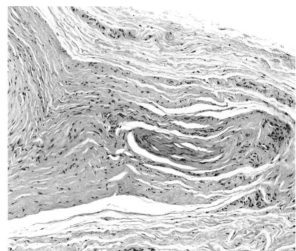

Figure 3-17

PACINIAN NEUROMA

These micrographs show a pacinian neuroma of irregular contour with a thickened capsule and somewhat disordered, sclerotic lamellae in the outer core (left). Its entering nerve is also affected (right).

the pacinian-like structures found in pacinian neurofibromas have the immunohistochemical and ultrastructural features of perineurial cells (49–51), it can be assumed that the lamellae of the hyperplastic pacinian corpuscles composing neuromas exhibit similar features.

Differential Diagnosis. Pacinian neuromas may be confused with either normal pacinian corpuscles or with neurofibromas containing

tactile body–like structures. Since the resection of a pacinian neuroma doesn't always result in relief of digital pain, questions arise as to the nature of the pacinian corpuscles commonly found in resection specimens. Findings favoring a diagnosis of pacinian neuroma over an incidentally discovered pacinian corpuscle include: 1) a history of local trauma; 2) point tenderness; 3) palpability of a lesion; 4) the operative findings of

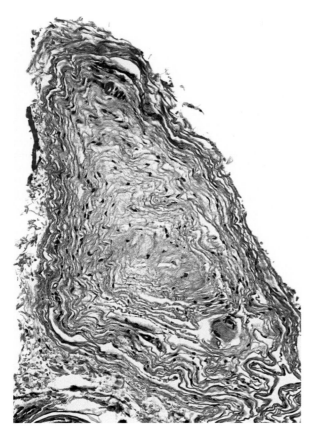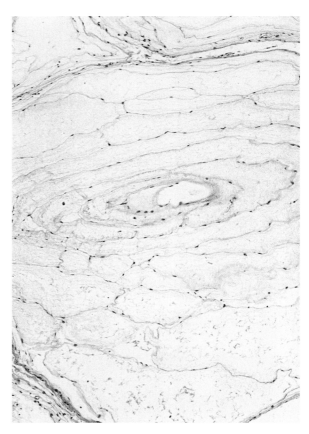

Figure 3-18

PACINIAN NEUROMA

Advanced degenerative changes include dense sclerosis of the entire corpuscle, a change best seen with a trichrome stain (left), as well as loss of the nerve fibers within the inner core (right).

nodule(s) variously related to a peripheral nerve; 5) corpuscle abnormalities such as large size, increased number, and abnormal shape; 6) degenerative microscopic changes such as fibrosis or loss of the inner core of the corpuscle(s); and 7) postoperative resolution of pain.

The neoplasm exhibiting tactile corpuscle-like differentiation most often linked to pacinian neuroma is the so-called pacinian neurofibroma. The term has been loosely applied to palpable masses of varied histology occurring at a variety of sites, usually ones only rarely affected by pacinian neuroma. Such tumors bear no resemblance to pacinian neuromas as discussed here. In retrospect, a number of purported pacinian neurofibromas can be reclassified as dermal nerve sheath myxoma (52–54) and neurothekeoma (55). Of the remainder, the numerous corpuscle-like structures occur

in association with proliferations resembling large nevi (56,57), neurofibromas (49–51,58,59), schwannomas (60), possible traumatic neuromas (61), or unclassifiable lesions (55). Some are unaccompanied by an underlying lesion (55). Distinguishing these processes from fully differentiated pacinian neuromas with their characteristic morphology and predictable localization usually poses no problem.

Morphologically, the tactile corpuscle-like differentiation usually seen in neurofibromas closely resembles Meissner corpuscles (62–64). Whether pacinian or meissnerian in nature, their features are similar (50,51,63,64), exhibiting a perineurial-like ultrastructure despite expression of S-100 protein immunoreactivity (64,65). Thus, such cells show hybrid features. We agree with Fletcher and Theaker (26) that true pacinian differentiation has never been convincingly demonstrated in benign or malignant nerve sheath neoplasms. Pacinian body–like structures have also been seen in experimentally induced nerve sheath tumors (66).

Treatment and Prognosis. Although initial excision is curative, the symptoms of pacinian neuroma occasionally persist, and are only relieved after resection of corpuscles not found at first surgery (31). Care must be taken to spare the parent nerve, particularly in type A neuromas in which corpuscles lie within the epineurium.

ORAL PSEUDOPERINEURIOMA

Definition. *Oral pseudoperineurioma* is an unusual, reactive-appearing perineurial proliferation characterized by pseudo-onion bulb formation and affecting the oral cavity (67).

General Features. The frequent localization of oral pseudoperineurioma at the border of the tongue and the variable collagen content strongly suggest a traumatic etiology. Oral pseudoperineuriomas represent 10 percent of oral nerve sheath lesions.

Clinical Features. Females are preferentially affected (2 to 1) and present at a mean age of 30 years. Most lesions involve the tongue (in one study [67]), 11 were lateral, 8 were tip, and 6 were dorsal), occasionally the lip, and rarely the buccal mucosa. Half occur in association with polypoid or nodular mucosal fibromas. Other rare associations include a traumatic neuroma component, an intimate association with granular cell tumor, or accompanying homolateral hemifacial hyperplasia.

Gross Findings. Oral pseudoperineuriomas form firm, elevated, plaque-like lesions on the mucosal surface (fig. 3-19). Although generally not ulcerated, the overlying mucosal surface may be thickened.

Microscopic Findings. Histologically, the affected fascicles vary in size and feature both pseudo-onion bulbs at various stages of development and a complete or incomplete perineurium (fig. 3-20A,B). A pseudo-plexiform pattern may be prominent (fig. 3-20C). Myelin loss is often seen. The fascicles are typically surrounded by zones of dense collagen that appear to encroach upon and compress them (fig. 3-20D). Normal nerves are occasionally seen in the vicinity.

Immunohistochemical Findings. The pseudo-onion bulbs are immunoreactive for

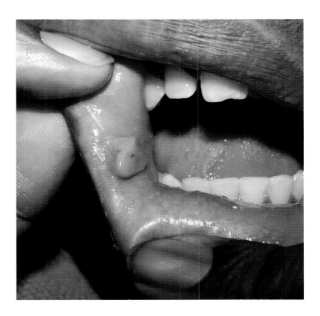

Figure 3-19

ORAL PSEUDOPERINEURIOMA

An elevated, firm, pale lesion is seen at the bite line. (Courtesy of Dr. I. G. Koutlas, Minneapolis, MN.)

EMA, glut-1, and claudin (fig. 3-21A). At their centers lie S-100 protein- and neurofilament protein-reactive nerve fibers (fig. 3-21B,C). No inflammation is evident but hyperplasia of the overlying mucosa is often seen.

Differential Diagnosis. Oral pseudoperineuriomas do not meet the histologic criteria of ordinary traumatic or amputation neuromas. They lack the nerve transection, axonal sprouting, and microfascicle formation. Furthermore, they represent a perineurial rather than Schwann cell response. Occasionally, pseudoperineuriomas are mistaken for simple or even plexiform neurofibromas. While there is little doubt that tumors reported to be intraoral soft tissue perineuriomas are such, some "intraneural perineuriomas" may in fact represent pseudoperineuriomas.

Treatment and Prognosis. Oral pseudoperineuriomas are considered reactive in nature and the result of repeated trauma, likely causing chronic compression and perhaps ischemia of nerve. Korthals et al. (68) observed a similar perineurial proliferation in experimentally induced acute ischemic injury of peripheral nerves.

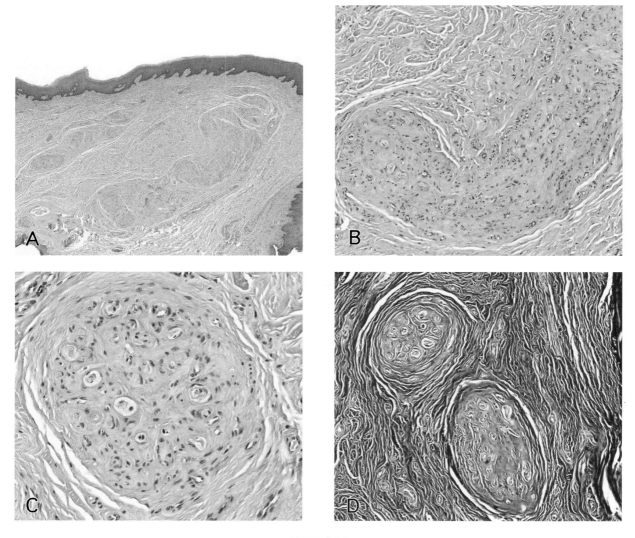

Figure 3-20

ORAL PSEUDOPERINEURIOMA

Two enlarged nerves (A), featuring hypercellularity (B) and, on cross section, well-formed pseudo-onion bulbs (C), are seen. The trichrome stain shows the marked collagen deposition, both within the nerves and in surrounding soft tissue (D). (Courtesy of Dr. I. G. Koutlas, Minneapolis, MN.)

INTRANEURAL INJURY NEUROMA

The capacity of the perineurium to undergo reactive proliferation is well known. Varying in degree and extent, it is seen in such non-neoplastic lesions as traumatic neuroma, LIN, and pacinian neuroma. Perineurial cells also variably contribute to a number of neoplasms, both benign (neurofibroma, nerve sheath myxoma, hybrid schwannoma-perineurioma, perineurioma) and malignant (perineurial malignant peripheral nerve sheath tumor) (69).

Best known of the *reactive perineurial proliferations* is the traumatic neuroma. In transection injury without reapproximation of the distal stump, nerve fiber outgrowth from the proximal stump results in the formation of microfascicles ensheathed by perineurium. This response may form a sizeable mass (see Traumatic Neuroma). More chronic and degenerative in nature, the plantar neuroma features lamellar fibrosis of the still EMA-immunoreactive perineurium surrounding degenerated nerve fascicles. Pacinian

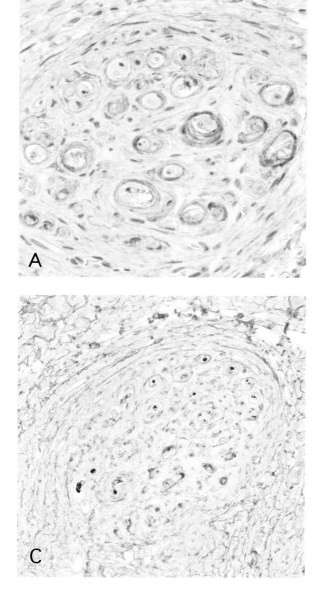

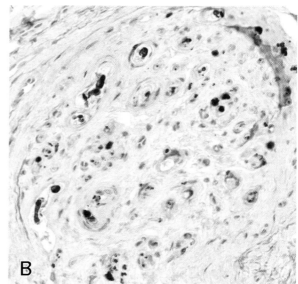

Figure 3-21

ORAL PSEUDOPERINEURIOMA

Immunohistochemistry shows the pseudo-onion bulbs to be EMA immunoreactive (A) and to surround nerve fibers, as readily evident on S-100 and neurofilament protein preparations (B,C). (Courtesy of Dr. I. G. Koutlas, Oral Pathology, University of Minnesota.)

neuromas, hyperplastic in nature, feature concentric lamellae of perineurial cells.

Perineurial reactions to ischemia and trauma have been studied experimentally (70). In one study (68), severe ischemic injury involving not only the center but also the periphery and perineurium of fascicles, resulted in the formation of pseudo-onion bulbs during the regenerative process in which small numbers of nerve fibers were surrounded by layers of perineurial cells (68). The injured perineurium was replaced by dense collagen. Interestingly,

the reaction observed was temporary (68,71), lasting in one model only 16 months (68). The reactions described are thought to be not only due to perineurial injury but to the result of the regeneration of nerves with Schwann cell injury and the disturbance of the endoneurial environment. It seems onion bulb formation by Schwann cells can also be induced by experimental compression of nerve (72). Similar results are observed in a nerve crush model where pseudo-onion bulbs are formed primarily at the periphery of fascicles (71). In the early

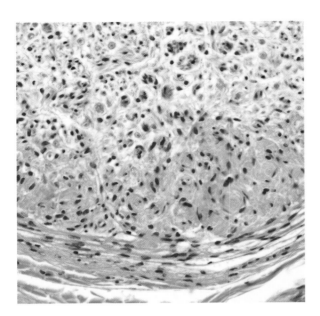
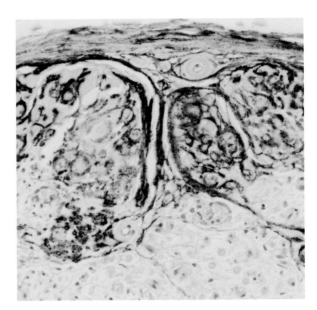

Figure 3-22

INTRANEURAL INJURY NEUROMA

The conspicuous, grossly inapparent reaction to remote injury involves the sciatic nerve of a late middle-aged woman who 10 years previously had sustained a closed injury to the nerve. Microscopically, it consists of multifocal pseudo-onion bulb formations contiguous with the perineurium (left) and composed of EMA-immunoreactive perineurial cells.

phase, the perineurial cells resemble fibroblasts. In a trauma model employing transection and close reapproximation of nerve stumps, such compartmentalization of regenerating units is more transient, and is replaced by normal architecture within 4 months (70). Reactive perineurial and Schwann cell proliferation in these settings varies in extent within affected fascicles but, unlike intraneural perineurioma, does not result in appreciable enlargement of the nerve. A clinical example of perineurial changes in chronic nerve injury is illustrated in figure 3-22.

EPITHELIAL SHEATH NEUROMA

Since the original description of four cases of a dermal lesion composed of squamous epithelial cuffs surrounding enlarged dermal nerves (73), a presumed neoplasm and named *epithelial sheath neuroma*, several additional cases have been published (74,75). All have presented in mid to late adulthood, originated on the back, formed a 0.5- to 2.0-cm erythematous dermal papule, and were unassociated with a prior lesion or surgery at the site.

The light microscopic features of these lesions are distinctive (fig. 3-23). The epithelial cuff is histologically benign, applied to the outer surface of the perineurium, with no connection with epidermis or adnexa. It stains variously for cytokeratins, but not for EMA or carcinoembryonic antigen. The ensheathed nerves lay within the superficial dermis and extend in various directions, an appearance reminiscent of traumatic neuroma but unassociated with significant fibroplasia. At least one example showed focal chronic inflammation, and some lesions featured centrally situated cysts lined by cornified epithelium.

These lesions show no proliferative activity in terms of mitoses or MIB-1 labeling, and there is no p53 immunoreactivity. Body site localization, age group, occasional evidence of chronic inflammation, and no reports of recurrence are more suggestive of a reactive than neoplastic process. The differential diagnosis includes direct extension by a metastatic carcinoma. Lack of cytologic malignancy and a nearby or associated systemic neoplasm, as well as an excellent prognosis unassociated with recurrence, all mitigate against that diagnosis (73–75).

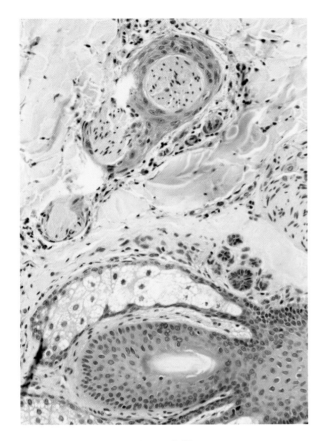

Figure 3-23

EPITHELIAL SHEATH NEUROMA

The nerves are encircled by benign-appearing squamous epithelium. The lesion is near a hair follicle.

GANGLION CYST OF NERVE

Definition. *Ganglion cyst of nerve* is a mucin-filled, nonepithelial-lined, uniloculate cyst involving a peripheral nerve and occasionally its branches. Synonyms include *nerve ganglion, intraneural ganglion, pseudocyst of nerve,* and *mucinous ganglion cyst.*

General Features. Cysts involving peripheral nerve are rare and occur as a linear, unilocular cyst, typically intimate and in parallel with the nerve. Most are fibrous walled and all are para-articular. Their location in areas subject to mechanical stress and chronic joint disease favors a traumatic etiology (76). In our experience, all arise from a joint from which they secondarily extend along nerve within the epineurium. It is questionable whether some originate in the nerve sheath. The most frequent location of nerves affected by ganglion cysts is the common peroneal nerve near the head of the fibula (77–80). In one review, this nerve was affected in 86 percent of cases (81). Other sites include the ulnar (82–85), median (86,87), posterior interosseous (88), suprascapular (89–91), tibial (92), and sural (93) nerves (figs. 3-24, 3-25).

The process of the formation of ganglion cysts of nerve, which has been controversial for two centuries, has recently been shown to follow a reproducible path of dissection of cyst fluid from a joint of origin along an articular branch to its parent nerve (85). For fibular (peroneal) nerve cysts, the most common form, the cyst arises from the anterior portion of the superior tibiofibular joint and extends along the articular branch, its "pedicle" (fig. 3-26). From there, it progresses into the deep fibular portion of the common fibular nerve, and at times into the sciatic nerve and the proximal portion of the tibial nerve. Such complex lesions may appear multifocal (fig. 3-27), but all can be shown to originate from joints rather than as a degenerative change intrinsic to nerve sheath (94). Proximal extension of cysts reaching the buttock has been reported (95,96); such examples arise from the superior tibiofibular joint (97). Analogous proximal extension of cysts has been demonstrated in other sites, including a tibial intraneural ganglion cyst arising from the posterior aspect of the superior tibiofibular joint (94,97,98) and a suprascapular intraneural cyst arising from the glenohumeral joint and extending to the neck (90).

The articular mechanism of intraneural ganglion cyst formation involves: 1) egress of cyst fluid from a capsular rent in a degenerative joint; 2) dissection along an articular branch to its parent nerve following the path of least resistance; and 3) propagation within compartments based on dynamic pressure fluxes (91). In a similar manner, extraneural ganglion cysts form when a joint capsule defect occurs, but at a location apart from a capsular-articular branch interface. Such cysts tend to be more globular in appearance, as they are not constrained by the configuration of a nerve. They may, however, compress neighboring nerves (99). Extraneural cysts are more common than intraneural cysts and have been described at many locations (89,100). Intraneural cysts may coexist with such extraneural cysts.

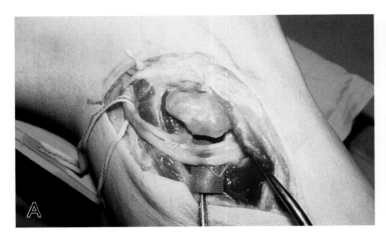
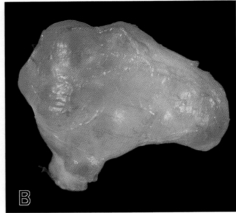
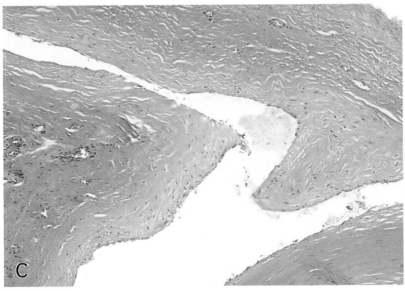

Figure 3-24

GANGLION CYST OF NERVE

The peroneal nerve is the most common site of nerve cysts. This example was related to local trauma 8 months before.

A: At surgery, the cyst was found to arise from the tibiofibular joint to which it was connected by a stalk. The anterior tibial nerve lies inferior to the cyst; markedly compressed and displaced, it was contiguous with the capsule. (A,B: Figs. 3.406 and 3.407 from Okazaki H, Scheithauer BW. Atlas of neuropathology. New York: Gower; 1988:181. With permission from the Mayo Foundation.)

B: Grossly, the cyst contained clear fluid and appeared thin-walled, distended, and translucent.

C: Microsections of another example show the typical features of a ganglion.

Clinical Features. Patients with ganglion cysts of nerve vary greatly in age from the first to the eighth decade (mean, 34 years) (79,101). Pediatric examples are uncommon (79). Approximately 80 percent of all nerve cysts occur in males (81). The lesions cause nerve compression with resultant motor dysfunction, sensory loss (81), or pain. Neurologic examination helps localize the lesions to nerve: for example, a peroneal nerve cyst may cause atrophy of the muscles of the anterior compartment of the leg, as well as pain on the anterolateral surface of the leg and dorsum of the foot; as a rule, sensory loss is slight (79). A tender and fluctuant mass may be present on palpation. Percussion of the lesion often elicits a positive Tinel sign, i.e., a tingling sensation radiating distally. Electromyograms demonstrate a neuropathy.

Radiologic Features. The diagnosis is suspected and frequently established by ultrasonography or magnetic resonance imaging (MRI) (102,103), which demonstrates not only the tubular cyst within the parent nerve, but also the cystic articular branch connecting it to the joint (fig. 3-28) (104).

Gross Findings. At surgery, the nerve is variably affected, being either locally displaced and compressed by a uniloculate cyst (fig. 3-24) or misshapen by multiple cystic dilations along its length (fig. 3-25). The lesions, measuring up to 30 cm in greatest dimension (knee to buttock), are actually uniloculate. Careful dissection shows nerve sheath

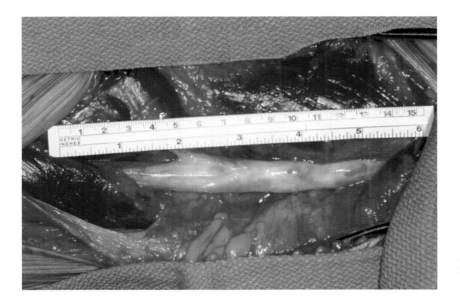

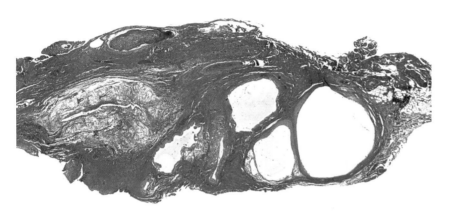

Figure 3-25

GANGLION CYST OF NERVE

Top: In this tibial nerve example, multiple cysts are distributed within a segment of epineurium.

Bottom: A longitudinal section of another example shows multiple cysts and segments of nearby, displaced nerve fascicles.

Figure 3-26

GANGLION CYST OF NERVE

In a schematic representation, the cyst originates from the joint, follows the articular branch of the popliteal nerve, and ascends along the parent nerve.

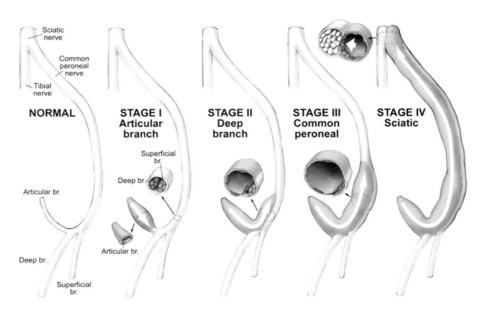

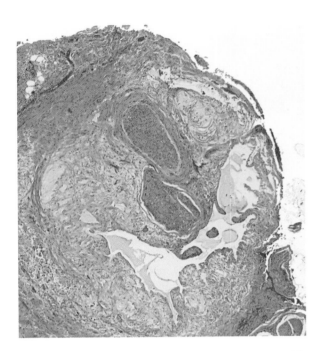
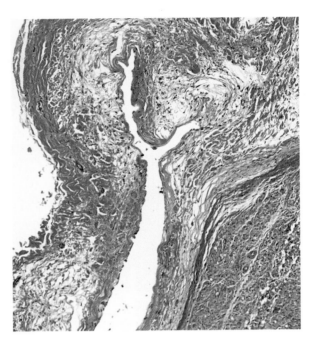

Figure 3-27

GANGLION CYST OF NERVE

On cross section, several nerve fascicles seem to lie within (left) or to abut (right) the cyst.

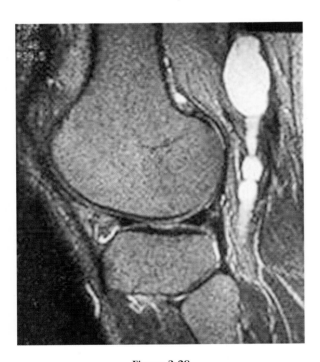

Figure 3-28

GANGLION CYST OF NERVE

Magnetic resonance imaging (MRI) shows a multilobular lesion originating from the tibial joint and following the popliteal nerve.

cysts to originate from a nearby joint via a stalk following the articular branch of the nerve (fig. 3-24A, B). Longitudinal section of the nerve may show beaded epineural expansions of the cyst (fig. 3-25). The lesion typically displaces nerve fascicles and, when ruptured, drains as clear to yellow, thin to viscous fluid.

Microscopic Findings. The walls of these cysts or the surrounding perineurium contain distorted nerve fascicles (fig. 3-27). The fibrous wall of the lesion lacks an epithelial lining (fig. 3-24C). Loose-textured mesenchymal cells cover the inner aspect of early examples, whereas compact collagen and occasional plump cells simulate a lining in chronic lesions (fig. 3-29). Occasional vacuolated histiocytes float in the mucoid or proteinaceous fluid filling the cyst. Mucin may accumulate in the endoneurium, presumably the result of local trauma (fig. 3-30), but does not indicate endoneurial involvement in the process.

Immunohistochemical Findings. Lacking the characteristics of nerve sheath, the cells comprising the nerve cyst wall stain for vimentin and perhaps actin, but are nonreactive for S-100 protein (79), EMA, or keratin.

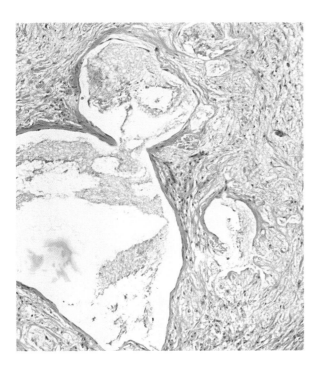 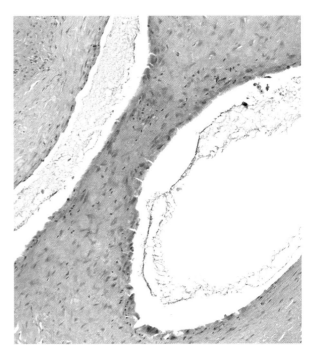

Figure 3-29

GANGLION CYST OF NERVE

Left: In the early phases of cyst development, the lining is thin.
Right: With time, fibrosis ensues and the inner aspect may assume a pseudoepithelial appearance.

Ultrastructural Findings. One ultrastructural study of the wall of a nerve cyst found the constituent cells to be myofibroblasts rather than synovial cells (81).

Differential Diagnosis. Extraneural ganglion cysts and synovial cysts derived from other joints can compress nerve roots (89,99,100,105,106). A popliteal or Baker cyst, as occurs in rheumatoid synovitis, can also cause nerve entrapment or compression and thus may simulate a ganglion cyst of nerve (107–109). A markedly cystic schwannoma with involvement of a grossly recognizable nerve is readily distinguished from a large, unilobular nerve cyst given the absence in the latter of tumor tissue, a biphasic Antoni A and B pattern, Verocay bodies, and reactivity for S-100 protein.

Treatment and Prognosis. Although the treatment of ganglion cyst of nerve is operative, historically there has been no uniform surgical approach. In the past, treatment varied from simple drainage, to marsupialization, to subtotal excision, and even complete resection of the cyst. Simple drainage is often followed by recurrence and complete excision sometimes results in severe or complete nerve deficit (79,110). Reported recurrence rates using prior methods of treatment are 7 (111) to 23 percent (110). A recently proposed, anatomically more meaningful approach has entirely eliminated intraneural recurrences. It addresses the underlying pathologic anatomy by disconnecting or ligating the articular branch of the nerve with limited decompression of the cyst (91,94). To avoid an extraneural recurrence, resection of the superior tibiofibular joint may be necessary.

ENDOMETRIOSIS OF SCIATIC NERVE

The most common cause of sciatic pain is vertebral disc prolapse, but when cyclic in nature and occurring in reproductive-age females, the differential diagnosis includes endometriosis. To date, few cases of *endometriosis affecting the sciatic nerve* have been reported (112,113). Previously, the diagnosis had only been suspected (114). It was not until 1955 that the first biopsy-

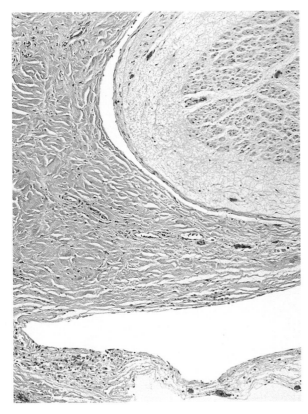

Figure 3-30

GANGLION CYST OF NERVE

Fascicles near a cyst show endoneurial accumulation of mucinous fluid.

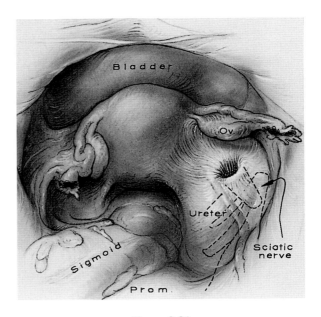

Figure 3-31

EVAGINATION OF PERITONEUM OF RIGHT BROAD LIGAMENT ("POCKET SIGN")

(Fig. 1 from Head HB, Welch JS, Mussey E, Espinosa RE. Cyclic sciatica: report of a case with introduction of new surgical sign. JAMA 1962;180:522.)

proven example was reported (115). Typical symptoms include pain, sensory motor deficits, and occasionally, foot drop. In classic cases, sciatica just precedes menses and persists several days after its cessation. With time, presumably with persistent reactive changes and fibrosis, the asymptomatic interval often becomes shorter. In some instances pain becomes constant. It is the right sciatic nerve that is most often affected, in that the position of the sigmoid colon prevents implantation of deposits of endometriosis on the left pelvic sidewall.

The diagnosis of endometriosis is suggested by the cyclic nature of the pain and is confirmed by relief of symptoms with suppressive hormone treatment. A normal gynecologic examination is the rule and does not exclude the diagnosis. Electromyography helps localize the lesion, distinguishing nerve root from peripheral nerve involvement. In most cases, imaging of the pel-

vic peritoneum demonstrates a characteristic "pocket sign" (116), a peritoneal evagination containing a mass of ectopic endometrial tissue (figs. 3-31, 3-32). It is unclear whether the pocket represents a fully developed preexisting structural abnormality (fig. 3-31) in which endometrial implants come to lie, or whether implantation and resulting tissue traction prompt its formation. In any event, careful intraoperative examination usually demonstrates the pocket and the endometrial tissue compressing or directly involving the sciatic nerve or its roots (fig. 3-33). Only rarely is no intrapelvic deposit seen, with the disease more directly affecting the nerve (117).

Therapy consists of total abdominal hysterectomy with bilateral salpingo-oophorectomy. When preservation of reproductive function is an issue, effective therapy involves meticulous resection of deposits from the sciatic nerve or its roots. Radiation therapy is also reportedly curative. Hormone suppression therapy has met with only limited success (117). Any resected tissue should be histologically examined since transformation to stromal sarcoma was reported in one instance (118).

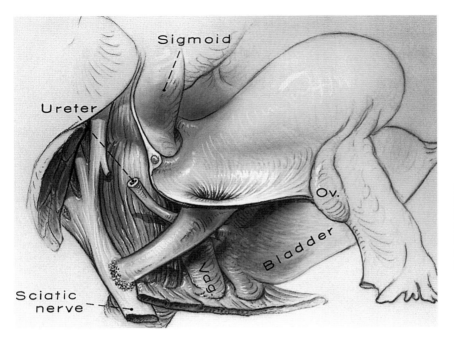

Figure 3-32

SCHEMATIC REPRESENTATION OF THE "POCKET SIGN" WITH ENDOMETRIOSIS AND SCIATIC NERVE INVOLVEMENT

Evagination of the pelvic peritoneum with endometriosis at its base is intimately associated with the sciatic nerve. (Fig. 2 from Head HB, Welch JS, Mussey E, Espinosa RE. Cyclic sciatica: report of a case with introduction of new surgical sign. JAMA 1962;180:522.)

Figure 3-33

ENDOMETRIOSIS OF SCIATIC NERVE

This typical deposit is within the sciatic nerve epineurium. Endometriotic tissue is associated with minute nerve branches.

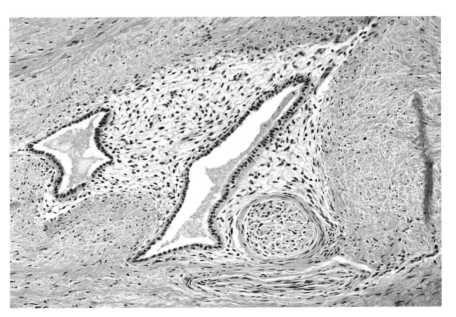

HETEROTOPIC OSSIFICATION OF NERVE (NEURITIS OSSIFICANS)

Definition. *Heterotopic ossification of nerve (neuritis ossificans) is a rare lesion that is similar to myositis ossificans. A similar process follows trauma or burns.*

General and Clinical Features. To date, only 11 well-documented examples of neuritis ossificans have been reported (119–125). In one case

(119), it presented as a palpable mass in a woman with a 9-year history of sensory abnormalities referable to an ulnar nerve, but no prior trauma. At surgery the hard, calcified mass was situated entirely within intact epineurium, separating but not directly involving its fascicles. Interfascicular neurolysis led to sacrifice of only a number of small fascicles and resulted in no appreciable neurologic deficits. We have observed an identical lesion

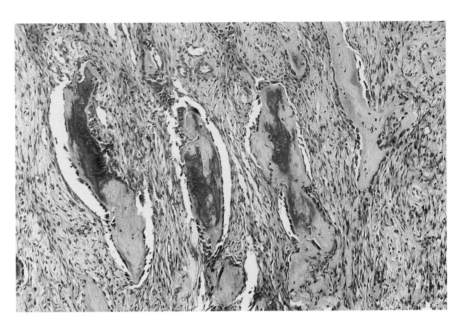

Figure 3-34

NEURITIS OSSIFICANS

The periphery of this epineurial lesion, occurring in a 16-year-old male without a prior history of trauma, shows an organized lamellar pattern of bone formation resembling that seen in myositis ossificans.

involving the tibial nerve of a 16-year-old male with a 4-week history of acute onset of painful pseudoparalysis and sensory loss. There was no history of prior trauma or of familial neurologic or metabolic disease. The lesion, partly calcified on plain X rays and measuring 4 cm, lay entirely within the nerve and was associated with edema in the surrounding soft tissue. Resection of the lobulated, peripherally ossified mass resulted in sacrifice of one third of the nerve fascicles but only minimal sensorimotor loss. The histologic features were similar to those of myositis ossificans (fig. 3-34).

As is often the case in myositis ossificans, no history of injury was elicited in the above-noted cases. Nonetheless, we suspect that neuritis ossificans represents heterotopic ossification as a reaction to local trauma. This is supported by the rare occurrence of somewhat similar, post-traumatic processes that vary in extent (126,127). These include: 1) localized plaque-like ossification of nerve sheath; 2) segmental ossification of nerve and an adjacent but separate major artery (126); 3) shell-like perineural ossification adherent to nerve; and 4) destructive lesions in which ossification and fibrosis replace an entire segment of nerve with no fascicles remaining.

Unlike one reported case in which mature lamellar bone lay enmeshed among fascicles of the median nerve (126), most lesions feature central ossification, often bone marrow associated and surrounding reactive fibrosis. The preoperative evolution of this spectrum of post-traumatic ossific lesions ranges from 7 months to 12 years. Heterotopic bone formation, typically with encasement of the ulnar nerve, also reportedly occurs as a complication of severe burns in the region of the elbow (128).

Differential Diagnosis. The differential diagnosis of neuritis ossificans is limited and includes ossification in a lipofibromatous hamartoma of nerve (129) and perhaps a peripheral nerve tumor. The latter is rare and usually occurs only in ancient schwannomas (130). Calcification of the perineurium in the setting of metabolic diseases, such as diabetes (131) and the CREST syndrome (calcinosis, Reynaud phenomenon, esophageal motility disorders, sclerodactyly, and telangiectasia) pose no differential diagnostic problem (132).

Treatment and Prognosis. The favorable outcome of neuritis ossificans in which the nerve is intact and unaffected by major trauma is attributable to a conservative, nerve-sparing, microsurgical approach to therapy (119).

REFERENCES

Traumatic Neuroma

1. Dyck PJ, Giannini C, Lais A. Pathologic alterations of nerves. In: Dyck PJ, Thomas PK, eds. Peripheral neuropathy. Philadelphia: WB Saunders; 1993:514-596.
2. Lundborg G. Nerve regeneration and repair. A review. Acta Orthop Scand 1987;58:145-169.
3. Nadim W, Anderson PN, Turmaine M. The role of Schwann cells and basal lamina tubes in the regeneration of axons through long lengths of freeze-killed nerve grafts. Neuropathol Appl Neurobiol 1990;16:411-421.
4. Giannini C, Dyck PJ. The fate of Schwann cell basement membranes in permanently transected nerves. J Neuropathol Exp Neurol 1990;49:550-563.
5. Harkin JC, Reed RJ. Tumors of the peripheral nervous system. Atlas of Tumor Pathology, 2nd Series, Fascicle 3. Armed Forces Institute of Pathology; 1969.
6. Shapiro L, Juhlin EA, Brownstein MH. "Rudimentary polydactyly": an amputation neuroma. Arch Dermatol 1973;108:223-225.
7. Elhag AM, al Awadi NZ. Amputation neuroma of the gallbladder. Histopathology 1992;21:586-587.
8. Rush BF Jr, Stefaniwsky AB, Sasso A, et al. Neuroma of the common bile duct. J Surg Oncol 1988;39:17-21.
9. Shumate CR, Curley SA, Cleary KR, et al. Traumatic neuroma of the bile duct causing cholangitis and atrophy of the right hepatic lobe. South Med J 1992;85:425-427.
10. Matsuoka J, Tanaka N, Kojima K, et al. A case of traumatic neuroma of the gallbladder in the absence of previous surgery and cholelithiasis. Acta Med Okayama 1996;50:273-277.
11. Sano T, Hirose T, Kagawa N, et al. Polypoid traumatic neuroma of the gallbladder. Arch Pathol Lab Med 1985;109:574-576.
12. Das Gupta TK, Brasfield RD. Amputation neuromas in cancer patients. N Y State J Med 1969;69:2129-2132.

Localized Interdigital Neuritis

13. Scotti TM. The lesion of Morton's metatarsalgia (Morton's toe). AMA Arch Pathol 1957;63:91-102.
14. Reed RJ, Bliss BO. Morton's neuroma. Regressive and productive intermetatarsal elastofibrosis. Arch Pathol 1973;95:123-129.
15. Wu KK. Morton's interdigital neuroma: a clinical review of its etiology, treatment, and results. J Foot Ankle Surg 1996;35:112-119; discussion 187-118.
16. Lassmann G, Lassmann H, Stockinger L. Morton's metatarsalgia. Light and electron microscopic observations and their relation to entrapment neuropathies. Virchows Arch A Pathol Anat Histol 1976;370:307-321.
17. Bennett GL, Graham CE, Mauldin DM. Morton's interdigital neuroma: a comprehensive treatment protocol. Foot Ankle Int 1995;16:760-763.
18. Young G, Lindsey J. Etiology of symptomatic recurrent interdigital neuromas. J Am Podiatr Med Assoc 1993;83:255-258.

Pacinian Neuroma

19. Cauna N, Mannan G. The structure of human digital pacinian corpuscles (corpus cula lamellosa) and its functional significance. J Anat 1958;92:1-20.
20. Keibel F, Mall FP. Materialien zur kenntnis der entwicklung des peripheren nerven-systems, Dissert, Moskow, 1903. In: Keibel F, Mall FP, eds. Manual of human embryology. Philadelphia: JB Lippincott; 1912:180-181.
21. Levi S. Osservazioni sullo sviluppo delle terminazioni nervose intraepiteliali, corpuscoli del Meissner e corpuscoli del Pacini. Arch Ital Anat Embriol 1933;32:149-170.
22. Woodruff JM. Tumors and tumorlike conditions of peripheral nerve. Contemporary Issues in Surgical Pathology 1991;18:205-228.
23. Bas L, Oztek I, Numanoglu A. Subepineural hyperplastic pacinian corpuscle: an unusual cause of digital pain. Plast Reconstr Surg 1993;92:151-153.
24. Brynildsen PJ. Painful digital subepineural pacinian corpuscles. Plast Reconstr Surg 1985;75:929-930.
25. Calder JS, Holten I, Terenghi G, et al. Digital nerve compression by hyperplastic pacinian corpuscles. A case report and immunohistochemical study. J Hand Surg Br 1995;20:218-221.
26. Fletcher CD, Theaker JM. Digital pacinian neuroma: a distinctive hyperplastic lesion. Histopathology 1989;15:249-256.
27. Fraitag S, Gherardi R, Wechsler J. Hyperplastic pacinian corpuscles: an uncommonly encountered lesion of the hand. J Cutan Pathol 1994;21:457-460.
28. Friedman HI, Nichter LS, Morgan RF, et al. Subepineural pacinian corpuscle: a cause of digital pain. Plast Reconstr Surg 1984;74:699-703.

29. Gama C, Franca LC. Nerve compression by pacinian corpuscles. J Hand Surg Am 1980;5:207-210.
30. Greider JL Jr, Flatt AE. Glomus tumor associated with pacinian hyperplasia—case report. J Hand Surg Am 1982;7:113-117.
31. Hart WR, Thompson NW, Hildreth DH, et al. Hyperplastic pacinian corpuscles: a cause of digital pain. Surgery 1971;70:730-735.
32. Jones NF, Eadie P. Pacinian corpuscle hyperplasia in the hand. J Hand Surg Am 1991;16:865-869.
33. McPherson SA, Meals RA. Digital pacinian corpuscle neuroma eroding bone: a case report. J Hand Surg Am 1992;17:476-478.
34. Patterson TJ. Pacinian corpuscle neuroma of the thumb pulp. Br J Plast Surg 1956;9:230-231.
35. Rhode CM, Jennings WD Jr. Pacinian corpuscle neuroma of digital nerves. South Med J 1975;68:86-89.
36. Sandzen SC, Baksic RW. Pacinian hyperplasia. Hand 1974;6:273-274.
37. Schuler FA 3rd, Adamson JE. Pacinian neuroma, an unusual cause of finger pain. Plast Reconstr Surg 1978;62:576-579.
38. Zweig J, Burns H. Compression of digital nerves by pacinian corpuscles. A report of two cases. J Bone Joint Surg Am 1968;50:999-1001.
39. Goldman F, Garner R. Pacinian corpuscles as a cause for metatarsalgia. J Am Podiatry Assoc 1980;70:561-567.
40. Toth SP. Vater-Pacinian corpuscle: A case report. J Am Podiatry Assoc 1975;65:247-249.
41. Sellyei M, Balo J. Pathologic changes in the pacinian corpuscles around the pancreas. Acta Morphol Acad Sci Hung 1964;13:75-82.
42. Stouder DJ, McDonald LW. Enlarged intra-abdominal pacinian corpuscles simulating tumor implants. Am J Clin Pathol 1968;49:79-83.
43. Dembinski AS, Jones JW. Intra-abdominal pacinian neuroma: a rare lesion in an unusual location. Histopathology 1991;19:89-90.
44. Bale PM. Sacrococcygeal developmental abnormalities and tumors in children. Perspect Pediatr Pathol 1984;8:9-56.
45. Bale PM. Sacrococcygeal paciniomas. Pathology 1980;12:231-235.
46. Pease DC, Quilliam TA. Electron microscopy of the pacinian corpuscle. J Biophys Biochem Cytol 1957;3:331-342.
47. Ariza A, Bilbao JM, Rosai J. Immunohistochemical detection of epithelial membrane antigen in normal perineurial cells and perineurioma. Am J Surg Pathol 1988;12:678-683.
48. Theaker JM, Fletcher CD. Epithelial membrane antigen expression by the perineurial cell: further

studies of peripheral nerve lesions. Histopathology 1989;14:581-592.
49. Schochet SS Jr, Barrett DA 2nd. Neurofibroma with aberrant tactile corpuscles. Acta Neuropathol 1974;28:161-165.
50. Smith TW, Bhawan J. Tactile-like structures in neurofibromas. An ultrastructural study. Acta Neuropathol 1980;50:233-236.
51. Weiser G. An electron microscope study of "Pacinian neurofibroma." Virchows Arch A Pathol Anat Histol 1975;366:331-340.
52. Fletcher CD, Chan JK, McKee PH. Dermal nerve sheath myxoma: a study of three cases. Histopathology 1986;10:135-145.
53. MacDonald DM, Wilson-Jones E. Pacinian neurofibroma. Histopathology 1977;1:247-255.
54. Owen DA. Pacinian neurofibroma. Arch Pathol Lab Med 1979;103:99-100.
55. Prichard RW, Custer RP. Pacinian neurofibroma. Cancer 1952;5:297-301.
56. Brogli M. Ein fall von rantenneurom mit tastkorperchen. Frankf Z Pathol 1931;41:595-610.
57. McCormack K, Kaplan D, Murray JC, et al. Multiple hairy pacinian neurofibromas (nerve-sheath myxomas). J Am Acad Dermatol 1988;18:416-419.
58. Enzinger FM, Weiss SW. Benign tumors of peripheral nerves. Soft tissue tumors. St. Louis: CV Mosby; 1983:580-624.
59. Toth BB, Long WH, Pleasants JE. Central pacinian neurofibroma of the maxilla. Oral Surg Oral Med Oral Pathol 1975;39:630-634.
60. Prose PH, Gherardi GJ, Coblenz A. Pacinian neurofibroma. AMA Arch Derm 1957;76:65-69.
61. Altmeyer P. [Histology of a plexiform neuroma with Vater-Pacini-lamellar-corpuscle-like structures]. Hautarzt 1979;30:248-252. [German]
62. Jurecka W. Tactile corpuscle-like structures in peripheral nerve sheath tumors in plastic embedded material. Am J Dermatopathol 1988;10:74-79.
63. Jurecka W, Lassmann H, Lassmann G, et al. Tactile corpuscle-like structures in a case of plexiform neurofibromatosis. Arch Dermatol Res 1979;266:43-50.
64. Watabe K, Kumanishi T, Ikuta F, et al. Tactile-like corpuscles in neurofibromas: immunohistochemical demonstration of S-100 protein. Acta Neuropathol 1983;61:173-177.
65. Shiurba RA, Eng LF, Urich H. The structure of pseudomeissnerian corpuscles. An immunohistochemical study. Acta Neuropathol 1984;63:174-176.
66. Rigdon RH. Neurogenic tumors produced by methylcholanthrene in the white Pekin duck. Cancer 1955;8:906-915.

Oral Pseudoperineuroma

67. Koutlas IG, Scheithauer BW. Reactive pseudo-onion bulb proliferation and intraneural perineurioma of the oral mucosa. Head Neck Pathol 2013. [Epub ahead of print]
68. Korthals JK, Gieron MA, Wisniewski HM. Nerve regeneration patterns after acute ischemic injury. Neurology 1989;39:932-937.

Intraneural Injury Neuroma

69. Erlandson RA. The enigmatic perineurial cell and its participation in tumors and in tumorlike entities. Ultrastruct Pathol 1991;15:335-351.
70. Mackinnon SE, Hudson AR, Hunter DA, et al. Nerve regeneration in the rat model: peripheral nerve repair and regeneration. Periph Nerve Repair Regen 1986;1:41-48.
71. Hirasawa Y, Saiki T, Katsumi Y. A correlative study of axonal and perineurial regenerations after crush nerve injury in rat sciatic nerve. Nippon Geka Hokan 1988;57:493-505.
72. Dyck PJ. Experimental hypertrophic neuropathy. Pathogenesis of onion-bulb formations produced by repeated tourniquet applications. Arch Neurol 1969;21:73-95.

Epithelial Sheath Neuroma

73. Requena L, Grosshans E, Kutzner H, et al. Epithelial sheath neuroma: a new entity. Am J Surg Pathol 2000;24:190-196.
74. Lin TY, Zhang AY, Bayer-Garner IB, et al. Epithelial sheath neuroma: a case report and discussion of the literature. Am J Dermatopathol 2006;28:216-219.
75. Husain EA, Al-Daraji WI. Epithelial sheath neuroma: be aware of benign perineural invasion! J Cutan Pathol 2009;36:570-572.

Nerve Cyst

76. Weller RO, Cervos-Navarro J. Pathology of peripheral nerves. London: Butterworth; 1977:153-154.
77. Cobb CA 3rd, Moiel RH. Ganglion of the peroneal nerve. Report of two cases. J Neurosurg 1974;41:255-259.
78. Krucke W. Pathologie der peripheran nerven. In: Olivecrona H, Tönnis W, Krenkel W, eds. Handbuch der neurochirugie, Vol 7, Part 3. Berlin: Springer-Verlag; 1974.
79. Nucci F, Artico M, Santoro A, et al. Intraneural synovial cyst of the peroneal nerve: report of two cases and review of the literature. Neurosurgery 1990;26:339-344.
80. Parkes AR. Intraneural ganglion of the lateral popliteal nerve (abstract). J Bone Joint Surg 1960;42B:652.

81. Scherman BM, Bilbao JM, Hudson AR, et al. Intraneural ganglion: a case report with electron microscopic observations. Neurosurgery 1981;8:487-490.
82. Bowers WH, Doppelt SH. Compression of the deep branch of the ulnar nerve by an intraneural cyst. Case report. J Bone Joint Surg Am 1979;61:612-613.
83. Gurdjian ES, Larsen RD, Lindner DW. Intraneural cyst of the peroneal and ulnar nerves. Report of two cases. J Neurosurg 1965;23:76-78.
84. Jenkins SA. Solitary tumours of peripheral nerve trunks. J Bone Joint Surg Br 1952;34-B:401-411.
85. Spinner RJ, Vincent JF, Wolanskyj AP, et al. Intraneural ganglion cyst: a 200-year-old mystery solved. Clin Anat 2008;21:611-618.
86. Hartwell AS. Cystic tumor of median nerve. Operation: restoration of function. Boston Med Surg J 1901;144:582-583.
87. Jaradeh S, Sanger JR, Maas EF. Isolated sensory impairment of the thumb due to an intraneural ganglion cyst in the median nerve. J Hand Surg Br 1995;20:475-478.
88. Hashizume H, Nishida K, Nanba Y, et al. Intraneural ganglion of the posterior interosseous nerve with lateral elbow pain. J Hand Surg Br 1995;20:649-651.
89. Iannotti JP, Ramsey ML. Arthroscopic decompression of a ganglion cyst causing suprascapular nerve compression. Arthroscopy 1996;12:739-745.
90. Spinner RJ, Amrami KK, Kliot M, et al. Suprascapular intraneural ganglia and glenohumeral joint connections. J Neurosurg 2006;104:551-557.
91. Spinner RJ, Mokhtarzadeh A, Schiefer TK, et al. The clinico-anatomic explanation for tibial intraneural ganglion cysts arising from the superior tibiofibular joint. Skeletal Radiol 2007;36:281-292.
92. Friedlander HL. Intraneural ganglion of the tibial nerve. A case report. J Bone Joint Surg Am 1967;49:519-522.
93. Herrin E, Lepow GM, Bruyn JM. Mucinous cyst of the sural nerve. J Foot Surg 1986;25:14-18.
94. Spinner RJ, Amrami KK, Wolanskyj AP, et al. Dynamic phases of peroneal and tibial intraneural ganglia formation: a new dimension added to the unifying articular theory. J Neurosurg 2007;107:296-307.
95. Harbaugh KS, Tiel RL, Kline DG. Ganglion cyst involvement of peripheral nerves. J Neurosurg 1997;87:403-408.
96. Wadstein T. Two cases of ganglia in the sheath of the peroneal nerve. Acta Orthop Scand 1932;2:221-231.

97. Spinner RJ, Hebert-Blouin MN, Rock MG, Amrami KK. Extreme intraneural ganglion cysts. J Neurosurg 2011;114:217-224.

98. Krishnan KG, Schackert G. Intraneural ganglion cysts: a case of sciatic nerve involvement. Br J Plast Surg 2003;56:183-186.

99. Spinner RJ, Atkinson JL, Tiel RL. Peroneal intraneural ganglia: the importance of the articular branch. A unifying theory. J Neurosurg 2003;99:330-343.

100. Seddon HJ. Surgical disorders of the peripheral nerves. Edinburgh: Churchill Livingstone; 1975:124-126.

101. Nicholson TR, Cohen RC, Grattan-Smith PJ. Intraneural ganglion of the common peroneal nerve in a 4-year-old boy. J Child Neurol 1995;10:213-215.

102. Ghossain M, Mohasseb G, Dagher F, Ghossain A. [Compression of the common peroneal nerve by a synovial cyst]. Neurochirurgie 1987;33:412-414. [French]

103. Masciocchi C, Innacoli M, Cisternino S, et al. Myxoid intraneural cysts of external popliteal ischiadic nerve. Report of 2 cases studied with ultrasound, computed tomography and magnetic resonance imaging. Eur J Radiol 1992;14:52-55.

104. Spinner RJ, Atkinson JL, Scheithauer BW, et al. Peroneal intraneural ganglia: the importance of the articular branch. Clinical series. J Neurosurg 2003;99:319-329.

105. Hsu KY, Zucherman JF, Shea WJ, et al. Lumbar intraspinal synovial and ganglion cysts (facet cysts). Ten-year experience in evaluation and treatment. Spine (Phila Pa 1976) 1995;20:80-89.

106. Kornberg M. Nerve root compression by a ganglion cyst of the lumbar anulus fibrosus. A case report. Spine (Phila Pa 1976) 1995;20:1633-1635.

107. Chang LW, Gowans JD, Granger CV, et al. Entrapment neuropathy of the posterior interosseous nerve. A complication of rheumatoid arthritis. Arthritis Rheum 1972;15:350-352.

108. DiRisio D, Lazaro R, Popp AJ. Nerve entrapment and calf atrophy caused by a Baker's cyst: case report. Neurosurgery 1994;35:333-334; discussion 334.

109. Fernandes L, Goodwill CJ, Srivatsa SR. Synovial rupture of rheumatoid elbow causing radial nerve compression. Br Med J 1979;2:17-18.

110. Orf G. [Intraneural ganglion cysts. Report on the clinicae aspects of the pseudotumor nervi]. Schweiz Arch Neurol Neurochir Psychiatr 1972;110:55-67. [German]

111. Robert R, Resche F, Lajat Y, et al. [Intraneural synovial cyst in the peroneal nerve. Case report (author's transl)]. Neurochirurgie 1980;26:135-143.

Endometriosis of Sciatic Nerve

112. Pham M, Sommer C, Wessig C, et al. Magnetic resonance neurography for the diagnosis of extrapelvic sciatic endometriosis. Fertil Steril 2010;94:351 e311-354.

113. Torkelson SJ, Lee RA, Hildahl DB. Endometriosis of the sciatic nerve: a report of two cases and a review of the literature. Obstet Gynecol 1988;71:473-477.

114. Schlicke CP. Ectopic endometrial tissue in the thigh. JAMA 1946;132:445-446.

115. Denton RO, Sherrill JD. Sciatic syndrome due to endometriosis of sciatic nerve. South Med J 1955;48:1027-1031.

116. Head HB, Welch JS, Mussey E, et al. Cyclic sciatica. Report of case with introduction of a new surgical sign. JAMA 1962;180:521-524.

117. Mannan K, Altaf F, Maniar S, et al. Cyclical sciatica: endometriosis of the sciatic nerve. J Bone Joint Surg Br 2008;90:98-101.

118. Lacroix-Triki M, Beyris L, Martel P, et al. Low-grade endometrial stromal sarcoma arising from sciatic nerve endometriosis. Obstet Gynecol 2004;104:1147-1149.

Heterotopic Ossification of Nerve

119. Catalano F, Fanfani F, Pagliei A, Taccardo G. [A case of primary intraneural ossification of the ulnar nerve]. Ann Chir Main Memb Super 1992;11:157-162. [French]

120. George DH, Scheithauer BW, Spinner RJ, et al. Heterotopic ossification of peripheral nerve ("neuritis ossificans"): report of two cases. Neurosurgery 2002;51:244-246; discussion 246.

121. Isla A, Perez-Lopez C, De Agustin D, et al. Neuritis ossificans of the sciatic nerve. Case illustration. J Neurosurg 2004;101:545.

122. Kemper CM, Rojas JC, Bauserman S. Neuritis ossificans of a cranial nerve. J Neurosurg 2010;113:1112-1114.

123. Trigkilidas D, Lidder S, Delaney D, et al. Neuritis ossificans of the common peroneal nerve: a case report. Skeletal Radiol 2009;38:1115-1118.

124. Villen GM, Canales V, Panisello JJ, et al. Ossifying neuropathy of the median nerve at level of the distal forearm and carpal tunnel in a patient with familial history of heterotopic calcification. Chir Main 2009;28:318-321.

125. Wasman JK, Willis J, Makley J, et al. Myositis ossificans-like lesion of nerve. Histopathology 1997;30:75-78.

126. Dal Monte A, Zanoli S. [On a case of ossification of the humeral artery and median nerve.]. Chir Organi Mov 1959;47:465-471.

127. Gui L. Ossificazioni post-traumatiche dei nervi periferici. Chir Org Mov 1948;32:241-270.

128. Vorenkamp SE, Nelson TL. Ulnar nerve entrapment due to heterotopic bone formation after a severe burn. J Hand Surg Am 1987;12:378-380.

129. Louis DS, Dick HM. Ossifying lipofibroma of the median nerve. J Bone Joint Surg Am 1973;55:1082-1084.

130. Sarma DP, Robichaux J, Fondak A. Ossified neurofibroma. J La State Med Soc 1983;135:22-23.

131. King RH, Llewelyn JG, Thomas PK, et al. Perineurial calcification. Neuropathol Appl Neurobiol 1988;14:105-123.

132. Polio JL, Stern PJ. Digital nerve calcification in CREST syndrome. J Hand Surg Am 1989;14:201-203.

4 INFLAMMATORY AND INFECTIOUS LESIONS SIMULATING TUMORS OF NERVE

Although uncommon, a variety of non-neoplastic conditions result in tumefactive enlargement of nerves. This chapter focuses upon several including: inflammatory pseudotumor, a rare lesion; sarcoidosis, the nature of which is unsettled; mycobacterial pseudotumor; and leprosy, the most common infection of nerve. We have seen massive examples of inflammatory pseudotumor that clinically simulated neoplasia. Although sarcoidosis, mycobacterial infection, and leprosy generally produce only limited, localized enlargement of nerve, they are discussed for the sake of completeness.

Nerves also become overrun and entrapped in benign fibroproliferative lesions, including extra-abdominal desmoid (fibromatosis); idiopathic processes, including mediastinal fibrosis, retroperitoneal fibrosis, and Riedel thyroiditis; and tumefactive fibroinflammatory lesions of the head and neck (1–4).

INFLAMMATORY PSEUDOTUMOR OF NERVE

Definition. *Inflammatory pseudotumor of nerve* is an idiopathic, localized, tumefactive fibroinflammatory process of nerve typically consisting of chronic inflammatory and reactive mesenchymal cells. Synonyms include *lymphoid hyperplasia, plasma cell granuloma*, and *inflammatory myofibroblastic tumor*.

General Features. The term inflammatory pseudotumor has been used to denote a heterogeneous group of tumor-like lesions of wide distribution with no known etiology (5). Composed of chronic inflammatory and fibrohistiocytic cells, examples at non-neural sites have variously been designated nodular lymphoid hyperplasia, plasma cell granuloma, and fibrous xanthoma. These varied terms reflect their broad range of appearances, particularly in terms of cellular composition (5). The various sites often affected by inflammatory pseudotumors include lung (6), lymph node (7), brain (8), orbit (9), and soft tissues. Many are present as mass lesions; some are clinically suggestive of malignancy. Also uncommon is mononeuropathy due to secondary involvement of nerve by fibroinflammatory processes primarily involving surrounding perineural soft tissues (3,4).

Clinical Features. To date, only nine cases of inflammatory pseudotumor originating in nerve have been reported. Three involved the sciatic nerve, one each the facial, and one each the ulnar, radial, greater auricular nerve, and peroneal nerve (10–12). In the largest series of five patients (13), all presented with a gradually progressive mononeuropathy characterized by weakness, sensory loss, and neuropathic pain. Symptom duration ranged from 3 to 36 months (median, 7 months). Electrodiagnostic studies revealed chronic axonal mononeuropathies with variable active denervation and reinnervation.

Radiologic Features. Magnetic resonance imaging (MRI) often demonstrates a large, irregular mass arising within nerve. Heterogeneous signal characteristics are noted on T1- and T2-weighted as well as postcontrast sequences (fig. 4-1).

Gross Findings. Affected nerves are segmentally enlarged and are either fusiform or nodular (fig. 4-2). The intact nerve is readily identified when the fibroinflammatory lesion is dissected free (fig. 4-2). Occasionally, perineurium and endoneurium are almost entirely spared. In reported cases, the process has largely been limited to epineurium.

Microscopic Findings. The histology varies but common features are those of a chronic reactive process with chronic inflammatory infiltrates, markedly increased fibrosis, an increase in vascular density, and obscuration of the nerve boundary due to expansion of epineurium. Aside from the presence of chronic inflammation, the cytologic composition of the infiltrates varies considerably, ranging from patchy chronic lymphoplasmacellular inflammation with a variable fibrous reaction (fig. 4-3), to germinal center

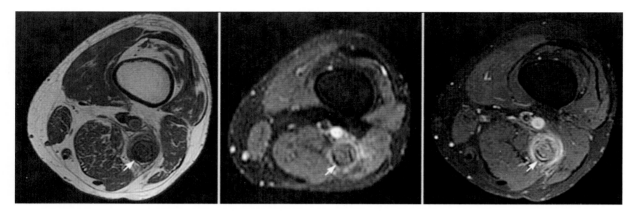

Figure 4-1

INFLAMMATORY PSEUDOTUMOR

Axial T1-weighted (left), T2-weighted (center), and T1-weighted postgadolinium magnetic resonance image (MRI) (right) demonstrate an irregular, large inflammatory pseudotumor involving and encasing the sciatic nerve of a 63-year-old male. There are heterogenous signal characteristics and enhancement. The dark signal on T1 suggests fibrosis and hemosiderin deposition. (Fig. 1G–I from Mauermann ML, Scheithauer BW, Spinner RJ, et al. Inflammatory pseudotumor of nerve: clinicopathological characteristics and a potential therapy. J Peripher Nerve Syst 2010;15:218.)

Figure 4-2

INFLAMMATORY PSEUDOTUMOR

A: The operative photograph shows the intact, grossly normal sciatic nerve as well as the pseudotumor, a layer of fibroinflammatory epineurial tissue (above) which was dissected free of the nerve. (Fig. 2 from Weiland TL, Scheithauer BW, Rock MG, Sargent JM. Inflammatory pseudotumor of nerve. Am J Pathol 1996;20:1214.)

B: The thick shell of affected epineurium, seen in cross section, chronically compressed the nerve with resultant near-total loss of neurologic function. (Figs. 4-2B and 4-5 are from case 2 from reference 12.)

C: This example affected the median nerve in a 51-year-old male. The epineurium is expanded by this demarcated, fusiform mass. (Fig. from Case 1 from Mauermann ML, Scheithauer BW, Spinner RJ, et al. Inflammatory pseudotumor of nerve: clinicopathological characteristics and potential therapy. J Peripher Nerv Syst 2010;15:216-226.)

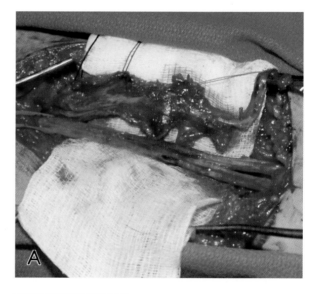

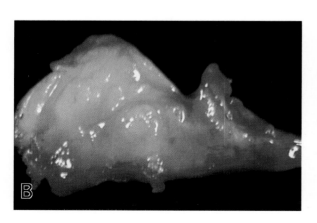

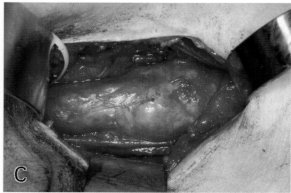

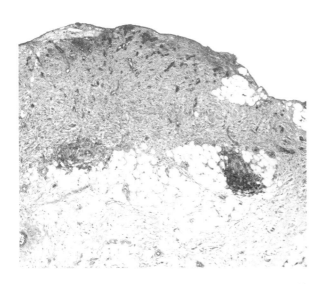 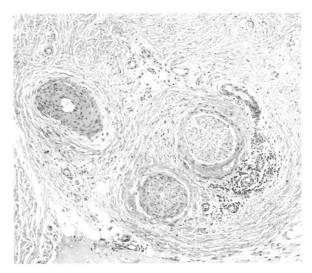

Figure 4-3

INFLAMMATORY PSEUDOTUMOR

Left: The surgical specimen consisted of inflamed epineurial fibroadipose tissue. At low magnification and in cross section, the markedly thickened epineurium shows extensive fibrosis and chronic inflammation. The smooth contour represents the perimeter of the epineurium.

Right: Composed of benign lymphocytes and occasional plasma cells, the inflammatory infiltrate entraps minute, otherwise normal-appearing nerve fascicles.

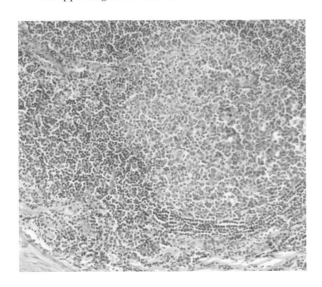 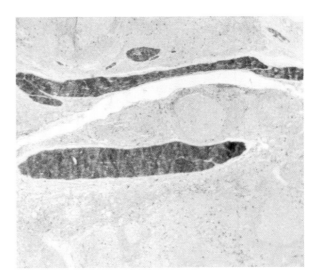

Figure 4-4

INFLAMMATORY PSEUDOTUMOR

This example, occurring in the greater auricular nerve of a 41-year-old male, featured nodular lymphoid hyperplasia limited to the epineurium. The intact, S-100 protein-positive nerve fascicles are encircled (right). Intrafascicular growth was a focal finding. (Courtesy of Dr. T. Beer, Gosport Hants, UK.)

formation, to dense nodular lymphoid hyperplasia (fig. 4-4). One unusual example was composed primarily of uninucleated and multinucleated histiocytes (fig. 4-5). Scattered giant cells are rarely encountered but formed granulomas are not seen (13). By definition, special stains for microorganisms, such as bacteria, tubercle bacilli, lepra bacilli, and fungi, are negative.

Table 4-1

INFLAMMATORY PSEUDOTUMOR OF NERVE: LITERATURE SUMMARY

Authors	Age/Sex	Nerve	Clinical
Keen et al. (11)	41/M	Right facial nerve and geniculate ganglion	Two episodes Bell palsy 5 years and 4.5 months prior; initial bout responsive to steroids and stellate ganglion block
Weiland et al. (case 1 [12])	35/M	Sciatic nerve	Two-year progression of idiopathic right lower leg weakness, numbness, and pain through atrophy to total sensorimotor loss in peroneal, tibial, sural nerves
Weiland et al. (case 2 [12])	18/F	Radial nerve	Three months; painful enlargement right distal radial nerve with associated radiation and dysesthesia to thumb, and index and middle fingers
Beer et al. (10)	41/M	Left greater auricular nerve	One year painful, mobile right neck mass; associated dental caries

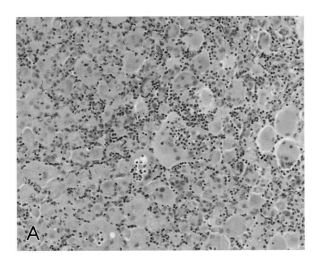

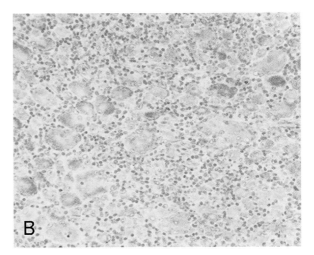

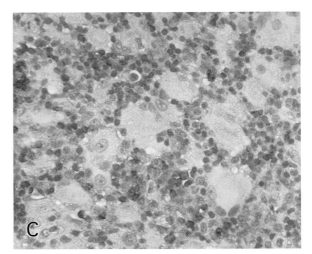

Figure 4-5

INFLAMMATORY PSEUDOTUMOR

A lesion of the radial nerve epineurium (A) consists of KP1-positive multinucleated giant cells (B), small CD45-reactive lymphocytes (C), and occasional eosinophils. (Case 2 from reference 12)

Table 4-1 (Continued)

INFLAMMATORY PSEUDOTUMOR OF NERVE: LITERATURE SUMMARY

Gross/Operative Findings	Surgery	Pathology	Follow-up
Hard, vascular mass involving geniculate ganglion, facial nerve, and tensor tympani muscle	Resection of mass and nerve	Epidural lesion; nerve surrounded by fibrotic granulation tissue with chronic inflammation	Total facial nerve palsy at 6 months, nerve function <5% at 2 years
Fusiform 16 x 2-cm enlargement of right sciatic nerve (see fig. 4-2)	Resection of epineurial mass encompassing the sciatic nerve	Epineurial T- and to a lesser extent B-lymphocyte infiltrate with fibrosis and loss of myelinated nerve fibers (see fig. 4-3)	Diminution in pain but persistent total sensori-motor loss; no recurrence at 4 years
Ovoid lipoma-like, 2.5-cm lesion involving right radial nerve	Resection of epineurial based lesion with sparing of nerve fascicles	Epineurial infiltrate of histiocytes, giant cells, and predominantly T lymphocytes (see fig. 4-5)	Neurologic recovery and no evidence of recurrence at 3 months follow-up
Mass affecting left greater auricular nerve; intact fascicles traversed the lesion	Resection with segment of nerve	Follicular lymphoid hyperplasia with primarily perifascicular growth; extension into one fascicle noted (see fig. 4-4)	Hypoesthesia of left face

Immunohistochemical Findings. In three reported cases, the lymphocytes were polyclonal and predominantly of T-cell type (10,12). In another instance (Table 4-1, case 2; figs. 4-2, 4-3), lymphocyte subtyping showed the infiltrate to be composed of a mixture of T and to a lesser extent B cells of normal phenotype. As expected, the occasional histiocytes and giant cells are immunoreactive for macrophage markers (fig. 4-5) and lack both S-100 protein and CD1a staining.

Differential Diagnosis. Although in clinical, radiographic, or operative terms, inflammatory pseudotumors may mimic benign and malignant peripheral nerve sheath tumors, the histologic distinction poses no problem. With the exception of schwannoma, particularly the cellular variant, which in our experience may show appreciable subcapsular and/or perivascular lymphocytic infiltrates, peripheral nerve tumors are infrequently inflamed. For unknown reasons, schwannomas rarely exhibit multiple noncaseating granulomas (see fig. 7-22, right). In such instances, stains for organisms are negative and the neoplastic nature of the underlying lesion is readily apparent.

The distinction of inflammatory pseudotumor from infection is based on negative histochemical stains for organisms as well as negative cultures. A discussion of the differential diagnosis with lymphoma is beyond the scope of this work. Nonetheless, lymphocytes of inflammatory pseudotumors lack cytologic atypia and are polytypic. Neither Langerhans cell histiocytosis nor Rosai-Dorfman disease cause tumor-like enlargement of nerve; unlike inflammatory pseudotumors rich in histiocytes, both these lesions are immunopositive for S-100 protein, the former also being CD1a and langerin reactive.

Treatment and Prognosis. Timely biopsy and nerve-sparing microsurgical resection afford a maximal chance of cure without neurologic deficit. We have observed only one instance of recurrence: regrowth of a lesion of the auricular nerve affecting proximal and distal nerve stumps 2 years after gross total resection. Successful therapy with corticosteroids has been reported in the largest clinical series (13); all patients so treated showed improvement on neurologic exam.

SARCOIDOSIS OF PERIPHERAL NERVE

Definition. *Sarcoidosis* is a systemic disorder characterized by idiopathic noncaseating granulomatous inflammation.

General Features. Sarcoidosis, a multisystem disorder of unknown etiology, shows a prevalence of 10 to 20 per 100,000 and clinically affects the nervous system in approximately 5 percent of cases (14). In many instances, involvement is largely or entirely of the peripheral or central nervous system. Indeed, in 10 to 20 percent or in 90 percent of cases, the disorder involves primarily peripheral nerve/muscle or the central nervous system/cranial nerves, respectively. Among cranial nerves, the 7th is most often involved (15). Patient age at the onset of peripheral neurosarcoidosis ranges from 10 to 40 years in 70 to 90 percent of cases. Females are more often affected. The disorder occurs in all races but shows a four-fold proclivity for blacks.

Clinical Features. Peripheral neurosarcoidosis presents in one of three forms: multiple mononeuropathy, radiculopathy, and polyneuropathy. Since significant nerve enlargement or hypertrophy is not a clinical feature of sarcoidal neuropathy, the lesions only rarely clinically mimic a neoplasm (16–18). Sarcoidosis may affect cranial and spinal nerves. Cranial polyneuritis is characterized by the occurrence of multiple fluctuating and remitting cranial nerve palsies, usually in young to middle-aged women, and may be associated with the uveoparotid form of sarcoidosis. Systemic symptoms are generally minimal. The facial nerve is most often affected. Lesions are usually bilateral but asynchronous. Although cranial and spinal nerves can be involved in isolation, the lesions frequently coexist. Often, affected nerves include the peroneal, median (19), radial (20), and phrenic (21) nerves, as well as the cauda equina (22). Sarcoidal polyneuropathy may be acute and indistinguishable from Guillain-Barré syndrome, or may present as a slowly progressive sensorimotor neuropathy. No specific clinical features distinguish progressive sarcoidal polyneuropathy from other forms of peripheral neuropathy.

A diagnosis of sarcoidosis may be made on biopsy of any accessible lesion, such as of skin, lymph node, muscle, scalene fat pad, gingiva, conjunctiva, bronchus, or liver. It may also be facilitated by a careful ophthalmologic examination, as well as by other, albeit less reliable, methods including: 1) the Kveim test, which yields a significant proportion of both false- positive and false- negative results; 2) measurement of serum levels of angiotensin-converting enzyme (ACE), which is often positive when the diagnosis is apparent; and 3) cerebrospinal fluid examination, which may demonstrate an elevated protein level, a slight increase in lymphocytes, and sometimes a decrease in glucose level.

Gross and Microscopic Findings. The peripheral neuropathy of sarcoidosis has been exhaustively studied (23). Affected nerves appear firm and thickened but do not resemble ordinary peripheral nerve tumors. Although not diagnostic, the histologic finding of a sarcoidal-type granuloma at any site is of clinical value. Typically, the noncaseating granulomas of sarcoidosis are sharply demarcated and consist, in varying proportion, of epithelioid histiocytes and multinucleated giant cells in association with only a small number of lymphocytes. Schaumann bodies are occasionally seen within giant cells. Although frank necrosis is lacking, fibrinoid material may be evident at the center of some granulomas. Sarcoidal granulomas often exhibit interstitial reticulin staining. Marked fibrosis is a common feature of chronic lesions. By definition, sarcoidal granulomas do not stain for microorganisms and are culture negative.

Neuropathy may result from granulomatous inflammation, but the mechanism of nerve injury in sarcoidal neuropathy is controversial. Diffuse involvement of the perineurium, epineurium, and endoneurium by sarcoidal granulomas is thought to mediate nerve fiber damage (fig. 4-6). Both nerve fiber compression and ischemia due to accompanying lymphocytic angiitis have been suggested as pathogenetic mechanisms (24,25). Clearly, axonal injury is far more frequent than demyelination (26). The pathologic basis of the acute sarcoidal polyradiculoneuropathy resembling Guillain-Barré syndrome is unclear.

Differential Diagnosis. The principal entities in the differential diagnoses are fungal and mycobacterial infections. The likelihood of infection is high in the face of necrotizing granulomas. Special stains, including silver preparations for fungi and acid fast or fluorescent stains for mycobacteria, are useful, but a negative reaction is no assurance that a lesion is noninfectious. Polymerase chain reaction similarly has suboptimal sensitivity and specificity for uncovering mycobacteria. Correlation with clinical data, skin tests, and culture results is mandatory. Other processes in the differential diagnosis are necrotizing vasculitis and lymphoma.

Treatment and Prognosis. Given its treatability, the outcome in sarcoidal neuropathy is favorable. Recoveries were documented even

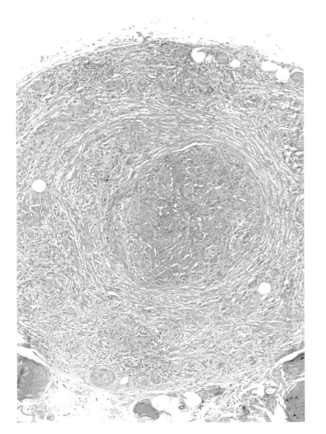
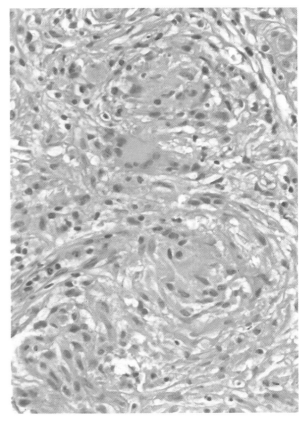

Figure 4-6

SARCOIDOSIS

This section of the sural nerve shows involvement of epineurium, perineurium, and endoneurium (left) by noncaseating granulomas (right). (Courtesy of Dr. C. Giannini and Dr. P.J. Dyck, Rochester, Minnesota).

prior to the introduction of steroid therapy. The latter has a beneficial effect upon cranial as well as spinal nerve disease (26), but relapses are common. Antitumor necrosis factor (TNF)-alpha therapy may also be useful (27). In general, the prognosis of patients with peripheral nervous system sarcoidosis is more favorable than for those with central nervous system involvement.

MYCOBACTERIAL PSEUDOTUMOR

Mycobacterial pseudotumor was initially described in an immunosuppressed patient (28). Today, particularly in the setting of acquired immunodeficiency syndrome (AIDS), mycobacterial pseudotumor involves not only lymph nodes but also subcutaneous soft tissue (28,29). As a result, a biopsy may be mistaken for neo-plasia on hematoxylin and eosin (H&E)-stained slides. The composition of spindle and epithelioid histiocytes arrayed in ill-defined fascicles may simulate schwannoma or leiomyoma (fig. 4-7A). Special stains show mycobacterial pseudotumors to contain numerous acid-fast- and Fite-positive *Mycobacterium avium intracellulare* (fig. 4-7B). Lymphocytes are generally few in number (30). Despite CD68 staining (fig. 4-7C), the similarity to schwannoma is furthered by S-100 protein immunoreactivity (fig. 4-7D). The mycobacteria are also known to show desmin staining; in leprosy, the same is true of *Mycobacterium leprae* organisms (see below) (29–32). Kaposi sarcoma, also in the differential diagnosis, is readily distinguished by its immunohistochemical profile (positive for CD34 and CD31; negative for S-100 protein and CD68) (29).

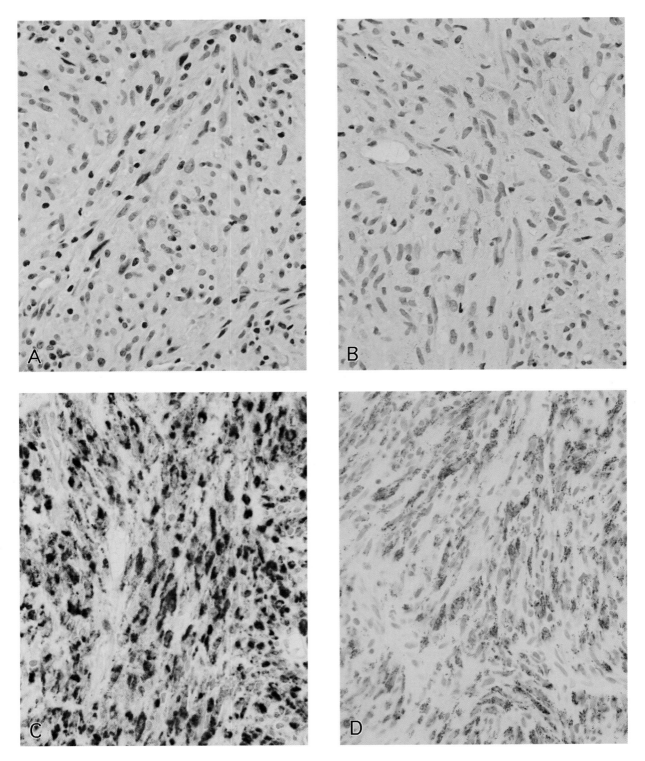

Figure 4-7

MYCOBACTERIAL PSEUDOTUMOR

This cellular soft tissue lesion consists of spindle cells and resembles schwannoma (A). The cells contain numerous acid-fast bacilli (B). The spindle cell histiocytes are CD68 immunoreactive (C). The organisms are positive for S-100 protein (D).

LEPROUS NEUROPATHY

General Features. *Leprosy,* the most common and treatable cause of peripheral neuropathy worldwide, is a chronic disease resulting from *Mycobacterium leprae* infection. It affects any part of the body, but shows a particular tendency to involve superficially situated nerves, as well as skin, eyes, respiratory tract, and testes. Bacterial invasion of peripheral nerve is noted in all cases.

Although the disease is most common in the tropics and subtropics, it also occurs in more temperate zones. Leprosy has been reported in association with human immunodeficiency virus (HIV) infection (33), although not to the extent that atypical mycobacterial infection occurs in this setting. The mechanism of spread is uncertain, but a respiratory route and direct inoculation into the skin appear most likely. Untreated patients are the major source of infection, but in North America infected armadillos also represent a potential reservoir. Only a minority of the population is susceptible to infection and children are more readily affected than adults (34).

M. leprae, the only bacterium that regularly invades peripheral nerve, is morphologically indistinguishable from *M. tuberculosis.* It consists of an acid-fast rod measuring 1 to 8 μm in length and up to 0.5 μm in diameter. Although the organism has not been cultured in vitro, the mouse foot pad (35) and the armadillo (36) serve as experimental models of infection. The optimal growth temperature of *M. leprae* is low (27° to 30° C).

Clinical Features. Patients with leprosy mainly present with peripheral neuropathy. Sensory loss often precedes other evidence of disease and manifests sequentially as loss of temperature, touch, pain, and pressure sensations. Affected nerves are more often the small, intracutaneous or subcutaneous nerves than the major peripheral nerve trunks (37). Depending upon the capacity of the patient to respond to the infection, three major clinicopathologic forms of leprosy are generally recognized: *tuberculoid, lepromatous,* and *borderline leprosy*, each of which features peripheral nerve involvement. Most patients fall into the borderline category, although it is preferable, both conceptually and in practical terms, to consider leprosy as a complete spectrum of host response to the pathogen rather than as a disease having various forms.

It is the nature of the cellular immune response that determines whether an exposed individual develops leprosy, as well as its subtype (38). In normal individuals, the organisms are taken up by macrophages which become activated by their interaction with T lymphocytes. The result is destruction of the bacillus. An abnormality of T-cell function probably plays a major role in the pathogenesis of leprosy, but the exact mechanisms are not understood. A minor excess in activity results in localized lesions (tuberculoid leprosy), whereas a more marked abnormality results in a major defect of cell-mediated immunity and the development of generalized disease (lepromatous leprosy). Patients with defects of intermediate severity develop the borderline form.

Gross and Microscopic Findings. *Tuberculoid Leprosy.* Presenting as localized disease, tuberculoid leprosy is characterized by asymmetric cutaneous lesions occurring over the extensor surfaces of the extremities, the face, or the buttocks. Microscopically, the lesions consist of epithelioid granulomas, only rarely associated with caseation, and a peripheral infiltrate of lymphocytes. The epithelioid histiocytes are numerous. The inflammatory process is concentrated about dermal appendages and to a great degree involves cutaneous and subcutaneous nerves (fig. 4-8A). Destruction of nerve fibers and loss of myelin are extensive. Although the fibers are invaded and destroyed, even a careful search under oil immersion reveals only rare Fite stain–positive organisms within epithelioid histiocytes and Langerhans-type giant cells.

The spread of tuberculoid leprosy to surrounding tissues is by direct extension, and animal models suggest that nerve trunks beneath cutaneous lesions are infected by hematogenous dissemination through the vasa nervorum (39). Transaxonal bacillary spread has not been proven to occur. Affected nerves are palpably enlarged (fig. 4-8A). Of the major sensorimotor nerves, those most frequently affected include the ulnar, median, peroneal, and facial; of sensory nerves, it is the cutaneous radial, digital, posterior auricular, and sural.

The inflammatory response to bacilli consists primarily of noncaseating granulomatous inflammation (fig. 4-8B,C). In cases with intense response to bacilli, necrosis may result in the

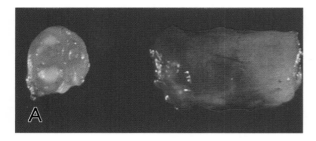

Figure 4-8

TUBERCULOID LEPROSY: NEUROPATHY

This form of the disease may markedly enlarge peripheral nerves (A). It features extensive noncaseating granulomatous inflammation (B) associated with nerve fibers and myelin loss (C). Necrosis of large nerves in advanced cases results in "cold abscess" formation that may grossly mimic tumor (D). (D, courtesy of Dr. P. Brand, Carville, Louisiana.)

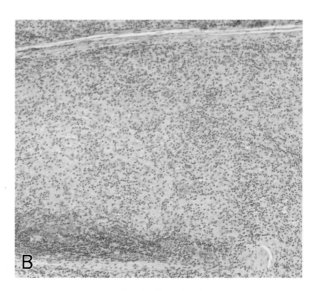

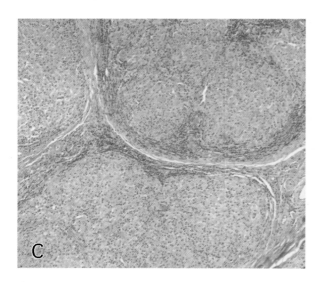

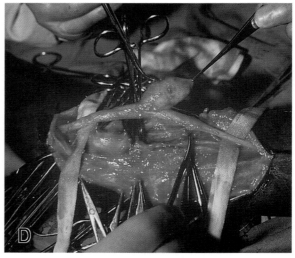

formation of a so-called cold abscess (fig. 4-8D) (40). Associated dystrophic calcification may occur and be radiographically apparent. Cold abscesses heal with time, resulting in widespread fibrosis of all nerve compartments. Microscopically, the changes resemble those occurring in smaller nerves. The infiltrate consists of epithelioid histiocytes and giant cells and, although concentrated within the epineurium and perineurium, may also extend to involve the endoneurium. Bacilli may not be demonstrable. Fascicular abnormalities are variable: some are destroyed and others are relatively spared.

Lepromatous Leprosy. In contrast to the tuberculoid variant, lepromatous leprosy is characterized by a florid proliferation of bacteria and their hematogenous dissemination. As in tuberculoid leprosy, superficial tissues are affected. In skin, the process is concentrated upon blood vessels, nerves, and adnexa. Gross infiltration of the skin of the face results in leonine facies, a feature of advanced disease. The upper respiratory tract, eyes, testes, and lymph nodes, particularly inguinal and epitrochlear nodes, may also be affected. A cutaneous biopsy in lepromatous leprosy shows an infiltrate of foamy histiocytes (Virchow cells) containing masses of bacilli, as well as scattered plasma cells. Unlike tuberculoid leprosy, the lepromatous form shows less inflammatory reaction and tissue destruction. Notably, most patients have tissue responses between the tuberculoid and

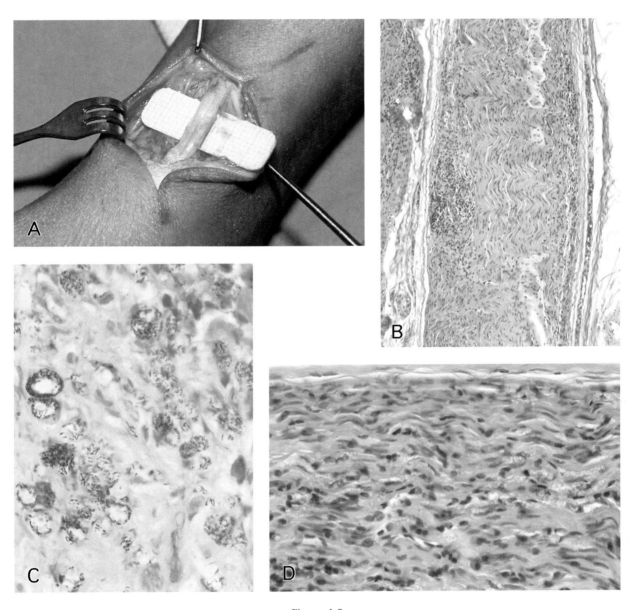

Figure 4-9

LEPROMATOUS LEPROSY: NEUROPATHY

A: This form of leprosy only occasionally produces nerve enlargement, in this case of a segment of the superficial radial nerve of an adult patient with a 5-year history of the disease.

B: Nerve involvement in yet another case features only mild chronic inflammation, primarily histiocytic infiltration of perineurium and peripheral endoneurium.

C: Cells contain masses of Fite stain-positive mycobacteria.

D: Bacilli-containing vacuoles within Schwann and perhaps endothelial cells are best seen in longitudinal sections of the nerve.

lepromatous extremes, in the broad category termed borderline leprosy.

Although nerve trunk involvement can occur in longstanding disease (fig. 4-9A), nerve enlargement is generally not as prominent a feature as in tuberculoid leprosy. Nonetheless, we have seen an example of nerve-centered lepromatous infection presenting as a palpable mass in the neck. It was regarded as a possible neoplasm of peripheral nerve by the referring pathologist.

The correct diagnosis was achieved only after the demonstration of acid-fast organisms. Affected nerves are architecturally preserved (fig. 4-9B), but bacteria-rich histiocytes involve the perineurium (fig. 4-9B), splitting it in an "onion skin" fashion. Fascicular involvement may be uneven. In addition to epineural and perineurial involvement, vacuoles containing abundant bacilli may be seen within the endoneurium (fig. 4-9C), particularly at its interface with the perineurial sheath. Longitudinal sections of the nerve show the bacilli-containing vacuoles seen in Schwann cells aligned along nerve fibers (fig. 4-9D). Endothelial cells within endoneurium may also contain bacilli. Wallerian degeneration and segmental demyelination may be seen (41). In longstanding cases, the endoneurium may undergo considerable fibrosis, but organisms are still demonstrable.

Differential Diagnosis. A complete discussion is beyond the scope of this work. The reader is referred to the excellent review by Sabin et al. (42). The diagnosis is predicated upon the demonstration of acid-fast- or Fite stain-positive microorganisms in the appropriate clinical setting.

Treatment and Prognosis. Specific antimicrobial therapy is curative, but in heavily infected patients the physical removal of dead organisms may take several years, during which immunological reactions may continue to cause clinical problems, including neuropathy. Neuropathic pain is occasionally encountered, both during treatment and even for years following completion of treatment (43).

REFERENCES

Introduction

1. Fanous MM, Margo CE, Hamed LM. Chronic idiopathic inflammation of the retropharyngeal space presenting with sequential abducens palsies. J Clinl Neuropathol 1992;12:154-157.
2. Wiseman JB, Arriaga MA, Houston GD, Boyd EM. Facial paralysis and inflammatory pseudotumor of the facial nerve in a child. Otolaryngol Head Neck Surg 1995;113:826-828.
3. Wold LE, Weiland LH. Tumefactive fibroinflammatory lesions of the head and neck. Am J Surg Pathol 1983;7:477-482.
4. Yanagihara N, Segoe M, Gyo K, Ueda N. Inflammatory pseudotumor of the facial nerve as a cause of recurrent facial palsy: case report. Am J Otol 1991;12:199-202.

Inflammatory Pseudotumor

5. Coffin CM, Watterson J, Priest JR, Dehner LP. Extrapulmonary inflammatory myofibroblastic tumor (inflammatory pseudotumor). A clinicopathologic and immunohistochemical study of 84 cases. Am J Surg Pathol 1995;19:859-872.
6. Matsubara O, Tan-Liu NS, Kenney RM, Mark EJ. Inflammatory pseudotumors of the lung: progression from organizing pneumonia to fibrous histiocytoma or to plasma cell granuloma in 32 cases. Hum Pathol 1988;19:807-814.
7. Davis RE, Warnke RA, Dorfman RF. Inflammatory pseudotumor of lymph nodes. Additional observations and evidence for an inflammatory etiology. Am J Surg Pathol 1991;15:744-756.
8. Figarella-Branger D, Gambarelli D, Perez-Castillo M, Garbe L, Grisoli F. Primary intracerebral plasma cell granuloma: a light, immunocytochemical, and ultrastructural study of one case. Neurosurgery 1990;27:142-147.
9. Diaz-Llopis M, Menezo JL. Idiopathic inflammatory orbital pseudotumor and low-dose cyclosporine. Am J Ophthalmol 1989;107:547-548.
10. Beer T, Carr NJ, Weller RO. Inflammatory pseudotumor of peripheral nerve. Am J Surg Pathol 1998;22:1035-1036.
11. Keen M, Conley J, McBride T, Mutter G, Silver J. Pseudotumor of the pterygomaxillary space presenting as anesthesia of the mandibular nerve. Laryngoscope 1986;96:560-563.
12. Weiland TL, Scheithauer BW, Rock MG, Sargent JM. Inflammatory pseudotumor of nerve. Am J Surg Pathol 1996;20:1212-1218.
13. Mauermann ML, Scheithauer BW, Spinner RJ, et al. Inflammatory pseudotumor of nerve: clinicopathological characteristics and potential therapy. J Peripher Nerv Syst 2010;15:216-226.

Sarcoidosis

14. Delaney P. Neurologic manifestations in sarcoidosis: review of the literature, with a report of 23 cases. Ann Intern Med 1977;87:336-345.
15. Silverstein A, Feuer MM, Siltzbach LE. Neurologic sarcoidosis. Study of 18 cases. Arch Neurol 1965;12:1-11.
16. Amrami KK, Felmlee JP, Spinner RJ. MRI of peripheral nerves. Neurosurg Clin N Am 2008;19:559-572, vi.

17. Dailey AT, Rondina MT, Townsend JJ, Shrieve DC, Baringer JR, Moore KR. Sciatic nerve sarcoidosis: utility of magnetic resonance peripheral nerve imaging and treatment with radiation therapy. J Neurosurg 2004;100:956-959.

18. Quinones-Hinojosa A, Chang EF, Khan SA, McDermott MW. Isolated trigeminal nerve sarcoid granuloma mimicking trigeminal schwannoma: case report. Neurosurgery 2003;52:700-705, discussion 704-705.

19. Kompf D, Neundorfer B, Kayser-Gatchalian C, Meyer-Wahl L, Ranft K. [Mononeuritis multiplex in Boeck's sarcoidosis]. Nervenarzt 1976;47:687-689. [German]

20. Cesaro P, Defer G, Barbizet J, Degos JD. [Sarcoidosis of the central and peripheral nervous system]. Ann Med Interne (Paris) 1984;135:144-148. [French]

21. Mayock RL, Bertrand P, Morrison CE, Scott JH. Manifestations of sarcoidosis. Analysis of 145 patients, with a review of nine series selected from the literature. Am J Med 1963;35:67-89.

22. Campbell JN, Black P, Ostrow PT. Sarcoid of the cauda equina. Case report. J Neurosurg 1977;47:109-112.

23. Matthews WB. Sarcoid neuropathy. In: Dyck PJ, Thomas PK, eds. Peripheral neuropathy, 3rd ed. Philadelphia: W. B. Saunders; 1993:1418-1423.

24. Bii SC, Otieno-Nyunya B, Siika A, Rotich JK. Self-reported adherence to single dose nevirapine in the prevention of mother to child transmission of HIV at Kitale District Hospital. East Afr Med J 2007;84:571-576.

25. Souayah N, Chodos A, Krivitskaya N, Efthimiou P, Lambert WC, Sharer LR. Isolated severe vasculitic neuropathy revealing sarcoidosis. Lancet Neurol 2008;7:756-760.

26. Burns TM, Dyck PJ, Aksamit AJ, Dyck PJ. The natural history and long-term outcome of 57 limb sarcoidosis neuropathy cases. J Neurol Sci 2006;244:77-87.

27. Hoitsma E, Faber CG, van Santen-Hoeufft M, De Vries J, Reulen JP, Drent M. Improvement of small fiber neuropathy in a sarcoidosis patient after treatment with infliximab. Sarcoidosis Vasc Diffuse Lung Dis 2006;23:73-77.

Mycobacterial Pseudotumor

28. Wood C, Nickoloff BJ, Todes-Taylor NR. Pseudotumor resulting from atypical mycobacterial infection: a "histoid" variety of Mycobacterium avium-intracellulare complex infection. Am J Clin Pathol 1985;83:524-527.

29. Logani S, Lucas DR, Cheng JD, Ioachim HL, Adsay NV. Spindle cell tumors associated with mycobacteria in lymph nodes of HIV-positive patients: 'Kaposi sarcoma with mycobacteri' and 'mycobacterial pseudotumor'. Am J Surg Pathol 1999;23:656-661.

30. Umlas J, Federman M, Crawford C, O'Hara CJ, Fitzgibbon JS, Modeste A. Spindle cell pseudotumor due to Mycobacterium avium-intracellulare in patients with acquired immunodeficiency syndrome (AIDS). Positive staining of mycobacteria for cytoskeleton filaments. Am J Surg Pathol 1991;15:1181-1187.

31. Mansfield RE. Histoid leprosy. Arch Pathol 1969;87:580-585.

32. Wade HW. The histoid variety of lepromatous leprosy. Int J Lepr 1963;31:129-142.

Leprous Neuropathy

33. Ponnighaus JM, Mwanjasi LJ, Fine PE, et al. Is HIV infection a risk factor for leprosy? Int J Lepr Other Mycobact Dis 1991;59:221-228.

34. Scollard DM, Adams LB, Gillis TP, Krahenbuhl JL, Truman RW, Williams DL. The continuing challenges of leprosy. Clin Microbiol Rev 2006;19:338-381.

35. Shepard CC. Experimental chemotherapy in leprosy, then and now. Int J Lepr Other Mycobact Dis 1973;41:307-319.

36. Scollard DM, Lathrop GW, Truman RW. Infection of distal peripheral nerves by M. leprae in infected armadillos; an experimental model of nerve involvement in leprosy. Int J Lepr Other Mycobact Dis 1996;64:146-151.

37. van Brakel WH, Nicholls PG, Wilder-Smith EP, et al. Early diagnosis of neuropathy in leprosy—comparing diagnostic tests in a large prospective study (the INFIR cohort study). PLoS Negl Trop Dis 2008;2:e212.

38. Adams LB, Krahenbuhl JL. Granulomas Induced by Mycobacterium leprae. Methods 1996;9:220-232.

39. Scollard DM, McCormick G, Allen JL. Localization of Mycobacterium leprae to endothelial cells of epineurial and perineurial blood vessels and lymphatics. Am J Pathol 1999;154:1611-1620.

40. Sehgal VN. Nerve abscesses in leprosy in Northern India. Lepr Rev 1966;37:109-112.

41. Gibbels E, Henke U, Klingmuller G, Haupt WF. Myelinated and unmyelinated fibers in sural nerve biopsy of a case with lepromatous leprosy—a quantitative approach. Int J Lepr Other Mycobact Dis 1987;55:333-337.

42. Sabin TD, Swift TR, Jacobson RR. Leprosy. In: Dyck PJ, Thomas PK, eds. Peripheral neuropathy, 3rd ed. Philadelphia: W. B. Saunders; 1993:1354-1379.

43. Hietaharju A, Croft R, Alam R, Birch P, Mong A, Haanpaa M. Chronic neuropathic pain in treated leprosy. Lancet 2000;356:1080-1081.

5 HYPERPLASTIC LESIONS

PALISADED ENCAPSULATED NEUROMA

Definition. *Palisaded encapsulated neuroma* (PEN), a form of true neuroma, is usually cutaneous and nodular or occasionally plexiform in appearance. It consists of Schwann cells as well as axons, all within a delicate perineurium-derived capsule. A synonym is *solitary circumscribed neuroma*.

General Features. First described by Reed et al. (1), many studies of PENs have since been published (2–6). PEN is a clinically and morphologically distinct form of true neuroma. Although underdiagnosed and often unrecognized, it is a common lesion. Originally considered a primary hyperplasia of nerve fibers or a hamartoma consisting of axons and their complement of Schwann cells, recent publications draw an analogy to traumatic neuroma (3,5). This analogy is weakened by the absence of scarring in surrounding dermal tissue. In any case, PEN can be viewed as one of several forms of true neuroma, a category that includes traumatic, intraneural perineurioma-like, pacinian, and mucosal neuromas.

Clinical Features. PENs are longstanding lesions. Approximately 90 percent affect the face, particularly the nose, cheek, forehead, and lips. Many lie in proximity to mucocutaneous junctions or even affect oral mucosa (fig. 5-1) (7–9). Although they occur from adolescence to old age, the peak incidence is the fifth to seventh decades, with a slight female predominance. Only occasional examples involve skin of the extremities. Most PENs are solitary, painless papules or nodules which, although not ballottable or hard, are firm. The overlying skin is usually smooth and intact, and lacks hair or hyperpigmentation. Clinically, most PENs resemble melanocytic nevi, basal cell carcinomas, or adnexal tumors. No association with neurofibromatosis or mucosal neuromatosis has been reported (4). Although there are no known predisposing factors, such as trauma, cutaneous PENs are associated with acne (5,10).

A recent series of 55 PENs affecting the oral cavity has been reported (11). All occurred in adults and showed a 2 to 1 male to female ratio. The majority (76 percent) affected the palate

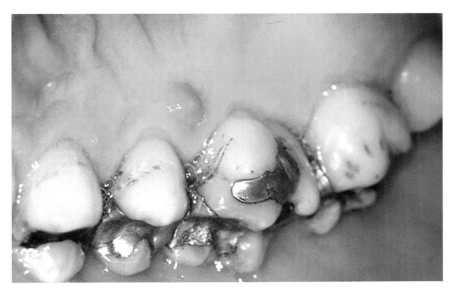

Figure 5-1

PALISADED ENCAPSULATED NEUROMA

A dome-shaped, somewhat erythematous lesion is near the gum line of the oral mucosa. (Courtesy of the Department of Oral Pathology, University of Minnesota, Minneapolis, MN.)

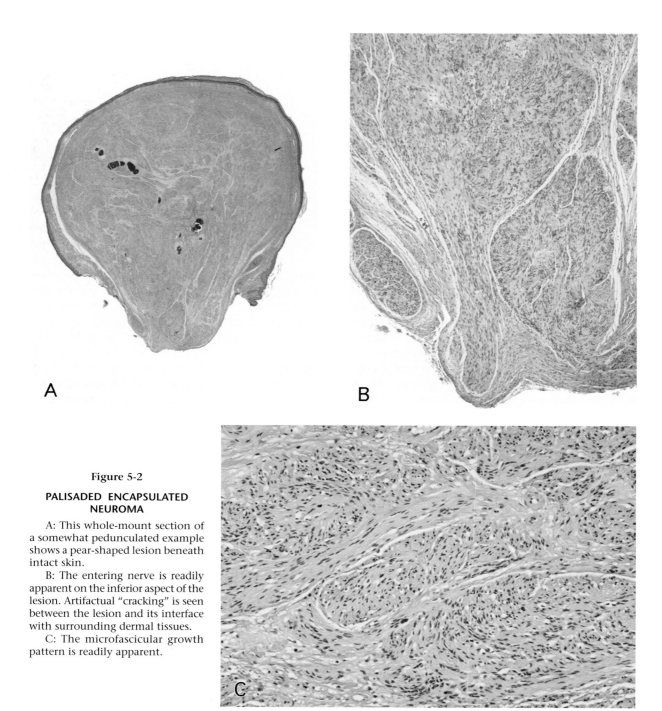

Figure 5-2

PALISADED ENCAPSULATED NEUROMA

A: This whole-mount section of a somewhat pedunculated example shows a pear-shaped lesion beneath intact skin.

B: The entering nerve is readily apparent on the inferior aspect of the lesion. Artifactual "cracking" is seen between the lesion and its interface with surrounding dermal tissues.

C: The microfascicular growth pattern is readily apparent.

and gingiva. Only 3 lesions were possibly trauma related. The authors stressed the importance of distinguishing these often plexiform (21 percent) or multilobular (8 percent) lesions from plexiform schwannoma.

Microscopic Findings. At low magnification, PENs appear circumscribed, smooth contoured,

and round or pear shaped; the largest or bulbous component is usually superficial (fungating pattern) (fig. 5-2). Many are multinodular (fig. 5-3, top) or even appear plexiform in configuration (3). Most PENs measure approximately 3 mm in diameter (range, 1 to 15 mm) and are situated in skin, centering upon the reticular

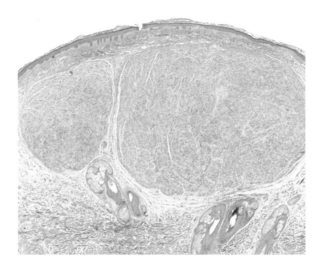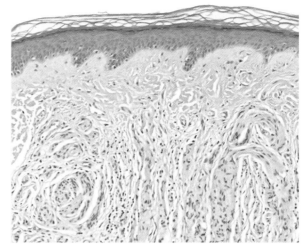

Figure 5-3

PALISADED ENCAPSULATED NEUROMA

Left: This multinodular lesion is dome-shaped. Despite the descriptive term "encapsulated," only a thin layer of perineurium and compressed connective tissue surrounds the process.

Right: Some lack of circumscription is apparent on the superficial aspect.

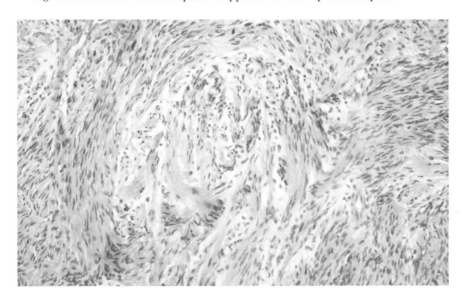

Figure 5-4

PALISADED ENCAPSULATED NEUROMA

Vague palisading, an uncommon feature, is noted.

dermis. Subcutaneous tissue is rarely involved. In approximately 20 percent of cases, a nerve of origin is microscopically apparent; serial sectioning increases the likelihood of finding the nerve, far more often at the base than at the apex of the lesion (fig. 5-2B). Despite the use of the descriptive terms "palisaded" and "encapsulated," PENs do not show significant palisading (fig. 5-4) and are often incompletely encapsulated. Most are only partially encapsulated by a

delicate, compact layer of perineurium. This, as well as the connective tissue surrounding PENs, is often lacking in superficial portions of the lesion where vertically aligned, minute, ragged fascicles may be seen (fig. 5-3, bottom). PENs situated entirely within the reticular dermis may appear totally encapsulated. A cracking artifact, presumably related to fixation, often surrounds them (fig. 5-2A) and/or produces slits between cell bundles (fig. 5-2B,C).

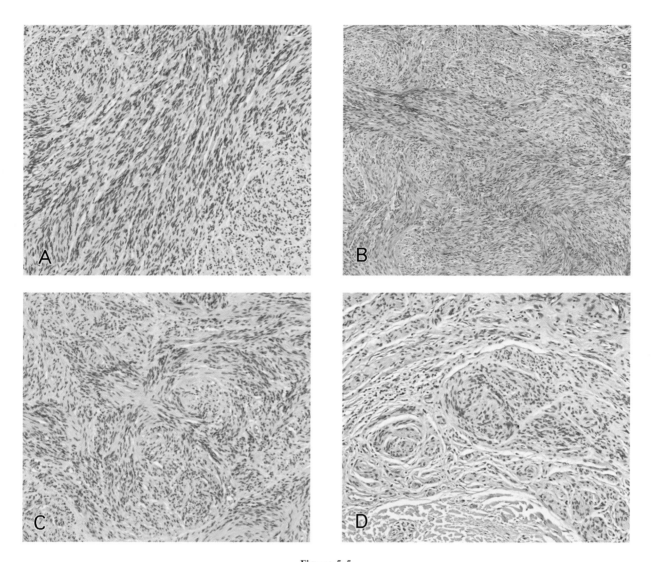

Figure 5-5

PALISADED ENCAPSULATED NEUROMA

Typically, the constituent cells show alignment (A), vague fasciculation, here accentuated with a trichrome stain (B), or random sweeping (C). Whorl formation is an inconspicuous feature (D), and palisading is only rarely observed.

At higher magnification, PENs consist largely of aligned and somewhat fasciculated, spindled-shaped Schwann cells coursing vertically or in various directions (figs. 5-2B,C; 5-3, bottom; 5-5A,B). On occasion, such cells form discrete whorls (figs. 5-3, bottom; 5-5C,D). The Schwann cells are normal in appearance, featuring a sinuous configuration and elongated, tapering nuclei (fig. 5-6A). Although not evident on hematoxylin and eosin (H&E)-stained slides, axons are seen with silver impregnations (Bodian and Bielschowsky stains); they appear variously distributed throughout the lesion and surrounded by bundles or micro-fascicles of aligned Schwann cells (fig. 5-6B). Axons are seen, but are concentrated in distinctly fascicular areas at the base of the lesion, where contiguity with nerve may be seen. They are also numerous in an occasionally traumatic neuroma element (fig. 5-6C). No atypia or mitotic activity is seen and stains for myelin are typically negative. Only a minority of lesions shows focal fibrosis, chronic inflammation, and stromal or mucin accumulation (fig. 5-6D)

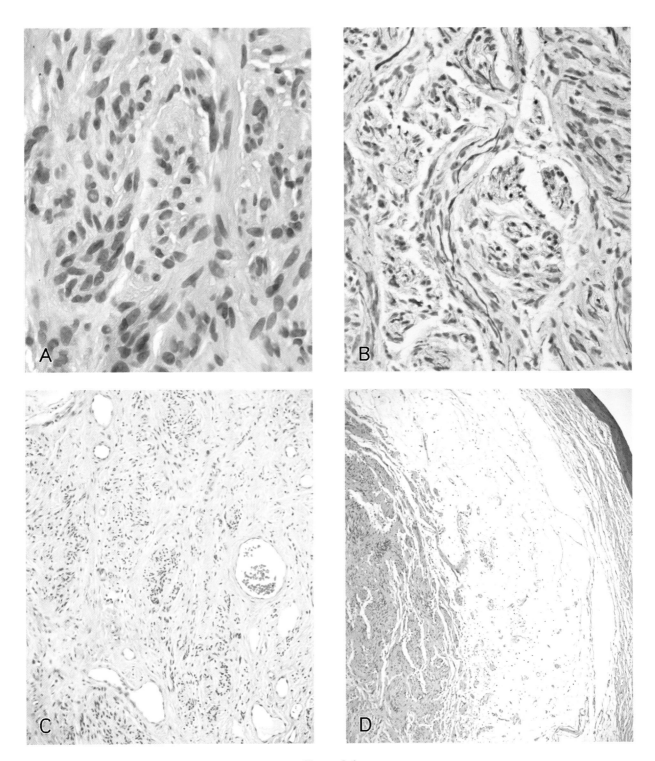

Figure 5-6

PALISADED ENCAPSULATED NEUROMA

The fascicles consist of typical, cytologically benign Schwann cells (A). Axons vary in number. Although inapparent with hematoxylin and eosin (H&E) stain, they are readily apparent with silver impregnation (B, Bodian stain). This view of the traumatic neuroma component demonstrates vague microfasciculation (C). Perilesional edema is an unusual feature (D).

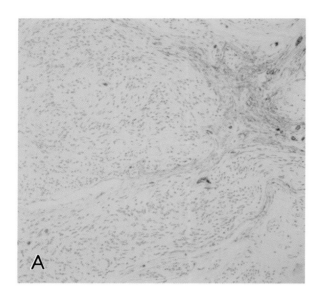

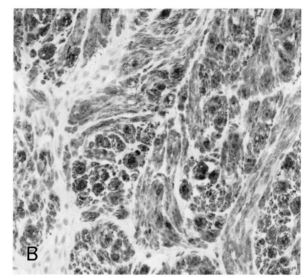

Figure 5-7

PALISADED ENCAPSULATED NEUROMA

Delicate partial ensheathment of the bilobed lesion is demonstrated by Glut-1 immunoreactive perineurial cells (A). The Schwann cells show generalized immunoreactivity for S-100 protein (B) while the axons are readily apparent with immunostains for neurofilament protein (C).

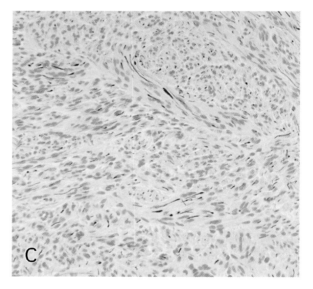

(3). Mast cells are infrequent. Overlying skin or mucosa occasionally shows mild hyperkeratosis but no hyperpigmentation.

Immunohistochemical Findings. Immunostains readily distinguish PEN from other, somewhat similar lesions. Epithelial membrane antigen (EMA) as well as Glut-1 highlight perineurial cells in varying numbers in the often incomplete, thin capsule of PENs, but not within their substance (fig. 5-7A). The Schwann cell component shows strong, uniform S-100 protein reactivity (fig. 5-7B). Staining for Leu-7 and even for myelin basic protein has been observed and type 4 collagen reactivity is the rule (12). Axons immunoreactive for neurofilament protein are seen in varying number (fig. 5-7C).

Ultrastructural Findings. PENs consist of well-differentiated Schwann cells often completely encircling axons and surrounded by basal lamina. Myelin sheath formation is minimal or focal at best (5).

Differential Diagnosis. Despite their frequency of occurrence, PENs are often misdiagnosed. Most are considered nerve sheath tumors of indeterminate type. Alternative diagnoses include schwannoma, neurofibroma, mucosal neuroma, traumatic neuroma, and angioleiomyoma (vascular leiomyoma).

At times, it is difficult to distinguish PEN from schwannoma. Unlike PENs, schwannomas usually affect subcutaneous tissue and only uncommonly arise in the dermis. Nonetheless, like PEN, cutaneous and mucosal schwannomas lack a distinct, fibrous capsule. In contrast to PEN, schwannomas show Antoni A and B patterns and generally lack all but isolated axons. Hyalinized thick-walled vessels similar to those seen in schwannoma may be seen in plexiform PEN (3).

In contrast to the compact architecture and coarse fasciculation of PEN, neurofibromas are typically loose textured, possess a mucin-rich stroma, and show a delicate fibrillary pattern of intercellular collagen deposition. Since most of the cells in PEN are normal Schwann cells, nuclear size is larger and more homogeneous than is seen in neurofibroma. As previously noted, there is no association of PEN with neurofibromatosis.

Although PEN only infrequently involves mucosae, those that do may prompt consideration of mucosal neuromatosis. Nerves in the latter are often multiple and exhibit a plexiform pattern of growth, a feature uncommon in PEN. The axons in mucosal neuromas are numerous and variably myelinated. Furthermore, a well-formed, intact perineurium is readily identified around each nerve. Many patients with mucosal neuromatosis show the stigmata of multiple endocrine neoplasia (MEN) type 2B. This inherited disorder includes medullary carcinoma of the thyroid gland and pheochromocytoma (see below) but is unassociated with PEN.

Compared with PEN, traumatic neuromas are architecturally complex (12), unencapsulated, and often associated with an obvious nerve. The microfascicles of fully developed traumatic neuromas are far better formed than are the vague fascicles of PEN. Each is ensheathed by an intact, circumferential layer of EMA-immunopositive perineurial cells. In PEN, such cells are largely limited to the lateral aspect of the poorly formed capsule. Furthermore, traumatic neuromas contain more axons and may exhibit some degree of myelination. They show greater degrees of stromal fibrosis and acidic mucin deposition. Chronic inflammation or foreign body reaction is occasionally seen in traumatic neuroma, but is not a feature of PEN.

Angioleiomyomas (vascular leiomyomas), unlike PEN, are circumscribed, cellular, dermal proliferations that lack intralesional perifascicular clefting, are more vascular, and are devoid of axons. Unlike Schwann cells, the smooth muscle cells of angioleiomyoma lack a sinuous configuration, exhibit blunt-ended nuclei and more defined cytoplasmic margins, and contain stainable phosphotungstic acid-hematoxylin (PTAH)-positive cytoplasmic fibrils. Immunostains show reactivity for smooth muscle antigens (smooth muscle actin, desmin) but not for uniform S-100 protein. If present, S-100 protein staining is usually patchy or weak. Unlike in PEN, hemosiderin deposits and extravasation of red blood cells are common features of angioleiomyoma.

Treatment and Prognosis. PENs are benign. Simple excision is curative. Recurrence is exceptional (4). No instances of malignant change or of metastasis have been described.

MULTIPLE ENDOCRINE NEOPLASIA 2B-ASSOCIATED MUCOSAL NEUROMA, MUCOSAL NEUROMATOSIS, AND INTESTINAL GANGLIONEUROMATOSIS

Definition. Well known to occur in the setting of multiple endocrine neoplasia (MEN) type 2B, this spectrum of lesions (*mucosal neuroma, mucosal neuromatosis,* and *intestinal ganglioneuromatosis*) results from hypertrophy of nerves and ganglia with resultant localized or extensive nerve plexus enlargement.

General Features. Since mucosal neuromas and intestinal ganglioneuromatosis are early markers of MEN 2B, it is important that pathologists be aware of their clinicopathologic features. Syndrome-affected patients are at risk of early death from medullary thyroid carcinoma, pheochromocytoma, and even the complications of intestinal ganglioneuromatosis (13–15). Like MEN 2A, subtype 2B is a multisystem disorder occurring either sporadically or in an inherited, autosomal-dominant manner. The disease is caused by germline mutations of the *RET* proto-oncogene (16). Affected patients often develop multicentric medullary thyroid carcinoma, parathyroid hyperplasia, and bilateral pheochromocytoma (17). Unlike MEN 2A, MEN 2B features mucosal neuromas, intestinal ganglioneuromatosis, and musculoskeletal

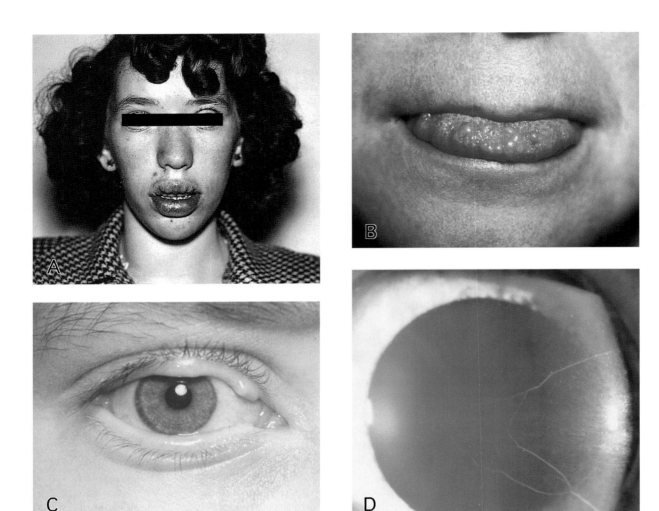

Figure 5-8

MULTIPLE ENDOCRINE NEOPLASIA (MEN) 2B

In addition to a long, narrow face, patients often have prominent bumpy lips (A), as well as nodularity of the anterolateral tongue (B) and eyelid margin (C) due to the presence of submucosal neuromas. On slit lamp examination enlarged corneal nerves are evident as delicate threads (D). Although greatly enlarged, the microanatomy of these affected nerves is essentially normal. (A and B, courtesy of Dr. J. A. Carney, Rochester, MN.)

abnormalities (18–22), and is associated with less pronounced parathyroid hyperplasia (13).

Mucosal neuromas often present in childhood and generally antedate the manifestations of thyroid or adrenal gland neoplasia. They often involve the tongue, lips, eyelids, eyes (conjunctiva, cornea), and, less often, the buccal mucosa, gingiva, palate, nose, larynx, or bronchi. Rarely, neuromas histologically similar to those of the oral cavity affect skin (13). Ganglioneuromatosis typically affects the intestines but may also involve the esophagus, salivary glands, pancreas, gallbladder, and

urinary bladder. Musculoskeletal abnormalities in MEN 2B resemble those of Marfan syndrome (fig. 5-8A) and include excessive length of the limbs, loose jointedness, scoliosis, anterior chest deformity, and a high arched palate (13,19,20). Muscular underdevelopment and hypotonia are frequent findings (13).

Clinical Features. A slight female predominance (56 percent) is noted among patients with MEN 2B (13). This is also the case for patients with mucosal neuromas and intestinal ganglioneuromatosis. Invariably, the lesions become

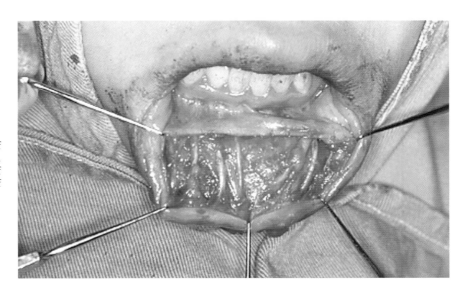

Figure 5-9

MUCOSAL NEUROMATOSIS IN MEN 2B

The submucosal nerves of the lower lip are prominent. (Courtesy of the Department of Oral Pathology, University of Minnesota, Minneapolis, MN.)

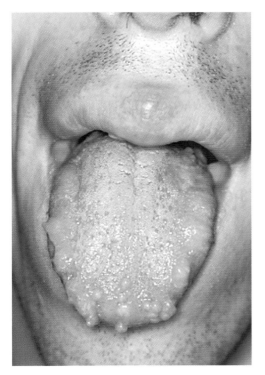

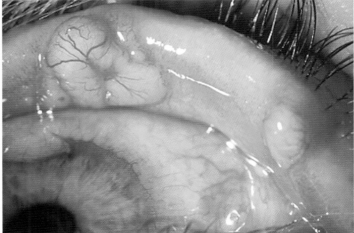

Figure 5-10

MUCOSAL NEUROMATOSIS IN MEN 2B

Left: The marked nodularity of the lateral border of the tongue and the thickened upper lip are due to the presence of numerous neuromas.

Above: Nodular submucosal neuromas are present in the upper eyelid. (Courtesy of the Department of Oral Pathology, University of Minnesota, Minneapolis, MN.)

manifest during the first three decades. As previously noted, common sites of involvement include the lips, tongue, and eyelids. Affected lips are diffusely enlarged, patulous, occasionally everted, and have a multinodular appearance (fig. 5-8A) (13,23). Their enlargement is obvious at surgery (fig. 5-9). The tongue is typically studded by hemispheric nodules at its tip, anterior one third, and occasionally lateral aspects. In

most instances, they range from pinhead size to a few millimeters in diameter (fig. 5-8B) (13,23). The eyelids may be similarly thickened by a diffuse process that results in eversion (fig. 5-8C). On occasion, these features are markedly expressed (fig. 5-10). Common but less obvious manifestations include broadening of the base of the nose, diffuse gingival hypertrophy, palatal nodules, and ocular changes including elevated

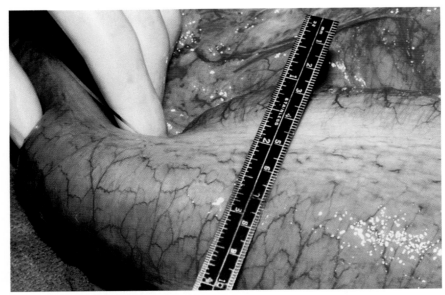

Figure 5-11

GANGLIONEUROMATOSIS OF THE COLON IN MEN 2B

Megacolon commonly results. The affected segment is dilated.

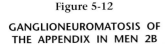

Figure 5-12

GANGLIONEUROMATOSIS OF THE APPENDIX IN MEN 2B

On occasion, the diagnosis is suspected at incidental appendectomy. The changes are identical to those in the colon (see figs. 5-15, 5-16).

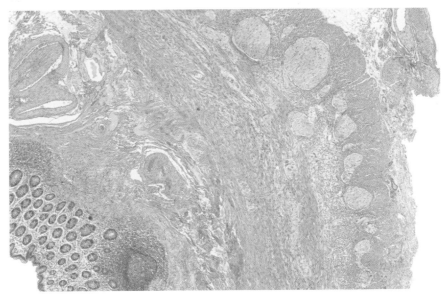

conjunctival lesions and thickened corneal nerves (19,24–27). The latter are best visualized by slit-lamp examination (fig. 5-8D).

Intestinal ganglioneuromatosis is common in MEN 2B and is often the earliest manifestation of the disorder (13,28,29). Associated features include constipation and diarrhea, generalized colonic diverticulosis, megacolon (fig. 5-11), and disturbance of esophageal motility (13,30). The diagnosis of MEN 2B is occasionally made when ganglioneuromatosis is seen in an incidentally removed appendix (fig. 5-12) or for presumed appendicitis.

Microscopic Findings. *Mucosal Neuromas.* Whether localized or diffuse, these are lesions that consist of markedly enlarged nerves. This is readily evident in the labial submucosa of the oral cavity and tongue, as well as in conjunctivae. Whether clinically polypoid, dome shaped, or diffuse, their morphologic features are the same (figs. 5-13, 5-14). Numerous, tortuous, highly branched, and loosely arrayed, the nerves vary in size. Less frequently, nerve bundles are compact and fascicular (17).

Microscopically, the perineurium of affected nerves is usually thickened. In addition, a

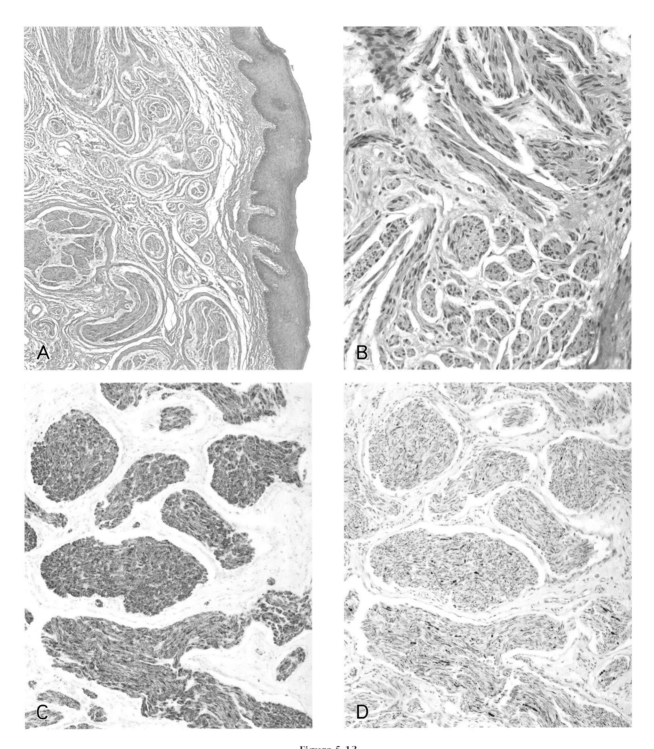

Figure 5-13

MUCOSAL NEUROMATOSIS OF THE LIPS IN MEN 2B

A: Hypertrophic submucosal nerves are unassociated with ganglion cells.

B: The increase of endoneurial mucin is a feature best seen at higher magnification.

C,D: The general normal microanatomy of the nerves is illustrated with immunostains for S-100 protein (C) and neurofilament protein (D).

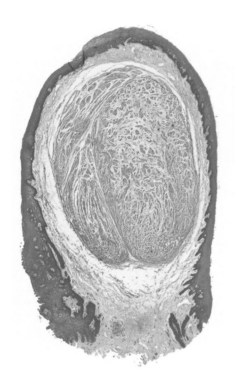
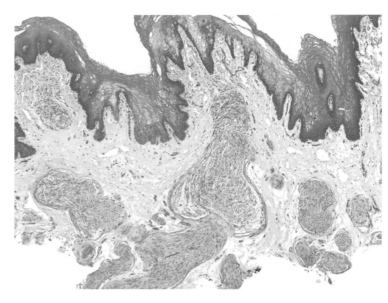

Figure 5-14

MUCOSAL NEUROMATOSIS OF THE TONGUE IN MEN 2B

The process varies from polypoid (left) to plexiform (above).

mucoid endoneurial matrix may separate nerve fibers (fig. 5-13B). Reactive perineural fibrosis is not a feature of mucosal neuromas. In contrast to the mass of affected nerves encountered at oral sites, corneal nerves feature linear thickening, mostly in the limbus (fig. 5-8D). The conjunctiva and iris are less often affected (31). Although proliferation of endoneurial cells is reported to occur in mucosal neuromas (13), at the ultrastructural level the ratio of Schwann cells to axons appears to be normal (31,32). Ganglion cells are lacking in mucosal neuromas, but have been noted in lingual and ciliary nerve examples (23,33,34), as well as in lesions at the root of the iris and in the uveal meshwork (31,32).

Intestinal Ganglioneuromatosis. This lesion affects the autonomic nervous system. It is characterized by band-like and nodular enlargement of both the submucosal and myenteric plexuses (figs. 5-15A,B; 5-16) (35). The process consists of an increase in all elements of the nerves, including ganglion cells (fig. 5-15). The latter may be arranged singly or in clusters. Their content of Nissl substance varies (fig. 5-16A,B). Whether there is actual ganglion cell hyperplasia is uncertain, since comparative studies have not been undertaken. Overall, the abnormalities are less pronounced in the submucosal plexus

(fig. 5-15B) than in the myenteric plexus (figs. 5-15A, 5-16). At the latter site, the enlarged nerve plexus forms an almost uninterrupted band between the longitudinal and circular muscle coats. In addition, hypertrophic neural tissue often lies dispersed within the muscularis propria and may even be seen in subserosal fat. Whereas increased neural tissue, with or without ganglion cells, may be seen within the lamina propria in patients with MEN 2B (fig. 5-15C), mucosal involvement is usually focal and is invariably associated with enlargement of the myenteric plexus. For practical purposes, ganglioneuromatous involvement of all layers of the intestine is seen only in patients with MEN 2B. Similar changes in neurofibromatosis type 1 (NF1) are rare (see fig. 5-22).

Immunohistochemical Findings. As expected, the cells of mucosal neuromas stain like normal nerve elements. Schwann cells and axons are strongly reactive for S-100 protein and neurofilament protein, respectively (fig. 5-13C,D), whereas the neoplastic ganglion cells are reactive for neuron-specific enolase (fig. 5-16C), neurofilament protein (fig. 5-16D), and synaptophysin.

Differential Diagnosis. Histologically, a limited biopsy of mucosal neuromas of MEN 2B

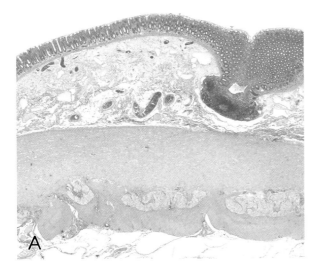

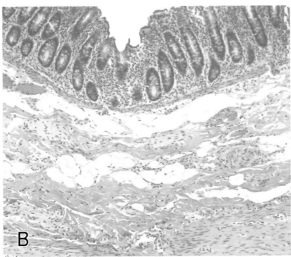

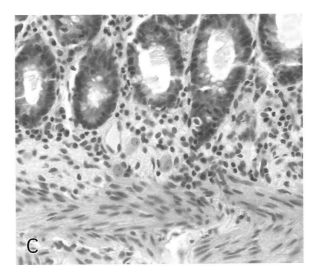

Figure 5-15

**GANGLIONEUROMATOSIS
OF THE COLON IN MEN 2B**

Massive, nearly continuous, band-like hypertrophy
of Auerbach myenteric plexus (A), hypertrophy of the
submucosal plexus (B), and lesser involvement of the lamina
propria (C) are seen.

may resemble either traumatic neuroma or
PEN, both of which occur in the lips and oral
mucosa (7). Plexiform schwannoma is also in
the differential diagnosis. Even normal labial
nerves may be sizable.

Cross sections of traumatic neuroma generally reveal a jumble of small, closely packed nerve
fiber bundles or fascicles ("microfascicles"),
smaller than their parent nerve. Varying in size,
shape, and maturity, the regenerating nerve
fiber groups show scant to definite perineurial
ensheathment, and lie in a background of reactive fibrosis, with or without associated chronic
inflammation. A readily recognized nerve is
often seen to enter and only occasionally to exit
the mass (traumatic neuroma in continuity).
In contrast, the mucosal neuromas of MEN 2B

represent a more orderly increase in discrete,
well-formed autonomic nerves in an otherwise
unremarkable submucosa.

Mucosal PEN, particularly multinodular
examples, may resemble mucosal neuroma of
MEN 2B. However, the compact, ill-defined
fascicles of PEN are very cellular, consist almost
entirely of Schwann cells, and contain fewer
axons than do mucosal neuromas. Further clues
to the distinction include the presentation of
mucosal PEN as solitary lesions occurring in an
older age group (middle age versus childhood
and adolescence) as well as the occasional finding of vaguely palisaded Schwann cells.

In contrast to mucosal neuromas, schwannomas affecting mucosa usually present as a discrete, unencapsulated lesion, some featuring

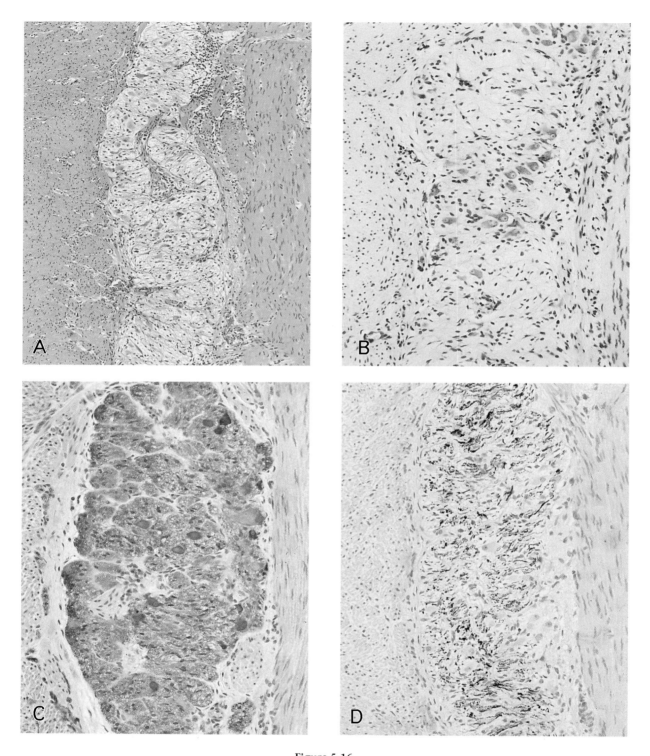

Figure 5-16

GANGLIONEUROMATOSIS OF THE COLON IN MEN 2B

The myenteric ganglia are markedly enlarged (A) but their cellular elements, Schwann cell-ensheathed axons, and ganglion cells are essentially normal with Nissl preparations (B), and neuron-specific enolase (C) and neurofilament protein (D) immunostains.

Antoni A and B tissue or tightly palisading tumor cells (Verocay bodies). Even when plexiform, schwannomas show a paucity of axons, either somewhat concentrated at the periphery of affected fascicles or scattered within their substance. A diagnosis of mucosal neuromatosis may be further aided by the identification of other manifestations of the MEN 2B syndrome, either in the patient or a relative.

Also to be considered in the differential diagnosis of ganglioneuromatosis of MEN 2B is focal or diffuse intestinal ganglioneuromatosis associated with other disorders. These include Cowden disease (36,37), juvenile polyposis (38–41), colonic adenoma and adenocarcinoma (41,42), and Hirschsprung disease (43–45). Isolated intestinal ganglioneuromatosis has also been reported (46–51). Unlike the intestinal ganglioneuromatosis of MEN 2B, the above-noted processes are usually focal and, with the exception of occasional extension into submucosa, do not involve deep layers of the intestinal wall. Far more difficult to distinguish from intestinal ganglioneuromatosis of MEN 2B are rare similar lesions occurring in NF1 (see below).

MEN 2B-UNASSOCIATED NEUROMA, GANGLIONEUROMA/ GANGLIONEUROMATOSIS, AND LOCALIZED HYPERTROPHIC NEUROPATHY

Unassociated with MEN 2B, these various lesions all consist of a hyperplastic/hypertrophic autonomic plexus, either localized and tumefactive or segmental as opposed to diffuse. As in MEN 2B, they are included under the broad category of true neuromas, lesions composed of all nerve elements, and are non-neoplastic. The processes include *neuroma, ganglioneuroma/ganglioneuromatosis*, and *localized hypertrophic neuropathy*. Diffuse ganglioneuromatosis associated with NF1 is separately discussed in chapter 14.

Neuroma

Appendiceal Neuroma. This commonly observed reactive lesion, also termed *mucosal neurogenic appendicopathy,* reportedly affects 10 to 27 percent of appendectomy specimens (52–54). Since its original description by Masson in the 1920s (55,56), a number of series have been reported (52–54,57–60). Examples causing luminal obstruction and symptoms simulating

acute appendicitis are rare (55,59,61). Grossly, most appendiceal neuromas are indistinguishable from fibrous obliteration of the appendiceal tip. On cross section, they appear gray and often glistening (54). Histologically, the appearance somewhat resembles that of traumatic neuroma. The key features are variable replacement of the appendiceal wall and luminal obliteration by loosely arranged, spindle-shaped cells possessing delicate eosinophilic processes (fig. 5-17A,B). Immunoreactivity for S-100 protein (fig. 5-17C), indicates that they are Schwann cells. Although nerve fibers are inapparent with H&E stains, they are demonstrable with silver impregnation (Bodian or Bielschowsky stain) and with immunostains for neurofilament protein. Unlike the ganglioneuromatous lesions previously discussed, appendiceal neuromas lack ganglion cells.

The three basic growth patterns of appendiceal neuroma are intramucosal, subserosal, and axial (53). Intramucosal examples expand the lamina propria, spread apart crypts, and depress the muscularis mucosae. The axial type, representing nearly half of all appendiceal neuromas, is most common (53). It is longitudinally oriented, involves the tip of the obliterated appendix, is encased by fibromuscular and adipose tissue, and only proximally contacts the mucosa. The boundary with adjacent, more normal lamina propria is often indistinct. Interestingly, appendiceal neuromas are often associated with argentaffin-positive neuroendocrine cells, both in the lamina propria (fig. 5-17D) and the neuromatous tissue. About 25 percent of neuromas show regressive changes, including atrophy of neurites, absence or loss of argentaffin cells, chronic inflammation, fibrosis, and sometimes stromal myxoid change (53).

Other Neuromas. Although neuromas also occur at other visceral sites, even bronchi, the intestinal tract (62) is most often affected, particularly the biliary tract and duodenum. Typical examples affect the wall of the gallbladder, common bile duct, or the second portion of the duodenum (fig. 5-18A,B). They arise from either the submucosal or myenteric plexus, and may be multinodular. They are devoid of ganglion cells and thus architecturally resemble traumatic neuroma (fig. 5-18B,C) (63). Not surprisingly, one example was reported as a "neurofibroma" (64), an error avoidable by the finding of abundant axons

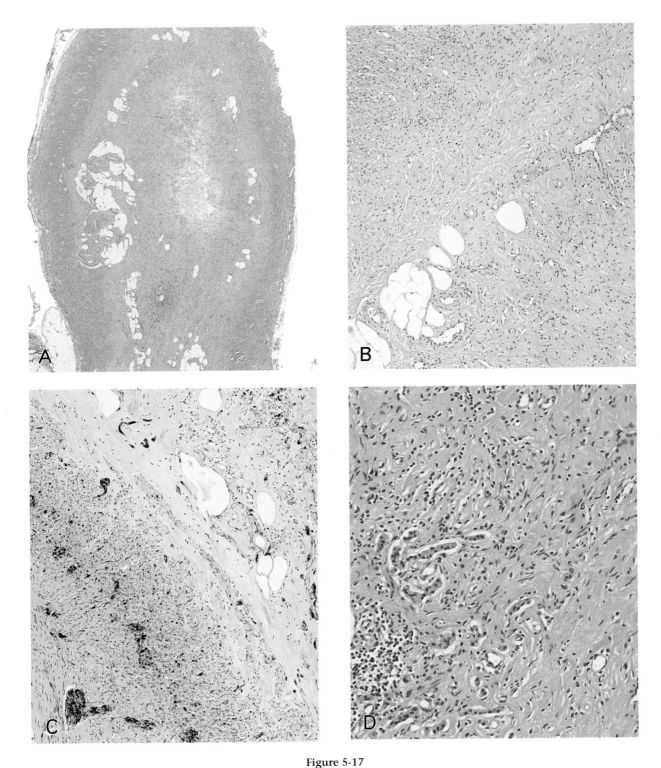

Figure 5-17

APPENDICEAL NEUROMA

The obliterated tip of the appendiceal lumen (A) is replaced by a tangle of hypertrophic nerve fibers which also involve the submucosa (B). Some single and others grouped, their Schwann sheaths immunoreact for S-100 protein (C). Clusters of neuroendocrine cells are a common finding within such neuromas (D).

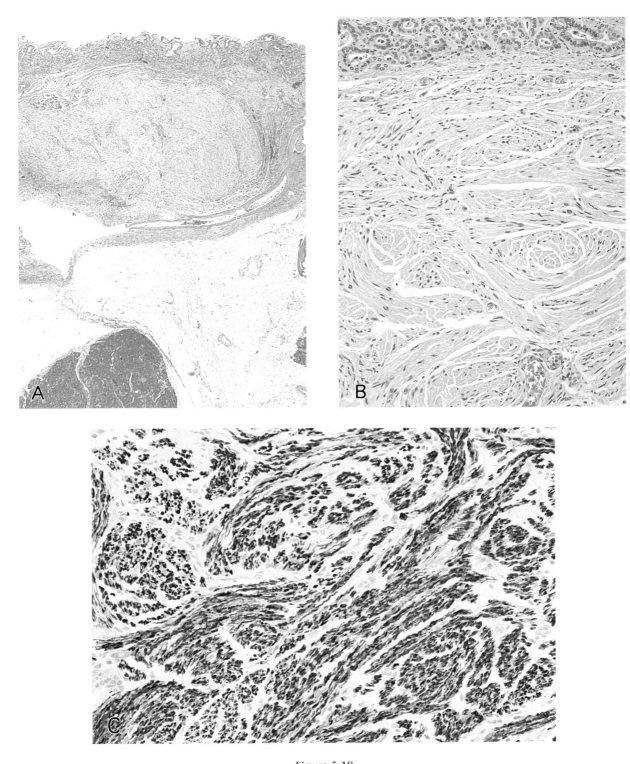

Figure 5-18

DUODENAL NEUROMA

This submucosal lesion (A) consists of spindle-shaped Schwann cells (B) associated with nerve fibers. Individual or disposed in fascicles, the Schwann sheaths and axons are immunoreactive for both neurofilament protein (C) and S-100 protein.

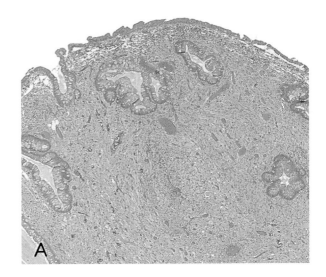

Figure 5-19

SOLITARY POLYPOID GANGLIONEUROMA

As isolated lesions such as this colonic example in a 50-year-old male (A), polypoid ganglioneuromas are of no clinical significance. Superficial in location, they expand the lamina propria and submucosa and consist of numerous mature ganglion cells and nerve fibers. The ganglion cells may be numerous (B) or, as in another example, sparse (C). (Courtesy of Dr. L. J. Burgart, Rochester, MN.)

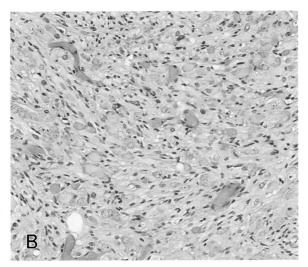

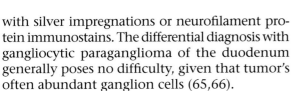

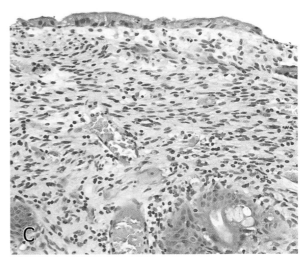

with silver impregnations or neurofilament protein immunostains. The differential diagnosis with gangliocytic paraganglioma of the duodenum generally poses no difficulty, given that tumor's often abundant ganglion cells (65,66).

Mucosal Ganglioneuroma and Ganglioneuromatosis

Solitary Polypoid Intestinal Ganglioneuroma. This usually incidental colonoscopic finding is unassociated with other conditions (fig. 5-19) (67). Measuring less than 2 cm, the majority are small, sessile or pedunculated polyps grossly resembling juvenile, hyperplastic, or adenomatous polyps. Their microscopic features vary from patchy involvement of the lamina propria (figs. 5-20, 5-21) to a nodular,

neurofibroma-like lesion involving both mucosa and submucosa (67). A combined pattern is also seen. Ganglion cells vary in number and cytology (fig. 5-19B,C). Shekitka and Sobin (67) showed no association with multiple tumors, NF1, or MEN 2B (68).

Ganglioneuromatosis. Consisting of hypertrophy of the diffuse autonomic plexus of the alimentary tract, this condition may occur in settings other than MEN 2B; for example, there are reports of intestinal ganglioneuromatosis in NF1 (67,69–71). Such lesions are rare (fig. 5-22) and, although usually limited to the submucosal plexus, can affect the myenteric plexus as well (69). In many instances, the changes are limited to the mucosa. In patients with NF1, the confusing term "ganglioneurofibromatosis" has crept

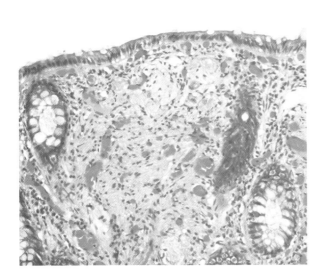 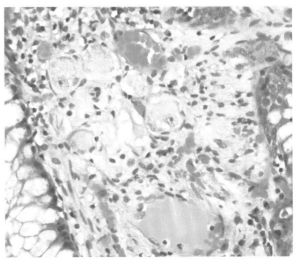

Figure 5-20

POLYPOID MUCOSAL GANGLIONEUROMA OF COLON

Left: The lamina propria is expanded by rare ganglion and spindle-shaped Schwann cells.

Right: At high power, six ganglion cells are present within the lamina propria and associated with somewhat spindle-shaped Schwann cells.

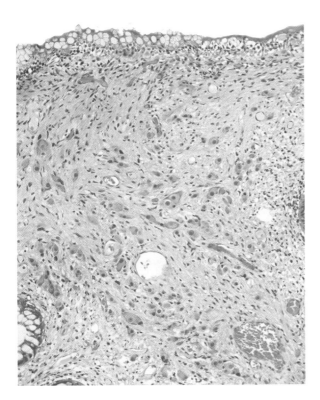 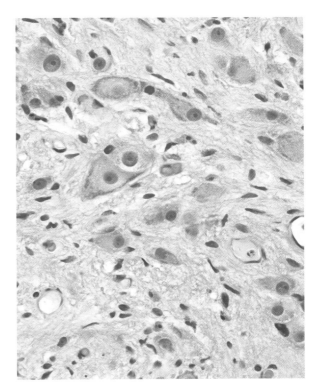

Figure 5-21

POLYPOID MUCOSAL GANGLIONEUROMA

Left: Dysmorphic ganglion cells are abundant within the lamina propria.

Right: A higher power view of the lesion clearly demonstrates the variation in size and shape of the numerous ganglion cells.

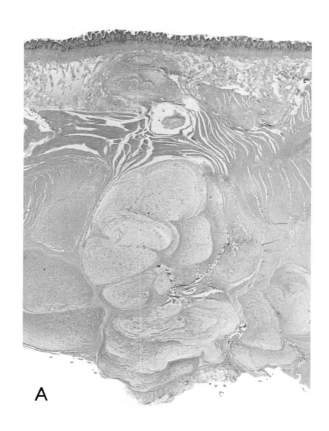

Figure 5-22

GANGLIONEUROMATOSIS IN NF1

In addition to plexiform neurofibroma affecting both the submucosa and serosa (A), ganglioneuromatous involvement of the submucosa (B) and mucosa (C) is seen. (Courtesy of Drs. L. Sobin, Washington, DC, and K. M. Shekitka, Annapolis, MD). (Also see figure 15-13.)

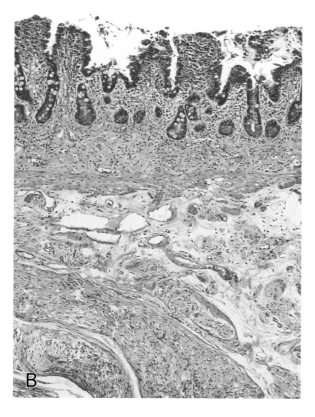

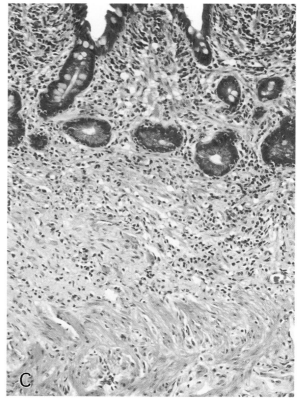

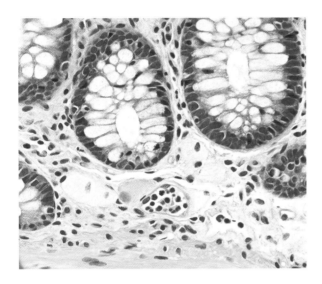

Figure 5-23

NORMAL COLONIC MUCOSA

A somewhat amphophilic ganglion cell is near the base of a crypt.

into use to describe a sprinkling of ganglion cells in the mucosa. We and others (70) do not consider this an entity and discourage the use of the designation. Indeed, ganglion cells may be seen in normal colorectal lamina propria (fig. 5-23), either singly or in clusters, particularly in females; in diverticular disease; and in inflammatory bowel disease (72,73).

In our experience, most reported examples of transmural hypertrophy of the autonomic plexus in patients with NF1 in part consist of plexiform neurofibroma (see chapter 15) (74–76). Subtle morphologic features distinguish such lesions from the intestinal ganglioneuromatosis of MEN 2B. The enlarged plexuses and discrete nodules noted in NF1 often include a mucoid matrix, a feature not seen in MEN 2B-associated ganglioneuromatosis. Affected nerves in NF1 are typically arranged both horizontally and vertically, whereas the enlarged plexuses of MEN 2B and only rarely of NF1, are solely horizontal in disposition.

Cowden syndrome is associated with mucosal ganglioneuromatosis (77). This systemic, autosomal dominantly inherited disorder involving *PTEN* mutations and having an incidence of 1 in 200,000 live births, is characterized by ectodermal, mesodermal, and endodermal abnormalities. These include mandibular hypoplasia; prominence of the forehead; facial trichilem-

momas (36,78); verruca-like cutaneous papules occurring in an acral distribution; squamous papules of the oral mucosa (78); small bowel polyposis (79); benign polyps of the colon (79); carcinoma of the thyroid (80), breast (81), and endometrium; and a variety of benign gastrointestinal lesions (36,79) including mucocutaneous neuromas (82). *Dysplastic gangliocytoma of the cerebellum* (*Lhermitte-Duclos disease*) is also a well-known association (83).

In addition to Cowden disease, *juvenile polyposis* (38–41), *colonic adenoma*, and *adenocarcinoma* (41,42) occasionally show hyperplasia of neural tissue of the intestinal mucosa, sometimes accompanied by ganglion cells. In these processes, mucosal ganglioneuromatosis is invariably an incidental finding. Mucosal ganglioneuromatosis occurring in these conditions takes the form of mucosal thickening due to the abundance of neural processes, their parent ganglion cells, and accompanying Schwann cells. When associated with benign polyps, the ganglioneuromatous proliferation involves either the polyps or the surrounding normal mucosa (41). In one case of colonic adenocarcinoma, the ganglioneuromatosis was diffuse, involving not only the region of the cecal tumor, but the vermiform appendix and terminal ileum as well (42). In yet another case of diffuse transmural ganglioneuromatosis, numerous rectal carcinoid tumors prompted an abdominoperineal resection (fig. 5-24) (84). Yet another association is with *familial gastrointestinal stromal tumor* (GIST). This autosomal dominant disorder, discussed in detail in chapter 13 (85), typically presents in mid adulthood and affects mainly the stomach and duodenum. It is characterized by involvement of the myenteric plexus by multiple tumors, typically of microscopic dimension. Lastly, ganglioneuromatosis on rare occasions affects the small bowel, where it may mimic Crohn disease (86).

Ganglioneuromatosis Polyposis. Multiple, innumerable ganglioneuromatous polyps are rarely associated with cutaneous lipomatosis (87) or with a coexisting aggressive adenocarcinoma (88).

LOCALIZED HYPERTROPHIC NEUROPATHY

Definition. *Localized hypertrophy of a peripheral nerve* is caused by onion bulb-like hyperplasia of Schwann cells with resultant fascicular enlargement.

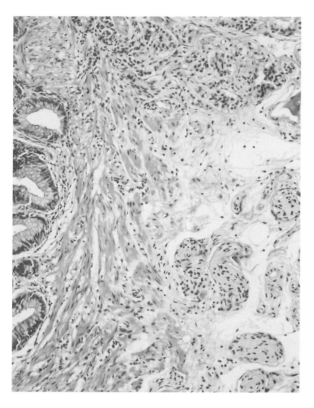

Figure 5-24

GANGLIONEUROMATOSIS OF COLON ASSOCIATED WITH CARCINOID TUMOR

This complex lesion was unassociated with MEN 2b. (Courtesy of Dr. M. Haraguchi, Nagasaki, Japan, and Y. Itoh, Fukuoka, Japan.)

General Features. The term localized hypertrophic neuropathy was once used to denote what is now recognized as two distinct lesions: the lesion under discussion, a nonhereditary, localized Schwann cell proliferation characterized by onion bulb formation, and a more common sporadic, intraneural tumor of perineurial cells engaged in pseudo-onion bulb formation. The latter is now designated *intraneural perineurioma*. Unlike some authors (89), we do not consider localized hypertrophic neuropathy to be a part of a lesion spectrum that includes perineurioma.

The nature and etiology of localized hypertrophic neuropathy are unclear, but the lesion is considered more a reactive than a neoplastic process. Since it involves isolated nerves, it should not be considered a variant of the two hereditary hypertrophic sensorimotor neuropathies, Dejerine-Sottas or Charcot-Marie-Tooth

disease. Onion bulb formation, the hallmark of Schwann cell hyperplasia, follows repeated episodes of demyelination and remyelination, and is seen in not only chronic inflammatory demyelinating neuropathy (90) but in other polyneuropathies as well.

Clinical Features. To date, only six examples of localized hypertrophic neuropathy have been described (89,91–93), all affecting adults. Although one patient had several cafe-au-lait spots, no association with NF1 has been reported. Since in one instance the process involved two nerves (93), the designation localized hypertrophic "mononeuropathy" should be avoided. Either cranial (89,91) or spinal (92,93) nerves may be affected. Both reported cranial nerve examples involved the trigeminal nerve. One spinal nerve example, a tibial nerve lesion, was associated with chronic inflammation (92). Yet another, a cauda equina example, involved two nerve roots and was associated with a sacral meningocele (93).

A clear distinction of localized hypertrophic neuropathy from perineurioma is essential when interpreting the literature. For example, one report of 146 peripheral non-nerve sheath tumors included 16 cases of loosely defined "localized hypertrophic neuropathy" inclusive of both Schwann cell and perineurial (perineurioma) lesions (94). Our finding of only six reported cases of strictly defined localized hypertrophic neuropathy underscores their infrequency relative to perineurioma.

Gross Findings. The six cases reported to date have involved nerves of differing size as well as cranial nerve ganglia. Grossly enlarged and yellow-gray, the affected nerves appeared fusiform with markedly enlarged fascicles. Maximal lesion length and diameter were 15 cm (92) and 2 cm (93), respectively. Adherence to normal surrounding roots was noted in the cauda equina example (93).

Microscopic Findings. Localized hypertrophic neuropathy is characterized by nerve fascicle enlargement (fig. 5-25A) due to the formation of "onion bulbs." These consist of whorls of uniform, cytologically normal Schwann cells encircling variably myelinated axons (fig. 5-25B). The onion bulbs contain collagen fibers (fig. 5-25C) and may appear to float in a loose, Alcian blue–positive matrix (fig. 5-25D). In some cases, the matrix is scant

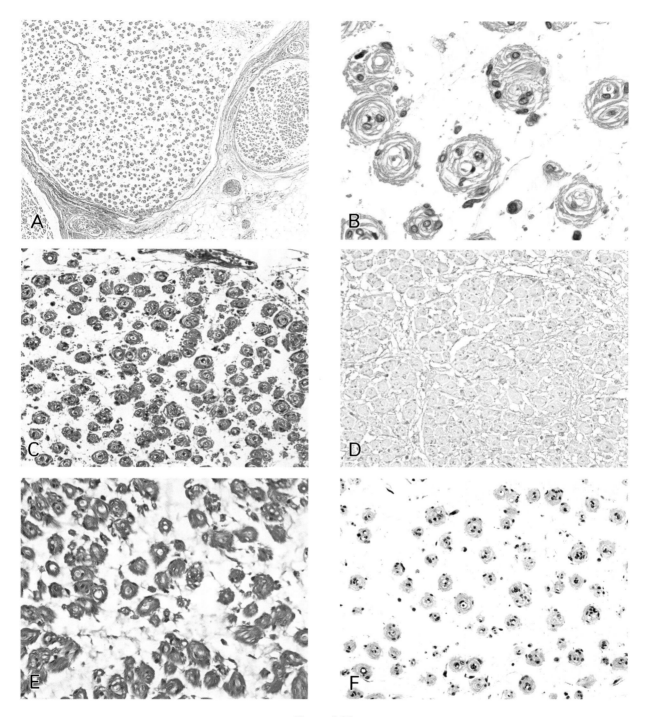

Figure 5-25

LOCALIZED HYPERTROPHIC NEUROPATHY

A: A portion of two affected fascicles shows the widely separated onion bulbs.
B: Onion bulbs consist of lamellae of Schwann cells surrounding a nerve fiber.
C: Considerable collagen accompanies the Schwann cells (trichrome stain).
D: The endoneurium contains Alcian blue-positive mucin.
E: Routine histochemical stains show myelin to be scant or lacking (Luxol-fast blue stain).
F: Axons are readily visible on silver preparation (Bielschowsky). (Courtesy of Dr. D. Horoupian, Palo Alto, CA.)

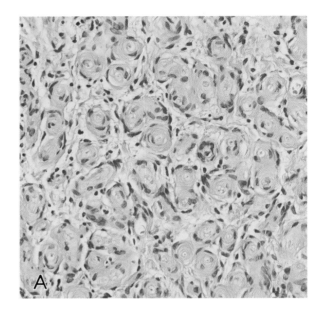

Figure 5-26

LOCALIZED HYPERTROPHIC NEUROPATHY

This example shows close approximation of numerous onion bulbs without significant stromal mucin.

A: H&E staining shows that perineurioma is closely mimicked.

B: The affected nerve is in longitudinal section. Note the similarity to the ropey appearance also seen in intraneural perineurioma (fig. 9-5A).

C: In poorly oriented sections, the onion bulbs are obscured. The accompanying myelinated nerve above is normal.

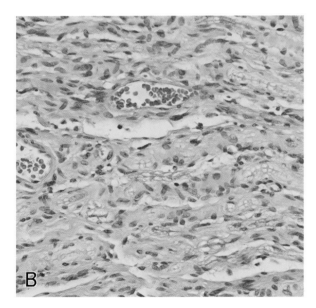

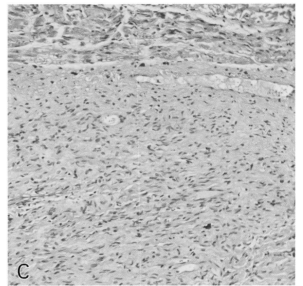

or lacking (fig. 5-26A), and the onion bulbs are inapparent on longitudinal (fig. 5-26B) or randomly oriented sections (fig. 5-26C). Stains show myelin to be scant (fig. 5-25E). Axons are readily demonstrated with silver preparations (Bodian, Bielschowsky) (fig. 5-25F).

Immunohistochemical Findings. Given their makeup of multilayered Schwann cells, onion bulbs are strongly S-100 protein immunoreactive (fig. 5-27A). Each surrounds a central, neurofilament protein–positive axon (fig. 5-27B). EMA reactivity is limited to the perineurium of affected nerve fascicles (fig. 5-27C).

Ultrastructural Findings. Individually, onion bulbs consist of multiple layers of Schwann cells encircling a variably myelinated axon. The layered Schwann cells exhibit loosely apposed cytoplasmic processes and possess a continuous surface basal lamina. Unlike the perineurial cells compressing pseudo-onion bulbs, Schwann cells lack numerous intercellular junctions, micropinocytotic vesicles, and interruption of basement membrane.

Differential Diagnosis. The main entity in the differential diagnosis of localized hypertrophic neuropathy is intraneural perineurioma, a

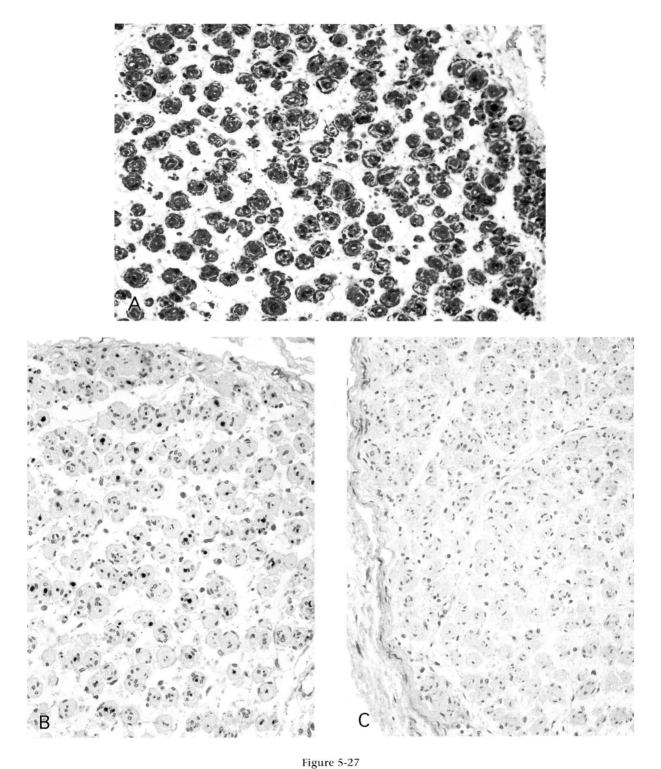

Figure 5-27

LOCALIZED HYPERTROPHIC NEUROPATHY

A: The Schwann cell nature of the cells comprising the onion bulb is evidenced by strong S-100 protein immunoreactivity.

B: The bulbs have central axons on neurofilament immunostain.

C: Staining for epithelial membrane antigen (EMA) is limited to normal perineurium.

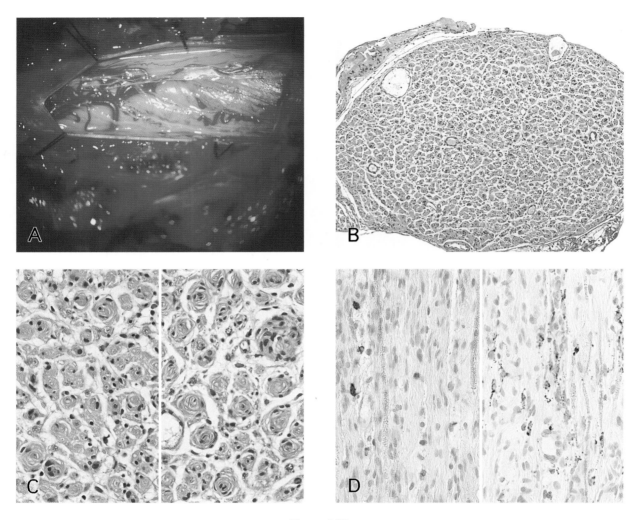

Figure 5-28

CHRONIC INFLAMMATORY DEMYELINATING POLYNEUROPATHY

This sporadic, often relapsing autoimmune condition varies in extent. This impressive example involved cranial and spinal nerve roots, including the cauda equina (A). The roots are markedly enlarged (A,B,) and show prominent onion bulb formation (C, left). Many fibers are affected, having lost their myelin (C, right; Luxol-fast blue), and are surrounded by hypertrophic Schwann cells. Inflammatory cells are few but include lymphocytes (D, left; CD45) and histiocytes (D, right; CD68).

lesion once included in the spectrum of localized hypertrophic neuropathy, but now considered a neoplasm rather than a reactive process (95). These perineuriomas affect major nerves and consist of proliferating, multilayered perineurial cells surrounding one or often more axons and their accompanying Schwann sheaths. The result is "pseudo-onion bulb" formation. Encirclement of adjacent pseudo-onion bulbs and of vessels may also be seen. Given their sheer number, the pseudo-onion bulbs fill the endoneurium. Intraneural perineuriomas differ

from localized hypertrophic neuropathy by being EMA immunoreactive. S-100 protein stains demonstrate only preexisting normal, centrally located Schwann sheaths. The ultrastructural features of the multilayered cells are those of well-differentiated perineurial cells, rather than of Schwann cells. A full description of the ultrastructure of intraneural perineurioma is presented in chapter 9.

Other disorders characterized by onion bulb formation, generalized rather than localized, include hereditary sensorimotor neuropathies

(Charcot-Marie-Tooth disease, Dejerine-Sottos disease) and chronic inflammatory demyelinating polyneuropathy (fig. 5-28). These conditions are readily distinguished from localized hypertrophic neuropathy on clinicopathologic grounds.

Treatment and Prognosis. Localized hypertrophic neuropathy is an indolent process. Only one example was actually tumefactive (89): a trigeminal lesion occupying the left cavernous sinus. The treatment is similar to that of intraneural perineurioma, which simply includes biopsy confirmation of the diagnosis followed by observation.

REFERENCES

Palisaded Encapsulated Neuroma

1. Reed RJ, Fine RM, Meltzer HD. Palisaded, encapsulated neuromas of the skin. Arch Dermatol 1972;106:865-870.
2. Argenyi ZB. Newly recognized neural neoplasms relevant to the dermatopathologist. Dermatol Clin 1992;10:219-234.
3. Argenyi ZB, Cooper PH, Santa Cruz D. Plexiform and other unusual variants of palisaded encapsulated neuroma. J Cutan Pathol 1993;20:34-39.
4. Dakin MC, Leppard B, Theaker JM. The palisaded, encapsulated neuroma (solitary circumscribed neuroma). Histopathology 1992;20:405-410.
5. Dover JS, From L, Lewis A. Palisaded encapsulated neuromas. A clinicopathologic study. Arch Dermatol 1989;125:386-389.
6. Fletcher CD. Solitary circumscribed neuroma of the skin (so-called palisaded, encapsulated neuroma). A clinicopathologic and immunohistochemical study. Am J Surg Pathol 1989;13:574-580.
7. Chauvin PJ, Wysocki GP, Daley TD, Pringle GA. Palisaded encapsulated neuroma of oral mucosa. Oral Surg Oral Med Oral Pathol 1992;73:71-74.
8. Koutlas IG, Scheithauer BW. Palisaded encapsulated ("solitary circumscribed") neuroma of the oral cavity: A review of 55 cases. Head Neck Pathol 2010;4:15-26.
9. Magnusson B. Palisaded encapsulated neuroma (solitary circumscribed neuroma) of the oral mucosa. Oral Surg Oral Med Oral Pathol Oral Radiol Endod 1996;82:302-304.
10. Argenyi ZB. Immunohistochemical characterization of palisaded, encapsulated neuroma. J Cutan Pathol 1990;17:329-335.
11. Koutlas IG, Scheithauer B. Reactive pseudo-onion proliferation and intraneural perineurioma of the oral mucosa. Head Neck Pathol 2013. [Epub ahead of print]
12. Argenyi ZB, Santa Cruz D, Bromley C. Comparative light-microscopic and immunohistochemical study of traumatic and palisaded encapsulated neuromas of the skin. Am J Dermatopathol 1992;14:504-510.

MEN 2B-Associated Neuroma

13. Carney JA, Sizemore GW, Hayles AB. Multiple endocrine neoplasia, type 2b. Pathobiol Annu 1978;8:105-153.
14. Frank K, Raue F, Gottswinter J, Heinrich U, Meybier H, Ziegler R. Importance of early diagnosis and follow-up in multiple endocrine neoplasia (MEN IIB). Eur J Pediatr 1984;143:112-116.
15. Norton JA, Froome LC, Farrell RE, Wells SA Jr. Multiple endocrine neoplasia type IIb: The most aggressive form of medullary thyroid carcinoma. Surg Clin North Am 1979;59:109-118.
16. Eng C, Smith DP, Mulligan LM, et al. Point mutation within the tyrosine kinase domain of the ret proto-oncogene in multiple endocrine neoplasia type 2B and related sporadic tumours. Hum Mol Genet 1994;3:237-241.
17. O'Riordain DS, O'Brien T, Crotty TB, Gharib H, Grant CS, van Heerden JA. Multiple endocrine neoplasia type 2B: More than an endocrine disorder. Surgery 1995;118:936-942.
18. Gorlin RJ, Mirkin BL. Multiple mucosal neuromas, pheochromocytoma, medullary carcinoma of the thyroid and marfanoid body build with muscle wasting. Syndrome of hyperplasia and neoplasia of neural crest derivatives—an unitarian concept. Z Kinderheilk 1972;113:313-325.
19. Gorlin RJ, Sedano HO, Vickers RA, Cervenka J. Multiple mucosal neuromas, pheochromocytoma and medullary carcinoma of the thyroid—a syndrome. Cancer 1968;22:293-299.

20. Khairi MR, Dexter RN, Burzynski NJ, Johnston CC, Jr. Mucosal neuroma, pheochromocytoma and medullary thyroid carcinoma: Multiple endocrine neoplasia type 3. Medicine (Baltimore) 1975;54:89-112.

21. Schimke RN, Hartmann WH, Prout TE, Rimoin DL. Syndrome of bilateral pheochromocytoma, medullary thyroid carcinoma and multiple neuromas. A possible regulatory defect in the differentiation of chromaffin tissue. N Engl J Med 1968;279:1-7.

22. Williams ED, Pollock DJ. Multiple mucosal neuromata with endocrine tumours: A syndrome allied to von Recklinghausen's disease. J Pathol Bacteriol 1966;91:71-80.

23. Carney JA, Sizemore GW, Lovestedt SA. Mucosal ganglioneuromatosis, medullary thyroid carcinoma, and pheochromocytoma: Multiple endocrine neoplasia, type 2b. Oral Surg Oral Med Oral Pathol 1976;41:739-752.

24. Braley AE. Medullated corneal nerves and plexiform neuroma associated with pheochromocytoma. Trans Am Ophthalmol Soc 1954;52:189-197.

25. Calmettes L, Bazex A, Deodati F, Dupre A, Bec P. Manifestations oculopalpebrales des neuromes myeliniques muqueux. Arch Ophthalmol (Paris) 1959;19:257-269.

26. Koke MP, Braley AE. Bilateral plexiform neuromata of the conjunctiva and medullated corneal nerves. Report of a case. Am J Ophthalmol 1940;23:179-182.

27. Robertson DM, Sizemore GW, Gordon H. Thickened corneal nerves as a manifestation of multiple endocrine neoplasia. Trans Sect Ophthalmol Am Acad Opthalmol Otolaryngol 1975;79:OP772-787.

28. Carney JA, Go VL, Sizemore GW, Hayles AB. Alimentary-tract ganglioneuromatosis. A major component of the syndrome of multiple endocrine neoplasia, type 2b. N Engl J Med 1976;295:1287-1291.

29. Carney JA, Hayles AB. Alimentary tract manifestations of multiple endocrine neoplasia, type 2b. Mayo Clin Pro 1977;52:543-548.

30. Cope R, Schleinitz PF. Multiple endocrine neoplasia, type 2b, as a cause of megacolon. Am J Gastroenterol 1983;78:802-805.

31. Spector B, Klintworth GK, Wells SA Jr. Histologic study of the ocular lesions in multiple endocrine neoplasia syndrome type IIb. Am J Ophthalmol 1981;91:204-215.

32. Riley FC Jr, Robertson DM. Ocular histopathology in multiple endocrine neoplasia type 2b. Am J Ophthalmol 1981;91:57-64.

33. Levy M, Habib R, Lyon G, Schweisguth O, Lemerle J, Royer P. [Neuromatosis and epithelioma with amyloid stroma of the thyroid in children.] Arch Fr Pediatr 1970;27:561-583. [French]

34. Reza MJ, Young RT, Van Herle AJ, DeQuattro V, Cole HS, Brown J. Multiple endocrine adenomatosis type II (sipple's syndrome) in twins. West J Med 1975;123:441-446.

35. d'Amore ES, Manivel JC, Pettinato G, Niehans GA, Snover DC. Intestinal ganglioneuromatosis: Mucosal and transmural types. A clinicopathologic and immunohistochemical study of six cases. Hum Pathol 1991;22:276-286.

36. Lashner BA, Riddell RH, Winans CS. Ganglioneuromatosis of the colon and extensive glycogenic acanthosis in Cowden's disease. Dig Dis Sci 1986;31:213-216.

37. Weary PE, Gorlin RJ, Gentry WC, Jr., Comer JE, Greer KE. Multiple hamartoma syndrome (Cowden's disease). Arch Dermatol 1972;106:682-690.

38. Donnelly WH, Sieber WK, Yunis EJ. Polypoid ganglioneurofibromatosis of the large bowel. Arch Pathol 1969;87:537-541.

39. Mendelsohn G, Diamond MP. Familial ganglioneuromatous polyposis of the large bowel. Report of a family with associated juvenile polyposis. Am J Surg Pathol 1984;8:515-520.

40. Pham BN, Villanueva RP. Ganglioneuromatous proliferation associated with juvenile polyposis coli. Arch Pathol Lab Med 1989;113:91-94.

41. Weidner N, Flanders DJ, Mitros FA. Mucosal ganglioneuromatosis associated with multiple colonic polyps. Am J Surg Pathol 1984;8:779-786.

42. Snover DC, Weigent CE, Sumner HW. Diffuse mucosal ganglioneuromatosis of the colon associated with adenocarcinoma. Am J Clin Pathol 1981;75:225-229.

43. Briner J, Oswald HW, Hirsig J, Lehner M. Neuronal intestinal dysplasia—clinical and histochemical findings and its association with hirschsprung's disease. Z Kinderchir 1986;41:282-286.

44. Puri P, Lake BD, Nixon HH, Mishalany H, Claireaux AE. Neuronal colonic dysplasia: An unusual association of Hirschsprung's disease. J Pediatr Surg 1977;12:681-685.

45. Scharli AF, Meier-Ruge W. Localized and disseminated forms of neuronal intestinal dysplasia mimicking Hirschsprung's disease. J Pediatr Surg 1981;16:164-170.

46. Brodey PA, Hoover HC. Polypoid gangliofibromatosis of the colon. Br J Radiol 1974;47:494-495.

47. Gleason IO, Beauchemin J, Bursk A. Polypoid ganglio-neuromatosis of the large bowel. Arch Neurol 1962;6:242-247.

48. Legros A, Leconte D, Huguet C. [Intestinal pseudo-obstruction due to ganglioneuromatosis (author's transl)]. Gastroenterol Clin Biol 1980;4:333-337. [French]

49. Masson P, Branch A. Gigantisme et ganglioneuromatose de l'appendice. Rev Canad Biol 1945;4:219-263.
50. Nezelof C, Guy-Grand D, Thomine E. [Megacolon with hyperplasia of the myenteric plexua. An anatomo-clinical entity, apropos of 3 cases.] Presse Med 1970;78:1501-1506. [French]
51. Rescorla FJ, Vane DW, Fitzgerald JF, West KW, Grosfeld JL. Vasoactive intestinal polypeptide-secreting ganglioneuromatosis affecting the entire colon and rectum. J Pediatr Surg 1988;23:635-637.

MEN 2B-Unassociated Neuroma

52. Höfler H, Kasper M, Heitz PU. The neuroendocrine system of normal human appendix, ileum and colon, and in neurogenic appendicopathy. Virchows Arch A Pathol Anat Histopathol 1983; 399:127-140.
53. Michalany J, Galindo W. Classification of neuromas of the appendix. Beit Pathol 1973;150:213-228.
54. Stanley MW, Cherwitz D, Hagen K, Snover DC. Neuromas of the appendix. A light-microscopic, immunohistochemical and electron-microscopic study of 20 cases. Am J Surg Pathol 1986;10:801-815.
55. Masson P. Carcinoids (argentaffin-cell tumors) and nerve hyperplasia of the appendicular mucosa. Am J Pathol 1928;4:181-212.19.
56. Masson P. Neural proliferations in the vermiform appendix. In: Penfield W, ed. Cytology and cellular pathology of the nervous system. New York: P. B. Hoeber, Inc; 1932:1094-1130.
57. Aubock L, Ratzenhofer M. "Extraepithelial enterochromaffin cell—nerve-fibre complexes" in the normal human appendix, and in neurogenic appendicopathy. J Pathol 1982;136:217-226.
58. Collins DC. 71,000 human appendix specimens. A final report, summarizing forty years' study. Am J Proctol 1963;14:265-281.
59. Millikin PD. Extraepithelial enterochromaffin cells and schwann cells in the human appendix. Arch Pathol Lab Med 1983;107:189-194.
60. Stephenson J, Snoddy WT. Appendiceal lesions. Observation in 4,000 appendectomies. Arch Surg 1961;83:661-666.
61. Isaacson NH, Blades B. Neuroappendicopathy. Review of the literature and report on fifty-two cases. AMA Arch Surg 1951;62:455-466.
62. Sugahara K, Yamamoto M, Iizuka H, Yoshioka M, Miura K. Spontaneous neuroma of the bile duct: a case report. Am J Gastroenterol 1985;80:807-809.
63. Rush BF Jr, Stefaniwsky AB, Sasso A, Dumitrescu I, Wexler D. Neuroma of the common bile duct. J Surg Oncol 1988;39:17-21.
64. Walsh MM, Drew M, Bleiweiss IJ. Neurofibroma of the common bile duct. A case report and review of the literature. Int J Surg Pathol 1997;4:245-247.
65. Kepes JJ, Zacharias DL. Gangliocytic paragangliomas of the duodenum. A report of two cases with light and electron microscopic examination. Cancer 1971;27:61-67.
66. Scheithauer BW, Nora FE, LeChago J, et al. Duodenal gangliocytic paraganglioma. Clinicopathologic and immunocytochemical study of 11 cases. Am J Clin Pathol 1986;86:559-565.
67. Shekitka KM, Sobin LH. Ganglioneuromas of the gastrointestinal tract. Relation to Von Recklinghausen disease and other multiple tumor syndromes. Am J Surg Pathol 1994;18:250-257.
68. Gibson JA, Hornick JL. Mucosal Schwann cell "hamartoma": clinicopathologic study of 26 neural colorectal polyps distinct from neurofibromas and mucosal neuromas. Am J Surg Pathol 2009;33:781-787.
69. Fuller CE, Williams GT. Gastrointestinal manifestations of type 1 neurofibromatosis (von Recklinghausen's disease). Histopathology 1991; 19:1-11.
70. Raszkowski HJ, Hufner RF. Neurofibromatosis of the colon: a unique manifestation of von Recklinghausen's disease. Cancer 1971;27:134-142.
71. Saul RA, Sturner RA, Burger PC. Hyperplasia of the myenteric plexus. Its association with early infantile megacolon and neurofibromatosis. Am J Dis Child 1982;136:852-854.
72. Oh HE, Chetty R. Intramucosal ganglion cells are common in diverticular disease. Pathology 2008;40:470-474.
73. Tunru-Dinh V, Wu ML. Intramucosal ganglion cells in normal adult colorectal mucosa. Int J Surg Pathol 2007;15:31-37.
74. Castleman B. Case records of the Massachusetts general hospital. Weekly clinicopathological exercises. Case 21-1974. N Engl J Med 1974;290:1248-1253.
75. Hochberg FH, Dasilva AB, Galdabini J, Richardson EP Jr. Gastrointestinal involvement in von Recklinghausen's neurofibromatosis. Neurology 1974;24:1144-1151.
76. Staple TW, McAlister WH, Anderson MS. Plexiform neurofibromatosis of the colon simulating Hirschsprung's disease. Am J Roentgenol Radium Ther Nucl Med 1964;91:840-845.
77. Lloyd KM, 2nd, Dennis M. Cowden's disease. A possible new symptom complex with multiple system involvement. Ann Intern Med 1963; 58:136-142.
78. Nuss DD, Aeling JL, Clemons DE, Weber WN. Multiple hamartoma syndrome (Cowden's disease). Arch Dermatol 1978;114:743-746.
79. Ortonne JP, Lambert R, Daudet J, Berthet P, Gianadda E. Involvement of the digestive tract in Cowden's disease. Int J Dermatol 1980;19:570-576.

80. Harach HR, Williams GT, Williams ED. Familial adenomatous polyposis associated thyroid carcinoma: a distinct type of follicular cell neoplasm. Histopathology 1994;25:549-561.
81. Rendler S. Cowden's disease. Curr Concepts Skin Dis 1981;2:7-11.
82. Schaffer JV, Kamino H, Witkiewicz A, McNiff JM, Orlow SJ. Mucocutaneous neuromas: an under-recognized manifestation of PTEN hamartoma-tumor syndrome. Arch Dermatol 2006;142:625-632.
83. Nelson J, Mena H, Ross KF, Martz KL. Lhermitte-Duclos disease (lDD): clinicopathologic features and association with Cowden's disease (CD). Lab Invest 1994;70:139A
84. Haraguchi M, Kinoshita H, Koori M, et al. Multiple rectal carcinoids with diffuse ganglioneuromatosis. World J Surg Oncol 2007;5:19.
85. Antonescu CR. Gastrointestinal stromal tumor (GIST) pathogenesis, familial GIST, and animal models. Semin Diagn Pathol 2006;23:63-69.
86. Lorenceau-Savale C, Savoye G, Pouzoulet J, et al. Ganglioneuromatosis: an unusual cause of ileal stricture mimicking Crohn's disease. Dig Dis Sci 2007;52:1806-1809.
87. Chan OT, Haghighi P. Hamartomatous polyps of the colon: ganglioneuromatous, stromal, and lipomatous. Arch Pathol Lab Med 2006;130:1561-1566.
88. Kanter AS, Hyman NH, Li SC. Ganglioneuromatous polyposis: a premalignant condition. Report of a case and review of the literature. Dis Colon Rectum 2001;44:591-593.

Localized Hypertrophic Neuopathy

89. Chang Y, Horoupian DS, Jordan J, Steinberg G. Localized hypertrophic mononeuropathy of the trigeminal nerve. Arch Pathol Lab Med 1993;117:170-176.
90. Suarez GA, Giannini C, Bosch EP, et al. Immune brachial plexus neuropathy: suggestive evidence for an inflammatory-immune pathogenesis. Neurology 1996;46:559-561.
91. Baskin DS, Townsend JJ, Wilson CB. Isolated hypertrophic interstitial neuropathy of the trigeminal nerve associated with trigeminal neuralgia. Case report of an entity not previously described. J Neurosurg 1981;55:987-990.
92. Chou SM. Role of macrophages in onion-bulb formation in localized hypertrophic mononeuritis (LHM). Clin Neuropathol 1991;10:112-121.
93. Yassini PR, Sauter K, Schochet SS, Kaufman HH, Bloomfield SM. Localized hypertrophic mononeuropathy involving spinal roots and associated with sacral meningocele. Case report. J Neurosurg 1993;79:774-778.
94. Kim DH, Murovic JA, Tiel RL, Moes G, Kline DG. A series of 146 peripheral non-neural sheath nerve tumors: 30-year experience at Louisiana State University Health Sciences Center. J Neurosurg 2005;102:256-266.
95. Emory TS, Scheithauer BW, Hirose T, Wood M, Onofrio BM, Jenkins RB. Intraneural perineurioma. A clonal neoplasm associated with abnormalities of chromosome 22. Am J Clin Pathol 1995;103:696-704.

6 LIPOMATOSIS AND NEUROMUSCULAR CHORISTOMA OF NERVE

LIPOMATOSIS OF NERVE

Definition. *Lipomatosis of nerve* (LN) is a benign overgrowth of epineurial fibroadipose tissue that most often affects the distal upper extremity and may be associated with macrodactyly. Synonyms include *lipofibromatous hamartoma, fibrolipomatous hamartoma, lipofibroma,* and *fibrolipomatosis.* The term *macrodystrophia lipomatosa* is applied when massive soft tissue overgrowth involves an entire limb.

General Features. First fully described by Silverman and Enzinger (1) under the designation lipofibromatous hamartoma, LN is a rare lesion. Well over 100 cases have been reported to date (1–9). Most are solitary lesions. Patients vary considerably in age. Occurring sporadically, there is no syndromic association, particularly with either form of neurofibromatosis. Nonetheless, one patient with involvement of two digits of one hand was reported to also have Klippel-Trenaunay syndrome, i.e., bony hyper-

trophy of the extremities with a concomitant vascular anomaly (2). Rare examples featuring epineurial and perineurial involvement are associated with Proteus syndrome (10,11).

The spectrum of adipose lesions directly or secondarily involving nerve is broad (see also chapter 11). Many occur in association with LN. Table 6-1 summarizes the comprehensive Mayo Clinic classification, which includes the full spectrum of LN and lipomas clinically encountered (11a).

Clinical Features. In addition to the sometimes clinically obvious mass, patients with LN often develop sensorimotor deficits. Involvement of the median nerve at the wrist may cause carpal tunnel syndrome. Females are twice as often affected as males. Most patients are adolescents or young adults; only occasional examples occur in the neonatal period or childhood (3,12) or in late adulthood (2). Distal peripheral nerves are most often affected; cranial nerve examples are rare (13). Lipomatosis of nerve affects the upper extremities

Table 6-1

CLINICOPATHOLOGIC CLASSIFICATION OF ADIPOSE LESIONS OF NERVE

Present Classification[a] (AFIP 1999, WHO 2000)	Modified Classification[b] (AFIP 2012)
Soft tissue lipoma (AFIP)	Lipoma Extraneural
Lipoma of nerve sheath (AFIP)	Intraneural
	Combined extraneural and intraneural

Lipofibromatous hamartoma (AFIP)
Lipomatosis of nerve (WHO)
	Lipomatosis
	    Lipomatosis of nerve
	    (single or multiple; with or without nerve territory overgrowth)
	        with associated intraneural lipoma
	        with extraneural lipoma
	            contiguous
	            independent (within or outside nerve territory)
	    Extraneural lipomatosis
	        Epineurial
	        Generalized
	            +/- lipomatosis of nerve
	            +/- intraneural lipoma

[a]Armed Forces Institute of Pathology (AFIP), 1999 and World Health Organization (WHO), 2000.
[b]AFIP, 2012.

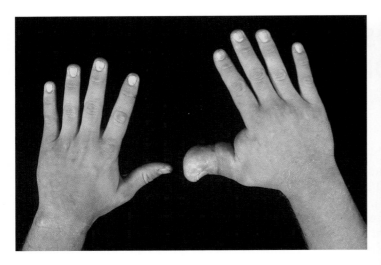

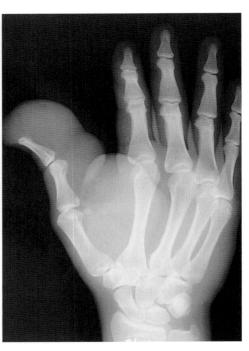

Figure 6-1

LIPOMATOSIS OF NERVE

Massive involvement of the thumb and thenar eminence (above) was radiographically unassociated with a skeletal abnormality (right). (Figs. 6-1, 6-4, and 6-5, right are from the same case.)

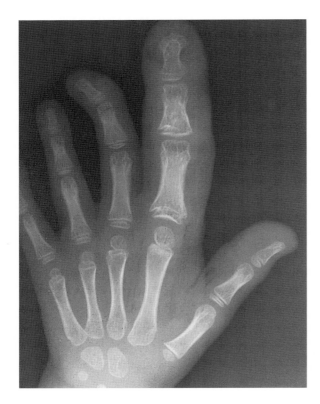

Figure 6-2

LIPOMATOSIS OF NERVE

This example, affecting the index finger, was associated with true macrodactyly and conforms to the "macro-dystrophia lipomatosa" variant.

three times more often than the lower limbs. Reported proximal lesions are few, and include one each of the ulnar nerve at the elbow (14), the sciatic nerve (15), and the whole of the brachial plexus (16). The median nerve is far more often involved than the ulnar or radial nerve. Only rare examples of LN are bilateral (2).

Digital enlargement due to an increase of soft tissue and skin commonly results (fig. 6-1). An association with true macrodactyly, i.e., enlargement of bone as well as soft tissue, is common (fig. 6-2). Since LN of the lower extremities is rarely associated with true macrodactyly, it has been suggested that a genetically determined abnormality in end-organ tissue responsiveness to trophic factors underlies the morphologic distinction from upper extremities examples (1). The non-neoplastic nature of LN is supported by the recent molecular genetic distinction of this lesion from true lipomas by a lack of *HMGA2* gene rearrangement (17).

Radiologic Features. The magnetic resonance imaging (MRI) features of LN are distinctive. MRI shows enlarged, serpiginous, T1- and T2-weighted low intensity nerves, the fascicles of which appear "spaghetti-like" on cross section (figs. 6-3, 6-4, top) and particularly on longitudinal section (fig. 6-4, bottom). Sonography may also aid in a preoperative diagnosis (18).

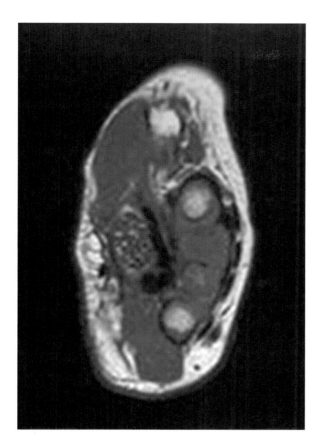

Figure 6-3

LIPOMATOSIS OF NERVE

Coronal section magnetic resonance image (MRI) of the wrist shows lipomatosis of nerve (LN) involving the median nerve. The nerve fascicles are separated by adipose tissue. (Courtesy of Dr. R. J. Spinner, Rochester, MN.)

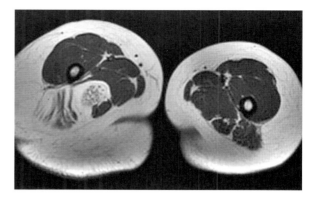
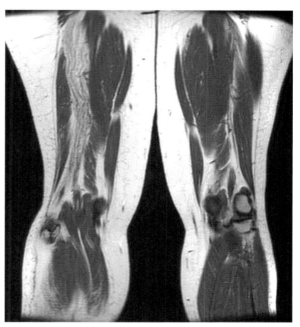

Figure 6-4

LIPOMATOSIS OF SCIATIC NERVE

Top: The affected nerve, as compared to the normal nerve, is marked enlarged.

Bottom: Longitudinal view of the enlarged sciatic nerve underscores the "spaghetti-like pattern" resulting from separation of fascicles by adipose tissue. (Courtesy of Dr. R. J. Spinner, Rochester, MN.)

Gross Findings. Nearly always solitary, LN manifests as a lobulated, yellow, sausage-like enlargement of a peripheral nerve and occasionally its branches by mature adipose tissue (fig. 6-5). As noted above, hypertrophy of the surrounding skin and soft tissue may also be seen, particularly in association with bony enlargement (true macrodactyly) (fig. 6-2). When totally resected, normal-appearing proximal and distal nerves are often identified (fig. 6-5). Ossification is rare (19,20).

Microscopic Findings. On transverse section, the optimal way to assess nerve lesions, the epineurium is expanded by adipose, and to a lesser extent, fibrous tissue (fig. 6-6). The process may affect branches of the nerve as well.

Proximal and distal portions of the lesion often exhibit a greater abundance of fibrous tissue. In addition to the LN itself, fibroadipose overgrowth is occasionally seen outside the vague, delicate confines of the epineurium (epineurial lipomatosis). Since small branches of a nerve can also be involved, a confident diagnosis may occasionally be made on a limited biopsy.

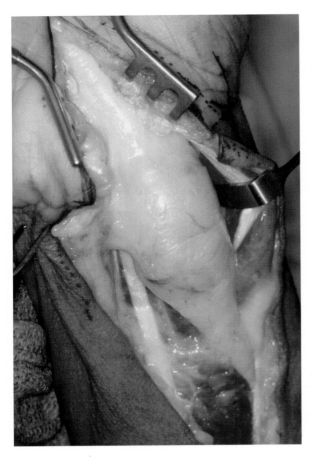 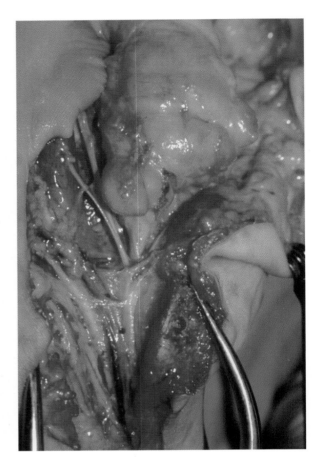

Figure 6-5

LIPOMATOSIS OF NERVE

Left: Operative view of LN of the median nerve after release of the transverse carpal ligament. The lesion occurred in a 63-year-old female with a 6-month history of weakness, numbness, and clumsiness of the right hand. The enormously swollen median nerve contained adipose tissue in the distal forearm and wrist. (Fig. 2 from Guthikonda M, Rengachary SS, Balko MG, van Loveren H. Lipofibromatous hamartoma of the median nerve: case report with magnetic resonance imaging correlation. Neurosurgery 1994;35:128.)

Right: Another more massive example shows more abrupt transition to normal nerve.

In addition to adipose tissue, the main element of the lesion, the encompassed nerve may also show alterations. These include perineurial septation of fascicles (fig. 6-7) (14,21), and pseudo-onion bulb-like hypertrophic change, a circumferential increase in perineurial cells around nerve fibers (fig. 6-6C,D). The latter should not be misinterpreted as intraneural perineurioma, a neoplasm discussed in detail in chapter 9. Other chronic intraneural alterations include collagen deposition and marked axonal loss (fig. 6-6F).

Immunohistochemical Findings. The key feature in many cases of LN is epithelial membrane antigen (EMA) expression in pseudo-on-

ion bulbs, and perineurial septa in the chronically compressed fascicles.

Ultrastructural Findings. Aside from the classic features of adipose cells and fibroblasts in the lipofibromatous element, the hypertrophic change in the entrapped nerves consists of multilayering of typical perineurial cells with their abundance of micropinocytotic vesicles and incomplete surface basal lamina (21). No significant changes are observed in enshrouded myelinated and unmyelinated axons and the accompanying Schwann cells.

Differential Diagnosis. Either intrinsic or extrinsic, a number of adipose lesions affect

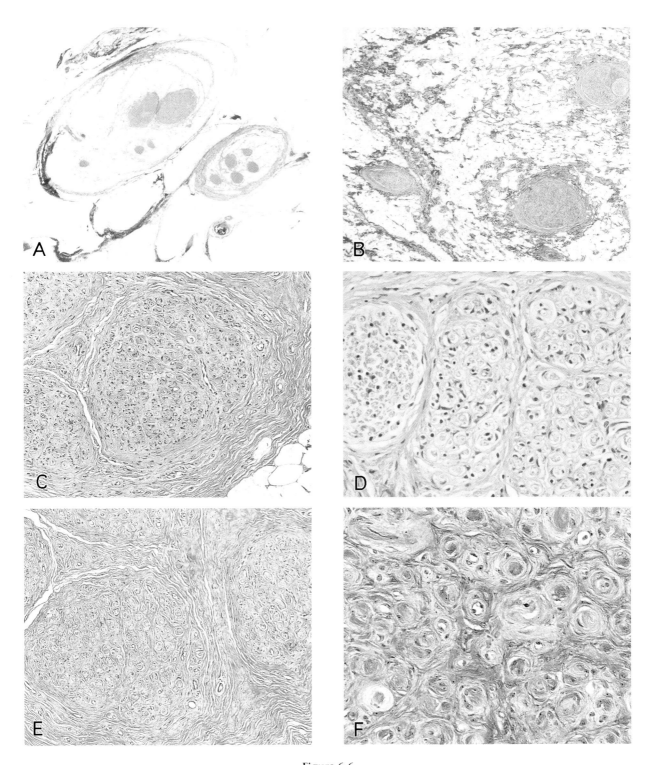

Figure 6-6

LIPOMATOSIS OF NERVE

Expansion of the epineurium of two nerve branches by adipose tissue (A). In another example, three fascicles lie within epineurial adipose tissue (B). Longstanding involvement is often associated with pseudo-onion bulb formation (C,D), collagen deposition (E), and severe axonal loss (F, Bielschowsky stain). (C,E,F: Courtesy of Dr. D. Horoupian, Stanford, CA.)

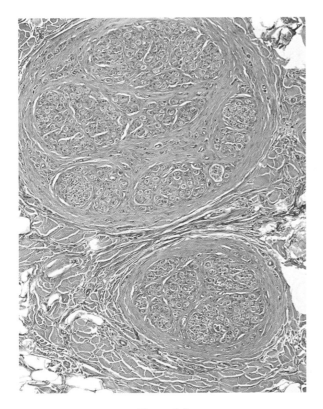

Figure 6-7

LIPOMATOSIS OF NERVE

Secondary, chronic changes in the nerve include microfasciculation.

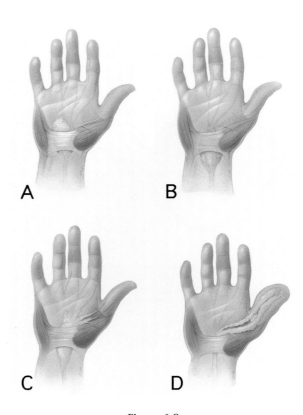

Figure 6-8

ADIPOSE LESIONS AFFECTING NERVE

A: Various lipomatous lesions occur in the forearm and hand. Soft tissue lipoma compresses the median nerve, with no intrinsic abnormality of the nerve.

B: Intraneural lipoma of the median nerve, a discrete and benign neoplasm, arises from adipose tissue within the epineurium and splays the median nerve fascicles.

C: A cleavage plane permits separation of the fascicles from the lipoma. The LN shows diffuse interfascicular and perifascicular infiltration by fibrofatty tissue, without a defined plane of cleavage between the lesion and nerve fascicles.

D: LN, macrodystrophia lipomatosa variant, with marked enlargement of a digit due to fatty infiltration of the epineurium and its surroundings, as well as hypertrophy of skin, subcutaneous tissue, and bone. (Fig. 4 from Guthikonda M, Rengachary SS, Balko MG, van Loveren H. Lipofibromatous hamartoma of the median nerve: case report with magnetic resonance imaging correlation. Neurosurgery 1994;35:129.)

nerve (Table 6-1; fig. 6-8) (6,11,21). Both soft tissue lipoma and lipoma of nerve sheath may compress nerves to produce neurologic symptoms. Their distinction from LN is readily made on imaging and at surgery. Composed entirely of adipose tissue, they are globular, delicately encapsulated, and lack a linear, encompassing association with a nerve and its branches. Furthermore, they show no association with macrodactyly. Intraneural lipomas are rare and occasionally associated with LN. Lipoma of soft tissue secondarily affecting nerve and epineurial lipoma are discussed in greater detail in chapter 11.

Treatment and Prognosis. The therapeutic approach to LN must consider both preservation of the affected nerve and debulking of frequently associated mesenchymal overgrowth. Older patients often show more significant neurologic deficits. Thus, approaches to therapy vary with age. As a rule, excision of the lesion

is not recommended (9). Nonetheless, having noted partial preservation of sensation despite nerve resection, some do recommend simple excision of the entire lesion (22,23), obviously a curative approach. Debulking of the lesion via microsurgical intraneural dissection of hamartomatous tissue is advocated by some (24) but may yield only limited success (2). Others have recommended no or only minimal surgical intervention (25). Despite therapy, occasional recurrence of symptoms, neuropathic pain, carpal tunnel syndrome, and even regrowth of the mass have been reported (2,4). In the presence of gross soft tissue overgrowth, particularly in adults, amputation may be considered (9).

NEUROMUSCULAR CHORISTOMA

Definition. *Neuromuscular choristoma* (NMC) is a non-neoplastic lesion consisting of an intimate admixture of mature skeletal or rarely smooth muscle and peripheral or cranial nerves. The key feature is the presence of myocytes lying distributed among nerve fibers within fascicles. A synonym is *neuromuscular hamartoma*.

General Features. The nature of NMC is unsettled. From the point of view of limb components, the once used designation neuromuscular hamartoma seems reasonable, but muscle of either skeletal or smooth type is not a normal component of nerve. Thus, the term choristoma is more appropriate when the process is viewed as intrinsic to nerve. The hamartoma concept is also hard to reconcile with the occurrence of morphologically similar lesions including skeletal and smooth muscle, but within the central nervous system (see below) (26,27).

The original suggestion of Orlandi (28) that NMC is malformative in nature and the result of entrapment of muscle into the substance of developing nerve, is indirectly supported by the report of a lipoma-associated example of NMC in the lumbar dural sac (26). Lipomas at this site and in the 8th nerve are considered malformative and often contain mesenchymal elements, such as skeletal or smooth muscle and cartilage. An alternative suggestion that NMCs represent hamartomas of muscle spindles is inviting (29), but the often strap-shaped myocytes with subplasmalemmal nuclei that comprise NMC more closely resemble normal striated muscle cells rather than the "bag and chain fibers" characteristic of muscle spindles. Lastly, Masson's (30) suggestion that neuroectoderm is capable of mesenchymal differentiation, the basis of the term "ectomesenchyme," may be relevant to the genesis of NMC. Examples of such differentiation in normal human embryogenesis include: 1) the development of iris

muscles from the eye cup (31); 2) the formation of cranial bones, soft tissue, and a portion of the leptomeninges from neuroectoderm (32); and 3) the occurrence of skeletal muscle "heterotopias" in leptomeninges (33) as well as in normal nerves of the larynx (34). The same mechanism has been used to explain the occurrence of skeletal muscle in a spinal nerve of a frog (35). The ectomesenchyme concept has also been used to explain the occurrence of skeletal muscle in benign (36) and malignant peripheral nerve sheath tumors (37,38), a subject discussed in detail in chapter 12. Which of these mechanisms, if any, underlies the development of NMC remains unresolved.

Clinical Features. Neuromuscular choristoma is a rare lesion. Its first description was as an incidental autopsy finding (28). Since then, few bona fide cases have been reported (11,26,27,29,39–46). Most present in early childhood, some are congenital, and some are encountered in adolescents. No gender predilection is noted. Most patients experience neurologic abnormalities, mainly sensorimotor deficits and muscle atrophy. Others have symptoms related to mass effect. Thus, lesion location and size determine the clinical manifestations.

NMC typically affects major nerve roots or trunks (47), however, exceptional examples affect smaller nerves, such as of the chest wall (41), head and neck (48), auditory canal, and maxilla (49). Even cranial nerves may be involved (27,50–53). NMCs are usually solitary lesions; only rare examples are multifocal (28,41). Associated malformations have included skeletal abnormalities and foot deformities (28,54) as well as an intimately associated spinal intradural lipoma (26). No association with the neurofibromatoses has been reported, but one laryngeal example occurred in a patient with Freeman-Sheldon syndrome (55).

The relationship of peripheral nerve NMC to ones affecting the optic nerve (56) is unsettled. In microanatomic terms, the optic nerve is a direct extension of the brain and lacks Schwann cells. Thus, it bears no resemblance to peripheral nerve.

Radiologic Features. Uncomplicated NMC presents as a fusiform to globular mass with the low T1-, and particularly, T2-weighted MRI signal characteristics of skeletal muscle. These images also demonstrate the enhancing nerve.

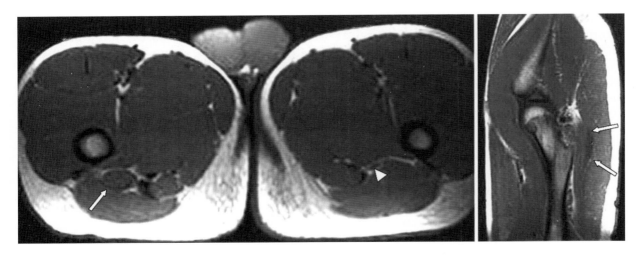

Figure 6-9

NEUROMUSCULAR CHORISTOMA

This coronal (left) and sagittal (right) MRI scan demonstrates expansion of the sciatic nerve by muscle within its substance. (Courtesy of Dr. R. J. Spinner, Rochester, MN.)

Figure 6-10

NEUROMUSCULAR CHORISTOMA

This intraoperative photograph shows a markedly expanded sciatic nerve (arrow) exhibiting red-brown coloration due to its content of skeletal muscle. Intraoperative stimulation of the lesion resulted in nerve contraction. (Courtesy of Dr. R. J. Spinner, Rochester, MN.)

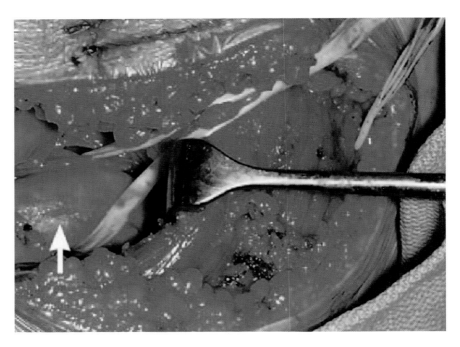

Associated atrophy of surrounding muscle may be seen (fig. 6-9) (57).

Gross Findings. NMCs are nodular, firm, gray-brown masses lying within or attached to a major nerve (fig. 6-10) (47). The nerve is often seen to enter and exit the demarcated or delicately encapsulated mass. On cut surface, the nodules of neuromuscular tissue are often separated by fibrous bands of varying thickness. Not surprisingly,

intraoperative electrical stimulation of the affected nerve results in its contraction.

Microscopic Findings. NMCs feature the presence of disordered skeletal muscle fibers within the peripheral nerve (fig. 6-11). Muscle fibers abound, lying within fascicles and occasionally in the epineurium as well. The fibers vary in size and are intimately associated with variably myelinated nerve fibers (fig. 6-11A,B).

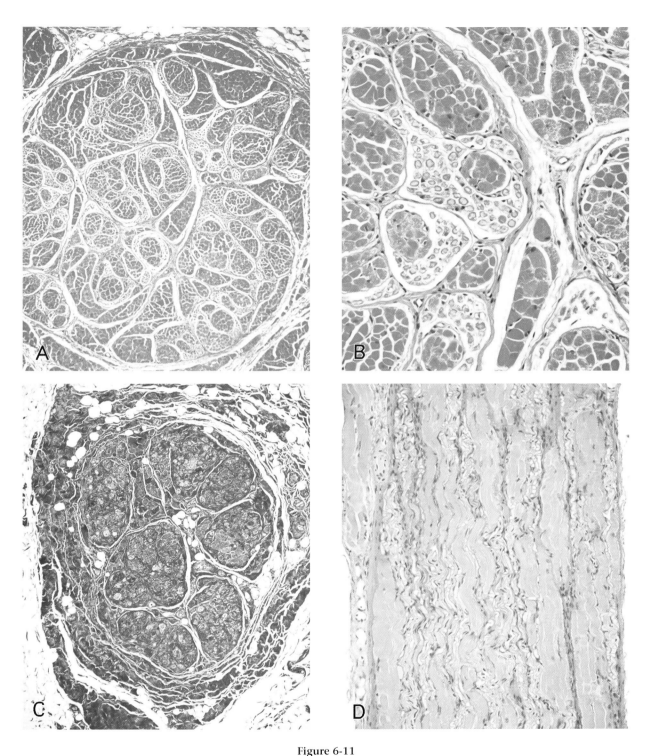

Figure 6-11

NEUROMUSCULAR CHORISTOMA

Cross sections of an affected sciatic nerve fascicle shows its enlargement by numerous skeletal muscle fibers (A), a feature best seen at higher power (B). Considerable interstitial collagen is evident with the Masson trichrome stain (C). Nerve and skeletal muscle fibers are also evident on longitudinal section (D), but their relationship is better appreciated with cross sections (A,B).

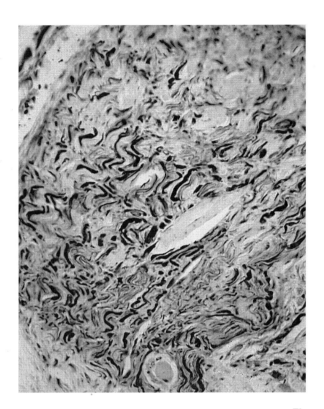
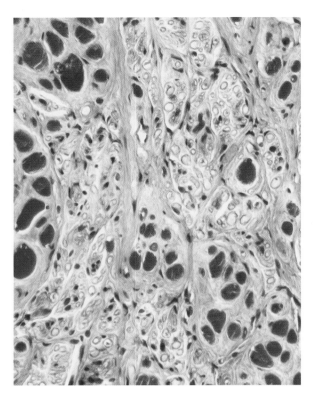

Figure 6-12

NEUROMUSCULAR CHORISTOMA

Left: Bodian stain for axons clearly shows black-staining nerve fibers separated by skeletal muscle fibers.
Right: A trichrome stain shows connective tissue septa separating neuromuscular bundles.

Despite their disarray, the skeletal muscle fibers appear cytologically normal, being strap shaped with multiple, often subplasmalemmal nuclei as well as cross striations. One rare example featured not only skeletal but smooth muscle fibers as well (46). Other examples have featured smooth muscle alone (46,50,52,53). The relative proportion of nerve and muscle varies, but myocytes usually predominate, particularly at the center of the nodules. Close scrutiny shows the myocytes to be situated both among nerve fibers within endoneurium and, to some, extent between fascicles as well (fig. 6-11). Nerve fibers are readily apparent with silver impregnation techniques for axons (Bielschowsky or Bodian preparations) (fig. 6-12, left) as myelin is variable with the Luxol-fast blue stain. The stroma takes the form of connective tissue septa separating nodules of neuromuscular tissue (fig. 6-12, right). Neither cytologic atypia nor mitoses are seen.

Not infrequently, a morphologically typical fibromatosis supervenes and becomes the major clinical problem (see fig. 6-17) (11,41,45). It and the NMC may be admixed. There was one report of a lymphangioma accompanying NMC (48).

Immunohistochemical Findings. The essential features of NMC include fascicles, their EMA-positive perineurium surrounding the endoneurial compartment (fig. 6-13A), and the unusual contents of the lesion (45). Neurofilament protein-reactive axons (fig. 6-13B) and S-100 protein-staining Schwann sheaths (fig. 6-13C) are intimately associated with the muscle fibers. To a minor extent, the muscular element may also be extrafascicular. The myocytes are immunoreactive for striated or smooth muscle markers, including desmin (fig. 6-13D), smooth muscle actin, HHF-35, sarcomeric actin, myogenin, and myoglobin.

Ultrastructural Findings. To date, only a single brief ultrastructural description of an unusual,

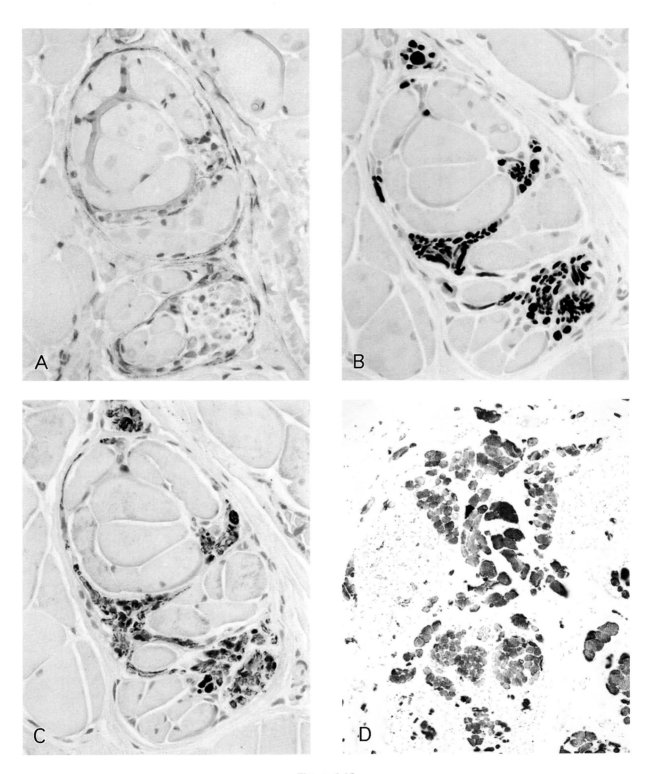

Figure 6-13

NEUROMUSCULAR CHORISTOMA

Cross sections of an affected fascicle are seen with immunostains for epithelial membrane antigen (EMA) (A), neurofilament (B), S-100 protein which highlights nerve fibers (C), and desmin which labels skeletal muscle fibers (D).

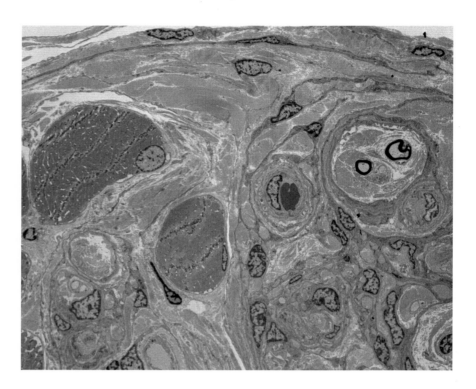

Figure 6-14

NEUROMUSCULAR CHORISTOMA

Ultrastructurally, this high-power illustration shows two muscle fibers within the substance of endoneurium where surrounding nerve fibers are clearly demonstrated.

smooth muscle-containing NMC has been published (46). In our experience, the perineurium-enshrouded fascicles show fully differentiated skeletal muscle fibers intimately associated with often myelinated axons (fig. 6-14).

Differential Diagnosis. Malignant peripheral nerve sheath tumor (MPNST) with myogenic differentiation (malignant triton tumor), the most common peripheral nerve sheath tumor featuring myogenic elements, presents little or no diagnostic problem. Such lesions, often associated with neurofibromatosis type 1 (NF1), feature cytologically malignant striated muscle typically in a patchy distribution and are usually high grade showing variable schwannian differentiation.

The term "benign triton tumor" has been inappropriately applied to NMC (29,39), a complex non-neoplastic lesion. NMCs differ from neurofibroma with a rhabdomyomatous component, the only legitimate form of "benign triton tumor" reported to date (36). Unlike neurofibromas, NMCs are not patternless and lack both loose-textured and mucin-rich matrix. Instead, both grossly and at low magnification, NMCs exhibit gross nodularity and microscopically feature overly abundant, intrafascicular mature skeletal muscle fibers among nerve fibers.

Rhabdomyoma and leiomyoma may abut nerve, but show no intraneural extension. Nonetheless, the high concentration of muscle cells at the center of NMC may simulate rhabdomyoma. An example is the trigeminal nerve lesion of Zwick et al. (27) in which a sparing removal of the choristoma revealed mainly skeletal muscle and only occasional nerve fibers. It could be argued that it, like the case of Gersdorff et al. (43), simply represented a rhabdomyoma, but the variable association with nerve argues otherwise, as does the occurrence of similar lesions containing small amounts of adipose tissue (58).

NMC may also be confused with muscle-containing lipomatous lesions enveloping or disrupting cranial nerve roots and ganglia (59). Although dubbed "cranial nerve lipoma" (60–62) (see chapter 11), such lesions may contain skeletal muscle (fig. 6-15). We have also seen an 8th cranial nerve example composed of smooth muscle and only minimal adipose tissue (fig. 6-16).

As has been reported in seven cases (11,40, 41,45), fibromatosis (desmoid tumor) may occur in association with NMC (fig. 6-17). This either coexists with and overshadows the NMC or postoperatively occurs in an otherwise

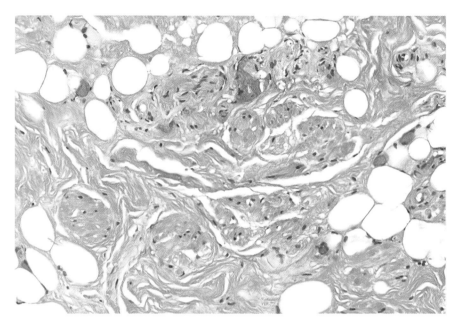

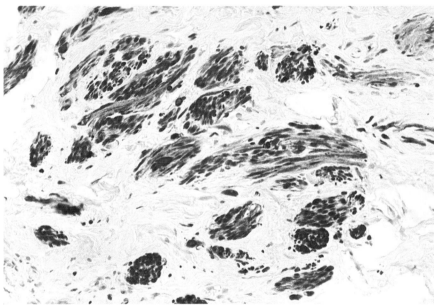

Figure 6-15

LIPOMA OF 8TH CRANIAL NERVE

Lipomas of the central nervous system that affect the cerebellopontine angle and cauda equina region may feature skeletal muscle components. This example (top) involving the entrapped nerve fascicles of the 8th cranial nerve contains bundles of myocytes. The latter are well seen with an immunostain for desmin (bottom).

uncomplicated NMC. Extensive sampling is of importance to establish a diagnosis of fibromatosis-associated NMC.

Treatment and Prognosis. NMCs are benign. Although resection is curative, incomplete excision or even biopsy is occasionally followed by spontaneous regression (44). Thus, treatment should be conservative and focused upon preservation of nerve function.

As noted above, fibromatosis may follow biopsies (11,40,41) and resection (11,45) of NMC. In instances in which the fibromatosis reoccurred, amputation resulted in cure.

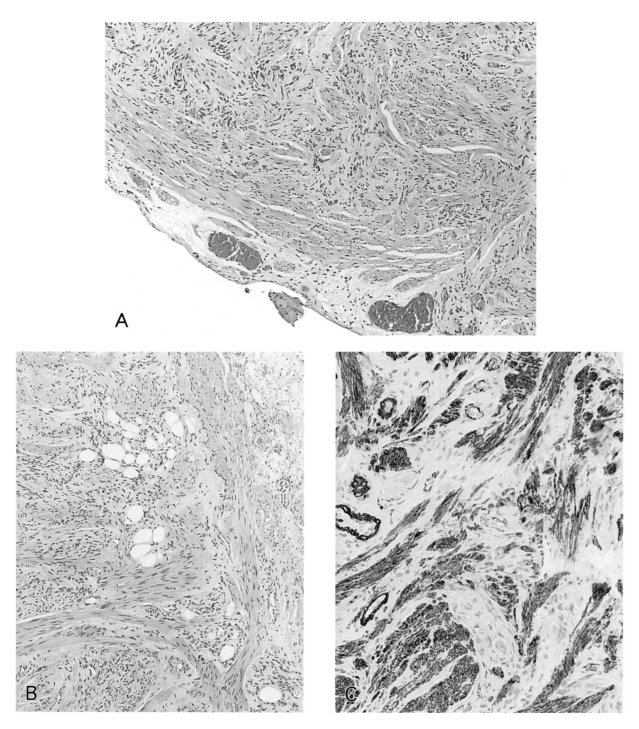

Figure 6-16

NEUROMUSCULAR CHORISTOMA OF 8TH NERVE AND GANGLION

The circumscribed, delicately encapsulated lesion consists primarily of smooth muscle intimately associated with Schwann cells and axon bundles as well as ganglion cells (A). A very minor adipose element is present (B). The components of the lesion are highlighted with stains for smooth muscle actin (C), S-100 protein (D), Luxol-fast blue for myelin (E), and neurofilament protein (F). Given the presence of a minor adipose component, the relationship of this lesion to lipoma of the 8th nerve is unclear. (Courtesy of Dr. R. Kalnins, Victoria, Australia)

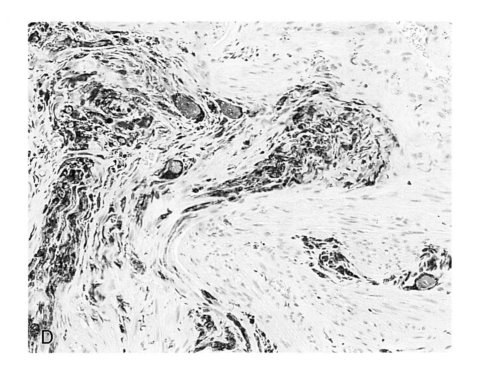

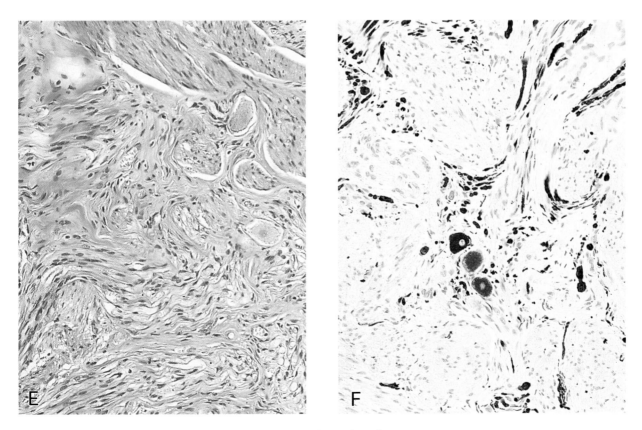

Figure 6-16, continued

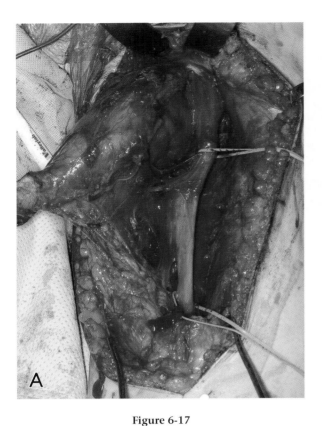

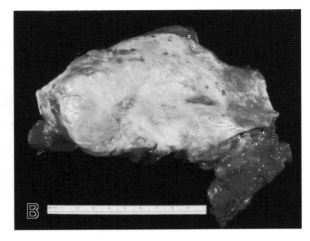

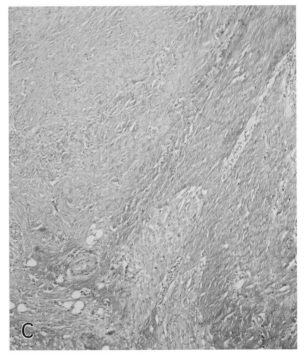

Figure 6-17

**FIBROMATOSIS SUPERVENING
UPON NEUROMUSCULAR CHORISTOMA**

A: This operative photo shows the involved segment of the sciatic nerve (center) to be red-brown due to the choristoma. At this site two branches of the nerve course leftward into the fibromatosis-affected hamstring muscle.

B: Cross section of the fibromatosis shows red-brown mottling reflecting its partial content of skeletal muscle.

C: The histologic section demonstrates fibromatosis (left) in association with skeletal muscle muscle (right). This intimate association may be present after a postoperative interval. (Courtesy of Dr. R. J. Spinner, Rochester, MN.)

REFERENCES

Lipomatosis of Nerve

1. Silverman TA, Enzinger FM. Fibrolipomatous hamartoma of nerve. A clinicopathologic analysis of 26 cases. Am J Surg Pathol 1985;9:7-14.
2. Amadio PC, Reiman HM, Dobyns JH. Lipofibromatous hamartoma of nerve. J Hand Surg Am 1988;13:67-75.
3. Bisceglia M, Vigilante E, Ben-Dor D. Neural lipofibromatous hamartoma: a report of two cases and review of the literature. Adv Anat Pathol 2007;14:46-52.
4. Chatillon CE, Guiot MC, Jacques L. Lipomatous, vascular, and chondromatous benign tumors of the peripheral nerves: representative cases and review of the literature. Neurosurg Focus 2007;22:E18.

5. Frykman GK, Wood VE. Peripheral nerve hamartoma with macrodactyly in the hand: Report of three cases and review of the literature. J Hand Surg Am 1978;3:307-312.

6. Guthikonda M, Rengachary SS, Balko MG, van Loveren H. Lipofibromatous hamartoma of the median nerve: case report with magnetic resonance imaging correlation. Neurosurgery 1994;35:127-132.

7. Johnson RJ, Bonfiglio M. Lipofibromatous hamartoma of the median nerve. J Bone Joint Surg Am 1969;51:984-990.

8. Patel ME, Silver JW, Lipton DE, Pearlman HS. Lipofibroma of the median nerve in the palm and digits of the hand. J Bone Joint Surg Am 1979;61:393-397.

9. Razzaghi A, Anastakis DJ. Lipofibromatous hamartoma: review of early diagnosis and treatment. Can J Surg 2005;48:394-399.

10. Choi ML, Wey PD, Borah GL. Pediatric peripheral neuropathy in proteus syndrome. Ann Plast Surg 1998;40:528-532.

11. Hebert-Blouin MN, Scheithauer BW, Amrami KK, Durham SR, Spinner RJ. Fibromatosis: a potential sequela of neuromuscular choristoma. J Neurosurg 2012;116:399-408.

11a. Spinner RJ, Scheithauer BW, Amrani KK, Wegner DE, Hebert-Blouin MN. Adispose lesions of nerve: the need for a mondified classificaiton. J Neurosurg 2012;116:418-431.

12. Taddie KL, Fallat LM. Lipofibromatous hamartoma of nerve. J Foot Ankle Surg 2007;46:116-119.

13. Berti E, Roncaroli F. Fibrolipomatous hamartoma of a cranial nerve. Histopathology 1994;24:391-392.

14. Gouldesbrough DR, Kinny SJ. Lipofibromatous hamartoma of the ulnar nerve at the elbow: brief report. J Bone Joint Surg Br 1989;71:331-332.

15. Marom EM, Helms CA. Fibrolipomatous hamartoma: pathognomonic on MR imaging. Skeletal Radiol 1999;28:260-264.

16. Price AJ, Compson JP, Calonje E. Fibrolipomatous hamartoma of nerve arising in the brachial plexus. J Hand Surg Br 1995;20:16-18.

17. Rodriguez FJ, Erickson-Johnson MR, Scheithauer BW, Spinner RJ, Oliveira AM. HMGA2 rearrangements are rare in benign lipomatous lesions of the nervous system. Acta Neuropathol 2008;116:337-338.

18. Toms AP, Anastakis D, Bleakney RR, Marshall TJ. Lipofibromatous hamartoma of the upper extremity: a review of the radiologic findings for 15 patients. AJR Am J Roentgenol 2006;186:805-811.

19. Drut R. Ossifying fibrolipomatous hamartoma of the ulnar nerve. Pediatr Pathol 1988;8:179-184.

20. Nogueira A, Pena C, Martinez MJ, Sarasva JG, Madrigal B. Hyperostotic macrodactyly and lipofibromatous hamartoma of the median nerve associated with carpal tunnel syndrome. Chir Main 1999;18:261-271.

21. Terzis JK, Daniel RK, Williams HB, Spencer PS. Benign fatty tumors of the peripheral nerves. Ann Plast Surg 1978;1:193-216.

22. Bergman FO, Blom SE, Stenstrom SJ. Radical excision of a fibro-fatty proliferation of the median nerve, with no neurological loss symptoms. Plast Reconstr Surg 1970;46:375-380.

23. Paletta FX, Senay LC Jr. Lipofibromatous hamartoma of median nerve and ulnar nerve: surgical treatment. Plast Reconstr Surg 1981;68:915-921.

24. Greene TL, Louis DS. Compartment syndrome of the arm—a complication of the pneumatic tourniquet. A case report. J Bone Joint Surg Am 1983;65:270-273.

25. Rowland SA. Case report: ten year follow-up of lipofibroma of the median nerve in the palm. J Hand Surg Am 1977;2:316-317.

Neuromuscular Choristoma

26. Chapon F, Hubert P, Mandard JC, Rivrain Y, Lechevalier B. [Spinal lipoma associated with a neuromuscular hamartoma. Report of one case]. Ann Pathol 1991;11:345-348. [French]

27. Zwick DL, Livingston K, Clapp L, Kosnik E, Yates A. Intracranial trigeminal nerve rhabdomyoma/choristoma in a child: a case report and discussion of possible histogenesis. Hum Pathol 1989;20:390-392.

28. Orlandi E. [A case of rhabdomyoma of the sciatic nerve.] Arch Sci Med (Torino) 1895;19:113-137. [Italian]

29. Markel SF, Enzinger FM. Neuromuscular hamartoma—a benign "triton tumor" composed of mature neural and striated muscle elements. Cancer. 1982;49:140-144.

30. Masson P. Tumeurs humaines: histologie, diagnostics et techniques. Paris: Librairie Maloine; 1956:973-975.

31. Moore KL. The developing human: clinically oriented embryology. Philadelphia: WB Saunders; 1973:339.

32. Weston JA. The migration and differentiation of neural crest cells. Adv Morphog 1970;8:41-114.

33. Ambler MW. Striated muscle cells in the leptomeninges in cerebral dysplasia. Acta Neuropathol 1977;40:269-271.

34. Zak FG, Lawson W. An anatomical curiosity: intra-neural striated muscle fibres in the human larynx. J Laryngol Otol 1975;89:199-201.

35. Anzil AP, Wernig A. Muscle cells in a nerve trunk of a frog muscle. Cell Tissue Res 1981;219:433-436.

36. Azzopardi JG, Eusebi V, Tison V, Betts CM. Neurofibroma with rhabdomyomatous differentiation: benign 'Triton' tumour of the vagina. Histopathology 1983;7:561-572.

37. Ducatman BS, Scheithauer BW. Malignant peripheral nerve sheath tumors with divergent differentiation. Cancer 1984;54:1049-1057.

38. Woodruff JM, Chernik NL, Smith MC, Millet WB, Foote FW Jr. Peripheral nerve tumors with rhabdomyosarcomatous differentiation (malignant "Triton" tumors). Cancer 1973;32:426-439.
39. Awasthi D, Kline DG, Beckman EN. Neuromuscular hamartoma (benign "triton" tumor) of the brachial plexus. Case report. J Neurosurg 1991;75:795-797.
40. Boman F, Palau C, Floquet A, Floquet J, Lascombes P. [Neuromuscular hamartoma]. Ann Pathol 1991;11:36-41. [French]
41. Bonneau R, Brochu P. Neuromuscular choristoma. A clinicopathologic study of two cases. Am J Surg Pathol 1983;7:521-528.
42. Chen KT. Neuromuscular hamartoma. J Surg Oncol 1984;26:158-160.
43. Gersdorff MC, Decat M, Duprez T. Neuromuscular hamartoma of the internal auditory canal. Eur Arch Otorhinolaryngol 1996;253:440-442.
44. Louhimo I, Rapola J. Intraneural muscular hamartoma: report of two cases in small children. J Pediatr Surg 1972;7:696-699.
45. Van Dorpe J, Sciot R, De Vos R, Uyttebroeck A, Stas M, Van Damme B. Neuromuscular choristoma (hamartoma) with smooth and striated muscle component: case report with immunohistochemical and ultrastructural analysis. Am J Surg Pathol 1997;21:1090-1095.
46. Maher CO, Spinner RJ, Giannini C, Scheithauer BW, Crum BA. Neuromuscular choristoma of the sciatic nerve. Case report. J Neurosurg 2002;96:1123-1126.
47. Tiffee JC, Barnes EL. Neuromuscular hamartomas of the head and neck. Arch Otolaryngol Head Neck Surg 1998;124:212-216.
48. Lassaletta L, Granell J, Patron M, Gavilan J. Smooth muscle choristoma of the internal auditory meatus. Eur Arch Otorhinolaryngol 2005;262:834-838.
49. Bassett GS, Monforte-Munoz H, Mitchell WG, Rowland JM. Cavus deformity of the foot secondary to a neuromuscular choristoma (hamartoma) of the sciatic nerve. A case report. J Bone Joint Surg Am 1997;79:1398-1401.
50. Galliani CA, Matt BH. Laryngomalacia and intra-neural striated muscle in an infant with the Freeman-Sheldon syndrome. Int J Pediatr Otorhinolaryngol. 1993;25:243-248.
51. Giannini C, Reynolds C, Leavitt JA, et al. Choristoma of the optic nerve: case report. Neurosurgery 2002;50:1125-1128.
52. Lai PH, Ho JT, Lin SL, et al. Neuromuscular hamartoma arising in the brachial plexus. Neuroradiology 2004;46:216-218.
53. Kawamoto S, Matsuda H, Ueki K, Okada Y, Kim P. Neuromuscular choristoma of the oculomotor nerve: case report. Neurosurgery 2007;60:E777-778; discussion E778.
54. Kushida Y, Haba R, Kobayashi S, Ishikawa M, Doi T, Kadota K. Ectopic hamartomatous thymoma: a case report with immunohistochemical study and review of the literature. J Cutan Pathol 2006;33:369-372.
55. Lena G, Dufour T, Gambarelli D, Chabrol B, Mancini J. Choristoma of the intracranial maxillary nerve in a child. Case report. J Neurosurg 1994;81:788-791.
56. Smith MM, Thompson JE, Thomas D, et al. Choristomas of the seventh and eighth cranial nerves. AJNR Am J Neuroradiol 1997;18:327-329.
57. Mitchell A, Scheithauer BW, Ostertag H, Seperhnia A, Sav A. Neuromuscular choristoma. Am J Clin Pathol 1995;103:460-465.
58. Vandewalle G, Brucher JM, Michotte A. Intracranial facial nerve rhabdomyoma. Case report. J Neurosurg 1995;83:919-922.
59. Apostolides PJ, Spetzler RF, Johnson PC. Ectomesenchymal hamartoma (benign "ectomesenchymoma") of the VIIIth nerve: case report. Neurosurgery 1995;37:1204-1207.
60. Burger PC, Scheithauer BW. Tumors of intracranial and intraspinal peripheral nerves. In: Burger PC, Scheithauer BW, eds. Tumors of the central nervous system. AFIP Atlas of Tumor Pathology, 4th Series, Fascicle 7. Washington, DC: American Registry of Pathology; 2007:446-447.
61. Kato T, Sawamura Y, Abe H. Trigeminal neuralgia caused by a cerebellopontine-angle lipoma: case report. Surg Neurol 1995;44:33-35.
62. Singh SP, Cottingham SL, Slone W, Boesel CP, Welling DB, Yates AJ. Lipomas of the internal auditory canal. Arch Pathol Lab Med 1996;120:681-683.

7 SCHWANNOMA

The classification of peripheral nerve sheath tumors (PNSTs), among which neuroectodermal tumors, schwannoma, and neurofibroma are the most frequent, is based upon which normal nerve sheath cell(s) the neoplastic cells resemble. Generally, a tumor's cell type is established by its immunohistochemical profile, ultrastructural features, or both; occasionally, recourse to some form of genetic evaluation is necessary. A tumor composed exclusively of neoplastic cells with differentiated or otherwise distinctly Schwann cell characteristics is designated schwannoma, and that with perineurial cell characteristics, perineurioma.

Recent genetic and immunophenotyping studies have suggested that a close relationship between neoplastic Schwann and perineurial cells exists. A hybrid tumor of intimately admixed schwannomatous and perineuriomatous cells has been labeled a hybrid schwannoma/perineurioma (1). Because on initial gross and microscopic evaluation this tumor is most commonly judged to be a soft tissue perineurioma, it is discussed in the chapter on perineurial cell tumors.

Neurofibroma, also Schwann cell derived, is least readily characterized in terms of its cellular makeup. Clinical differences exist between conventional schwannoma and neurofibroma and are usually sufficient to permit their ready distinction (Table 7-1). Although the existence of a schwannoma with a neurofibroma component was initially postulated because schwannomas, unlike neurofibromas, were thought not to contain intratumoral nerve fibers (2), subsequent studies demonstrating the presence of variable numbers of such axons in schwannomas invalidated the histologic basis for this conclusion (3–6).

An offshoot of the more recent finding of a significant percentage of schwannoma-bearing axon segments, as identified by neurofilament protein immunostaining, has been the suggestion that schwannomas have a mixed population of cells more similar to neurofibroma cells than previously believed (5); however, there is abundant evidence that the tumor cells in most conventional schwannomas have a strictly differentiated Schwann cell ultrastructure. A more plausible explanation rests with axonal entrapment by an expansile tumor. The axons found in schwannomas usually are haphazardly distributed, individual truncated filaments or not grouped, and linearly arranged as in many neurofibromas. The significance of the alternative combination of neurofibroma with schwannoma, as represented by some mainly plexiform neurofibromas found to contain solitary or multiple minischwannomas (7), is a subject of continuing analysis (see chapter 8).

Schwannoma is a generic designation covering two major tumor forms: *conventional schwannoma*, defined in part by the absence of melanin production by tumor cells, and *melanotic schwannoma* (8), by its presence. The two differ genetically and clinically. Two clinically significant variants of conventional schwannoma are recognized: *cellular* and *plexiform schwannomas*.

CONVENTIONAL SCHWANNOMA

Definition. *Conventional schwannoma* is a tumor composed entirely of nonmelanotic cells which, although variable in their light microscopic appearance, possess the immunohistochemical and ultrastructural characteristics of differentiated Schwann cells. The tumor is encapsulated by perineurial cells and almost uniformly benign.

General Features. Conventional schwannoma was the earliest form of PNST to be defined. It has a monomorphous, differentiated cellular makeup, and limited capacity to undergo divergent differentiation. An appreciation of the morphologic variability and clinical behavior of conventional schwannoma and the related cellular and plexiform variants is basic to our understanding of other PNSTs.

Conventional schwannomas have been referred to as *neurinomas, schwannogliomas,* and *neurilemomas* (9,10). The identification of other schwannoma variants is a relatively recent

Table 7-1

CLINICOPATHOLOGIC DISTINCTION OF CONVENTIONAL SCHWANNOMA AND NEUROFIBROMA

Conventional Schwannoma	Neurofibroma
Sporadic/occasional NF2 association[a]	NF1 association/sporadic
Altered gene, NF2	Altered gene, NF1
Extremities> trunk	Trunk> extremities
Usually solitary	Most often solitary
Originating nerve often identified	Originating nerve infrequently identified
Discrete expansive tumor pushing aside uninvolved nerve fascicles	Incorporates nerve
Most often globoid	Fusiform, globoid or diffuse and not uncommonly plexiform
Commonly encapsulated	Nonencapsulated
Cut surface nonmucoid, firm to soft	Cut surface mucoid, firm, pliable
Varied appearance: tan, gray, often focally yellow and hemorrhagic	Uniform appearance: gray-tan, glistening
Occasionally cystic	Noncystic
High cellularity	Generally low cellularity
Biphasic Antoni A and B patterns	Usually of uniform low cellularity
Scant or no stromal mucus	Myxoid rich matrix
Some intratumoral axons in almost half of tumors	Intratumoral axons often present
Palisades and Verocay bodies	No palisades; occasionally Wagner-Meissner–like corpuscles
Composed of differentiated, nonmelanotic Schwann cells and intracapsular perineurial cells	Composed of differentiated Schwann cells, perineurial-like cells, some perineurial cells, and fibroblasts
Mast cells infrequent	Mast cells frequent
Uniform S-100 protein staining	Scattered S-100 protein staining
Malignant transformation extremely rare	Malignant transformation rare, most often arising from deep-seated plexiform tumors

[a]NF2 = neurofibromatosis type 2.

development. Stout, uncertain as to the tumor's cell type, based the term neurilemoma on the Greek word "eilema," a closely applied sheath or covering. A mistaken belief by some that the base word was "lemma," a loosely applied sheath or bark, led to the frequent use of the alternative spelling "neurilemmoma" (11). Subsequent work supported a Schwann cell origin for this tumor (12). As a reflection of this cellular make up, the designation schwannoma is now preferred.

Genetics. The development of conventional schwannomas is causally related to the loss of expression of the neurofibromatosis type 2 (NF2) tumor-suppressor gene product (13,14). Termed merlin (or schwannomin), the product is a 595-amino acid member of the ezrin-radixin-moesin family of cytoskeleton proteins (15,16). When present, merlin has a growth inhibitory effect.

Underlying the loss of merlin expression is inactivation of the *NF2* tumor suppressor gene, located at 22q12. Whether sporadic or *NF2*-derived, most schwannomas show aberrations of chromosome 22 (17,18). This takes the form of partial or complete monosomy of the chromosome (19–21), or *NF2* gene (22q12) mutations (15,22), which in most instances are truncating (15). In a study of 30 vestibular schwannomas, Sainz et al. (13) demonstrated loss or mutation of both *NF2* alleles in seven cases. Monosomy of chromosome 22 has also been found in the cellular schwannoma variant (23). Less frequently reported has been chromosome 17 changes in the forms of monosomy of the chromosome in a small number of cases studied cytogenetically (24) and losses on 17p and 17q in approximately 20 to 30 percent of soft tissue conventional schwannomas studied by comparative genetic hybridization (25). In the only genetic study thus far of gastrointestinal schwannomas, loss of heterozygosity (LOH) for *NF2* was less frequent (1 of 20) than in nonintestinal conventional schwannomas (4 of 10) (26). There was also a lack of inactivating *NF2* mutations in 13 gastrointestinal tumors examined, and a higher LOH at *NF1* (50 percent) than found among other conventional schwannomas (33 percent). The study used formalin-fixed, paraffin-embedded, archival tissue.

Predisposing Factors. As currently understood, these consist of two syndromes (NF2 and Gorlin-Koutlas syndromes), a multiple schwannoma disorder (schwannomatosis), and radiation-related tumor induction. The first three have a strong proclivity for schwannoma development in that their signature feature is the formation of multiple such lesions.

Most conventional schwannomas are sporadic in occurrence. Although rare examples are encountered in patients with NF1, by far the strongest association is with NF2, an autosomal dominant genetic disorder characterized by nervous system lesions and caused by a germline loss of function of the *NF2* gene situated on chromosome 22q12 (15,16). Principal among the lesions of NF2 are multiple conventional schwannomas, meningiomas, and ependymomas. A high proportion of NF2-associated schwannomas are multiple (27), particularly those affecting vestibular or spinal nerves roots. So-called acoustic tumors actually arise from the vestibular nerve. Bilateral involvement of this nerve by schwannoma, a finding in about 95 percent of adults with NF2 (28), is regarded as the diagnostic hallmark of the disorder (see chapter 15).

Schwannomatosis is the second most frequent schwannoma-associated disorder underlying tumor development and found in 2.4 to 5.0 percent of all patients requiring resection (29). It clinically simulates NF2 and is causally related. By definition, the disorder results in the formation of multiple conventional or, less often, plexiform schwannomas, but without bilateral vestibular nerve involvement (29,30) (see chapter 15).

The *Gorlin-Koutlas syndrome* is a syndrome in which multiple conventional schwannomas appear in both male and female members of an extended family who also develop multiple nevocytic nevi and vaginal leiomyomas (31). The

nevi are congenital and the earliest manifestation of the disorder, and the schwannomas and leiomyomas do not appear until adulthood. Other than exhibiting an autosomal dominant pattern of inheritance, the precise genetic defect underlying the disorder is presently unknown.

Aside from genetic factors predisposing to the development of conventional schwannomas, irradiation has also been implicated (32–34). Over 150 *radiation-induced intracranial* and *peripheral schwannomas* have been reported, their mean latency period being about 20 years. Only a few are multiple.

Conventional Schwannoma and Variants. The clinical and morphologic spectrum of conventional schwannomas is broad. With the exception of rare malignant examples (see chapter 12) (35), all are benign. Since a number of basic features are shared by all nonmelanotic schwannomas, the most common conventional form is given first consideration.

Cellular and *plexiform schwannomas* deserve separate mention since these variants histologically mimic malignant peripheral nerve sheath tumors (MPNSTs) (36,37) and, if subtotally excised, show a higher likelihood of recurrence than common conventional schwannomas (38).

While most conventional schwannomas are globular, uninodular masses, some, most often dermal tumors, have a plexiform or multinodular growth pattern. Unlike plexiform neurofibromas, such tumors are unassociated with NF1 (39–41). Both this tumor and the cellular schwannoma are separately discussed in detail below.

Clinical Features. Conventional schwannomas occur in individuals of all ages, but show a peak incidence between the third and sixth decades, with an earlier age of presentation for those that are NF2 associated. No sex predilection is evident, but females are twice as often affected by central nervous system examples; radiation-induced schwannomas most often occur in males (32).

The most common sites of occurrence of peripheral nerve schwannomas are the head and neck region and the flexor surfaces of the extremities. Of tumors involving sizable nerves, sensory cranial and spinal nerve roots are predominantly affected. Motor roots (42,43) and sympathetic nerve tumors are uncommon.

Table 7-2

CONVENTIONAL SCHWANNOMA, CELLULAR SCHWANNOMA, AND MPNST[a]: DIFFERENTIAL DIAGNOSIS

Findings	Conventional Schwannoma	Cellular Schwannoma	MPNST
Gross	Usually globoid encapsulated tumor that has abundant homogeneous tan tissue, and may be cystic or hemorrhagic and show yellow patches	Usually globoid encapsulated tumor, firmer than classic schwannoma and homogeneous tan; occasional patches of yellow, but no gross necrosis	Fusiform or globoid, pseudoencapsulated (infiltrative of surrounding tissues), firm cream-tan, often grossly necrotic tumor
Microscopic	Antoni A and B areas with Verocay bodies and commonly hyalinized thick-walled blood vessels and lipid-laden histiocytes; mitotic figures infrequent; rarely seen malignant transformation	Mainly hypercellular Antoni A tissue; cells arranged in fascicles or whorls and may show marked hyperchromasia and nuclear pleomorphism; notable are lymphoid deposits in capsule or perivascular area; often find thick-walled blood vessels and collections of lipid-laden histiocytes; rare foci of necrosis; mitoses not uncommon but usually number no more than 4/10 HPF	Markedly hypercellular, fasciculated, spindle cell tumor generally consisting of uniformly slender cells; pronounced hyperchromasia; geographic necrosis and mitotic counts in excess of 4/10 HPF[b] are common; epithelioid cells predominate in <5 percent of tumors and about 15 percent show heterologous glandular or sarcomatous elements
Immunohistochemical	Diffuse and strong expression of S-100 protein, except in capsule which contains EMA-positive cells	Diffuse and strong expression of S-100 protein, except in capsule which contains EMA-positive cells	S-100 protein expression in scattered cells of 50-70 percent of cases
Electron Microscopy	Well-differentiated cells with long, often interlacing cytoplasmic processes coated by basal lamina on their free surfaces; intercellular long-spacing collagen common	Similar to classic schwannoma; increased cellularity; more nuclear atypia and occasional residual arrays of long, basal lamina-coated cytoplasmic processes; long-spacing collagen less common	Poorly differentiated cells with more pleomorphic nuclei, thick cytoplasmic processes, and occasionally patchy basal lamina; long-spacing collagen rarely seen
Clinical	May cause bone erosion and can recur if incompletely excised; some reported examples of malignant transformation that followed a malignant clinical course	May cause bone erosion and recur if incompletely excised; thus far no clinically malignant examples	Prone to invade and destroy nearby soft tissues, recur locally, and metastasize distantly (most often to lung); about 85 percent are high-grade lesions

[a]MPNST = malignant peripheral nerve sheath tumor.
[b]HPF = high-power fields; EMA = epithelial membrane antigen.

The tumors, most often solitary, grow slowly over a period of years. Their size varies from microscopic (fig. 7-1A,B), through those that are barely palpable, to larger lesions which on physical examination are mobile (figs. 7-1C,D, 7-2, 7-3). As with most benign nerve sheath tumors, schwannomas resist movement along the longitudinal axis of their parent nerve. Only rare examples affect viscera and fewer still are primary in bone (44).

Patients with schwannomas are often asymptomatic but may present with pain. This is particularly true in the setting of schwannomatosis. Cutaneous schwannomas are commonly small, grossly unassociated with a nerve, and rare,

except in the setting of NF2 (28). Mediastinal, retroperitoneal, and sacral examples are well known for their large size (fig. 7-4A) and usually come to attention on the simple basis of mass effects. Paraspinous tumors usually present with sensory disturbance, whereas those with a significant intraspinal component may compress the spinal cord to produce motor signs (figs. 7-5B,C; 7-6A).

Radiographic Features. On ordinary radiographs, schwannomas generally appear as sharply circumscribed masses (fig. 7-4A). Computerized tomographic (CT) scans show circumscribed, low-attenuation masses (fig. 7-6B) that exhibit uniform or heterogeneous

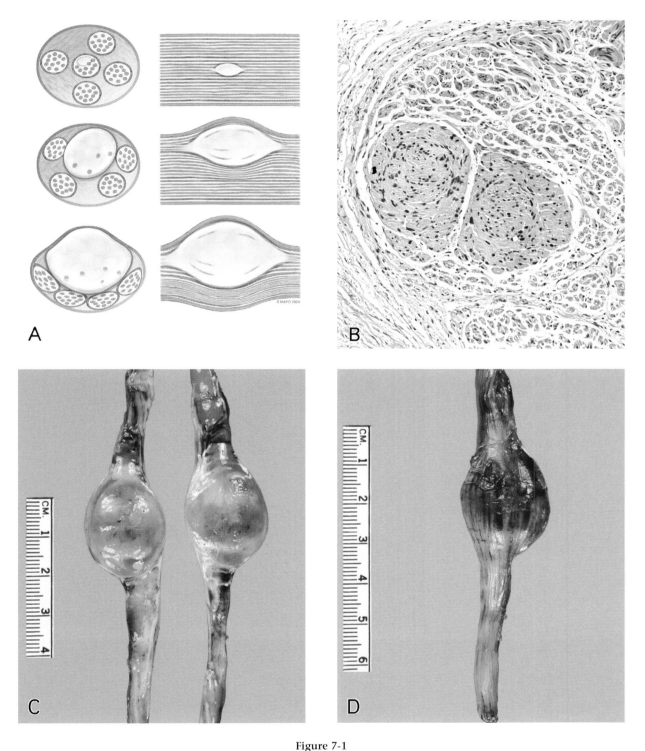

Figure 7-1

CONVENTIONAL SCHWANNOMA AND MANNER OF GROWTH

Conventional schwannomas originate from one or a group of nerve fibers (A,B), and in their initial (B) and subsequent growth (A,C) form a cohesive cell mass that displaces surrounding nerve fibers and fascicles and commonly comes to lie eccentric to uninvolved nerve fascicles (A,B). The side of this affected nerve opposite to protrusive schwannonma (C) shows uninvolved fascicles splayed over the tumor's base (D). In A, fascicles are blue-gray or green, and schwannoma is light tan.

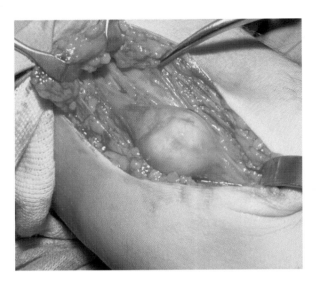
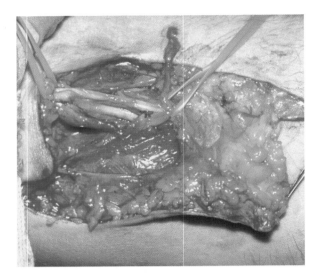

Figure 7-2

SCHWANNOMA

Due to their encapsulation and eccentric growth (left), sizable schwannomas lend themselves to gross total resection with sparing of the parent nerve (right).

Figure 7-3

SCHWANNOMA

Most conventional schwannomas are solitary, globular, and encased by a smooth capsule (A,B), from which a parent nerve may or may not be observed to protrude. Tumor elongation (C) and bosselation in schwannoma are uncommon. The hemorrhagic area seen in A is the biopsy site.

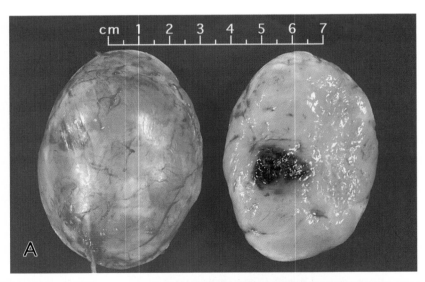

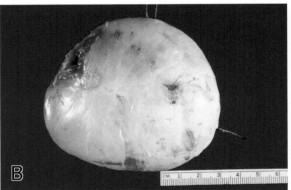
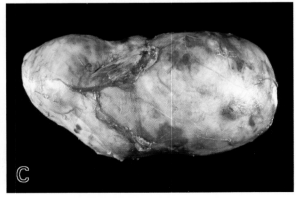

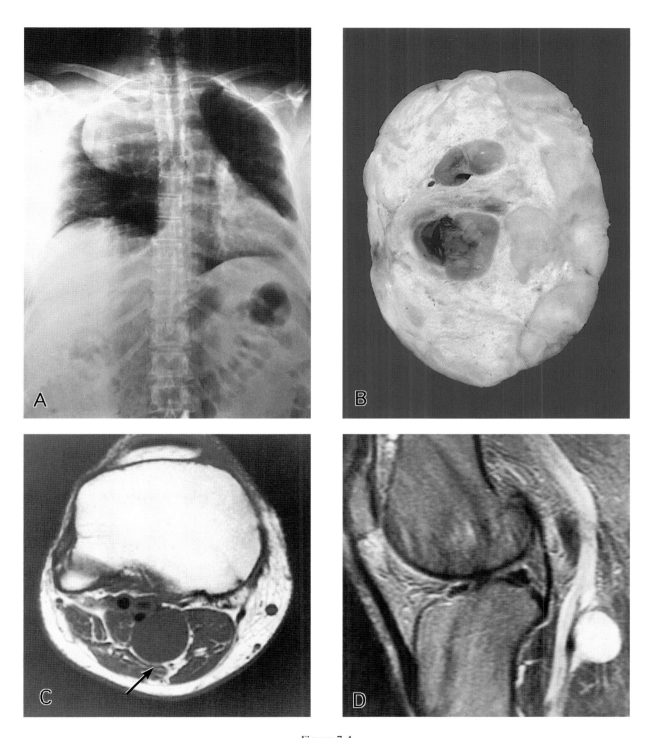

Figure 7-4

SCHWANNOMA

A: On ordinary radiographs, schwannomas generally appear as sharply circumscribed and solid or partly cystic masses.

B: Gross appearance of cystic tumor in A.

C: This axial T1-weighted computerized tomography (CT) image of a schwannoma (arrow) shows a low signal beneath the bright tibial plateau.

D: On a sagittal T2 study, the uniformly bright signal clearly demonstrates a solid tumor attached to a nerve.

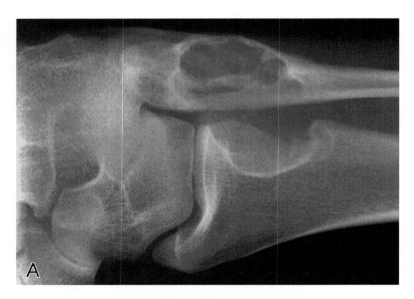

Figure 7-5

SCHWANNOMA: BONE REMODELING AND DESTRUCTION

A: The impression of smooth contoured bone is produced by this schwannoma arising between the distal tibia and fibula.

B,C: A giant sacral schwannoma, here seen on sagittal T1- and T2-weighted images, expands the sacral canal, displaces and in part destroys the sacrum, and emerges in the presacral space via intervertebral foramina. Central cystic change is indicated by a bright signal on the T2 image (C).

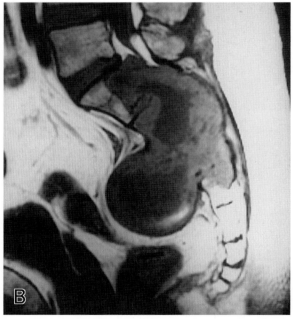

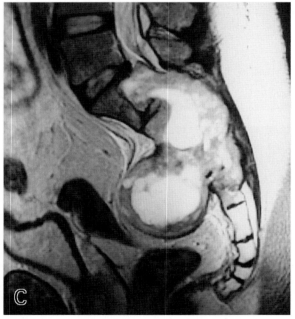

contrast enhancement. Magnetic resonance imaging (MRI) shows low to intermediate signal intensity on T1-weighted images, enhancement with contrast administration, and a high T2-weighted signal (fig. 7-4B,C). In a correlative MRI and histopathologic study, imaging characteristics were related not only to proportions of Antoni A and B tissue, but to superimposed degenerative changes as well (45). On both CT and MRI, large tumors often feature cystic changes (fig. 7-5B,C). If in the vicinity of bone (figs. 7-5A–C; 7-6B), the tumor causes compressive remodeling, usually with a smooth tumor-bone interface. Frank destruction of bone is far less common: examples include intraspinal schwannomas, which often straddle and expand a spinal foramen to assume a dumb-bell shape (fig. 7-6A–C), and so-called giant sacral schwannomas (fig. 7-5B,C) (46). In contrast to schwannoma, active invasion of bone by MPNST often leads to an irregular, lytic rather than sclerotic boundary between tumor and bone (see fig. 12-11). On CT scan, intestinal schwannomas differ from peripheral schwannomas by their

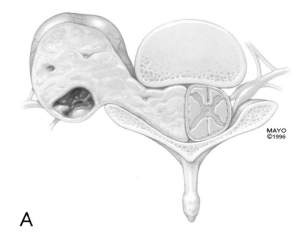

A

Figure 7-6

**DUMBBELL-SHAPED
SCHWANNOMA OF NERVE ROOT**

A: By intraspinal and paraspinal growth, spinal examples may assume a "dumbbell" configuration. The spinal cord is displaced and there is focal cystic degeneration of tumor.

B: An axial CT study of such a lesion shows unilateral expansion of a spinal foramen and extension of tumor into the paraspinous space. The spinal cord is compressed.

C: Axial CT study of a more destructive dumbbell-shaped schwannoma shows considerable bone remodeling and loss.

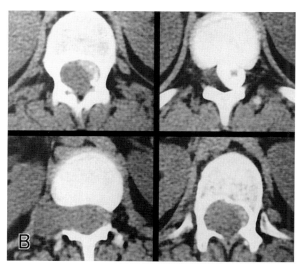

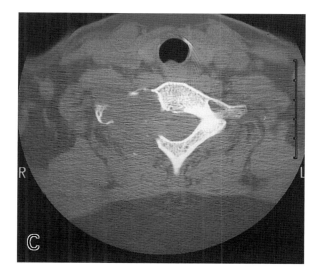

homogeneity and lack of foci of low attenuation that reflect the cystic changes resulting from hemorrhage or degeneration. These features also serve as points of distinction with gastrointestinal tumors (47).

Schwannomas can be conveniently subdivided according to location into intracranial, intraspinal, peripheral, and visceral tumors. *Intracranial schwannomas* arise from nerve roots distal to their transition zone, a region in which central portions of a nerve root become peripheral nerve. The transition is associated with a change in myelination by oligodendrocytes to Schwann cells (48). Sensory nerves are far more often involved than motor nerves. When arising in the 8th nerve, the vestibular portion is most often affected. Such lesions typically expand the internal auditory meatus

in a nipple-like fashion but only rarely focally destroy bone. Large examples often compress the brain stem and cerebellum as well as one of the peduncles. Similarly, large schwannomas of the trigeminal nerve often extend into the middle cranial fossa. Involvement of motor or other cranial nerves, such as the 9th and 10th, is more likely to occur in the setting of NF2. Multiple schwannomas are uncommon; again, many occur in the setting of NF2 (see figs. 15-25, 15-26). Bilateral vestibular schwannomas are diagnostic of NF2 (see fig. 15-25) and often occur in association with gliomas and meningiomas. On rare occasion, an intracranial schwannoma arises within the cavernous sinus (49), dura, or even the sella (50).

Uncommon are parenchymal schwannomas arising in the substance of the brain or

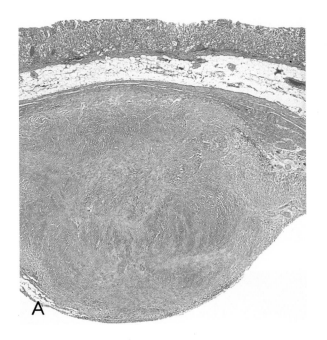

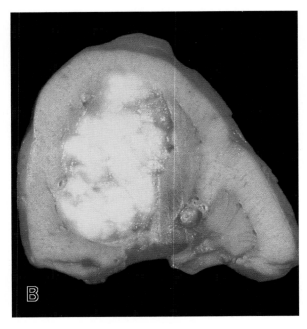

Figure 7-7

VISCERAL-MUCOSAL SCHWANNOMA

A: Visceral tumors are infrequent and most often affect the gastrointestinal tract, such as stomach.

B–D: Involvement of kidney (B,C), nose, or paranasal sinuses (D) is also uncommon. In each instance, a well-formed capsule is lacking. Limited extension into the surrounding tissue should not be interpreted as evidence of malignancy.

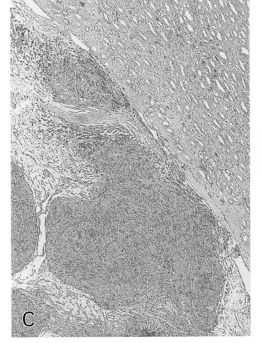

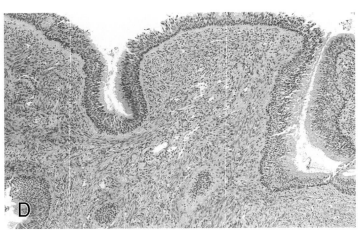

within the ventricular system (51,52). Such lesions presumably arise from nerves innervating vessels within the Virchow-Robin space or choroid plexus or, alternatively, from Schwann cell nests. Parenchymal schwannomas occur primarily in males. Since both conventional and cellular schwannomas arise at intracranial sites, the finding of increased cellularity and occasional mitoses should not prompt a reflex diagnosis of malignancy.

Intraspinal schwannomas far more often arise from sensory than from motor nerve roots. Whether intradural, extradural, or both, intraspinal schwannomas occur at any level.

Sporadic tumors are most often lumbar in location, whereas those occurring in NF2 show a predilection for cervicothoracic roots (1). Most solitary examples are sporadic. When multiple, consideration should be given to both NF2 and schwannomatosis (1,17,30). Spinal schwannomas with intradural and paraspinal components ("dumbbell tumors") usually arise in the cervicothoracic region (fig. 7-6). Cauda equina lesions are often sausage-shaped, lie distal to the conus medullaris, and displace surrounding nerve roots of the cauda equina (see fig. 7-8B). Schwannomas arising within the spinal cord are rare (53).

Peripheral schwannomas affect nerves of all sizes including cutaneous and subcutaneous nerves, and frequently present on the flexor aspect of the extremities, at the level of the elbow, wrist, or knee. Alternatively, large examples arise in nerves within the posterior mediastinum (fig. 7-4A), retroperitoneum (fig. 7-3C), or pelvis. Many of these examples partly extend into an intervertebral or sacral foramen. Unlike neurofibromas, peripheral schwannomas infrequently affect superficial nerves of the trunk. An unusual site of peripheral nerve involvement by schwannoma is the oral cavity, particularly the tongue, palate, and larynx. As previously noted, intraosseous schwannomas are rare (44). Sites of osseous schwannoma include the maxilla and, less frequently, a vertebral body (54). Examples affecting the mandible arise not within the bone but in the dental foramen.

Visceral schwannomas are rare and usually sporadic. Most reported examples arise in the gastrointestinal tract, a site at which accurately ascertaining an incidence is difficult because of the close histologic resemblance of some examples to the gastrointestinal tumor (GIST). Essentially all gastrointestinal schwannomas and about 5 percent of GISTs are immunopositive for S-100 protein (55). For this reason, a definitive diagnosis of schwannoma in this setting rests upon the lack of reactivity for CD117 or DOG1 (56), in addition to an expected diffuse staining for S-100 protein. In a series of 83 gastrointestinal schwannomas derived from five studies of at least five cases each (57–61), 78 percent of the tumors were gastric in origin (fig. 7-7A). Among large bowel tumors, the second most common location, the cecum and sigmoid colon were the sites most often affected. Pre-

sentation as a polypoid intraluminal mass was common. The esophagus was affected only once and the small bowel not at all. In other studies, however, additional bowel schwannomas have been reported (62,63). Immunohistochemical evaluation of the above 83 tumors showed all except one positive for S-100 protein, but only 52 were stained for CD117, all of which were nonreactive (59). Schwannomas only rarely affect other organs, such as the heart (64), lung (65), and kidney (66).

Gross Findings. Most schwannomas are solitary, globular, and smooth surfaced, and measure less than 10 cm in greatest dimension (figs. 7-1C, 7-2, 7-3A,B). A few are bosselated (fig. 7-8A), assume an oblong (fig. 7-3C) or sausage shape (fig. 7-8B), or take the form of multiple tumors that are closely apposed (fig. 7-8C). Oblong shapes likely result from the compressive effect of surrounding tissues at particular anatomic sites on tumor growth. Lobulation and multinodularity are particularly common in bilateral NF2-associated 8th nerve tumors and are also reported in schwannomatosis. A more extensive discussion of plexiform and multinodular schwannomas is presented in a later section. Least common are widely separated tumors on a single nerve (fig. 7-8D), and thin-walled, almost entirely (fig. 7-8E) or entirely cystic examples. Gross identification of a nerve of origin is not always apparent. A fibrocollagenous capsule, varying from thick to thin, and sometimes focally discontinuous, is evident in most tumors. Schwannomas of the central nervous system, mucosal sites such as the nose and nasopharynx (67), and the viscera often lack a capsule (fig. 7-7) (58). No capsules are grossly evident in gastrointestinal examples. The largest schwannomas are encountered in the mediastinum (fig. 7-4A), retroperitoneum (figs. 7-3C, 7-9D), and pelvis.

The above gross presentations are the result of progressive growth of an initially small lesion arising from Schwann cells in one or more nerve fibers of a fascicle (fig. 7-1A). As growth proceeds, the enlarging tumor forms an expansile mass of cohesive cells that more often peripherally displaces than incorporates surrounding nerve fibers (fig. 7-1B). With further growth, the tumor extends beyond its fascicle of origin, pushing aside uninvolved fascicles and

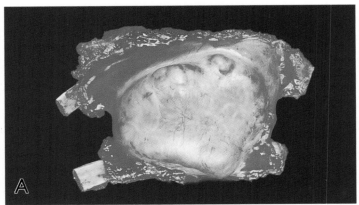

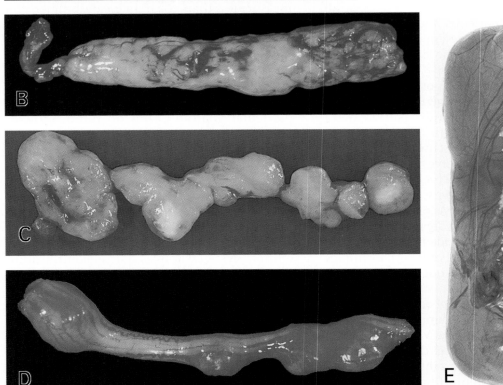

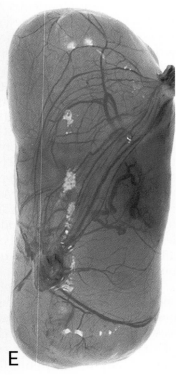

Figure 7-8

SCHWANNOMA

A: Tumor configuration may vary. This bosselated intercostal nerve example was misshapen by surrounding osseous structures.

B: Due to their axial orientation, tumors arising in the lumbar intradural space are often sausage-shaped.

C,D: Multiple tumors may be closely apposed (C) or more separated as in this intradural lumbar lesion (D).

E: This oblong soft tumor was a transilluminated, cystic intradural schwannoma.

coming to lie beside them (fig. 7-1A,C). This process underlies what has been referred to in the literature as schwannoma growing eccentric to the nerve (66,68). To the best of the authors' knowledge, no one has provided evidence for or suggested that schwannomas arise directly from the surface of a nerve. The shift of tumor to an eccentric position becomes obvious in some multi-fascicle nerves, where uninvolved fascicles become splayed over the tumor (fig. 7-1D) (68). At the time of resection, displacement of uninvolved fascicles allows for their preservation by blunt dissection of tumor along its capsule, i.e., the tumor-nerve interface (fig. 7-2) (68).

The cut surface of conventional schwannomas is most often smooth but sometimes somewhat lobulated. Its color, when evaluated within three minutes of sectioning, varies from a homogeneous tan (figs. 7-1C, 7-3A) to tan with gray, white, and yellow patches (fig. 7-9). Histologically, tan areas represent unaltered Antoni A tissue and gray, Antoni B tissue. Yellow patches, deposits of lipid-containing cells, are usually located in Antoni B areas. White areas correlate

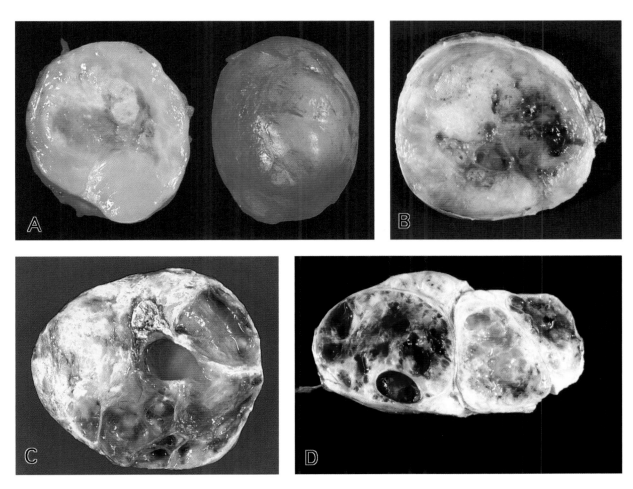

Figure 7-9

SCHWANNOMA

On cut section, the most recognizable schwannomas are mainly solid and homogeneously tan (A). The tan areas represent Antoni A tissue. In many tumors they are mixed with gray (Antoni B tissue) (B), yellow (lipid deposition) (C), and white (fibrosis) areas, and hemorrhage (C). Cyst formation with extensive hemorrhage is common in large schwannomas (C,D), and can produce a diagnostically confusing mottled gross appearance. The cut surface of the retroperitoneal tumor seen in figure 7-3C is illustrated (D).

with fibrosis. In addition to adipose tissue and fat, degenerative changes include cyst formation and hemorrhage, which in sizeable tumors may be extensive (fig. 7-9C,D) (69). Calcification may also occur. The two most striking results of degeneration grossly are diffuse calcification (fig. 7-10A) and total or near total cystification of a schwannoma (fig. 7-10B). In the latter case, the sectioned tumor can present as a bag of grumous material lined externally by a thin fibrous band overlying a narrow rim of residual tan and yellow Antoni A tissue (68). Large, symptomatic cystic schwannomas present most often in the retroperi-toneum and pelvis. In some cases, the presence of a few minute fragments of Antoni A tissue is the only clue to the diagnosis (fig. 7-10C,D). Such tumors, when subject to needle aspiration, pose a significant diagnostic challenge.

Microscopic Findings. A common feature of most adequately sampled schwannomas is a well-formed fibrous capsule (fig. 7-11A,B). Properly oriented sections often show it to contain fascicles of the displaced parent nerve (fig. 7-11C). Extensions of this nerve may become embedded in the subcapsular region of the tumor, and recently it has been found that, excepting

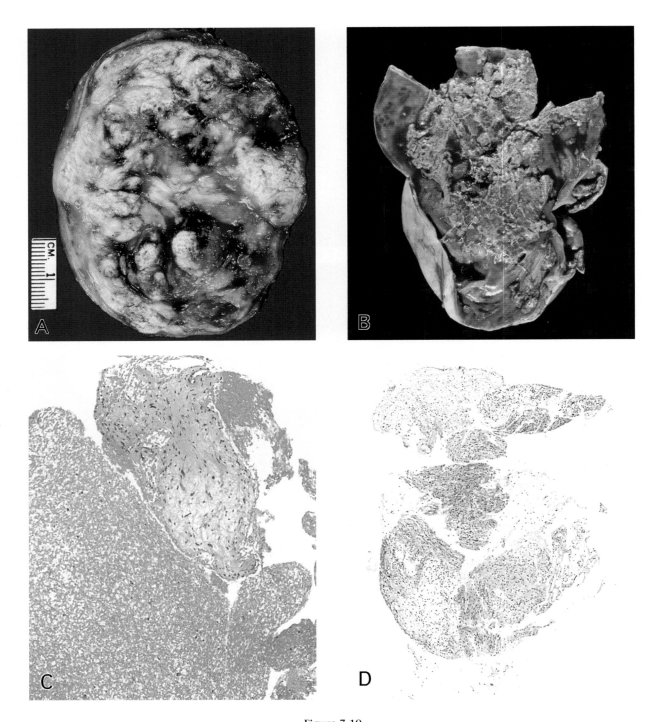

Figure 7-10

SCHWANNOMA: DEGENERATIVE CHANGES

A: The internal aspects of a globoid, bosselated and hard, extensively calcified subrenal schwannoma are seen.

B: This bag-like mass, from the psoas muscle and distended by grumous material, was a cystic hemorrhagic schwannoma.

C: Needle aspiration biopsy of a mass in the adrenal region of a woman with a history of mammary carcinoma.

D: Since only rare fragments of a possible schwannoma were identified, an immunostain for S-100 protein was performed to confirm the diagnosis.

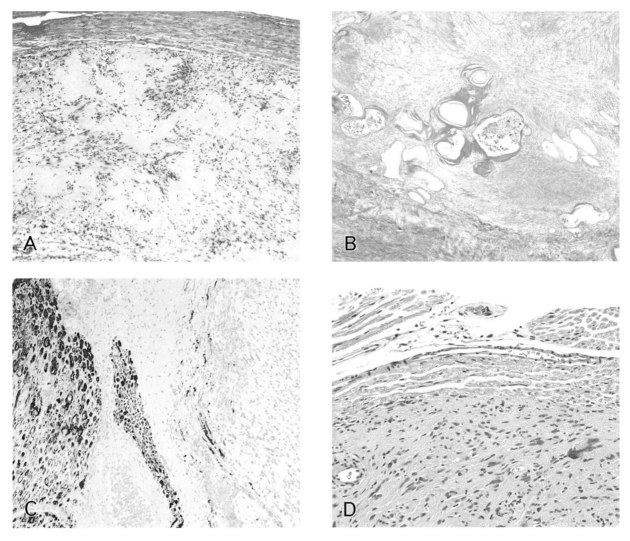

Figure 7-11

SCHWANNOMA

A: Schwannomas of peripheral nerve typically possess a thick hyaline capsule.

B: This feature is highlighted with a trichrome stain, as are the hyalinized vessels.

C: It is within the capsule that remnants of the parent nerve are most often found (neurofilament protein immunostain).

D: Intradural tumors such as this cauda equina lesion and schwannomas arising within the brain or spinal cord often lack a thick capsule.

intestinal examples, almost half of conventional schwannomas (inclusive of "ancient schwannomas") contain some intratumoral axons (see below) (4,5). For intradural tumors, the capsule is often very thin and may be lacking (fig. 7-11D). Gastrointestinal schwannomas, tumors generally situated in the muscularis propria and contiguous with the myenteric plexus from which they are thought to arise, are almost

uniformly unencapsulated (57,59), but also usually devoid of identifiable intratumoral axon filaments (4). Frequent features of intestinal schwannomas and ones shared with cellular schwannomas are a peripheral cuff of lymphoid cells with or without germinal center formation (see fig. 7-36D) and dense intratumoral perivascular lymphoid deposits. Occasional schwannomas overrun a nearby ganglion; these include

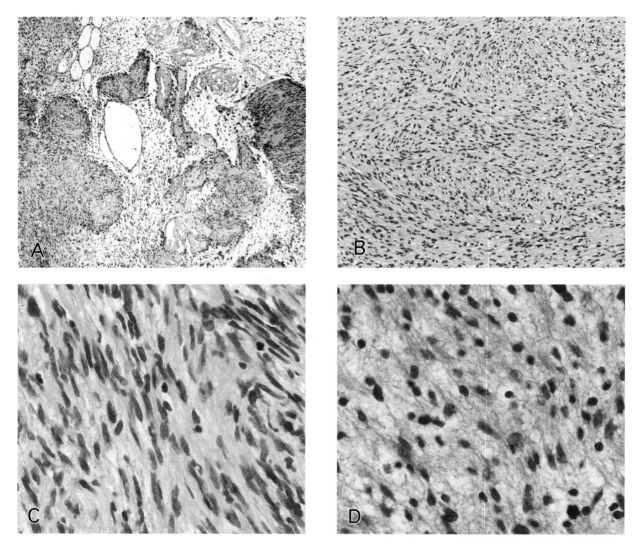

Figure 7-12

SCHWANNOMA

A: The low-magnification appearance of conventional schwannoma is characterized by a mingling of compact Antoni A and loose-textured Antoni B areas.

B–D: Antoni A (B,C) and Antoni B (D) areas at higher magnification.

a dorsal root ganglion in spinal examples and Scarpa ganglion in vestibular tumors (70).

Most conventional schwannomas have two intermingled, histologically different tissue aggregates. They are designated Antoni A and B tissues (fig. 7-12A). Their relative proportions vary widely. Their interface generally is fairly well demarcated, and is highlighted by differences in histochemical staining, collagen being more abundant in Antoni A and mucopolysaccharides in Antoni B areas.

Antoni A tissue predominates in tumors of the spinal canal and the intestines, and in cellular schwannomas (see below). It consists of compact elongated cells with tapered, spindle-shaped nuclei; while most often bland, the cells show varied chromasia, ample pink cytoplasm (fig. 7-12B), and indiscernible cell membranes (fig. 7-12C). The nuclei are larger than those of neurofibroma. On histologic sections and in smears, intranuclear cytoplasmic inclusions may be seen (fig. 7-13), but nucleoli, with rare exception (fig.

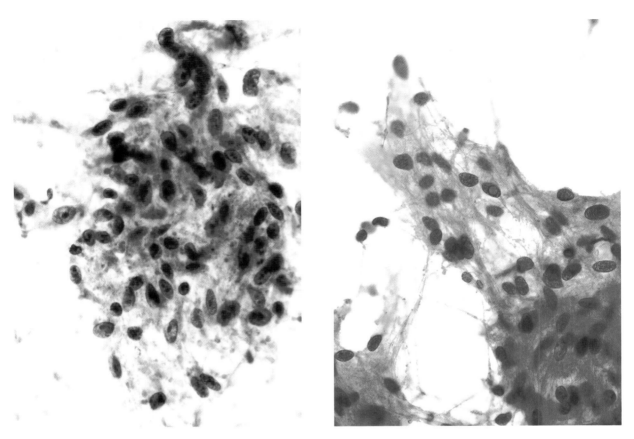

Figure 7-13

SCHWANNOMA

Left: The constituent cells possess elongated to ovoid nuclei with stippled chromatin, inconspicuous nucleoli that here are more prominent than usual, and delicate wispy cell processes of varying length.

Right: Nuclear cytoplasmic pseudoinclusions are also seen.

7-13, left), are inconspicuous (fig. 7-12C). The cells in Antoni A areas are most often disposed in sheets, interlacing fascicles (fig. 7-12B), and palisades (fig. 7-14A). The most frequent palisaded arrangement consists of double rows of nuclei that are separated by a densely eosinophilic zone (fig. 7-14B–D), shown on electron microscopy to be packed with alternating horizontally aligned Schwann cell processes and basal lamina (71). Termed Verocay bodies, they often lie distinct from their surroundings. Verocay bodies vary in frequency. Although uncommon in 8th nerve schwannomas, and absent in a majority of gastrointestinal cases, they are frequently found in intraspinal examples. Verocay body–rich tumors (figs. 7-14D, 7-15B) are rare.

Antoni B tissue is readily distinguished from Antoni A tissue by its contrasting hypocel-lularity and vascularity (fig. 7-12A). Here the neoplastic Schwann cells form a loose-textured meshwork of cells bearing multipolar processes embedded in a variably mucinous background (figs. 7-12A,D; 7-16A–C). The loose texture of the tissue often gives way to cyst formation. The Schwann cells have ovoid to tapered, occasionally hyperchromatic nuclei that may contain cytoplasmic inclusions. They are most often aligned haphazardly or roughly parallel (fig. 7-16B), but sometimes assume a honey-comb arrangement (62,66,68) in which tumor cells enwrap puddles of mucin (fig. 7-16C), a formation referred to by some as microcysts (62). Both arrangements sometimes appear side-by-side in the same microscopic field (fig. 7-16C). The vascularity, often prominent, takes the form of vessels that are thick walled or

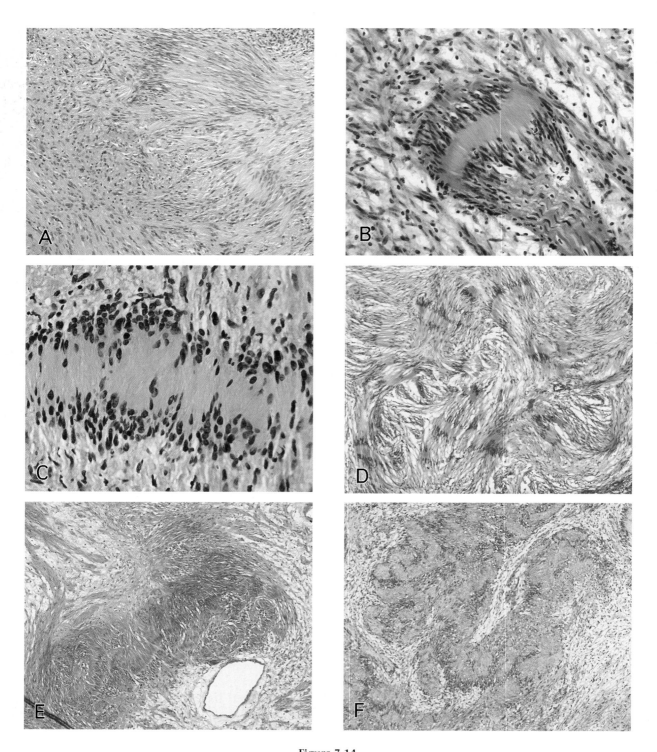

Figure 7-14

SCHWANNOMA: VEROCAY BODIES

A distinctive feature of schwannoma is the tendency to cellular regimentation which varies from indistinct (A), to the formation of tight, occasionally discrete aggregates termed Verocay bodies (B,C). Verocay bodies may be numerous in intraspinal schwannomas (D). The strong periodic acid–Schiff (PAS) staining (E) and S-100 protein immunoreactivity (F) in Verocay bodies result from compaction of basement membranes and cell processes.

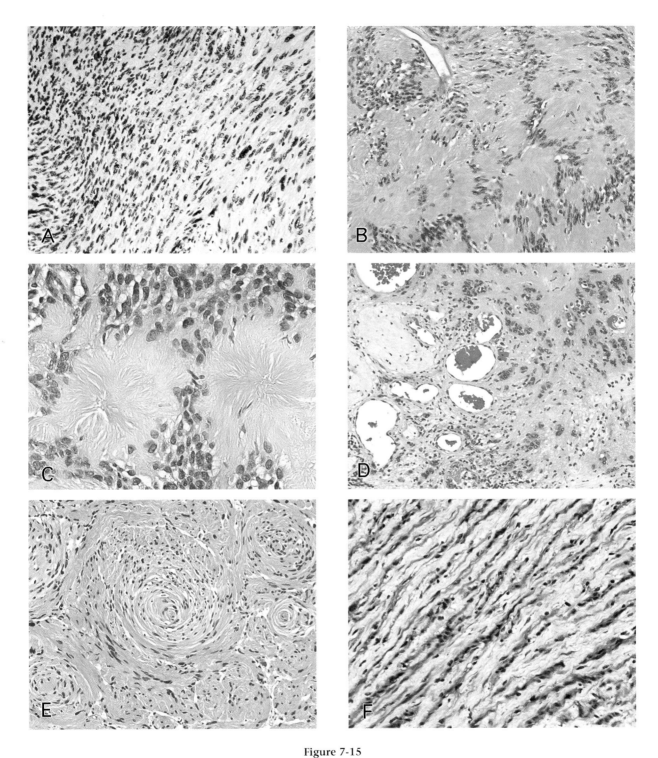

Figure 7-15

SCHWANNOMA: UNCOMMON ANTONI A FEATURES

Uncommon histologic features that may cause diagnostic confusion are: marked hyperchromasia (A); coalescence of Verocay bodies (B); Verocay bodies with centrally radiating cell processes, thus simulating Homer-Wright rosettes (C); and tight clover leaf-like clusters of Schwann cell nuclei (D). Whorl formation may be seen, even more so in neurofibromatosis (NF)2-associated schwannomas (E); and many intestinal schwannomas feature a trabecular growth pattern (F).

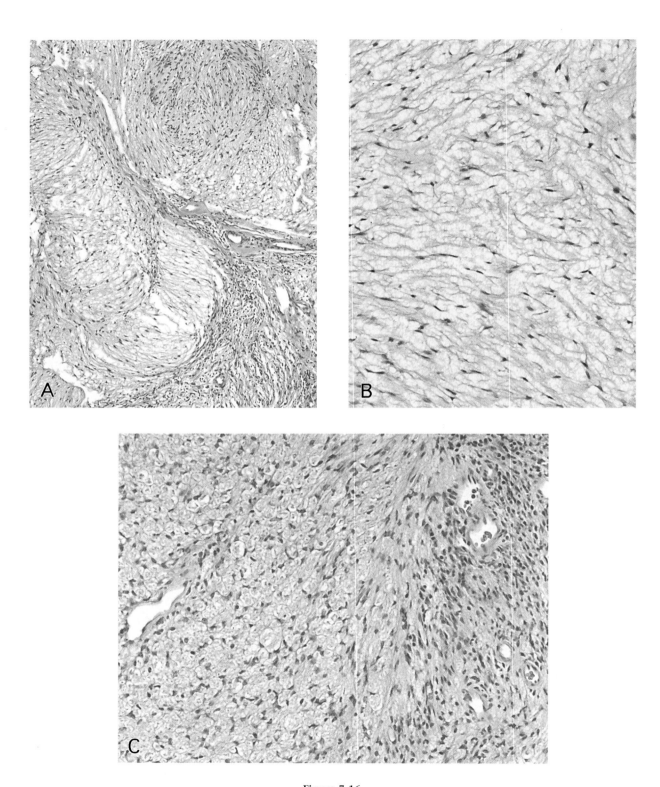

Figure 7-16

ANTONI B TISSUE AND MICROCYSTIC/RETICULAR SCHWANNOMA

A meshwork of tumor cells with multipolar processes set in a variably myxoid stroma is common (A–C). Most often irregularly arrayed, in some areas the cells surround puddles of mucin (C).

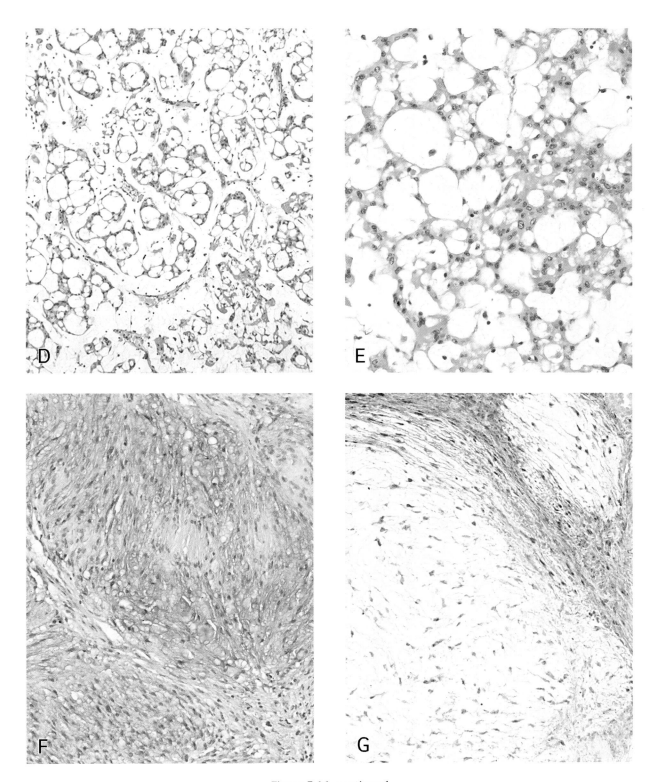

Figure 7-16, continued
A net-like reticular cellular arrangement with pooled mucin is a prominent feature of the recently described microcystic/ reticular schwannoma (D,E), a tumor with a predilection for visceral sites. Mucin-rich schwannomas are strongly Alcian blue positive (F) and uniformly S-100 protein expressive (G). (D,E: courtesy of Dr. C. Fletcher, Boston, MA.)

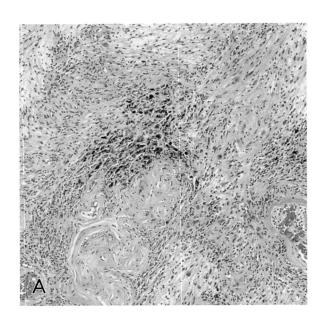

Figure 7-17

SCHWANNOMA: VASCULAR FINDINGS

These commonly consist of some thick-walled and hyalinized blood vessels (A), and less often, thin-walled and ectatic vessels (B). Such vessels tend to undergo thrombosis and micro-hemorrhage. The latter accounts for hemosiderin deposits (A) and iron deposition (see fig. 7-18E), and probably underlies the occasional microscopic finding of nonpalisading necrosis (C).

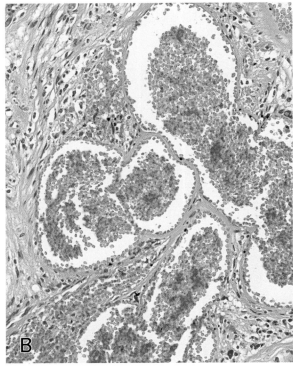

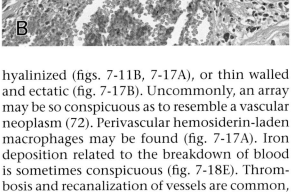

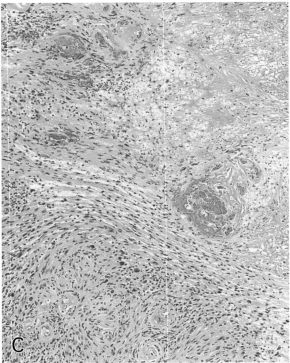

hyalinized (figs. 7-11B, 7-17A), or thin walled and ectatic (fig. 7-17B). Uncommonly, an array may be so conspicuous as to resemble a vascular neoplasm (72). Perivascular hemosiderin-laden macrophages may be found (fig. 7-17A). Iron deposition related to the breakdown of blood is sometimes conspicuous (fig. 7-18E). Thrombosis and recanalization of vessels are common,

and on occasion, there may be small patches of nonpalisaded, infarct-like necrosis (fig. 7-17C). An important feature, notable for its usefulness in distinguishing nonmelanotic schwannoma from other tumors of the peripheral nerve, is the frequent presence of foamy cells. These are arranged in sheets (fig. 7-18B) or in small clusters in or at the perimeter of Antoni B tissue

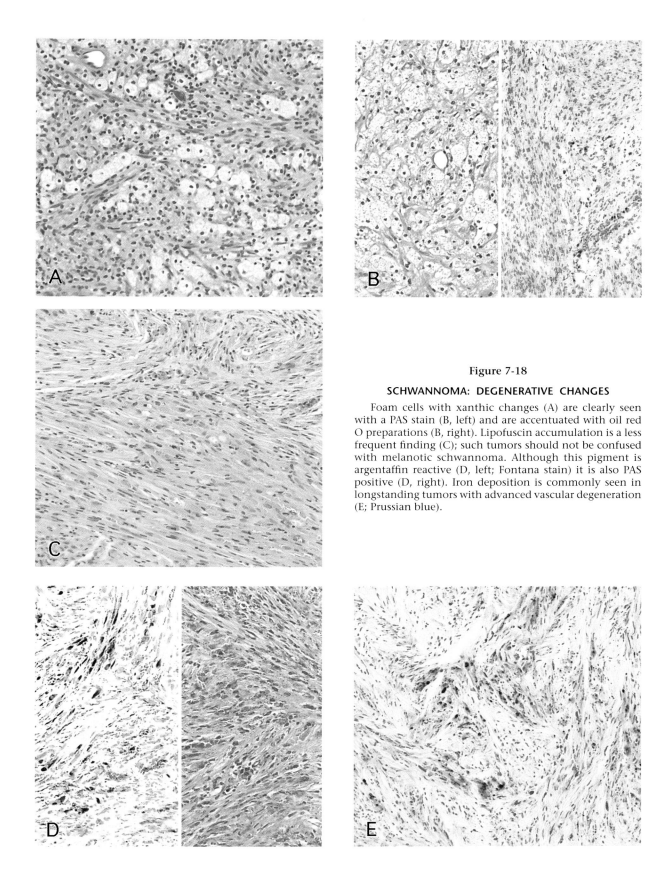

Figure 7-18

SCHWANNOMA: DEGENERATIVE CHANGES

Foam cells with xanthic changes (A) are clearly seen with a PAS stain (B, left) and are accentuated with oil red O preparations (B, right). Lipofuscin accumulation is a less frequent finding (C); such tumors should not be confused with melanotic schwannoma. Although this pigment is argentaffin reactive (D, left; Fontana stain) it is also PAS positive (D, right). Iron deposition is commonly seen in longstanding tumors with advanced vascular degeneration (E; Prussian blue).

(fig. 7-18A). They are particularly common in 8th cranial nerve examples. The foam cells are delicately periodic acid–Schiff (PAS) positive and lipid laden (oil red O reactive) (fig. 7-18B).

There are exceptions to the patchwork of Antoni A and B tissue seen in conventional schwannomas. These include examples distorted by extensive hemorrhage and lipid deposition or those with, or possibly with, predominant or exclusive growth of either Antoni A or Antoni B tissue. In this latter group is the cellular schwannoma, a variant composed predominantly or exclusively of Antoni A tissue. Evidence for possibly an exclusively Antoni B schwannoma may have recently been provided: 10 examples, reported by Liegl et al. (62) and designated *microcystic/reticular schwannoma*, were characterized by anastomosing and intersecting strands of spindle cells with ill-defined eosinophilic cytoplasm, set in a myxoid to collagenous stroma. Conspicuous was the presence of microcystic or reticular structures containing myxoid material and sometimes fibrillary collagen (fig. 7-16 D,E). Each tumor strongly expressed S-100 protein. The identification of the tumors as schwannomas was aided by the presence in two tumors of areas of conventional schwannoma, inclusive of hyalinized vessels, a feature absent in the remaining examples. Foam cells were usually missing. Mainly citing a lack of the usual spindle cell component, myxoid stroma, and hyaline vessels of Antoni B tissue in the microcystic/reticular areas, the authors chose to view their tumor as not one of Antoni B tissue but as a new schwannoma variant. Although few examples of cystic/reticular schwannoma have thus far been reported, those that have been differ clinically from other conventional schwannomas in that they present at an older average age and have a predilection for viscera, notably the intestines (62). Due to their uncommon growth characteristics, both microcystic/reticular and cellular schwannomas pose a diagnostic challenge for pathologists. Examples of the former thus far described, however, have not shared with the latter the presence of worrisome histologic features or the tendency to locally recur, features potentially prompting an erroneous malignant diagnosis.

Other unusual histologic features are found in conventional schwannomas, any of which may cause diagnostic confusion. Most present in Antoni A areas. The neoplastic Schwann cells may show marked hyperchromasia, with or without accompanying mitotic figures (fig. 7-15A). A confluence of Verocay bodies may cause confusion (fig. 7-15B). Rarely, circular or oval Verocay bodies form that superficially resemble Homer-Wright rosettes of neuroblastoma (fig. 7-15C) (73,74), and in some instances, neoplastic Schwann cells are arranged in tight cloverleaf-like or asymmetrical clusters (fig. 7-15D). Antoni A cells may be arranged in whorls (fig. 7-15E), and in intestinal examples, may show a trabecular or wiry growth pattern (fig. 7-15F). Another finding peculiar to many intestinal conventional schwannomas is the presence of peripheral lymphoid cuffs. The authors have seen an example of this with such a large lymphoid deposition as to mislead the pathologist into making a diagnosis of schwannoma of lymph node origin, a site of origination yet to be described.

Epithelioid-appearing cells are occasionally seen in otherwise conventional schwannomas, but only rare schwannomas are composed largely of epithelioid cells (fig. 7-19). Commonly termed *epithelioid schwannomas*, most are subcutaneous and behave as ordinary schwannomas (75). The presence of mild to moderate nuclear atypia should not be interpreted as a malignant change.

Special stains provide diagnostically useful information regarding the microanatomy of schwannomas. In longstanding tumors, trichrome stains often reveal considerable collagen formation in both the Antoni A and B components. Compared to the abundance of mucopolysaccharide-rich matrix in neurofibromas, Alcian blue stains for mucin are usually only mildly reactive in schwannomas. Reticulin stains in a dense pericellular pattern in the Antoni A component, highlighting not only intercellular collagen bundles but the pericellular distribution of basement membrane so typical of Schwann cells. As recently demonstrated, in addition to the earlier known presence of fibers of the parent nerve in the capsule of tumors (fig. 7-11C), some neurofilament-positive axons may be identified within the substance of many sporadic and NF2-associated schwannomas (2–5). Mast cells are often seen, particularly in the Antoni B component.

Although uncommon, metaplasia of cartilage, bone, and even adipose tissue may be seen

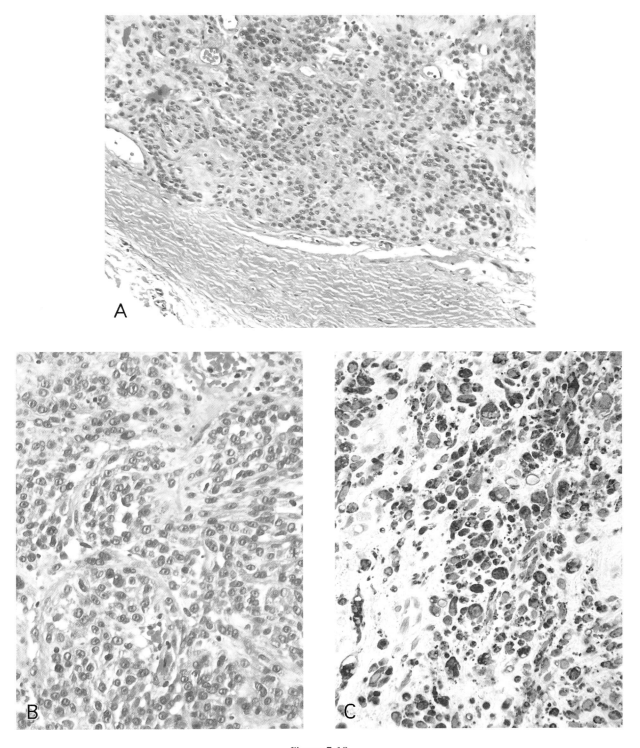

Figure 7-19

EPITHELIOID SCHWANNOMA

A: A benign, typically encapsulated, epithelioid schwannoma.
B: The cells usually have ample eosinophilic cytoplasm and slightly pleomorphic and hyperchromatic nuclei.
C: The tumors are diffusely S-100 protein positive.

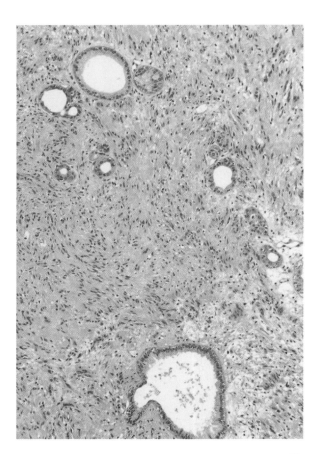 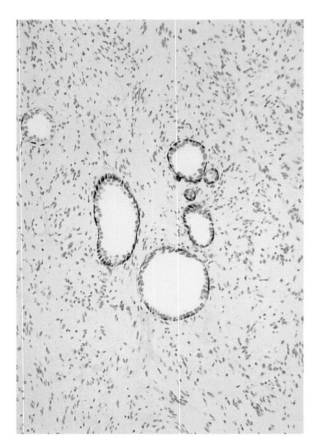

Figure 7-20

CUTANEOUS SCHWANNOMA WITH ENTRAPPED SWEAT GLAND

So-called glandular schwannomas are schwannomas that in their growth incorporate sweat gland tissue that mimics glandular differentiation. An immunostain for muscle common actin (right) shows "glands" surrounded by myoepithelial cells, a finding consistent with sweat glands.

in schwannomas (76–79). It is doubtful whether schwannomas ever show true epithelial (glandular or squamous) differentiation. Most purported examples were located in skin, a site in which the presence of epithelium can be explained by entrapment of cutaneous adnexa (80). No evidence is found of a myoepithelial cell layer surrounding glands in glandular PNSTs arising at noncutaneous sites. In contrast, those in "cutaneous glandular schwannomas" (fig. 7-20, left) are invested by myoepithelial cells (fig. 7-20, right), a feature of the coiled secretory portions of sweat glands (81). Sometimes mistaken for glands in schwannoma are single or multiple microcysts lined by compacted eosinophilic, S-100 protein–reactive Schwann cells superficially resembling epithelium (fig. 7-21) (82).

The histologic changes in schwannomas that in the past raised unnecessary concern about malignant change include marked hyperchromasia (fig. 7-15A) and the presence of mitoses (fig. 7-12C). As previously noted, infarct-like necrosis unassociated with palisaded cells may be seen, particularly in large tumors (fig. 7-17C). None of these findings is of prognostic significance.

Lymphoplasmacellular infiltrates are found in approximately 5 percent of schwannomas (fig. 7-22, left) and occasionally accompany other degenerative changes. Noncaseating microgranulomas of unknown etiology and significance are rarely seen in otherwise typical schwannomas (fig. 7-22, right).

Longstanding schwannomas often show not only extensive stromal and vascular

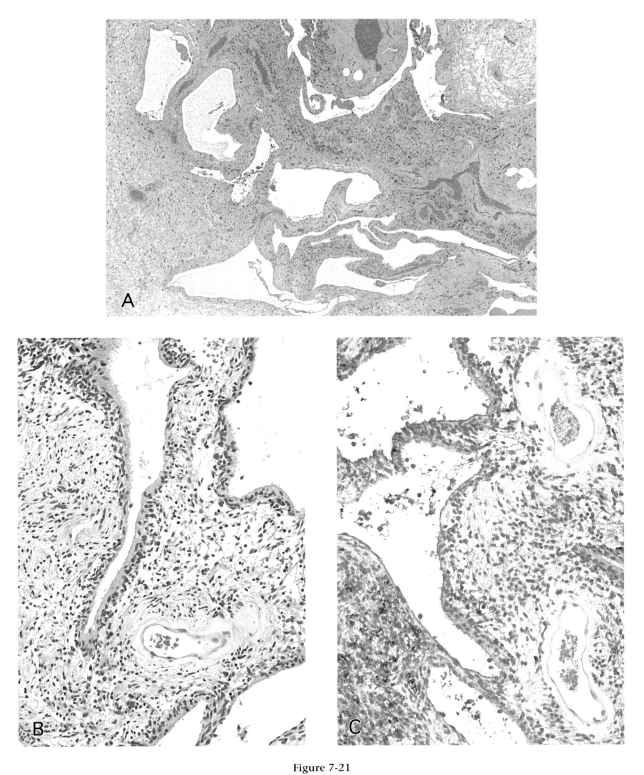

Figure 7-21

SCHWANNOMA: PSEUDOGLANDS

The occasional formation of microcysts (A) with a pseudoepithelial lining of Schwann cells (B) is considered a degenerative change. The lining cells are S-100 protein immunoreactive and lack immunoreactivity for epithelial markers (C).

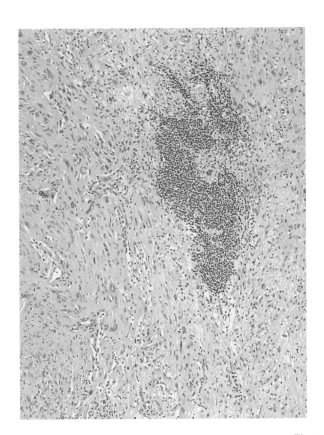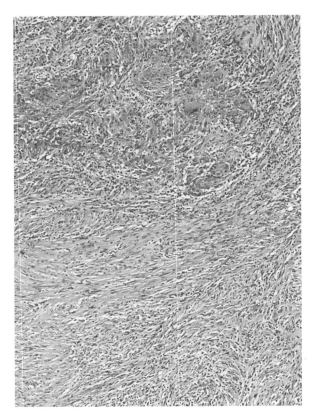

Figure 7-22

SCHWANNOMA: INFLAMMATORY CHANGES

Left: The often found chronic inflammation consists primarily of lymphoid cells.
Right: Noncaseating granulomas are rare and of unknown significance.

degenerative changes, including tissue loss (fig. 7-23A,B), organization of remote hemorrhage, widespread hyalinization (fig. 7-23C), and some calcification, but degenerative nuclear changes characterized by marked hyperchromasia, pleomorphism, and nuclear cytoplasmic pseudoinclusions (fig. 7-23D). Once termed "ancient schwannomas" (83), tumors with these findings are in no way clinically distinctive. We recognize such lesions, but do not consider them a specific variant of schwannoma.

With regard to vestibular tumors, certain histologic features are more common in the NF2-associated schwannomas than in sporadic cases. These include a lobular "grape-like" pattern of growth, foci of hypercellularity, more Verocay bodies (84), a tendency to whorl formation (fig. 7-15E), and the presence of deeply embedded nerve fibers (3). Rarely, there is also a peripheral ingrowth of exuberant, peritumoral arachnoid

tissue. On occasion, the latter progresses to a blending of schwannoma and meningioma tissue (84,85).

Immunohistochemical Findings. The immunophenotype of schwannomas is highly distinctive. Staining for S-100 protein is very useful in identifying schwannomas: all optimally fixed tumors are diffusely immunopositive for this antigen (87–89). The rare lack of reactivity may be attributed to problems with tissue fixation or processing. Staining for S-100 protein is often stronger in Antoni A tissue than in the less cellular Antoni B areas (figs. 7-14F, 7-16G, 7-24A). Less frequent and more variable staining is seen with Leu-7 (fig. 7-24B) (87). Myelin basic protein (MBP) staining has been reported by some (90), but most studies report no reactivity for this antigen (87,91). Negative results are not surprising, since MBP has not been biochemically demonstrated in schwannomas (92).

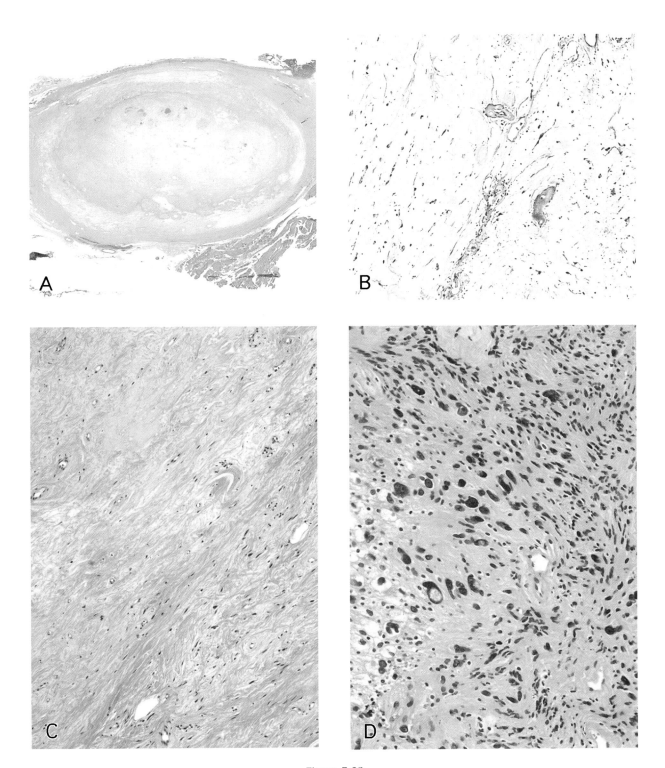

Figure 7-23

"ANCIENT SCHWANNOMA"

Schwannomas known or presumed to be longstanding often show degenerative changes, including central tissue loss (A,B), widespread hyalinization (C), focal calcification, and degenerative nuclear atypia (D). (A.B: Courtesy of Dr. D. Horoupian, Stanford, CA.)

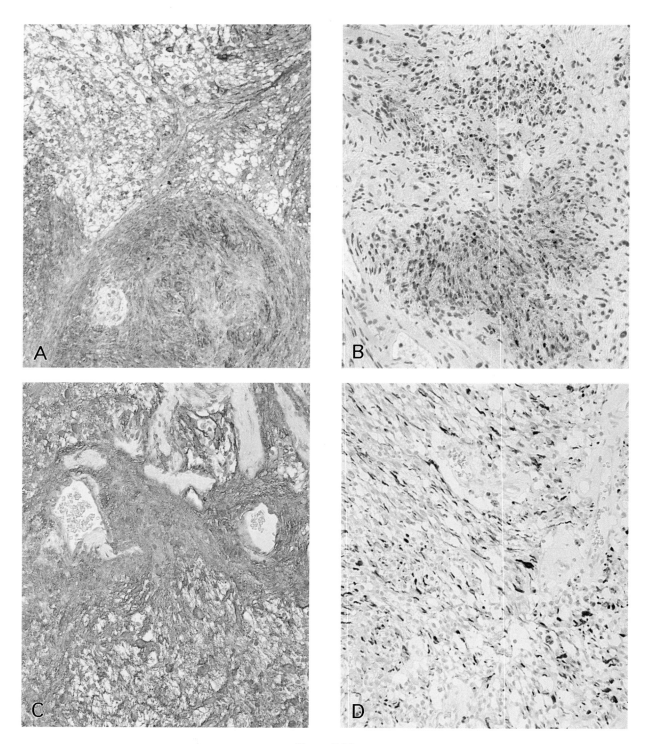

Figure 7-24

SCHWANNOMA: IMMUNOPROFILE

The immunoprofile of schwannoma includes staining of Antoni A and B tissues for vimentin as well as for S-100 protein (A). Stains for Leu-7 are variably positive (B). Reactivity for glial fibrillary acidic protein is commonly seen (C), but is usually patchy. Collagen 4 reactivity corresponds to pericellular basal lamina (D). Neurofilament protein-positive axons, if present within the substance of schwannomas, are most often identified in the subcapsular region (see fig. 7-11C).

Immunoreactivity for glial fibrillary acidic protein (GFAP) may be seen in a significant number of schwannomas (fig. 7-24C) (87,93–95), including gastrointestinal cases (26). The frequency and degree of staining vary with the source of the antibody. The reaction is thought to detect a GFAP-like substance distinct from that found in the glial cells of the central nervous system. Such reactivity is of practical diagnostic significance, since benign nerve sheath tumors are more often GFAP reactive than are malignant ones, which are either nonreactive (88,94) or only sparsely reactive (93). Unlike neurofibroma, wherein CD34-positive cells may be seen throughout, schwannomas show reactivity only in Antoni B tissue, usually nearby the capsule (96). Despite the demonstration of CD68 staining in schwannoma (fig. 7-24D), we have not seen widespread granular cell change in this tumor.

Basement membrane staining for collagen 4 (fig. 7-24D) and laminin shows a pattern corresponding to that of reticulin (97). Both are particularly strong in Antoni A tissue and among the aligned, compact cells and processes that comprise areas of palisading and Verocay body formation. The types of collagen represented vary somewhat. Antoni A regions are collagen 4 immunoreactive, whereas Antoni B areas reportedly stain for collagen types 1, 3, and 4 (98).

Stains for neurofilament protein (NFP) are useful in assessing the relationship of a schwannoma to its parent nerve, the fibers of which reside in the capsule (fig. 7-11C) and in the substance of the lesion. Immunostaining for NFP is more sensitive in demonstrating nerve fibers than the Bodian and Bielschowsky silver impregnation methods. Two recent studies of NFP positivity in conventional schwannomas found a higher number of axons than previously thought. In a study of 31 schwannomas of the skin looking for axons inside and not at the periphery of the tumors, Wechsler et al. (5) found them in 4 of 12 schwannomatosis-associated, and 3 of 7 NF2-associated schwannomas; none were noted in 12 solitary schwannomas. In a second study, Nascimento and Fletcher (4) identified intratumoral axon filaments in 11 of 20 conventional and 7 of 20 ancient schwannomas: in the former group they were most often rare, focal, or multifocal, and almost equally

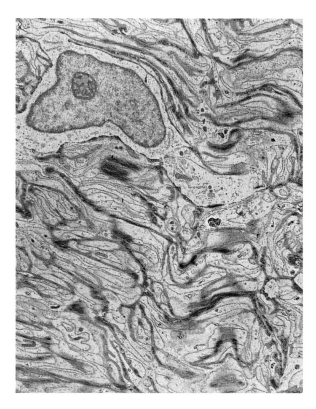

Figure 7-25

SCHWANNOMA: ANTONI A TISSUE

Ultrastructurally, Antoni A tissue consists of closely packed neoplastic Schwann cell processes that are coated on their free surfaces by basal lamina substance.

peripherally and centrally situated; in the latter group they were rare, focal, or multifocal, with a majority peripherally located.

While staining for vimentin is of little diagnostic utility, a positive reaction serves as evidence of immunoviability. Vimentin staining is strong in schwannomas, as well as in other nerve sheath tumors (99). Given the striking histologic similarity to GIST, suspected gastrointestinal schwannomas should be nonreactive for CD117 (100).

Ultrastructural Findings. Although electron microscopy usually is not required for the routine diagnosis of schwannoma, a working knowledge of the ultrastructural features of this lesion is useful in the differential diagnosis. Antoni A tissue is composed of neoplastic Schwann cells having prominent, long cytoplasmic processes, often complexly entangled (fig. 7-25) and joined by widely scattered rudimentary cell junctions (66,71,101–103). Their smooth-contoured

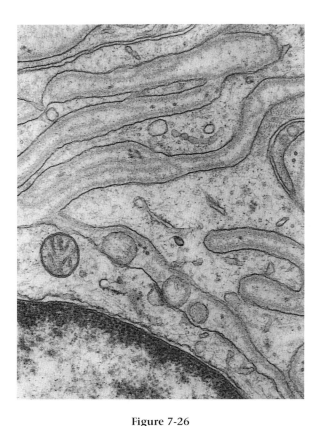

Figure 7-26

SCHWANNOMA: ANTONI A TISSUE

A detail of neoplastic Schwann cell processes. Occasionally, there is replication of basal lamina in the intercellular spaces.

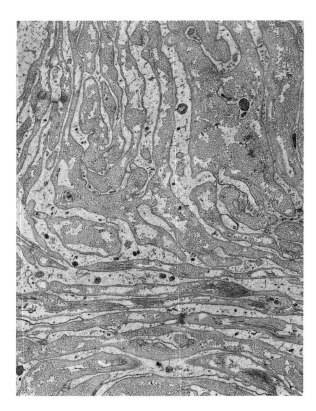

Figure 7-27

SCHWANNOMA: VEROCAY BODY

The central portion of a Verocay body consists of generally straight Schwann cell processes with prominent intervening collagen/basal lamina stroma.

nuclei are elongated and contain delicate, dispersed chromatin and one or two micronucleoli. The perinuclear cytoplasm features a small Golgi apparatus, scattered mitochondria, short profiles of rough endoplasmic reticulum, ribosomes and polysomes, primary and secondary lysosomes, and occasional small lipid droplets (fig. 7-26). The prominent, intertwined cell processes generally contain few organelles other than scattered arrays of intermediate filaments and microtubules, as well as small vesicles (fig. 7-26). The architecture of the Verocay bodies is distinctive: their central anucleate portions are composed of closely packed, long, parallel cell processes covered by basement membrane substance and separated by collagen fibrils (fig. 7-27) (71). The main constituents of the generally sparse stroma include reduplicated basement membrane, bundles of ordinary collagen fibrils (7-26), and often bundles of long-spacing

(130-nm periodicity) collagen referred to as Luse bodies (fig. 7-28).

In contrast, Antoni type B tissue is less cellular and consists of dispersed neoplastic Schwann cells with convoluted cell processes, separated by a flocculent matrix of low electron density and scattered collagen fibrils (fig. 7-29). The Schwann cell nuclei in Antoni B areas often are somewhat pleomorphic and may contain more clumped chromatin than do those in Antoni A tissue. The frequent finding of secondary lysosomes and myelin figures may reflect cell degeneration (fig. 7-30) (104). The blood vessels of schwannoma characteristically exhibit a thickened basement membrane (102,104,105) and are fenestrated (106).

Differential Diagnosis. A number of lesions enter into the differential diagnosis of conventional schwannoma. Principal among these are cellular schwannoma (see below), neurofibroma, nerve

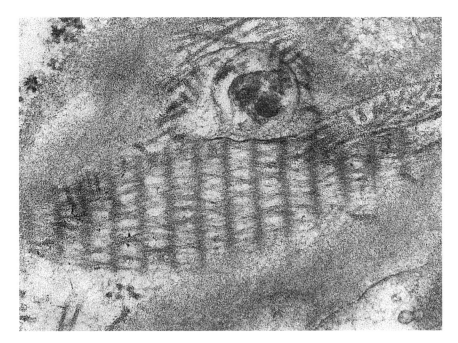

Figure 7-28

SCHWANNOMA

A portion of the intercellular stroma contains a Luse body, typical collagen fibrils, and basal lamina substance.

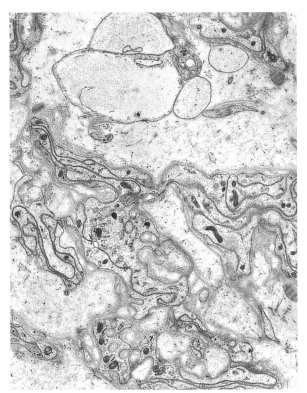

Figure 7-29

SCHWANNOMA: ANTONI B TISSUE

Schwann cell processes in a prominent stroma contain sparse basal lamina substance and collagen fibrils. Some Schwann cell processes are dilated.

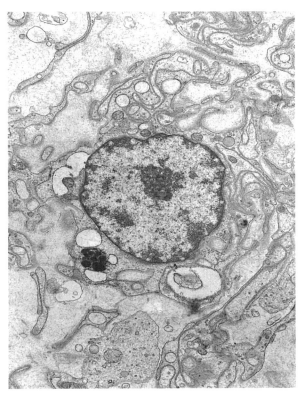

Figure 7-30

SCHWANNOMA: ANTONI B TISSUE

There is a cluster of lysosomes in the perinuclear cytoplasm and in the dilated rough endoplasmic reticulum (RER) cisternae.

sheath myxoma, and MPNST. Other lesions to be considered are ganglioneuroma, leiomyoma, palisaded myofibroblastoma, pleomorphic hyalinizing angioectatic tumor of soft parts, and GIST. Two central nervous system tumors, meningioma and pilocytic astrocytoma, can also be histologically confused with schwannoma.

Distinguishing schwannoma from neurofibroma usually poses no problem (see Table 7-1); confusion may occur because the loose-textured Antoni B tissue of schwannoma sometimes closely mimic neurofibroma (66). Attention to the overall architectural and immunocytochemical features usually resolves the issue. Neurofibromas are surrounded by a variably thickened perineurium and epineurium, but lack the thick, collagenous capsule of most schwannomas. Furthermore, many neurofibromas, notably plexiform examples, diffusely infiltrate surrounding soft tissue. Neurofibromas lack the Antoni A and B patterns of schwannoma, but rare plexiform examples contain nodules of neoplastic Schwann cells resembling mini-schwannomas (see chapter 8). Unlike most schwannomas, neurofibromas often possess a widely distributed mucinous matrix readily appreciated with the hematoxylin and eosin (H&E) stain and contain abundant axons. Immunoreactivity for S-100 protein is seen in only a portion of the cells comprising neurofibroma, whereas reactivity is usually uniform throughout schwannoma. Neurofibromas also show cellular heterogeneity at the ultrastructural level. In contrast to the homogeneous composition of schwannomas, neurofibromas contain not only Schwann cells but fibroblasts and perineurial-like cells.

Schwannomas rich in mucopolysaccharide matrix (see fig. 7-16) may simulate nerve sheath myxoma (see chapter 10). The latter is unencapsulated, does not exhibit Antoni A and B patterns, and lacks Verocay bodies. Immunohistochemistry is of little use since both lesions are composed of Schwann cells.

Unlike most schwannomas, MPNSTs commonly invade surrounding tissues. The thickened fibrous tissue surrounding most MPNSTs is a reaction to invasive tumor cells and therefore represents a pseudocapsule, not a true capsule. Adjacent skeletal muscle grossly found to be adherent or microscopically incorporated

into the fibrous periphery of a MPNST may be part of the pseudocapsule. As previously noted, visceral schwannomas and those occurring at mucosal sites, such as in the nose or paranasal sinuses (67), often lack a capsule (fig. 7-7). In these settings, limited infiltration should not be overinterpreted as evidence of malignancy. The same is true of schwannomas associated with osseous destruction, as seen in giant sacral schwannoma. Their erosive effects upon bone are due to compression, not to permeative growth (44,101), which is a feature of MPNST. Hyalinized vasculature accompanied by histiocytes and hemosiderin deposition, characteristic of schwannoma, are not usually found in the MPNST. Aside from rare examples arising directly from a schwannoma, MPNSTs lack distinctive Antoni A and B patterns as well as Verocay bodies. The degenerative nuclear atypia in some schwannomas, which includes pleomorphism, smudgy hyperchromasia, and cytoplasmic intranuclear inclusions, is readily distinguished from the monotonously uniformly sized spindle cells with hyperchromatic nuclei characterizing most MPNSTs. Unlike schwannoma, occasional MPNSTs contain multinucleated tumor giant cells, and areas of necrosis are often ringed by palisaded tumor cells. Immunohistochemistry helps distinguish schwannoma from most MPNSTs since the latter generally show dispersed S-100 protein and Leu-7 staining. Reactivity for GFAP, a common feature of schwannomas and other benign PNSTs (95), is rare in MPNSTs (45,93,94).

Leiomyoma is considered primarily in tumors of skin, deep soft tissue, and gynecologic tract. Leiomyomas are unassociated with nerve and lack the thick capsule and hyalinized vasculature of schwannoma. Although smooth muscle tumors do not feature well-formed Antoni and B components, nuclear palisades may be seen, notably in some uterine examples where regimented palisades (sometimes reminiscent of zebra stripes) simulate Verocay body formation (fig. 7-31A). The nuclei of smooth muscle tumors, especially leiomyomas, are often blunt-ended rather than tapered. Smooth muscle cells also have a more densely eosinophilic cytoplasm and, unlike neoplastic Schwann cells, often feature distinct cell borders. Trichrome and phosphotungstic acid-hematoxylin (PTAH) stains often show red and

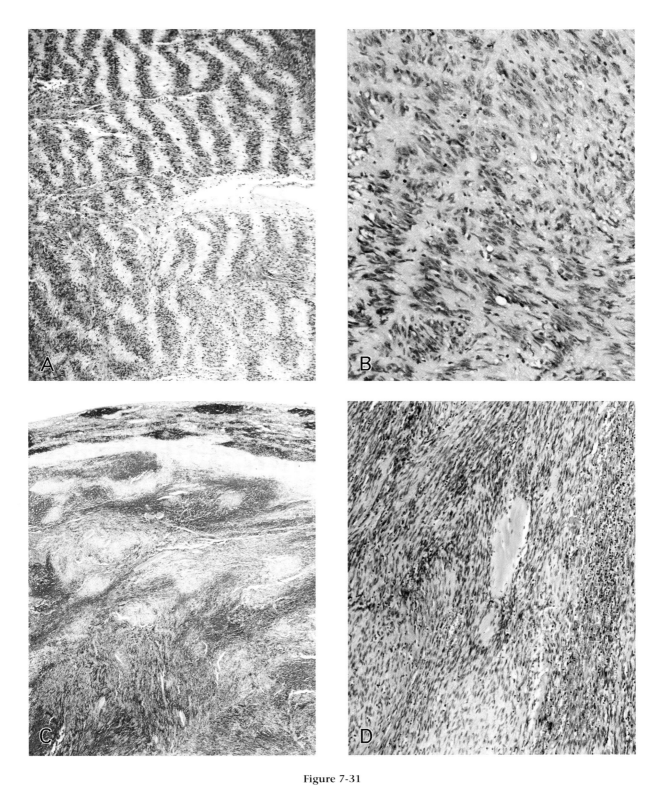

Figure 7-31

SCHWANNOMA SIMULATORS

Cellular growth patterns seen in some examples of uterine leiomyoma (A), gastrointestinal stromal tumor (GIST) (B), and palisaded myofibroblastoma (C,D) mimic those found in conventional schwannoma.

blue, longitudinally oriented cytoplasmic fibrils, a feature lacking in cells of schwannoma. These fibrils are less discernible with H&E stains, but immunohistochemistry readily settles the issue. Smooth muscle tumors, with some exceptions (107,108), lack S-100 protein staining and Leu-7 reactivity. Instead, they are reactive for myogenic markers, such as smooth muscle actin and sometimes desmin. The ultrastructure of smooth muscle tumors is highly distinctive. Their cells usually are bounded by a basement membrane, and they often contain parallel arrays of cytoplasmic microfilaments (actin) with interspersed fusiform dense bodies, subplasmalemmal attachment plaques, and pinocytotic vesicles.

The distinction of schwannoma from ganglioneuroma (chapter 10) only becomes an issue if the schwannoma, usually a paraspinous example, overruns or arises from a dorsal root ganglion. The anatomic distribution and uniform cytology generally distinguish normal ganglion cells of residual dorsal root ganglia from the haphazardly arrayed, often dysmorphic (multinucleated, vacuolated) ganglion cells that typify ganglioneuroma. Since ganglion cells in ganglioneuroma are surrounded by varying numbers of satellite Schwann cells, the simple presence of the latter does not distinguish ganglioneuroma from either schwannoma or neurofibroma involving a ganglion. The spindle cell component of ganglioneuroma is usually less cellular than that of schwannoma and more closely resembles neurofibroma. Ganglioneuromas are rich in unmyelinated axons, structures generally lacking in conventional schwannoma and neurofibroma. Axons are readily identified on immunostains for neurofilament protein. Myelinated axons are a prominent feature of normal and overrun dorsal root ganglia. Grossly, ganglioneuromas, unlike the globoid shape assumed by most schwannomas, are more pancake shaped. The cut surface also more closely resembles that of neurofibroma than schwannoma.

A diagnosis of GIST should always be considered when dealing with a possible gastrointestinal schwannoma. This is crucial in view of the frequent malignant behavior by GIST (109), and the necessity for specific treatment with the receptor tyrosinase inhibitor, imatinib mesylate (see chapter 13) (110). Most GISTs are composed

of uniform, somewhat syncytial-appearing spindle cells with pale eosinophilic cytoplasm, arranged in short fascicles or whorls. These findings are only suggestive of schwannoma. Real confusion with schwannoma arises when a GIST shows nuclear palisading. But, unlike in schwannoma, the palisading is sinuous and disordered (fig. 7-31B). Additional confusion results from the presence of patches of eosinophilic, periodic acid–Schiff (PAS)-positive, skeinoid fibers in some GISTs which may suggest the core of a Verocay body. GIST cells sometimes feature prominent paranuclear vacuoles. Gastrointestinal schwannomas, in contrast to GISTs have peripheral lymphoid cuffs and an occasional wire-like or microtrabecular growth pattern. Immunohistochemistry is of great help in the distinction. Intestinal schwannomas, in contrast to GISTs, usually express S-100 protein, often GFAP, but not CD117 (55,58). The marker nestin is not helpful in distinguishing the two tumors (58).

By its content of Verocay-like bodies and patchy hemorrhage, palisaded myofibroblastoma mimics schwannoma (111). Its location, typically in lymph nodes (fig. 7-31C), usually of the inguinal region, is diagnostically useful since unequivocal lymph node involvement by schwannoma has yet to be convincingly described. Cell palisading in the tumor is vague, and what at first glance appear to be eosinophilic centers of Verocay bodies are in actuality patches of amainthoid collagen fibers (fig. 7-31D) (112). Palisaded myofibroblastomas do not express S-100 protein but may show smooth muscle actin staining. Fibroblastic or myofibroblastic processes that may be mistaken for schwannoma can readily be distinguished by a lack of immunoreactivity for S-100 protein.

The pleomorphic hyalinizing angiectatic tumor of soft parts is a distinctive lesion arising mainly in the subcutaneous tissue of the lower extremity in adults (113). The tumor shares several features with conventional schwannoma, such as a spindle cell composition, with some degree of nuclear pleomorphism and nuclear-cytoplasmic inclusions as well as ectatic vasculature with partial hyalinization (fig. 7-32). Not surprisingly, of the 14 cases originally described, 3 had been misdiagnosed as schwannomas. In contrast to conventional schwannoma, pleomorphic hyalinizing angioectatic tumor

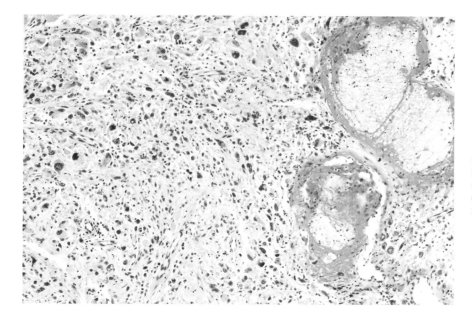

Figure 7-32

SCHWANNOMA SIMULATOR

The pleomorphic hyalinizing angioectatic tumor of soft parts, illustrated here, in contrast to conventional schwannoma lacks encapsulation and immunoreactivity for S-100 protein.

of soft parts is unencapsulated, lacks Antoni A and B areas, grows in an infiltrative fashion, sometimes forming satellite nodules, and lacks S-100 protein reactivity.

Among tumors of the central nervous system, meningioma, especially the fibrous type, is the chief histologic pitfall in the diagnosis of schwannoma. Both tumors have spindle cell growth patterns, may show cellular whorls, and are S-100 protein positive. However in meningioma the cellular whorls are tight not loose, and staining for S-100 is infrequent and only patchy. More significant is strong and diffuse epithelial membrane antigen (EMA) immunoreactivity of meningioma cells which, in addition, lack basement membranes, as demonstrable ultrastructurally and when stained for collagen 4 and laminin. Meningiomas are also reticulin negative. A less common problem is a pilocytic astrocytoma jutting into the cerebellopontine angle and presenting in a biopsy of a presumed schwannoma. Both schwannoma and pilocytic astrocytoma share expression for S-100 protein and are reactive for GFAP but, but unlike the former, the latter is devoid of a reticulin network (114).

Treatment and Prognosis. Optimal treatment of schwannomas is gross total resection with sparing of the parent nerve, when one is identified (see fig. 7-2). Although conventional schwannomas are benign, incompletely excised examples are capable of slow recurrence. So-called giant sacral schwannomas are especially prone to do so (46). As a result, the parent nerve may have to be sacrificed. On balance, however, the overall favorable outcome of schwannoma permits a conservative approach, such as "gutting" or enucleation with nerve sparing.

A recent clinicopathologic study found that NF2 patients with symptomatic schwannomas not only present with more severe neurologic deficits, but experience little postoperative improvement and a higher rate of recurrence (115). There is no evidence supporting the notion that schwannomas undergo accelerated growth during pregnancy (116). Lastly, malignant transformation of schwannoma is an exceedingly rare event (see chapter 12). When found, it thus far has almost always involved non-NF2-associated sporadic conventional biphasic schwannomas. We have reviewed the slides of a single NF2-associated schwannoma that underwent malignant transformation (68,117). We are unaware of any schwannomatosis-associated or gastrointestinal schwannoma having similarly transformed.

CELLULAR SCHWANNOMA

Definition. *Cellular schwannoma* is a schwannoma variant characterized by a largely persistent initial growth phase histology: high cellularity, a mostly Antoni A pattern, an absence of well-formed Verocay bodies, and often mitotic activity.

General Features. This is a variant of conventional schwannoma that is histologically often misinterpreted by pathologists as a conventional MPNST. Since its clinicopathologic characterization in 1981 (118), and despite initial reservations (119–122), several studies have confirmed that this schwannoma variant is benign (123–127). While they may recur, they lack metastatic potential. Slow clinical progression, lack of a significant association with NF1 (127), and failure to metastasize all distinguish this tumor from conventional MPNST. Ironically, when malignant change does rarely occur in conventional schwannoma it assumes a form other than a spindle cell tumor, and is most likely to develop in a classic biphasic conventional schwannoma. The recognition of cellular schwannoma permits nerve-sparing resection and obviates both radical surgery and unnecessary adjuvant radiation or chemotherapy for a tumor once regarded as malignant in about one fourth of cases (127).

Clinical Features. With rare exceptions (123,127), cellular schwannomas are solitary lesions. In the Mayo Clinic experience, they represent approximately 5 percent of benign PNSTs (123), and females are twice as often affected. Although they occur over a wide age range, with a maximal incidence in the fourth decade (127), nearly 5 percent present in childhood and adolescence (123). A similar small proportion (2 to 4 percent) occur in individuals who also have NF1 (123,125,127).

Cellular schwannomas grow slowly, some enlarging imperceptibly over a period of as many as 20 years. Most present as painless, palpable masses, but a minority produce neurologic symptoms including pain, paresthesia, and weakness. Occasional examples are incidentally encountered on physical examination or at radiography. Cellular schwannomas show a tendency to involve either the paravertebral region of the mediastinum, retroperitoneum, or pelvis, or the intraspinal space (123). Of the latter, approximately one third have a dumbbell configuration, and a similar number show bone erosion. In one large series, nearly 10 percent were intracranial, some affecting cranial nerves 5 and 8 (123). Other favored sites include the head and neck as well as the extremities (127). Tumors involving the limbs rarely occur distal

to the wrists and ankles (143). Dermal lesions are similarly rare (fig. 7-33D) (123). Resectability is in large part dependent upon tumor location. As mentioned, recurrences are few and slow to present; no metastases have been described.

Gross Findings. Like conventional schwannomas, cellular schwannomas are well circumscribed, encapsulated, lie eccentric to the nerve of origin, and most commonly are globular (fig. 7-33). Approximately one third arise from a recognizable nerve (127). They lack the fusiform shape common to MPNSTs, but on occasion are multinodular (fig. 7-34) or assume a plexiform configuration (see fig. 7-44B). Cellular schwannomas range in size from 1 to 20 cm (mean, 5 cm). Typically rubbery and mostly tan (fig. 7-33) with sometimes minor gray-white or yellow areas, only a small number show grossly evident cystic degeneration (fig. 7-33C). Foci of hemorrhage occasionally may be found but, unlike in MPNST, gross necrosis is not a feature. A smooth tumor margin is present, even in areas of bone erosion. Radiographic or operative evidence of the latter is most frequently seen in tumors of the lumbosacral region (127). A partial lack of a capsule is unusual (127).

Microscopic Findings. Microscopically, the close relationship of the cellular variant to conventional schwannoma is confirmed by several features, most fundamentally the presence in all instances of identical cytology and immunostaining characteristics (fig. 7-35). Additional supportive features are a well-formed capsule (fig. 7-36A), hyalinization of tumor vasculature (fig. 7-36B), and, less frequently, collections of lipid-laden histiocytes (fig. 7-36C). Architecturally, they differ from conventional schwannoma by their higher cellularity; more uniform pattern; frequent presence of capsular, subcapsular, and perivascular lymphocytic infiltrates (fig. 7-36D); and infrequent occurrence of hemosiderin deposits. All examples are dominated by Antoni A tissue (fig. 7-35) (118,127). An Antoni B pattern, although focally present in nearly two thirds of cases in one series (123), generally occupies no more than 10 percent of the tumor area and is often subcapsular (127).

Nearly one fourth of the tumors exhibit microcyst formation (123). Microfoci of necrosis are rare (see fig. 7-38C) (127), and are usually solitary. Such foci commonly consist of

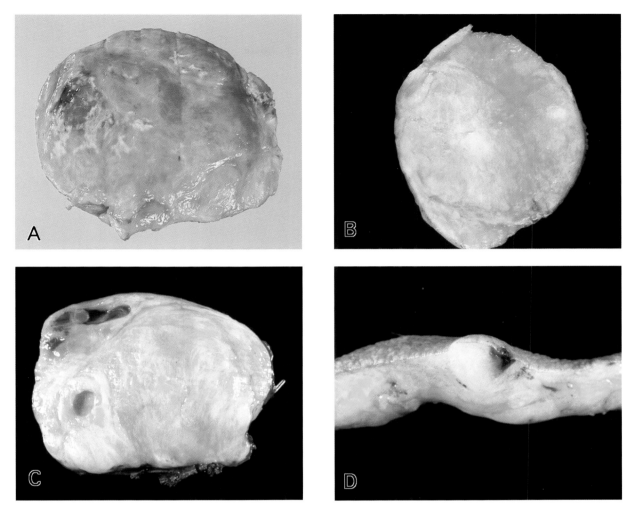

Figure 7-33

CELLULAR SCHWANNOMA

On sectioning, the cellular variant of schwannoma is firm and mostly tan to light tan (A–D). Lipid degeneration (A), small cysts (C), and a minor Antoni B component are occasionally found. Cutaneous examples are infrequent (D).

circumscribed areas of pale-staining tissue devoid of nuclear detail and, unlike the geographic necrosis of MPNST, are not sharply demarcated and lack pseudopalisaded cells. In some instances, the presence of necrosis is related to prior trauma (127). On close inspection, H&E-stained sections show the presence of residual nerve within the capsule in approximately 15 percent of cases (123). Focal tumor infiltration of nearby normal tissue is unusual (128).

The predominant Antoni A component of cellular schwannomas consists of sheets of interlacing spindle cells, with intertumoral and intratumoral variations in the degree of hypercellularity (figs. 7-35, 7-37). The cells have thin tapered nuclei (fig. 7-39A) with frequent but not invariable hyperchromasia. The cytoplasm is eosinophilic and afibrillar, and cell borders are indistinct (fig. 7-39A,B). Some nuclear pleomorphism may be present (fig. 7-39C) but generally does not approach that seen in ancient schwannomas (see fig. 7-23C). In some cases, focal features include vague storiform (figs. 7-35, left; 7-40A), ill-defined fascicular (fig. 7-40B), and whorled (fig. 7-40C,D) patterns. Among schwannomas, cellular whorls are most common in the cellular variant. Nuclear palisading in the form of single files of

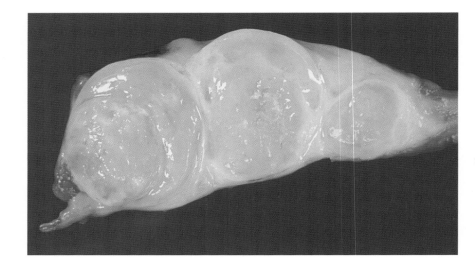

Figure 7-34

CELLULAR SCHWANNOMA

Gross multinodularity is an uncommon feature.

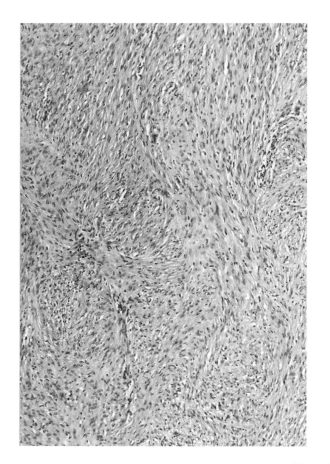

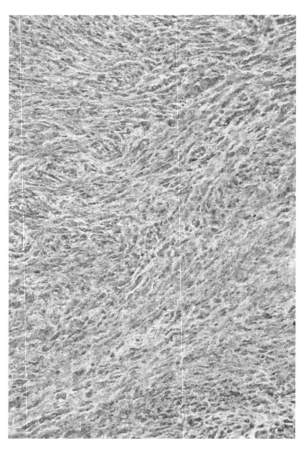

Figure 7-35

CELLULAR SCHWANNOMA

The two essential features are cellular Antoni A tissue with an absence of any formed Verocay bodies (left) and diffuse reactivity for S-100 protein (right).

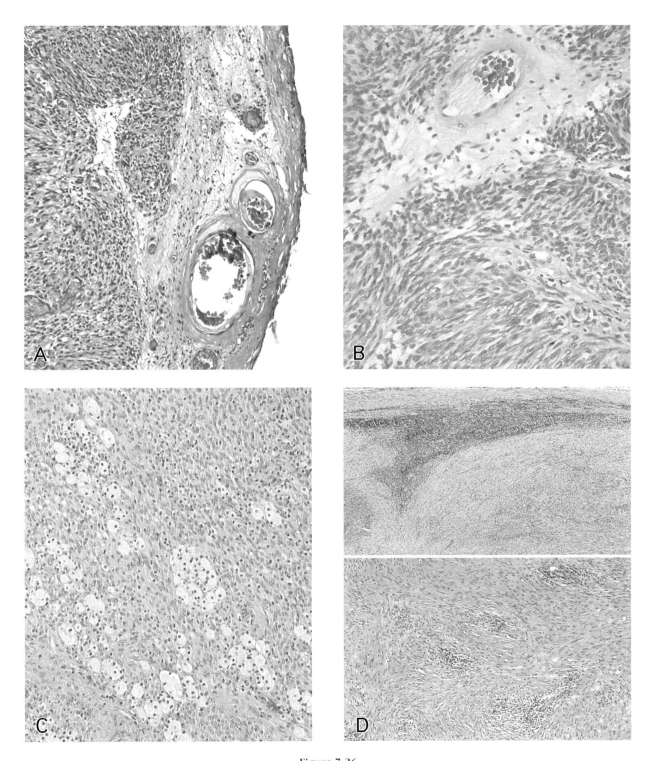

Figure 7-36

CELLULAR SCHWANNOMA

The tumors are typically encapsulated (A), here highlighted with a trichrome stain. There may be vascular hyalinization (B) and patchy histiocyte accumulation (C). Subcapsular (D, top) and perivascular (D, bottom) collections of chronic inflammatory cells are common findings.

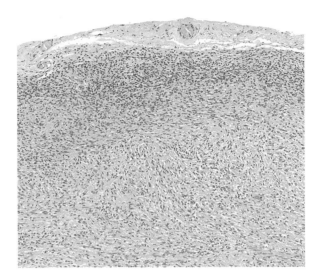 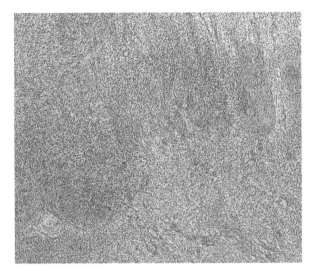

Figure 7-37

CELLULAR SCHWANNOMA

Hypercellularity may be uniform (left) or varying in degree (right).

nuclei (fig. 7-38A) is seen in 10 to 15 percent of cases (123,127), but well-formed Verocay bodies are not (127). As in conventional schwannoma, nuclei aggregated into irregularly shaped clusters are occasionally present (fig. 7-38B). Foci of loose-textured myxoid stroma superficially resembling that of neurofibroma are noted in approximately 10 percent of cases (123,127,128).

Most tumors show mitotic figures (fig. 7-39B), generally in the range of 1 to 4 per 10 high-power fields. In one large series (123), half of the tumors exhibited an average of 1 mitotic figure per 10 high-power fields. Although examples with as many as 8 mitoses per 10 high-power fields have been reported in the adult (127), we have occasionally encountered tumors with even higher proliferative indices (fig. 7-39D), notably in the pediatric age group (see below). Thus, we do not agree with those who believe that brisk mitotic activity is indicative of malignancy in these tumors.

Immunohistochemical Findings. As with conventional schwannomas, cellular schwannomas nearly always show strong, uniform S-100 protein immunoreactivity (fig. 7-35) (123–125,127). In contrast, Leu-7 staining is seen in only a third to half the cases and is irregular and patchy (fig. 7-41B). GFAP staining is evident in nearly half of tumors (123) and may be strong (fig. 7-41C). The presence of a

basement membrane is reflected in pericellular collagen 4 or laminin reactivity (fig. 7-41D), a finding anticipated by the result of a reticulin stain (fig. 7-41A). Unlike perineurioma, cellular schwannomas do not stain for EMA. The scant capsular reactivity for this antigen noted in half of cellular schwannomas simply reflects the presence of residual normal perineurium (129). Usually, the parent nerve within the capsule and sometimes in the subcapsular region is identifiable in conventionally stained material (123,124), but search for intratumoral axons is best conducted using stains for neurofilament protein (fig. 7-41E). Intratumoral axons, in the form of rare, focal or multifocal axon filaments, were found by Nascimento and Fletcher (130) in 15 of 20 cellular schwannomas.

Proliferation markers, including proliferating cell nuclear antigen (PCNA) and MIB-1 (Ki-67 antigen), have been studied in a large series of cellular schwannomas (123). Nuclear labeling for both proliferation markers varied widely; median values were 6 and 8 percent, respectively (fig. 7-41F). One recent series compared PCNA and MIB-1 staining in benign PNSTs, including conventional and cellular schwannomas, to that of MPNST (131). Whereas nearly all MPNSTs showed MIB-1 labeling indices in the range of 5 to 65 percent, neither conventional nor cellular schwannoma had indices exceeding 1 percent.

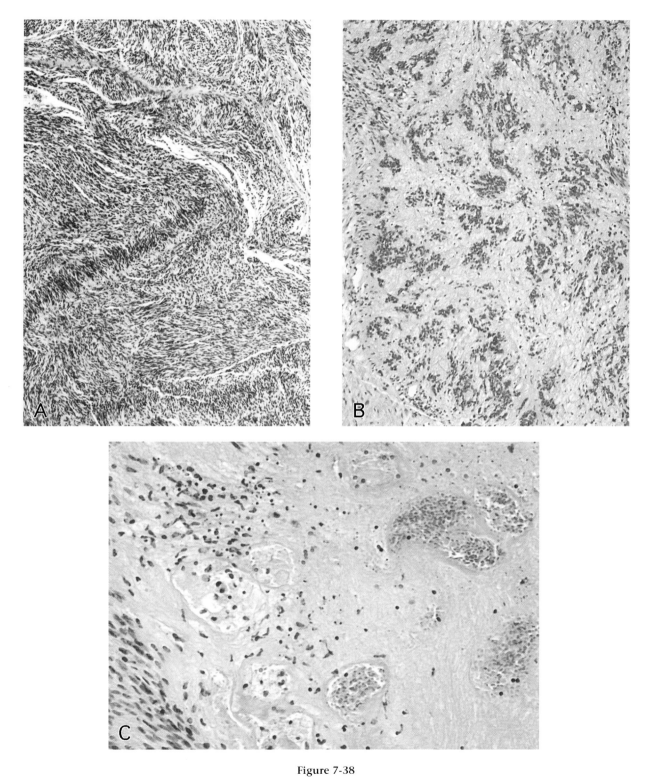

Figure 7-38

CELLULAR SCHWANNOMA

Unusual features of cellular schwannoma include regimentation of nuclei that take the form of single palisades (A) and focal nuclear clusters (B). Uncommonly, foci of nonpalisading necrosis, in some cases secondary to trauma, are found (C).

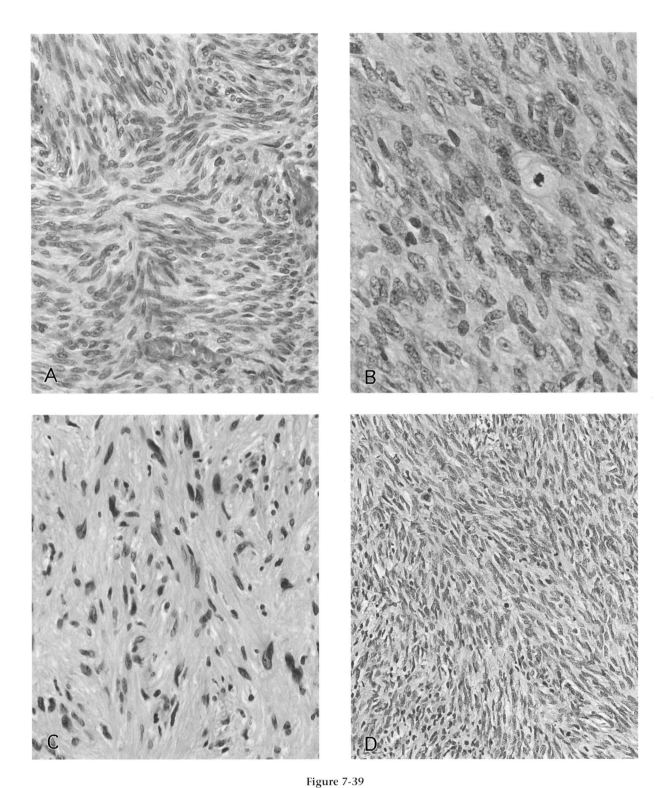

Figure 7-39

CELLULAR SCHWANNOMA

Nuclear uniformity is most often found (A), but slight nuclear pleomorphism (B) and smudgy degeneration (C) may be present. Mitoses vary from scant to occasional in most cases (C), but in some are conspicuous (D).

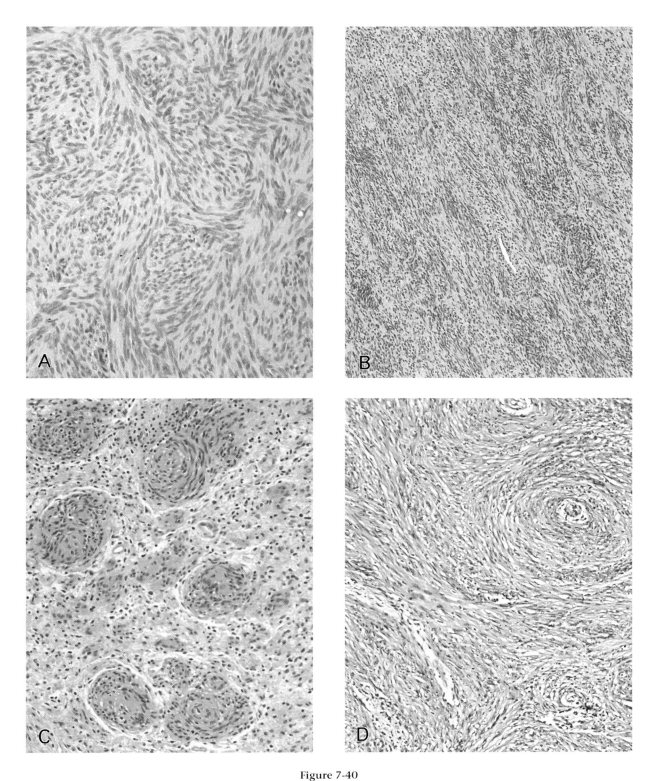

Figure 7-40

CELLULAR SCHWANNOMA

Although Antoni A tissue comprises most if not all of these tumors, the histologic pattern varies and includes curved fascicles (A), straight fascicles (B), and compact or loose cellular whorls (C,D).

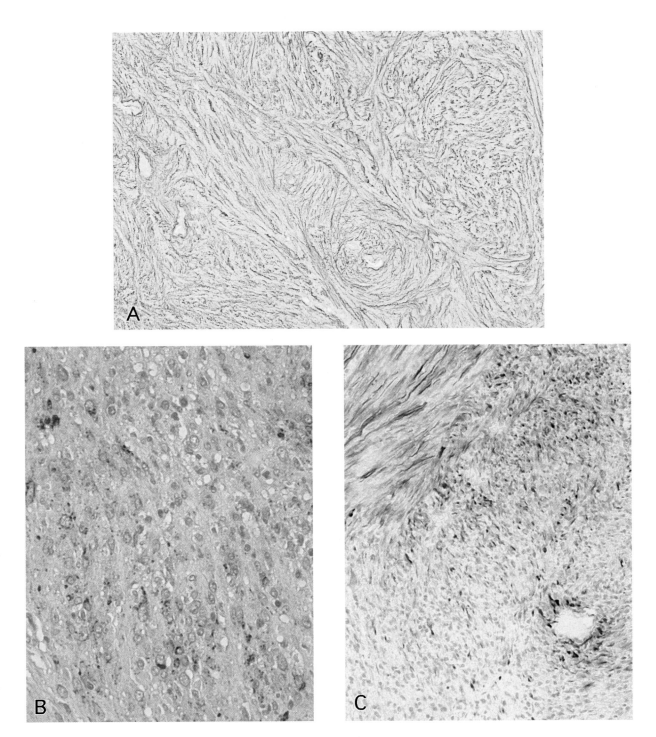

Figure 7-41

CELLULAR SCHWANNOMA

Due to the presence of pericellular basal lamina, like conventional schwannoma, the cells of cellular schwannoma are individually surrounded by reticulin (A). Similarly, there is patchy Leu-7 staining (B), frequent staining for glial fibrillary acidic protein (C), usually uniform pericellular reactivity for laminin or collagen 4 (D), and occasional residual neurofilament-positive axons in the subcapsular portion of the lesion or intratumorally (E). Stains for the proliferation marker M1B-1 often show moderate labeling indices (F).

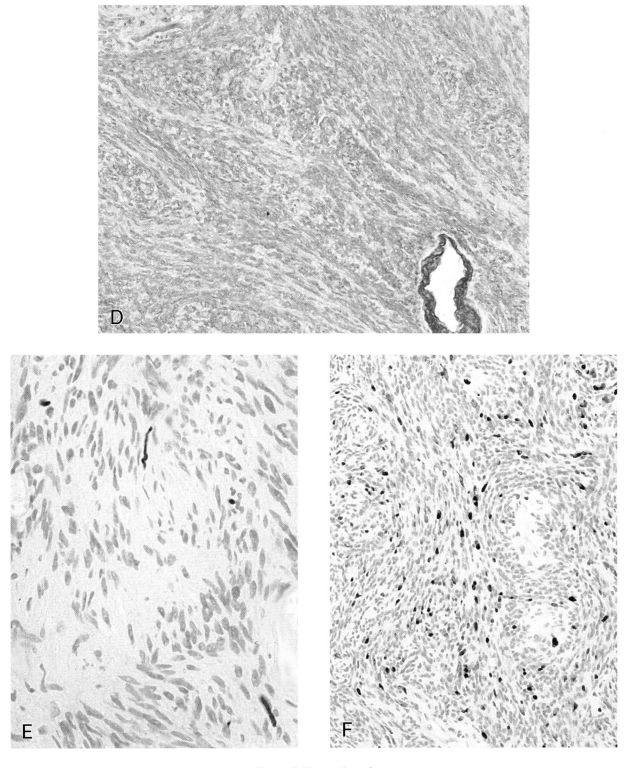

Figure 7-41, continued

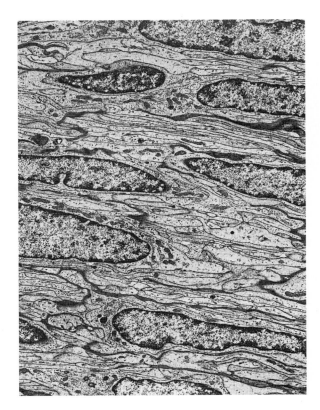

Figure 7-42

CELLULAR SCHWANNOMA

Ultrastructurally, nuclei are more abundant in cellular than in conventional schwannomas.

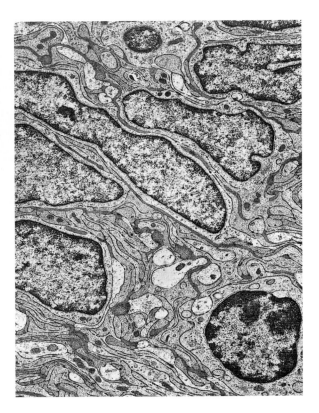

Figure 7-43

CELLULAR SCHWANNOMA

Nuclear pleomorphism, marginated chromatin, and tortuous arrays of Schwann cell processes are seen.

The indices of schwannoma and MPNST overlap considerably, and the most reliable cutoff value is 75 percent.

Ultrastructural Findings. Electron microscopy plays an important role in distinguishing cellular schwannoma from light microscopically similar tumors. Although it has been suggested that cellular schwannomas may be less fully differentiated than conventional schwannomas (132), we view them as well-differentiated neoplasms showing the full spectrum of Schwann cell features (118,123–125,133,134). Most conspicuous are elongated, interlacing processes covered with a continuous, occasionally duplicated basement membrane and joined by poorly developed intercellular junctions. As previously noted, the nuclei are more abundant and often more atypical than those of conventional schwannoma (fig. 7-42). This is manifested by irregularities in nuclear contour, an increase in heterochromatin, and larger nucleoli (fig. 7-43).

Abortive mesaxon formation, around bundles of stromal collagen, is less commonly seen than in conventional schwannoma. The cytoplasm is moderate in quantity and contains scattered nonspecific organelles, small numbers of intermediate filaments, and occasional microtubules. If sampling includes an Antoni B component, scattered lysosomes and cytoplasmic lipid droplets may be seen. The intercellular matrix varies in quantity, particularly in terms of its collagen content. Long-spacing collagen Luse body formation—a patch of long-spacing collagen—is less commonly observed in cellular schwannomas than in conventional tumors (123,127).

DNA Flow Cytometry. A study of the DNA flow cytometric characteristics of cellular schwannoma found two thirds to be diploid and the remainder equally divided among tetraploid and aneuploid examples (123). S-phase determinations ranged from 1 to 26 percent (mean, 6.6 percent); values for diploid, tetraploid, and aneuploid tumors were 5.5, 5.5, and 11.5 percent, respectively. No differences in S-phase determinations were noted among nonrecurring and recurring tumors.

Differential Diagnosis. Of foremost concern is the distinction of a possible cellular schwannoma from a differentiated MPNST. Salient features of each are summarized in Table 7-2. Unlike patients with cellular schwannoma, over half of those with MPNST have NF1 or tumors arising within a neurofibroma (see chapter 12). The gross presentation of an MPNST also differs from that of cellular schwannoma in that the former more often originates in large nerves, is frequently fusiform, and is not covered by a well-formed collagenous capsule but rather most often by a pseudocapsule. MPNST is gray-tan on cut surface, often exhibiting zones of necrosis. A definitive distinction generally rests upon microscopic findings. Cells of differentiated MPNST are equally as large as those of cellular schwannoma but, in contrast, are usually more uniform in size and shape and degree of hyperchromasia. Microfoci of necrosis in MPNST are typically geographic and often bordered by palisaded malignant cells. Vascular hyalinization, perivascular lymphocytic infiltrates, collections of lipid-laden histiocytes, hemosiderin deposits, and minor Antoni B components, common in cellular schwannoma, are lacking in MPNSTs. Mitotic activity, often is in excess of 10 per 10 high-power fields, is higher than in cellular schwannoma. Divergent differentiation, a rare occurrence in schwannomas of any type, may be present in MPNST. The uniform S-100 protein reactivity of cellular schwannomas differs from that of differentiated MPNST, where it is most commonly scattered or nonuniform. A notable exception is a small, diagnostically troublesome subgroup of well-differentiated MPNSTs that are diffusely and strongly S-100 protein positive. We have seen a few examples of this type which on biopsy material could not be confidently distinguished from cellular schwannoma. In such a case, staining for EMA and claudin-1, markers of perineurial cells present in the capsule of schwannomas but not in the pseudocapsule of MPNSTs, may provide a resolution. Although rare well-differentiated MPNSTs also exhibit limited GFAP reactivity (135), staining is far more often seen in benign

than in malignant nerve sheath tumors (136). The same is true of immunoreactivity for collagen 4 or laminin. Ultrastructurally, the uniform Schwann cell differentiation seen in cellular schwannoma is lacking in most MPNSTs, where cells are usually less well to poorly differentiated and exhibit only patchy basement membrane formation (133,137).

Cellular schwannomas on occasion exhibit foci resembling neurofibroma (128). Such lesions pose a diagnostic problem in that neurofibromas can give rise to MPNST whereas schwannomas only rarely do so. The distinction from neurofibroma rests with the greater cellularity of cellular schwannoma, the larger less uniform size and shape of its nuclei, and the common presence of some thick-walled vessels and perivascular lymphoid deposits. Unlike in neurofibroma, S-100 protein reactivity in cellular schwannoma involves virtually all cells, even those in neurofibroma-like areas. Lastly, sections stained for neurofilament protein generally show more residual axons in neurofibromas than in schwannomas.

Unlike cellular schwannoma, leiomyosarcoma lacks a fibrous capsule, and on cut surface grossly exhibits a distinctive whorled pattern. No nerve association is evident. Nuclei often are blunt-ended rather than pointed like those of most schwannomas. The cells of leiomyosarcoma have more distinct cell borders and denser eosinophilic cytoplasm, which, with optimal fixation, is fibrillated. Such fibrils are highlighted with trichrome or PTAH stains by which they appear red or blue, respectively. Immunostains for actin are frequently positive, but desmin stains are less often so. With an occasional exception, S-100 protein reactivity is lacking in leiomyosarcoma (138). Ultrastructurally, the cytoplasm of leiomyosarcoma cells is microfilament (actin) rich, especially in well-differentiated examples. On careful study, fusiform dense bodies, subplasmalemmal attachment plaques, and pinocytotic vesicles may be found. Basement membrane formation is common to both Schwann cell and smooth muscle tumors, but the latter lack Luse bodies.

Some fibrosarcomas have areas simulating cellular schwannoma. A clear distinction between the two most often rests upon the absence in cellular schwannoma of the herringbone pattern of some fibrosarcomas and failure of fibrosarcomas in general to stain for S-100 protein. Ultrastructurally, fibrosarcomas feature a well-developed, dilated and branching rough endoplasmic reticulum; a prominent Golgi apparatus; and an absence of basement membrane. The latter may, however, be focally present in myofibroblastic tumors.

Cellular schwannomas must also be distinguished from meningiomas, particularly those occurring in the posterior fossa, at the skull base, or in the intraspinal space. Unlike schwannoma, a nerve-associated tumor, meningiomas are dura based. Enlargement of the spinal foramen is a common feature of schwannoma but is infrequent in meningioma. Microscopically, meningiomas lack the fibrous capsule of a schwannoma, as well as Antoni A and B pattern variation. Although a hyaline vasculature is common to both, schwannomas more often show perivascular collections of lymphocytes. Collagen disposition in schwannoma is generally reticular, diffuse, and intercellular, whereas in meningioma it takes the form of bands or blocks. A dense intercellular pattern of reticulin staining is characteristic of schwannoma but not of ordinary meningioma or even the fibrous variant. Although both tumors may have cell whorls, such whorls are not as discrete and tightly wound in meningioma. Psammoma bodies, a common feature of meningioma, are limited among schwannomas to the melanotic form. At the immunohistochemical level, schwannomas are readily recognized by their diffuse, strong S-100 protein reaction. In contrast, only 20 percent of meningothelial or transitional meningiomas exhibit patchy S-100 protein reactivity (139), although extensive staining may be seen in fibrous meningiomas (140). A membrane pattern of staining for EMA is characteristic of meningiomas, and is not seen in cellular schwannomas. Reactivity for GFAP may be seen in central and peripheral nervous system schwannomas (123,141) but not in meningioma. Ultrastructure readily distinguishes schwannoma from meningioma. Schwannomas exhibit long entangled processes covered by basement membrane whereas meningiomas feature interdigitation of cell membranes and well-formed desmosomes, but lack basement membranes.

Treatment and Prognosis. Given the benign nature of cellular schwannoma, therapy should be conservative and directed toward sparing the parent nerve. Depending upon tumor location, the extent of tumor resection varies considerably among reported series. In studies dealing primarily with peripherally situated tumors, 90 percent were amenable to gross total removal, with a recurrence rate of 5 percent (129). In contrast, cellular schwannomas affecting the intracranial space, spinal canal, and paravertebral region are more often debulked; the frequency of their gross total removal is only 10 percent (142). The overall rate of recurrence in one series in which central lesions were numerous averaged 16 percent; recurrence was particularly high in intraspinal (33 percent), sacral (37 percent), and intracranial (40 percent) lesions (123). The rate of tumor growth, whether of primary or recurrent lesions, is slow. In the three largest series, the mean time to recurrence was 7 years (123,127,131). Occasional tumors undergo multiple recurrences. In some cases, the interval to recurrence may be as long as two decades. Although there is no statistically significant association between recurrence and PCNA or MIB-1 labeling indices, a statistically significant association with mitotic index has been reported (123).

We have seen only one cellular schwannoma that underwent a focal but extensive malignant change (143). Another tumor thought possibly to be an example because of the presence of prominent cellular whorls was so extensively necrotic that it could not be conclusively distinguished from a classic biphasic conventional schwannoma (141). In both tumors, the malignant element had epithelioid cell characteristics, a finding in keeping with cellular schwannoma being a variant of conventional schwannoma. No follow-up was provided in either case. The subject is further discussed in chapter 12.

PLEXIFORM SCHWANNOMA

Definition. *Plexiform schwannoma* is a tumor composed exclusively of differentiated neoplastic Schwann cells and exhibiting a plexiform, most often intraneural, growth pattern.

General Features. Schwannomas of the conventional or cellular variety are occasionally plexiform (144–155). Until the 1980s, there was a tendency to regard cellular examples as plexiform neurofibromas or MPNSTs. These tumors most commonly affect young adults.

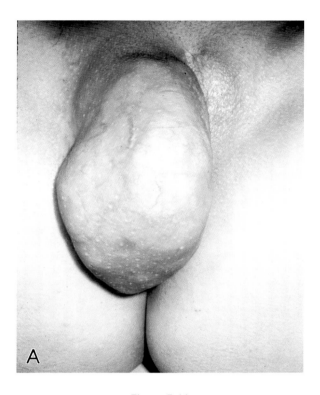

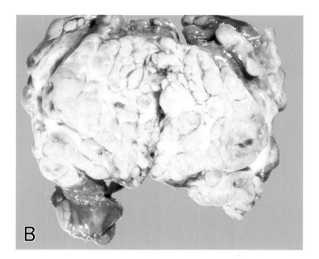

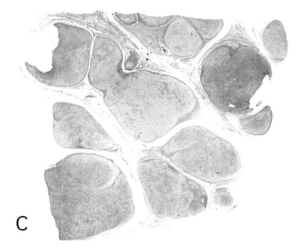

Figure 7-44

PLEXIFORM CELLULAR SCHWANNOMA

A: A gourd-shaped, 15 x 10 x 4 cm plexiform cellular schwannoma arose in the vulva of a 26-year-old woman.

B: The cut surface shows many nodules of varying size.

C: Macroscopically, the nodules were sharply circumscribed, uniformly tan, firm, sometimes interconnected, and thinly encapsulated.

Clinical Features. There is a wide age range for patients, from newborns to 80 years. About 75 percent occur in the first four decades. No gender predilection is noted. Only a small number of patients have been reported to have NF1 (152,154,156) and NF2 (151,157). Congenital examples have also been reported (145,148,154,158). Often, the mass is present for years before diagnosis. Only occasional tumors are painful or tender (152). Most plexiform schwannomas arise in the dermis or subcutaneous tissue. Most affect the head and neck or an extremity, followed by the trunk. Rare examples present in the oral mucosa (146,147), vulva (fig. 7-44), vagina (158), and penis (153). Visceral examples are also rare (fig. 7-45) (150). Multicentricity is infrequent (152,156,157).

Gross Findings. Plexiform schwannomas are usually circumscribed lesions which, on cut surface, are composed of tan or gray-tan interconnected nodules that may or may not appear to be nerve associated. Rarely are they suspected grossly (figs. 7-44A,B; 7-45A; 7-46A); most are similar macroscopically (figs. 7-44C, 7-47). Average dimensions range from 1.2 to 2.4 cm. Unless traumatized, tumor hemorrhage and necrosis are not grossly evident. As in conventional schwannoma, the occasional finding of compressive bone erosion is of no prognostic significance (see fig. 7-53).

Microscopic Findings. Microscopically, the tumors consist of oval to irregularly shaped nodules of roughly similar size (figs. 7-44C, 7-46B, 7-47). The nodules most commonly are surrounded by a thin fibrous capsule, but some appear unencapsulated; those in a few tumors are cystic (fig. 7-47). The number of nodular profiles comprising a tumor ranges

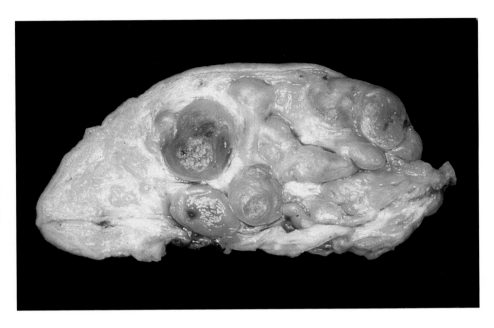

Figure 7-45

PLEXIFORM SCHWANNOMA

A large example growing from the skin and subcutaneous tissue of the hip of a 78-year-old man had been present for over 50 years. Plexiform growth imparts the appearance of a bag of worms.

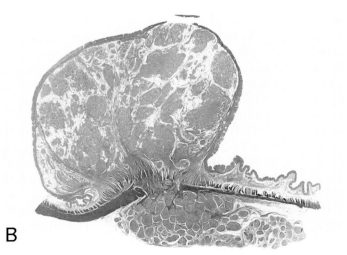

Figure 7-46

PLEXIFORM SCHWANNOMA

A: This large visceral example arose from the enteric nerve plexus in the colon of a 54-year-old man without neurofibromatosis.

B: Seen are the polypoid intraluminal and serosal components.

C: Microsections show the typical schwannoma features including some Verocay bodies.

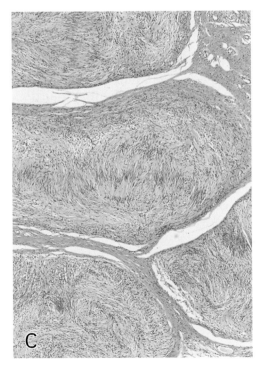

180

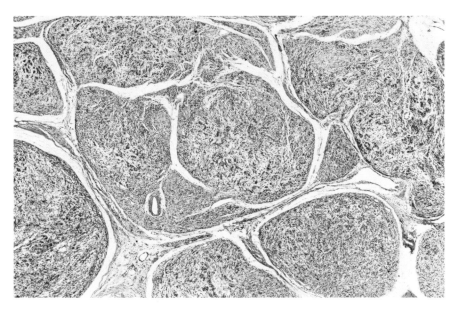

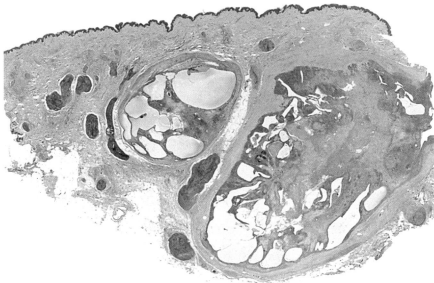

Figure 7-47

PLEXIFORM SCHWANNOMA

Top: Macroscopic view of a cutaneous example.

Bottom: A sizable cutaneous and subcutaneous tumor growing as interconnected nodules with cystic change.

from 2 to at least 50 (148,155). It generally requires serial sections to show that the nodular, puzzle piece-shaped profiles are interconnected (fig. 7-47). The tumors are composed entirely of compact cellular Antoni A tissue or have features of conventional schwannoma. Verocay body formation is uncommon (fig. 7-46C). More common are disordered arrays of palisaded nuclei (fig. 7-48A) and single nuclear palisades. The cytologic features of plexiform schwannomas are identical to those of conventional schwannoma (fig. 7-48B), with occasional examples dominated

by neval-like cells (fig. 7-48C). Degenerative nuclear atypia may be seen but mitoses are rare and necrosis is absent. The majority are sufficiently cellular to warrant the designation of plexiform schwannoma.

Immunohistochemical Findings. Plexiform schwannomas are diffusely reactive for S-100 protein (fig. 7-49) (152,153) and in most cases for GFAP (152). As in other Schwann cell tumors, reactivity for S-100 protein is both nuclear and cytoplasmic (153). Consistent but weak reactivity for neuron-specific enolase has been reported, but staining for MBP has

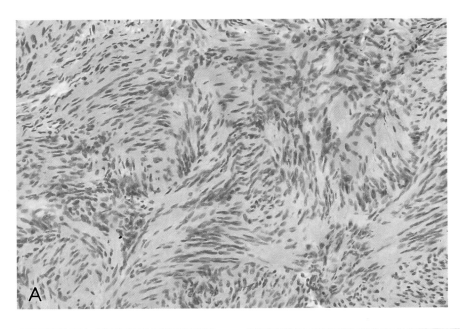

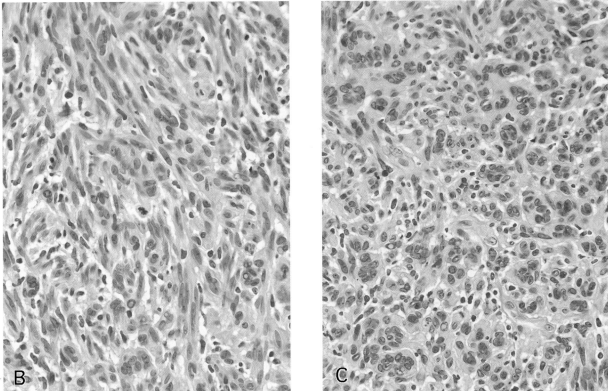

Figure 7-48

PLEXIFORM SCHWANNOMA

A: Some examples may feature nuclear palisading.

B: In most cases the cytologic features, which include spindle cells with dense eosinophilic cytoplasm, are those of conventional Antoni A tissue.

C: Exceptions feature neval-like cells.

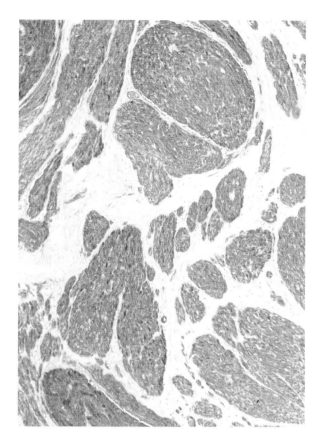 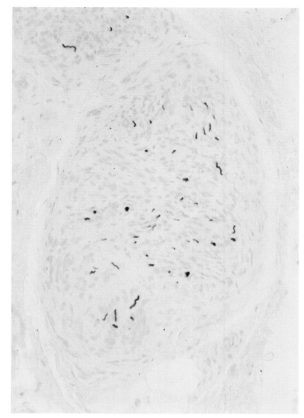

Figure 7-49

PLEXIFORM SCHWANNOMA

Left: The tumor cells are diffusely and strongly immunopositive for S-100 protein.
Right: Scant neurofilament-positive fibers are sometimes found.

not (152). Neurofilament protein stains show small numbers of residual axons within tumor nodules (fig. 7-49), a finding reported by Nascimento and Fletcher (159) in 3 of 10 cases.

Ultrastructural Findings. The fine structural features of plexiform schwannoma are identical to those of conventional and cellular schwannomas (figs. 7-26–7-30, 7-43, 7-50) (150, 155,160).

Differential Diagnosis. The differential diagnosis includes "true neuromas," such as palisaded encapsulated neuroma (PEN) and traumatic neuroma, and two neoplasms, plexiform neurofibroma and cutaneous leiomyoma. Plexiform schwannomas are most closely simulated by PEN. The latter, although usually uninodular, is occasionally multinodular and features vague microfasciculation, little or no well-formed nuclear palisades, no Verocay bodies, but far more abundant axons. Intralesional axons

are more prominent in traumatic neuroma, a process lacking the circumscription and nuclear palisading of plexiform schwannoma. In addition, a small obvious parent nerve is often seen in traumatic neuroma.

The distinction from plexiform neurofibroma is based upon the uniform appearance of ovoid to spindled nuclei in neurofibroma, ones smaller and more widely spaced than those of plexiform schwannoma. Furthermore, the cells of neurofibroma are often separated by large collagen bundles and lie within an abundant mucinous matrix. Unlike the uniform staining of schwannoma, S-100 protein preparations are reactive in only a portion of neurofibroma cells. Cutaneous leiomyoma is composed of cells with more dense, fibrillated cytoplasm, and may readily be distinguished from plexiform schwannoma by staining for muscle markers

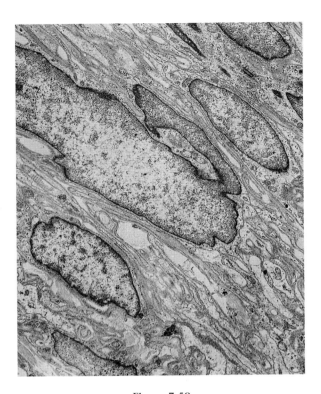

Figure 7-50

PLEXIFORM SCHWANNOMA

At the ultrastructural level, this tumor shows features typical of neoplastic Schwann cells, including cytoplasmic intermediate filaments and processes covered by basal lamina.

such as HHF35 (muscle common actin), smooth muscle actin, and desmin.

Treatment and Prognosis. The prognosis for patients with ordinary plexiform schwannoma is excellent following simple excision alone. Local recurrence may be a problem, however. This is exemplified by the largest plexiform schwannoma yet reported, a 15 x 10 x 4-cm tumor removed from the vulva of a 26-year-old woman (fig. 7-44A,B) (155). Focally, it had a mitotic count of 8 mitoses per 10 high-power fields. After two local recurrences, measuring 3 and 5 mm in greatest dimension, the patient was alive and well at 3 years. Treatment of congenital and childhood plexiform cellular schwannomas is more complex. Complicating the treatment are: establishing the correct diagnosis on an often small biopsy featuring histology which, to some pathologists is suggestive of a sarcoma; the difficulty during resection in obtaining tumor-free margins with respect to subcutaneous tumors because irregular

multinodularity obscures tumor limits and thin encapsulation invites tumor disruption; and parental pressure for aggressive resection of all recurrences in their child, even though most measure only millimeters in size.

Congenital and Childhood Plexiform (Multinodular) Cellular Schwannoma

This is a recently identified subset of plexiform schwannoma that was initially thought to be a possible congenital neural hamartoma (145), and later a plexiform MPNST of infancy and childhood (154). We subsequently reported 6 patients, and by combining data with that from the earlier reports, accumulated 14 cases on the basis of which we were able to establish the clinicopathologic features of this tumor (158). No gender preference was apparent. Slightly more than half of the tumors presented in infancy and, remarkably, 43 percent were congenital. In multiple cases, the congenital nature of a tumor only became evident on retrospective review of the pediatrician's findings recorded at the time of the child's birth. Most tumors involved skin and subcutaneous tissue, but the retro-orbital space and pelvis (fig. 7-51A) were also affected. Tumor size ranged from 1.5 to 9.0 cm, and one third were 5 cm or larger.

Grossly, the tumors were multinodular, thinly encapsulated (fig. 7-51B), and on cross section appeared uniformly tan, lobulated, non-necrotic, nonlipid-containing, and firm to rubbery (fig. 7-51C). The predominant histologic features were a hypercellularity of variably hyperchromatic spindle cells (fig. 7-51D,E) that were uniformly decorated by antibodies to S-100 protein (figs. 7-51F, 7-52B). These were arranged in fascicles, sheets, and patches; dispersed micronodules (fig. 7-52A); and lobules separated by thin fibrous tracts (fig. 7-51E). EMA immunostaining at the periphery of "infiltrative" micronodules (fig. 7-52C) indicated tumor extension along a nerve plexus. Mitoses were routinely found, and in areas of greatest proliferative activity, they ranged from 4 to 31 per 10 high-power fields. MIB-1 immunoreactivity of at least 30 percent was noted in three cases (fig. 7-52D). In terms of growth pattern, half of the tumors were well-circumscribed (fig. 7-51A,C), while the others had mixed, pushing and infiltrative margins or were purely infiltrative (fig. 7-52B).

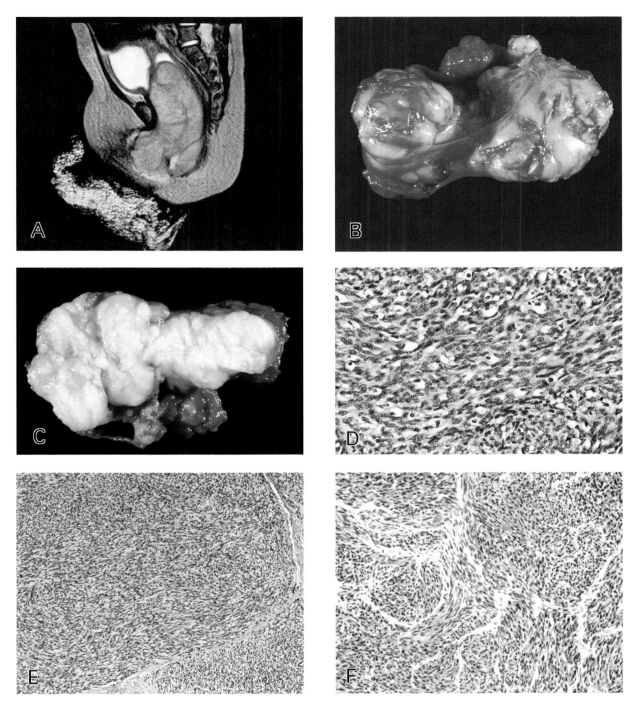

Figure 7-51

CONGENITAL AND CHILDHOOD PLEXIFORM CELLULAR SCHWANNOMA

A: Magnetic resonance image (MRI) shows a large, well-circumscribed congenital example in the pelvis of a 5-month-old girl.

B,C: Grossly, the tumor was thinly encapsulated (B), lobulated (B,C), and uniformly tan (C).

D: On biopsy, the tumor cells were crowded and hyperchromatic.

E: Resected tissue revealed compact, variably chromatic spindle cells that were divided into lobules by fibrous septa.

F: There was diffuse and strong S-100 protein immunoreactivity. The similarity to adult plexiform cellular schwannoma is clear.

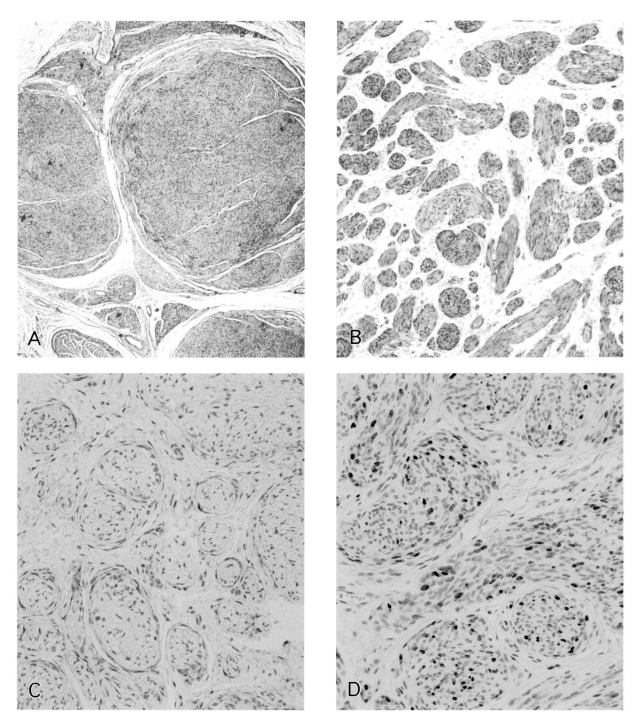

Figure 7-52

CONGENITAL AND CHILDHOOD PLEXIFORM CELLULAR SCHWANNOMA

A: This multinodular example arose in the calf of a 15-month-old girl and like the tumor in figure 7-51 was initially thought to be malignant.

B: The infiltrative component of such tumors consists of strongly S-100 protein-positive micronodules.

C: The peripheral lining cells stain for epithelial membrane antigen.

D: High MIB-1 immunoreactivity is seen.

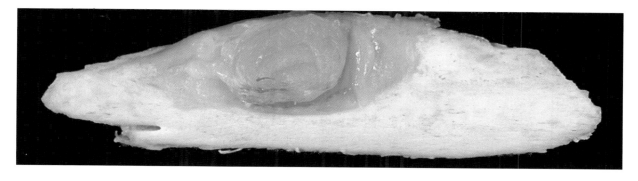

Figure 7-53

CONGENITAL AND CHILDHOOD PLEXIFORM CELLULAR SCHWANNOMA

Tibial bone erosion by the fourth recurrence of a subcutaneous tumor, originating in the calf of a 15-month-old girl and first resected 29 months earlier.

Local recurrence was almost the rule: of 11 children followed, 10 had recurrent or persistent tumors. No tumor metastasized, but one child died, an infant who at age 2 months had undergone exenteration of an orbital schwannoma, followed by a partial course of radiotherapy (8 Gy). His death, subsequently found due to an intercurrent infection (158), occurred 6 months after the exenteration and shortly after the discovery of a local recurrence.

Factors that early suggest that the tumors might be malignant include their high cellularity, hyperchromasia, and brisk mitotic activity; aggressive local recurrence, with one tumor on its third recurrence extending into adjacent cortical bone (fig. 7-53); and the above-mentioned fatality, initially attributed to tumor. Arguments for a benign neoplastic process include: the tumor's histologic resemblance to initial growth phase schwannoma (fig. 7-1B) and to adult plexiform schwannoma (figs. 7-44C; 7-47, top); lack of epithelioid cell change, anaplasia, and necrosis; tumors instead possessing the immunohistochemical and ultrastructural findings of entirely well-differentiated neoplastic Schwann cells (145,158); infiltrative tumors that take the form of delicately encapsulated nodules rather than individual cells, and are not pseudoencapsulated; and no recorded fatality directly resulting from primary tumor growth or spread.

MELANOTIC SCHWANNOMA

Definition. *Melanotic schwannoma* is a commonly circumscribed nerve sheath tumor of melanin-producing Schwann cells.

General Features. The tumor was originally described by Millar in 1932 (161) as a "malignant melanotic tumor of sympathetic ganglion cells". In 1961, Hodson (162) suggested that it was a form of schwannoma. Its clinical presentation, syndrome association, genetics, pathology, ultrastructure, and clinical course point to it being a distinct clinicopathologic entity (163). The lesion is classifiable as a PNST due to its frequent association with neurologic signs and symptoms, tendency to involve somatic and autonomic nerves as well as sympathic ganglia, and uniform composition of Schwann cells. Among schwannomas, melanotic schwannomas are unique because of their melanin pigmentation. Pigment production is attributable to the differentiating potential retained by cells of neural crest lineage.

The cells of melanotic schwannomas are predominately spindled and epithelioid, and are consistently immunoreactive for S-100 protein. Collagen 4 variably surrounds single or clustered cells. The ultrastructural features are also consistent with Schwann cell differentiation and include elongated cell processes lined by continuous or discontinuous basement membrane, as well as intercellular aggregates of long-spacing collagen. Dissimilarities with conventional schwannoma include the absence of clear-cut Antoni A and B tissue as well as Verocay bodies, the frequent presence of epithelioid cells, the more than occasional psammoma bodies and adipose tissue components, and ultrastructural evidence of melanin synthesis by tumor cells.

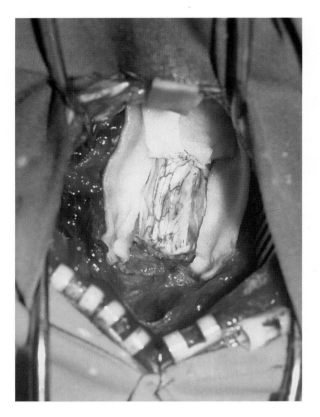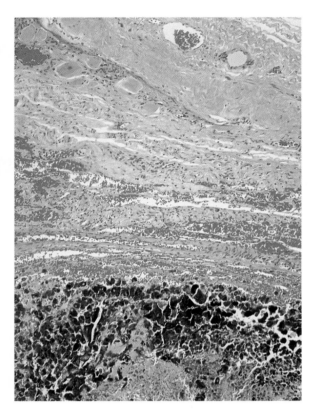

Figure 7-54

SPINAL MELANOTIC SCHWANNOMA

Left: At surgery, this deeply pigmented spinal tumor arose in a T5 nerve root, but was seen to be partially embedded within the spinal cord.

Right: More common are examples arising in nearby sympathetic ganglia; seen here is an affected ganglion adjacent to a heavily pigmented tumor.

Psammoma bodies are observed in approximately 40 to 50 percent of melanotic schwannomas. Over half such tumors, termed *psammomatous melanotic schwannomas*, occur in the setting of Carney complex (CNC) (see below). The nonoccurrence of conventional schwannoma in patients with CNC and of melanotic schwannoma in patients with NF2 underscore the fundamental difference between these two forms of schwannoma. A further difference is that malignant change in conventional schwannoma is rare; in contrast, between 10 and 15 percent of all melanotic schwannomas are malignant.

Clinical Features. Melanotic schwannomas occur in patients 10 to 84 years of age, but their peak incidence is in the fourth decade (mean age, 37 years). There is a slight female predominance (ratio, 1.4 to 1.0). Although widely distributed, about half (46 percent) show spinal nerve involvement, particularly at the cervical and thoracic levels (fig. 7-54). A minority involve autonomic nerves of the alimentary tract (stomach, sigmoid colon, rectum, and esophagus). Spinal nerves are more commonly involved by nonpsammomatous tumors, whereas most alimentary tract tumors are of the psammomatous type. Tumors of the trigeminal ganglion, acoustic nerve, sympathetic ganglia, and eye have been reported. Unusual sites include the heart, liver, bronchus, soft tissues, bone, and soft palate.

The symptoms at presentation relate to involvement of a nerve (pain or sensory abnormality) or to mass effect within an organ or soft tissue. Bone erosion may be noted, particularly in spinal nerve root tumors, the expansile growth of which affects vertebral foramina. Destruction of bone is more often a feature of malignant examples.

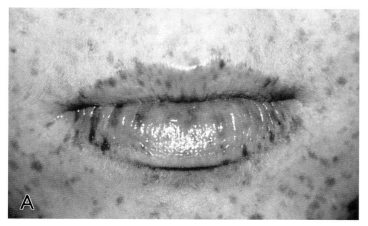

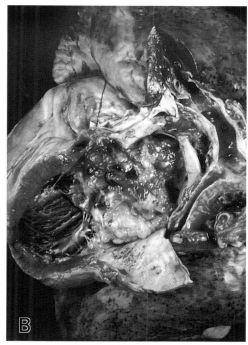

Figure 7-55

CARNEY COMPLEX

Aside from psammomatous melanotic schwannoma, a feature of many but not all cases of Carney complex, the disorder includes lentiginous pigmentation, here seen to conspicuously involve the face and lips (A); myxoma of the heart (B) or other sites; and endocrine overactivity, often Cushing syndrome due to pigmented multinodular adrenocortical disease (C,D). (Courtesy of Dr. J. A. Carney, Rochester, MN.)

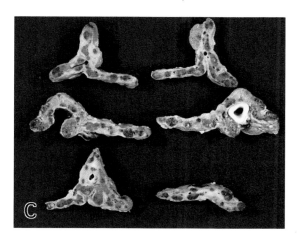

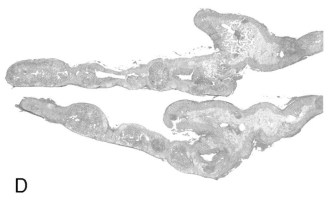

D

About half (55 percent) of the patients with psammomatous melanotic schwannomas have CNC (164). This is an autosomal dominant multiple endocrine and lentiginosis syndrome featuring a variety of tumors, among which melanotic schwannoma is common (165,166). Approximately half of CNC cases are familial. The mean age at diagnosis of patients with CNC and psammomatous melanotic schwannoma is 22.5 years, a full decade earlier than that of patients with melanotic schwannoma but without the complex. In addition to the melanotic schwannomas, which affect primarily posterior spinal nerve roots, upper alimentary tract, bone, and skin, the key features of CNC include: lentiginous pigmentation (65 percent); myxomas of the heart (65 percent) (fig. 7-55B), skin (25 percent), or breast (20 percent); endocrine overactivity (10 percent); blue nevi (10 percent) (164,165,167); and a most recently described congenital osteochondromyxoma (168). Pigmentation (fig. 7-55A) involves primarily skin and mucosae of the face (lips, lacrimal caruncle, conjunctival semilunar fold) and, in females, the external genitalia. Endocrinopathy includes adrenocorticotrophic hormone (ACTH)-independent Cushing syndrome caused by primary pigmented nodular adrenocortical disease (PPNAD) (fig. 7-55C,D), sexual precocity resulting from large cell Sertoli cell tumors of the testis, and acromegaly due to pituitary adenoma. The blue nevi affect primarily the extremities and trunk, are typically multiple, and may be either of conventional or epithelioid type (167).

Minimal criteria for a diagnosis of CNC have been published (168). The complex is genetically heterogenous. Two genetic loci have been identified, one on chromosome 17q22–24 (CNC1) (169) and the other on chromosome 2p16 (CNC2) (170). The former is the site of the *PRKAR1A* gene, which codes for the type 1 alpha regulatory subunit of the protein kinase A (PKA) haloenzyme, a critical component of numerous cellular signaling systems (171,171a). *PRKAR1A* is a tumor suppressor gene, and molecular studies have shown that it is mutated in about half of the CNC kindreds (171a,172). More consistent changes have been found for the CNC2 region on chromosome 2. These include amplification and deletion, separate or together, in 87 percent of tumor samples from CNC patients with and without germline, inactivating *PRKAR1A* mutations (173).

Some nonpsammomatous melanotic schwannomas are multiple; at least three individuals have been reported to have four or more tumors (164,174,175). The incidence of such tumors is unknown, however, that of the psammomatous variant is 19 percent (164). The majority of patients with multiple psammomatous melanotic schwannomas, 83 percent in one series (164), have the Carney complex.

Gross Findings. Melanotic schwannomas range from 0.5 to 26.0 cm (164,176); most are 5 cm or larger. Most are circumscribed and, rather than being encapsulated, are enveloped by a thin fibrous membrane, which may, in part, be interrupted by tumor infiltration (fig. 7-56, top) (164). Their configuration varies from round to ovoid or sausage shaped. Lesions affecting spinal nerve roots are often dumbbell shaped (164). Large tumors are occasionally lobulated (164).

On cut surface, melanotic schwannomas are usually solid and only infrequently cystic (164,177,178). Their texture is variously described as soft, firm, rubbery, or hard (164,179,180), and in some heavily pigmented cases, have the consistency of dried tar (181). The cut surface shows black-blue, brown, or gray pigmentation which may be uniform or unevenly distributed (fig. 7-56). Some feature

areas of hemorrhage (164,176,180,182) or necrosis (164,177). Occasional psammomatous tumors have gross subcapsular calcification and metaplastic bone formation (164). When seen, the bone destruction is generally associated with malignancy (fig. 7-56, bottom).

Microscopic Findings. Most melanotic schwannomas are quite cellular and are composed of spindle-shaped and epithelioid cells (figs. 7-57–7-59). Generally closely packed, the cells are usually arranged in lobules, short fascicles, or groups of curvilinear arrays (figs. 7-57A–E, 7-58). Palisades and microcyst formation are rare (fig. 7-58). The cells possess abundant eosinophilic to amphophilic cytoplasm. The outlines of the spindle cells may be indistinct, whereas those of epithelioid cells are often well defined. Scattered multinucleated cells are often present (fig. 7-57F). Less frequent are cells with vacuolated cytoplasm (fig. 7-60C) or clear cells (figs. 7-60C, 7-61E) (164). The nuclei are often round and contain delicate, evenly distributed chromatin and a small, distinct nucleolus. Pink nuclear-cytoplasmic pseudoinclusions are commonly seen (figs. 7-60C, 7-62C). Melanin pigment, in the form of brown to black granules, is present in varying amounts within both spindled and epithelioid cells (figs. 7-59, 7-62B,C). In some instances the Fontana-positive pigment obscures nuclear details. Other cells encountered include heavily pigmented macrophages (melanophages) (fig. 7-57A,C) and small collections of lymphocytes (fig. 7-60C). Potassium permanganate bleaching of melanin may be required to reveal the cytologic features of the pigmented cells (183), although some tumors feature only scant, patchy pigmentation. Occasional tumors show myxoid change or stromal fibrosis (fig. 7-59).

Psammomatous Melanotic Schwannoma. In addition to showing the histologic and cytologic features noted above, psammomatous melanotic schwannomas are characterized by the presence of laminated calcospherites (fig. 7-60A,B) (164). Often a focal finding, these spherical to oval, PAS-positive bodies range from few to numerous (164). Another feature, one evident in nearly 60 percent of the tumors, is the presence of cytoplasmic vacuoles having the appearance of mature adipose tissue (fig. 7-60B). Unlike in conventional and cellular schwannomas, the vessels are thin walled rather than thickened

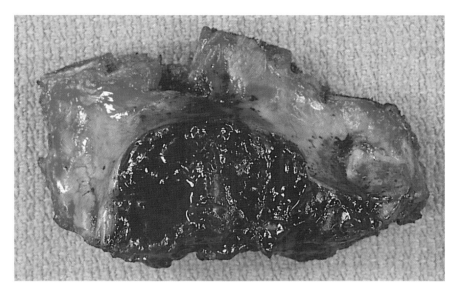

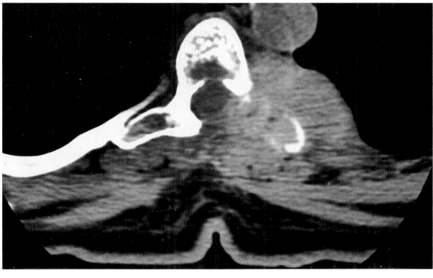

Figure 7-56

MALIGNANT PSAMMOMATOUS MELANOTIC SCHWANNOMA

This unencapsulated, paravertebral tumor, which on gross examination resembled dry tar (top), arose in the T6 nerve root, destroyed adjacent vertebral bone and a rib (bottom), and gave rise to multifocal pulmonary metastases.

and hyalinized. Local hemorrhage is noted in many instances, and focal necrosis in some. Infrequently, osseous metaplasia is seen at the periphery of the tumor.

Malignancy in Melanotic Schwannoma. In contrast to conventional schwannoma, a small percentage of melanotic schwannomas follow a clinically malignant course, usually after an initial local recurrence (figs. 7-61, 7-62). Of these, about one quarter metastasize (184), and of those, 15 percent cause death (164). Although the histologic criteria for malignancy in melanotic schwannomas have not been clearly formulated, the features common to clinically malignant tumors include large, vesicular nu-

clei with scant chromatin and very prominent eosinophilic or violaceous macronucleoli (fig. 7-62D); increased mitotic activity, including abnormal mitoses; and broad zones of necrosis (fig. 7-61C). While these features vary in combination in tumors that metastasize, none in isolation permits a firm diagnosis of malignancy. For example, macronucleoli may be seen in tumors that do not metastasize (164). On the other hand, metastases of malignant melanotic schwannoma may consist of uniform, unremarkable spindle cells having little or no melanin pigmentation, thus inviting a broad differential diagnosis. Figure 56.42 from Antonescu and Woodruff (181) illustrated such an amelanotic example involving

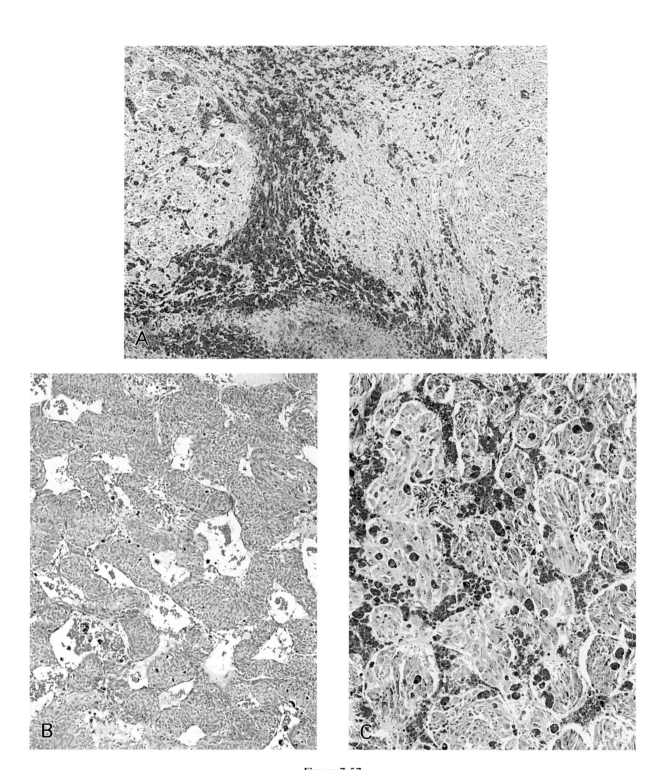

Figure 7-57

MELANOTIC SCHWANNOMA

The microscopic architecture may vary, but most tumors grow in sheets (A) or lobules (B). Although pigmentation is generally obvious, especially in macrophages (A center, C), sampling may show portions of the tumor to be nearly devoid of melanin (D). Uniform spindle to epithelioid (E) cells predominate, but bizarre hyperchromatic multinucleated cells may be seen (F). The latter are not diagnostic of malignancy.

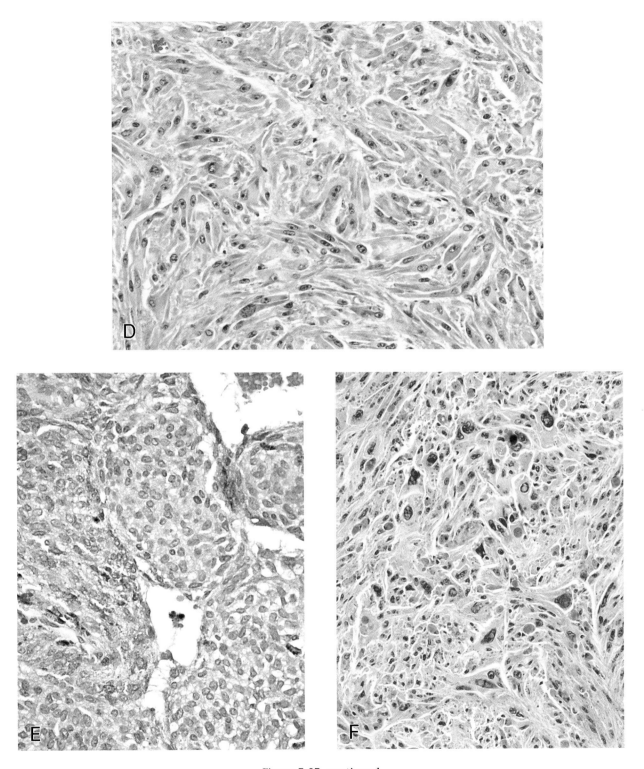

Figure 7-57, continued

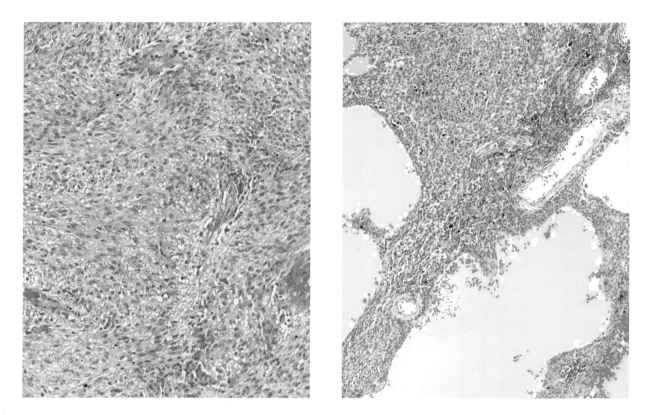

Figure 7-58

MELANOTIC SCHWANNOMA

Left: This gastric example features plump spindle cells with scant pigmentation.
Right: Portions of the tumor show microcystic change.

Figure 7-59

MELANOTIC SCHWANNOMA

Extensive collagen deposition in a spinal nerve root example.

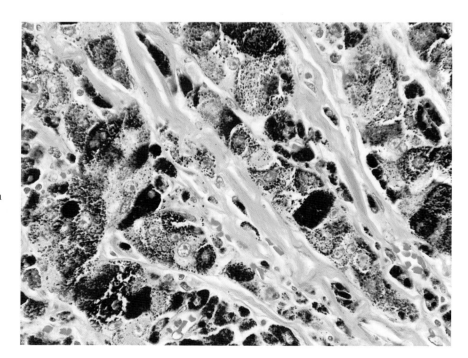

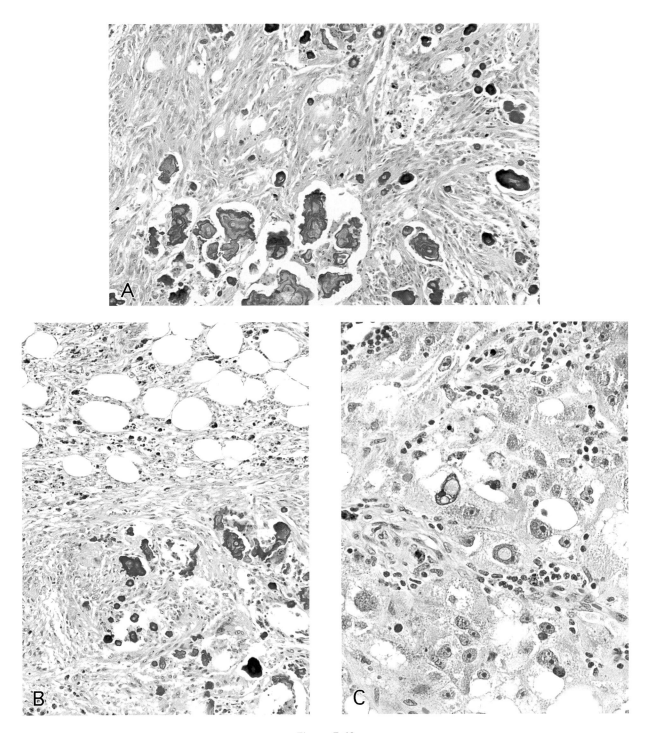

Figure 7-60

PSAMMOMATOUS MELANOTIC SCHWANNOMA

A,B: This example, occurring in a patient with Carney complex, has psammoma bodies of varying shape (A) as well as adipose-like cells (B).

C: Like conventional melanotic schwannomas, such tumors show cytologic variation ranging from spindle to epithelioid, with cytoplasmic vacuoles displacing nuclei that have open chromatin, nucleolar prominence, atypia, and nuclear-cytoplasmic pseudoinclusions.

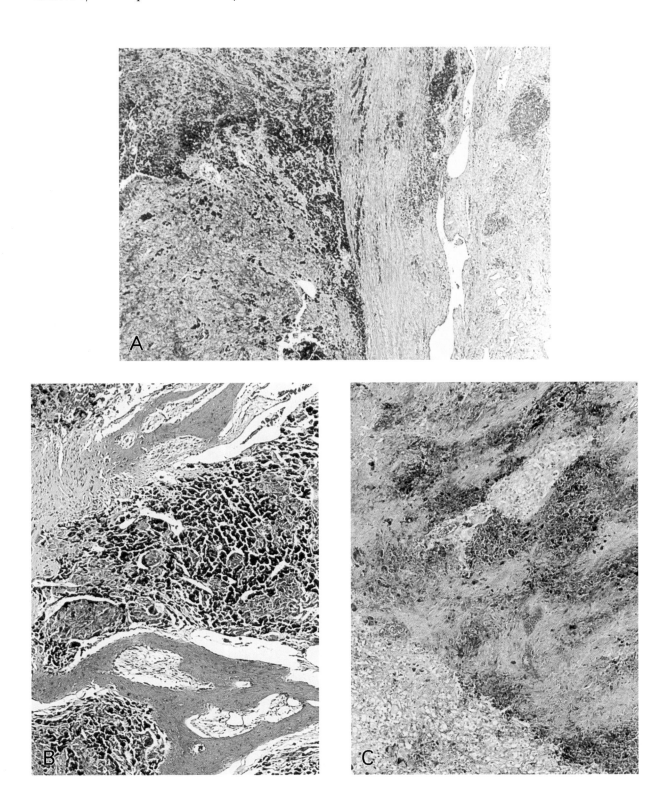

Figure 7-61

MALIGNANT PSAMMOMATOUS MELANOTIC SCHWANNOMA

This example invades peritumoral soft tissue (A), infiltrates bone (B), is necrotic (C), and has readily evident nucleoli and mitotic activity (D), clear cell change (D,E), and pulmonary metastases (F).

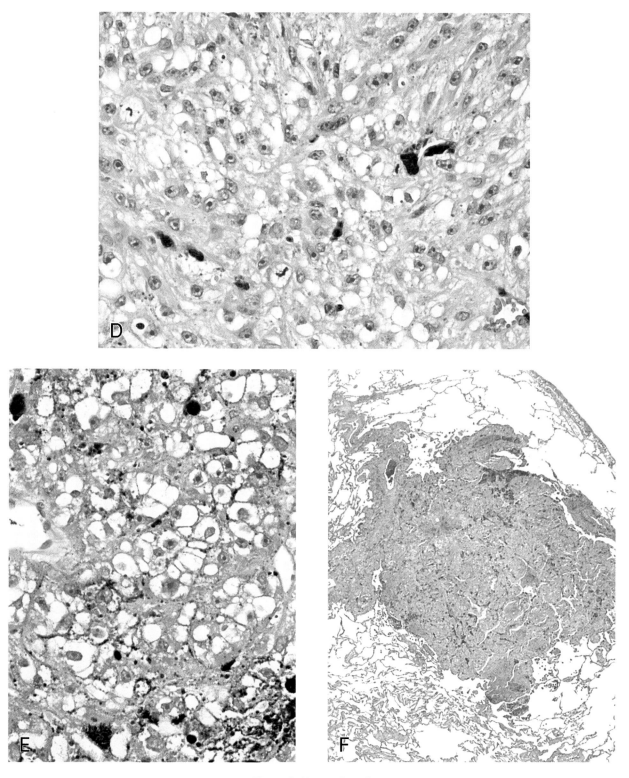

Figure 7-61, continued

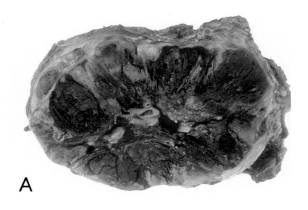

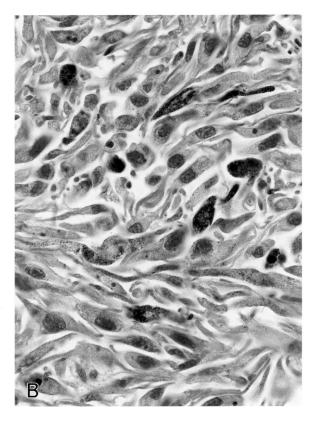

Figure 7-62

**MALIGNANT PSAMMOMATOUS
MELANOTIC SCHWANNOMA**

Histologic features of this pitch black example that arose from a spinal sympathetic ganglion (A) include cells that are plump and spindled (B,C), sometimes with prominent nuclear pseudoinclusions (C), and epithelioid with large violaceous nucleoli (D). The tumor metastasized widely and resulted in death two years after resection. (Courtesy of Dr. S. McClure, Akron, Ohio.)

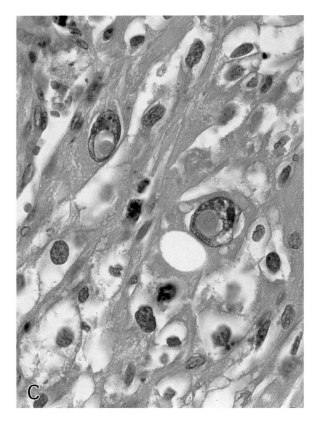

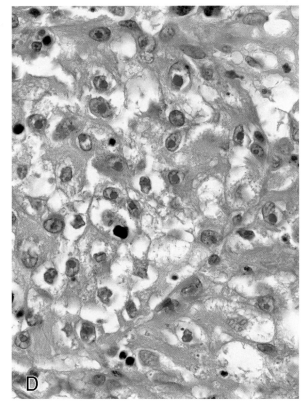

a metacarpal bone in a young adult woman. The tumor, containing a few psammoma bodies, presented as a solitary lesion of uncertain type. Subsequently, a history of Carney complex and an earlier resected spinal primary melanotic schwannoma came to light.

Cytopathologic Findings. Cytologic preparations may be of diagnostic assistance in the prebiopsy evaluation or in the assessment of a possible recurrence or metastasis. Based on three published reports, the key cytologic features were loosely cohesive clusters and isolated spindle cells with ill-defined borders and long, branching processes reminiscent of dendritic cells; elongated and pleomorphic nuclei with finely granular chromatin, sometimes prominent nucleoli and intranuclear inclusions; and cytoplasmic pigment ranging from delicate to coarsely granular and variable in amount (fig. 7-63) (185–187). A finding simulating adenocarcinoma is tumor cells with vacuoles peripherally displacing the nucleus and imparting a signet ring cell appearance (185). This cellular alteration is the counterpart of the adipose-like appearance seen histologically in many psammomatous melanotic schwannomas (figs. 7-60C, 7-61D).

Immunohistochemical Findings. The often bipolar, spindled and epithelioid Schwann cells comprising both benign and malignant melanotic schwannomas are immunoreactive for vimentin, S-100 protein (fig. 7-64A), and HMB45 (fig. 7-64B) (164,178,179,182,188–190). Additional reactivity is noted for the melanocytic cell marker melan A, microphthalmia transcription factor (MiTF), and melanoma cell adhesion molecule (Mel-CAM) (191). The basement membrane markers laminin (189) and collagen type 4 (fig. 7-64C) are also positive. There has been a single report of tumor staining for GFAP (189).

Ultrastructural Findings. Studies of melanotic schwannoma, primarily spinal nerve and sympathetic ganglion examples, have shown them to be composed of clusters of spindle-shaped or plump cells with long, often interdigitating cytoplasmic processes. The latter are joined by occasional rudimentary cell junctions and coated on their free surfaces by a continuous, often reduplicated, basement membrane (figs. 7-65, 7-66). In addition to these typical schwannian features (183), conspicuous melanosomes in all stages of maturation, most

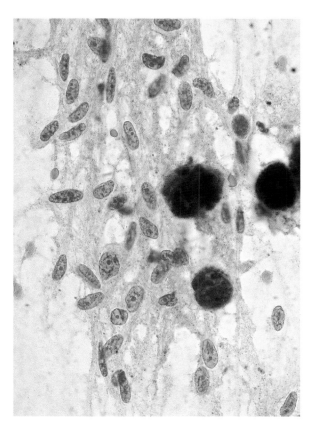

Figure 7-63

MALIGNANT PSAMMOMATOUS MELANOTIC SCHWANNOMA

This Papanicolaou-stained smear shows macronucleoli. The pigmentation varies and is most abundant in melanophages. (Courtesy of Dr. P. B. Illei, New York, NY.)

often stages II to IV, are readily found within the cytoplasm of the tumors cells (figs. 7-65, 7-66) (178,179,182,188,189,193–196). Nonspecific ultrastructural features include extracellular long-spacing collagen (182,195), variable numbers of surface micropinocytotic vesicles (188,195,196), and cytoplasmic intermediate filaments (188).

Differential Diagnosis. The differential diagnosis of melanotic schwannoma includes conventional schwannoma and pigmented lesions, such as pigmented neurofibroma, meningeal melanocytoma, metastatic melanoma, and clear cell sarcoma of soft parts.

Melanotic schwannomas are readily distinguished from conventional schwannomas. The former lack a distinct capsule, clear-cut Antoni

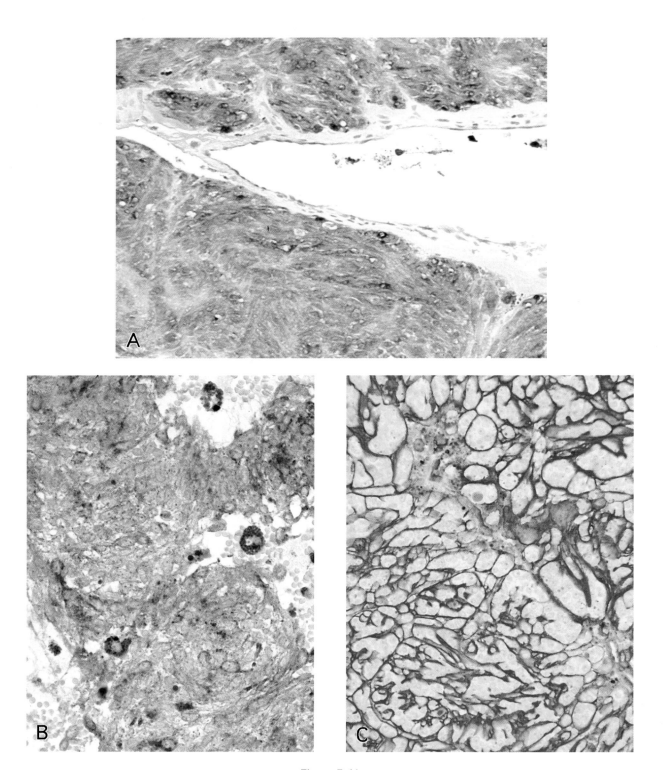

Figure 7-64

MELANOTIC SCHWANNOMA

The tumors are immunoreactive for S-100 protein (A) and HMB45 (B), thus sharing some features with melanoma. Prominent lobular collagen 4 staining (C) reflects the presence of pericellular basal lamina around nests of tumor cells (a feature also found in conventional schwannomas), an unusual finding in melanoma.

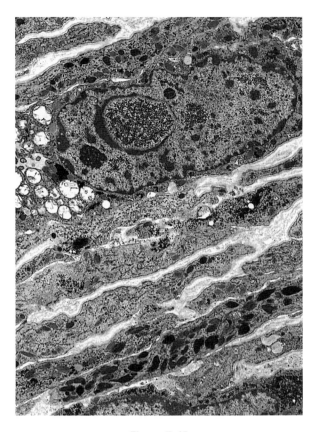

Figure 7-65

MELANOTIC SCHWANNOMA

The spindle-shaped neoplastic Schwann cells contain numerous electron-dense melanosomes as well as clusters of glycogen particles. There is reduplicated basal lamina in the intercellular spaces.

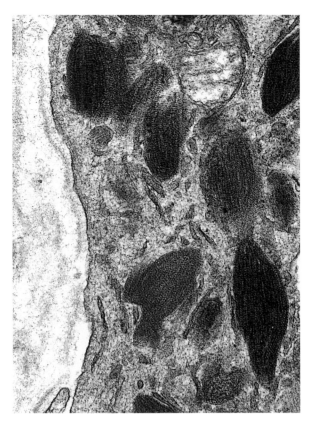

Figure 7-66

MELANOTIC SCHWANNOMA

Details of a melanosome-containing neoplastic Schwann cell process and basal lamina in the intercellular space.

A and B areas, and Verocay bodies. In contrast, conventional schwannomas lack melanin, psammoma bodies, and fat. The gray-brown granular pigment occasionally seen in ordinary schwannomas represents not true melanin but lipofuscin.

The distinction of melanotic schwannoma from pigmented neurofibroma (197) is more difficult. Such neurofibromas are often of the diffuse type, vary in size, show only microscopic pigmentation, and lack both psammoma bodies and fat. Their nuclei are small and often elongated, whereas those of melanotic schwannoma tend to be round with delicate chromatin and a distinct central nucleolus. The cytoplasm of melanotic schwannoma cells is generally abundant, whereas that of neurofibroma is usually scant. Immunostaining for S-100 protein is nonuniform in neurofibroma. The ultrastructural

heterogeneity of the cell types in neurofibroma also contrasts with the homogeneity of melanotic schwannomas.

Also in the differential diagnosis of melanotic schwannoma is melanocytoma, a central nervous system tumor with primarily melanocytic features. As more of these two tumors are critically studied, they may be found to represent a lesion continuum. Melanocytomas typically arise in the cranial or spinal leptomeninges (198–202), are largely demarcated and compressive of their surroundings, and consist of often heavily pigmented, polygonal to somewhat elongated or occasionally dendritic-appearing cells with vesicular nuclei and distinct nucleoli. Mitoses are scant to absent. The immunoprofile resembles that of melanotic schwannoma, although staining for collagen type 4 is less abundant and

201

often perilobular rather than intercellular. The distinction of melanocytoma from melanotic schwannoma may require electron microscopy. Features common to both tumors include melanosomes in variable stages of development, occasional intermediate junctions, and basement membrane production. Melanocytomas are devoid of psammoma bodies and adipose-like cells. In our experience, melanocytomas do not exhibit pericellular basement membranes, but membrane envelopment of cell lobules. Long-spacing collagen is also lacking. Lastly, tumor location is a factor in distinguishing the two lesions: we have never seen a melanotic schwannoma arising in the meninges.

Of greatest clinical importance is the distinction of melanotic schwannoma from metastatic melanoma. A paraspinal site is extremely rare for metastatic melanoma. Metastatic melanomas are rarely totally black, are soft or pliable in consistency, and lack the feel of dried tar often seen in melanotic schwannoma. Unlike the majority of melanotic schwannomas, most metastatic melanomas are obviously cytologically malignant. With respect to histology, Carney (164) refers to the dendritic appearance of cells of melanotic schwannoma, a feature uncommonly seen in metastatic melanoma. Melanoma cells are also devoid of fat as well as psammoma bodies, if the report of a melanoma with extensive calcification is excluded (203). At the immunohistochemical and ultrastructural levels, melanomas only rarely exhibit basement formation (204,205).

Clear cell sarcomas (soft tissue melanomas) (207,207) show a predilection for soft tissues, are both macroscopically and microscopically invasive, and are composed of cytologically malignant cells with little or no pigment production. Devoid of psammoma bodies and fat, they also lack evidence of basement membrane formation. Two features specific for clear cell sarcoma are scattered multinucleated giant cells with peripherally aligned nuclei and an underlying t(12;22) translocation (208,209).

Treatment and Prognosis. Most melanotic schwannomas are benign, slowly growing tumors, albeit ones that may erode bone. Among malignant examples, death due to disease, often metastatic, is as frequent with conventional as with psammomatous tumors. Of all reported patients with melanotic schwannoma, approximately 15 percent of those with conventional tumors (174,193,210–213) and 15 percent of those with psammomatous tumors have died of tumor (164). Melanotic schwannomas may be multiple and distinguishing between a second primary lesion and a metastasis may be difficult (164). Surgical excision with tumor-free margins is the treatment of choice for both melanotic schwannoma variants. Some patients with CNC experience additional morbidity and mortality due to associated cardiac myxomas or endocrinopathy.

REFERENCES

Conventional Schwannoma

1. Halliday AL, Sobel RA, Martuza RL. Benign spinal nerve sheath tumors: their occurrence sporadically and in neurofibromatosis types 1 and 2. J Neurosurg 1991;74:248-253.
2. Hamada Y, Iwaki T, Fukui M, Tateishi J. A comparative study of embedded nerve tissue in six NF2-associated schwannomas and 17 nonassociated NF2 schwannomas. Surg Neurol 1997;48:395-400.
3. Jaaskelainen J, Paetau A, Pyykko I, Blomstedt G, Palva T, Troupp H. Interface between the facial nerve and large acoustic neurinomas. Immunohistochemical study of the cleavage plane in NF2 and non-NF2 cases. J Neurosurg 1994;80:541-547.
4. Nascimento AF, Fletcher CD. The controversial nosology of benign nerve sheath tumors: neurofilament protein staining demonstrates intratumoral axons in many sporadic schwannomas. Am J Surg Pathol 2007;31:1363-1370.
5. Wechsler J, Lantieri L, Zeller J, Voisin MC, Martin-Garcia N, Wolkenstein P. Aberrant axon filaments in schwannomas associated with phacomatoses. Virchows Arch 2003;443:768-773.
5a. Feany MB, Anthony DC, Fletcher CD. Nerve sheath tumors with hybrid feautres of neurofibroma and schwannoma: a conceptual challenge. Histopathology 1998;32:405-410.
6. Hornick JL, Bundock EA, Fletcher CD. Hybrid schwannoma/perineurioma. Clinicopathologic analysis of 42 distinctive benign nerve sheath tumors. Am J Surg Pathol 2009;33:1554-1561.
7. Michal M, Kazakov DV, Belousova I, Bisceglia M, Zamecnik M, Mukenshabl P. A benign neoplasm with histologic features of both schwannoma and retiform perineurioma (benign schwannoma-perineurioma): a report of six cases of a distinctive soft tissue tumor with a predilection for the fingers. Virchows Arch 2004;445:347-353.
8. Erlandson RA. Melanotic schwannoma of spinal nerve origin. Ultrastruct Pathol 1985;9:123-129.
9. Stout A. The peripheral manifestations of the specific nerve sheath tumor (neurilemoma). Am J Cancer 1935;24:751-796.
10. Verocay J. Zur kenntnis der "neurofibrome," Beitr Pathol Anat 1910;48:1-68.
11. Stout A. Case 5. Neurilemoma of the sciatic nerve. Cancer Seminar 1950;1:8-9.
12. Murray M, Stout AP, Bradley CF. Schwann cell versus fibroblast as the origin of the specific nerve sheath tumor. Observations upon normal nerve sheaths and neurilemomas in vitro. Am J Pathol 1940;16:41-60.
13. Sainz J, Huynh DP, Figueroa K, Ragge NK, Baser ME, Pulst SM. Mutations of the neurofibromatosis type 2 gene and lack of the gene product in vestibular schwannomas. Hum Mol Genet 1994;3:885-891.
14. Stemmer-Rachamimov AO, Xu L, Gonzalez-Agosti C, et al. Universal absence of merlin, but not other ERM family members, in schwannomas. Am J Pathol 1997;151:1649-1654.
15. Rouleau GA, Merel P, Lutchman M, et al. Alteration in a new gene encoding a putative membrane-organizing protein causes neuro-fibromatosis type 2. Nature 1993;363:515-521.
16. Trofatter JA, MacCollin MM, Rutter JL, et al. A novel moesin-, ezrin-, radixin-like gene is a candidate for the neurofibromatosis 2 tumor suppressor. Cell 1993;72:791-800.
17. Jacoby LB, MacCollin M, Louis DN, et al. Exon scanning for mutation of the NF2 gene in schwannomas. Hum Mol Genet 1994;3:413-419.
18. Seizinger BR, Martuza RL, Gusella JF. Loss of genes on chromosome 22 in tumorigenesis of human acoustic neuroma. Nature 1986;322:644-647.
19. Bello MJ, de Campos JM, Kusak ME, et al. Clonal chromosome aberrations in neurinomas. Genes Chromosomes Cancer 1993;6:206-211.
20. Bijlsma EK, Brouwer-Mladin R, Bosch DA, Westerveld A, Hulsebos TJ. Molecular characterization of chromosome 22 deletions in schwannomas. Genes Chromosomes Cancer 1992;5:201-205.
21. Couturier J, Delattre O, Kujas M, et al. Assessment of chromosome 22 anomalies in neurinomas by combined karyotype and RFLP analyses. Cancer Genet Cytogenet 1990;45:55-62.
22. Louis DN, Ramesh V, Gusella JF. Neuropathology and molecular genetics of neurofibromatosis 2 and related tumors. Brain Pathol 1995;5:163-172.
23. Lodding P, Kindblom LG, Angervall L, Stenman G. Cellular schwannoma. A clinicopathologic study of 29 cases. Virchows Arch A Pathol Anat Histopathol 1990;416:237-248.
24. Mitelman F. Catalog of chromosome aberrations in cancer, 6th ed. New York: Wiley-Liss; 1998.
25. Koga T, Iwasaki H, Ishiguro M, Matsuzaki A, Kikuchi M. Frequent genomic imbalances in chromosome 17, 19 and 22q in peripheral nerve tumors detected by comparative genomic hybridization analysis. J Pathol 2002;197:98-107.
26. Lasota J, Wasag G, Dansonka-Mieszkowska A, et al. Evaluation of NF2 and Nf2 tumor suppressor genes in distinctive gastrointestinal nerve sheath tumors traditionally diagnosed as benign schwannomas: a study of 20 cases. Lab Invest 2003;83:1361-1371.

27. Izumi AK, Rosato FE, Wood MG. Von Recklinghausen's disease associated with multiple neurolemomas. Arch Dermatol 1971;104:172-176.

28. Evans DG, Huson SM, Donnai D, et al. A genetic study of type 2 neurofibromatosis in the United Kingdom. I. Prevalence, mutation rate, fitness, and confirmation of maternal transmission effect on severity. J Med Genet 1992;29:841-846.

29. MacCollin M, Chiocca EA, Evans DG, et al. Diagnostic criteria for schwannomatosis. Neurology 2005;64:1838-1845.

30. MacCollin M, Woodfin W, Kronn D, Short MP. Schwannomatosis: a clinical and pathologic study. Neurology 1996;46:1072-1079.

31. Gorlin RJ, Koutlas IG. Multiple schwannomas, multiple nevi, and multiple vaginal leiomyomas: a new dominant syndrome. Am J Med Genet 1998;78:76-81.

32. Salvati M, Ciappetta P, Raco A, Capone R, Artico M, Santoro A. Radiation-induced schwannomas of the neuraxis. Report of three cases. Tumori 1992;78:143-146.

33. Shore-Freedman E, Abrahams C, Recant W, Schneider AB. Neurilemomas and salivary gland tumors of the head and neck following childhood irradiation. Cancer 1983;51:2159-2163.

34. Sznajder L, Abrahams C, Parry DM, Gierlowski TC, Shore-Freedman E, Schneider AB. Multiple schwannomas and meningiomas associated with irradiation in childhood. Arch Intern Med 1996;156:1873-1878.

35. Woodruff JM, Selig AM, Crowley K, Allen PW. Schwannoma (neurilemoma) with malignant transformation. A rare, distinctive peripheral nerve tumor. Am J Surg Pathol 1994;18:882-895.

36. White W, Shiu MH, Rosenblum MK, Erlandson RA, Woodruff JM. Cellular schwannoma. A clinicopathologic study of 57 patients and 58 tumors. Cancer 1990;66:1266-1275.

37. Woodruff JM, Godwin TA, Erlandson RA, Susin M, Martini N. Cellular schwannoma: a variety of schwannoma sometimes mistaken for a malignant tumor. Am J Surg Pathol 1981;5:733-744.

38. Casadei GP, Scheithauer BW, Hirose T, Manfrini M, Van Houton C, Wood MB. Cellular schwannoma. A clinicopathologic, DNA flow cytometric, and proliferation marker study of 70 patients. Cancer 1995;75:1109-1119.

39. Fletcher CD, Davies SE. Benign plexiform (multinodular) schwannoma: a rare tumour unassociated with neurofibromatosis. Histopathology 1986;10:971-980.

40. Hirose T, Scheithauer BW, Sano T. Giant plexiform schwannoma: a report of two cases with soft tissue and visceral involvement. Mod Pathol 1997;10:1075-1081.

41. Woodruff JM, Marshall ML, Godwin TA, Funkhouser JW, Thompson NJ, Erlandson RA. Plexiform (multinodular) schwannoma. A tumor simulating the plexiform neurofibroma. Am J Surg Pathol 1983;7:691-697.

42. Celli P, Ferrante L, Acqui M, Mastronardi L, Fortuna A, Palma L. Neurinoma of the third, fourth, and sixth cranial nerves: a survey and report of a new fourth nerve case. Surg Neurol 1992;38:216-224.

43. Santoreneos S, Hanieh A, Jorgensen RE. Trochlear nerve schwannomas occurring in patients without neurofibromatosis: case report and review of the literature. Neurosurgery 1997;41:282-287.

44. Emory TS, Unni KK. Intraosseous neurilemoma: a clinicopathologic study of 26 cases [Abstract]. Am J Clin Pathol 1993;100:328-329.

45. Gomez-Brouchet A, Delisle MB, Cognard C, et al. Vestibular schwannomas: correlations between magnetic resonance imaging and histopathologic appearance. Otol Neurotol 2001;22:79-86.

46. Abernathey CD, Onofrio BM, Scheithauer BW, Pairolero PC, Shives TC. Surgical management of giant sacral schwannomas. J Neurosurg 1986;65:286-295.

47. Levy AD, Quiles AM, Miettinen M, Sobin LH. Gastrointestinal schwannomas: CT features with clinicopathologic correlation. AJR Am J Roentgenol 2005;184:797-802.

48. Burger PC, Scheithauer BW. Tumors of the central nervous system. AFIP Atlas of Tumor Pathology, 4th series, Fascicle 7. Washington, DC: American Registry of Pathology; 2007.

49. Inoue T, Fukui M, Matsushima T, Hasuo K, Matsunaga M. Neurinoma in the cavernous sinus: report of two cases. Neurosurgery 1990;27:986-990.

50. Goebel HH, Shimokawa K, Schaake T, Kremp A. Schwannoma of the sellar region. Acta neurochir (Wien) 1979;48:191-197.

51. Casadei GP, Komori T, Scheithauer BW, Miller GM, Parisi JE, Kelly PJ. Intracranial parenchymal schwannoma. A clinicopathological and neuroimaging study of nine cases. J Neurosurg 1993:79:217-222.

52. Stefanko SZ, Vuzevski VD, Maas AI, van Vroonhoven CC. Intracerebral malignant schwannoma. Acta Neuropathol 1986;71:321-325.

53. Ross DA, Edwards MS, Wilson CB. Intramedullary neurilemomas of the spinal cord: report of two cases and review of the literature. Neurosurgery 1986;19:458-464.

54. Polkey CE. Intraosseous neurilemmoma of the cervical spine causing paraparesis and treated by resection and grafting. J Neurol Neurosurg Psychiatry 1975;38:776-781.

55. Fletcher CD, Berman JJ, Corless C, et al. Diagnosis of gastrointestinal stromal tumors: A consensus approach. Hum Pathol 2002;33:459-465.

56. Liegl B, Hornick JL, Corless CL, Fletcher CD. Monoclonal antibody DOG1 shows higher sensitivity than KIT in the diagnosis of gastrointestinal stromal tumors, including unusual subtypes. Am J Surg Pathol 2009;33:437-446.

57. Daimaru Y, Kido H, Hashimoto H, Enjoji M. Benign schwannoma of the gastrointestinal tract: a clinicopathologic and immunohistochemical study. Hum Pathol 1988;19:257-264.

58. Hou YY, Tan YS, Xu JF, et al. Schwannoma of the gastrointestinal tract: a clinicopatological, immunohistochemical and ultrastructural study of 33 cases. Histopathology 2006;48:536-545.

59. Miettinen M, Shekitka KM, Sobin LH. Schwannomas in the colon and rectum: a clinicopathologic and immunohistochemical study of 20 cases. Am J Surg Pathol 2001;25:846-855.

60. Prevot S, Bienvenu L, Vaillant JC, de Saint-Maur PP. Benign schwannoma of the digestive tract: a clinicopathologic and immunohistochemical study of five cases, including a case of esophageal tumor. Am J Surg Pathol 1999;23:431-436.

61. Sarlomo-Rikala M, Miettinen M. Gastric schwannoma—a clinicopathological analysis of six cases. Histopathology 1995;27:355-360.

62. Liegl B, Bennett MW, Fletcher CD. Microcystic/reticular schwannoma: a distinct variant with predilection for visceral locations. Am J Surg Pathol 2008;32:1080-1087.

63. Miettinen M, Kopczynski J, Makhlouf HR, et al. Gastrointestinal stromal tumors, intramural leiomyomas, and leiomyosarcomas in the duodenum. A clinicopathologic, immunohistochemical, and molecular genetic study of 167 cases. Am J Surg Pathol 2003;27,625-641.

64. Factor S, Turi G, Biempica L. Primary cardiac neurilemoma. Cancer 1976;37:883-890.

65. Silverman JF, Leffers BR, Kay S. Primary pulmonary neurilemoma. Report of a case with ultrastructural examination. Arch Pathol Lab Med 1976;100:644-648.

66. Scheithauer B, Woodruff JM, Erlandson RA. Tumors of the peripheral nervous system. AFIP Atlas of Tumor Pathology, 3rd Series,, Fascicle 24. Washington, DC: American Registry of Pathology; 1999.

67. Hasegawa SL, Mentzel T, Fletcher CD. Schwannomas of the sinonasal tract and nasopharynx. Mod Pathol 1997;10:777-784.

68. Antonescu CR, Woodruff JM. Primary tumors of cranial, spinal and peripheral nerves. In: Russell and Rubinstein's pathology of tumors of the nervous systems. London: Hodder Arnold; 2006:787-835.

69. Goetting MG, Swanson SE. Massive hemorrhage into intracranial neurinomas. Surg Neurol 1987;27:168-172.

70. Neely JG. Hearing conservation surgery for acoustic tumors—a clinical-pathologic correlative study. Am J Otol 1985 Suppl:143-146.

71. Erlandson RA, Woodruff JM. Peripheral nerve sheath tumors: an electron microscopic study of 43 cases. Cancer 1982;49:273-287.

72. Kasantikul V, Netsky MG. Combined neurilemmoma and angioma. Tumor of ectomesenchyme and a source of bleeding. J Neurosurg 1979;50:81-87.

73. Fisher C, Chappell ME, Weiss SW. Neuroblastoma-like epithelioid schwannoma. Histopathology 1995;26:193-194.

74. Goldblum JR, Beals TF, Weiss SW. Neuroblastoma-like neurilemoma. Am J Surg Pathol 1994;18:266-273.

75. Kindblom LG, Meis-Kindblom JM, Havel G, Busch C. Benign epithelioid schwannoma. Am J Surg Pathol 1998;22:762-770.

76. Graham DI, Bond MR. Intradural spinal ossifying schwannoma. Case report. J Neurosurg 1972;36:487-489.

77. Kasantikul V, Brown WJ, Netsky MG. Mesenchymal differentiation in trigeminal neurilemmoma. Cancer 1982;50:1568-1571.

78. Ou YC, Yang DY, Chang CG. Ossification within a thoracic neurilemoma—a case report. Zhonghua Yi Xue Za Zhi (Taipei) 1988;42:143-146.

79. Plaza JA, Wakely PE Jr, Suster S. Lipoblastic nerve sheath tumors: report of a distinctive variant of neural soft tissue neoplasm with adipocytic differentiation. Am J Surg Pathol 2006;30:337-344.

80. Woodruff JM, Christensen WN. Glandular peripheral nerve sheath tumors. Cancer 1993;72:3618-3628.

81. Fawcett D. Bloom and Fawcett: a textbook of histology. New York: Chapman & Hall; 1994.

82. Ferry JA, Dickersin GR. Pseudoglandular schwannoma. Am J Clin Pathol 1988;89:546-552.

83. Ackerman LV, Taylor FH. Neurogenous tumors within the thorax. A clinicopathological evaluation of forty-eight cases. Cancer 1951;4:669-691.

84. Sobel RA. Vestibular (acoustic) schwannomas: histologic features in neurofibromatosis 2 and in unilateral cases. J Neuropathol Exp Neurol 1993;52:106-113.

85. Geddes JF, Sutcliffe JC, King TT. Mixed cranial nerve tumors in neurofibromatosis type 2. Clin Neuropathol 1995;14:310-313.

86. Mautner VF, Lindenau M, Baser ME, Kluwe L, Gottschalk J. Skin abnormalities in neurofibromatosis 2. Arch Dermatol 1997;133:1539-1543.

87. Johnson MD, Glick AD, Davis BW. Immunohistochemical evaluation of Leu-7, myelin basic-protein, S100-protein, glial-fibrillary acidic-protein, and LN3 immunoreactivity in nerve sheath tumors and sarcomas. Arch Pathol Lab Med 1988;112:155-160.

88. Kawahara E, Oda Y, Ooi A, Katsuda S, Nakanishi I, Umeda S. Expression of glial fibrillary acidic protein (GFAP) in peripheral nerve sheath tumors. A comparative study of immunoreactivity of GFAP, vimentin, S-100 protein, and neurofilament in 38 schwannomas and 18 neurofibromas. Am J Surg Pathol 1988;12:115-120.

89. Weiss SW, Langloss JM, Enzinger FM. Value of S-100 protein in the diagnosis of soft tissue tumors with particular reference to benign and malignant Schwann cell tumors. Lab Invest 1983;49:299-308.

90. Penneys NS, Mogollon R, Kowalczyk A, Nadji M, Adachi K. A survey of cutaneous neural lesions for the presence of myelin basic protein. An immunohistochemical study. Arch Dermatol 1984;120:210-213.

91. Clark HB, Minesky JJ, Agrawal D, Agrawal HC. Myelin basic protein and P2 protein are not immunohistochemical markers for Schwann cell neoplasms. A comparative study using antisera to S-100, P2, and myelin basic proteins. Am J Pathol 1985;121:96-101.

92. Pfeiffer SE, Sundarraj N, Dawson G, Kornblith PL. Human acoustic neurinomas: nervous system specific biochemical parameters. Acta Neuropathol 1979;47:27-31.

93. Giangaspero F, Fratamico FC, Ceccarelli C, Brisigotti M. Malignant peripheral nerve sheath tumors and spindle cell sarcomas: an immunohistochemical analysis of multiple markers. Appl Pathol 1989;7:134-144.

94. Gray MH, Rosenberg AE, Dickersin GR, Bhan AK. Glial fibrillary acidic protein and keratin expression by benign and malignant nerve sheath tumors. Hum Pathol 1989;20:1089-1096.

95. Memoli VA, Brown EF, Gould VE. Glial fibrillary acidic protein (GFAP) immunoreactivity in peripheral nerve sheath tumors. Ultrastruct Pathol 1984;7:269-275.

96. Chaubal A, Paetau A, Zoltick P, Miettinen M. CD34 immunoreactivity in nervous system tumors. Acta Neuropathol (Berl) 1994;88:454-458.

97. McComb RD, Bigner DD. Immunolocalization of laminin in neoplasms of the central and peripheral nervous systems. J Neuropathol Exp Neurol 1985;44:242-253.

98. Oda Y, Kawahara E, Minamoto T, et al. Immunohistochemical studies on the tissue localization of collagen types I, III, IV, V and VI in schwannomas. Correlation with ultrastructural features of the extracellular matrix. Virchows Arch 1988;56:153-163.

99. Gould VE, Moll R, Moll I, Lee I, Schwechheimer K, Franke WW. The intermediate filament complement of the spectrum of nerve sheath neoplasms. Lab Invest 1986;55:463-474.

100. Sarlomo-Rikala M, Kovatich AJ, Barusevicius A, Miettinen M. CD117: a sensitive marker for gastrointestinal stromal tumors that is more specific than CD34. Mod Pathol 1998;11:728-734.

101. de la Monte SM, Dorfman HD, Chandra R, Malawer M. Intraosseous schwannoma: histopathologic features, ultrastructure and review of the literature. Hum Pathol 1984;15:551-558.

102. Erlandson RA. Diagnostic transmission electron microscopy of tumors. New York: Raven Press; 1994.

103. Lassmann H, Jurecka W, Lassmann G, Gebhart W, Matras H, Watzek, G. Different types of benign nerve sheath tumors. Light microscopy, electron microscopy and autoradiography. Virchows Arch A Pathol Anat Histol 1977;375:197-210.

104. Sian CS, Ryan SF. The ultrastructure of neurilemoma with emphasis on Antoni B tissue. Hum Pathol 1981;12:145-160.

105. Kasantikul V, Glick AD, Netsky MG. Light and electron microscopic observations of blood vessels in neurilemoma. Arch Pathol Lab Med 1979;103:683-687.

106. Hirano A, Dembitzer HM, Zimmerman HM. Fenestrated blood vessels in neurilemoma. Lab Invest 1972;27:305-309.

107. Swanson PE, Manivel JC, Wick MR. Immunoreactivity for Leu-7 in neurofibrosarcoma and other spindle cell sarcomas of soft tissue. Am J Pathol 1987;126:546-560.

108. Swanson PE, Stanley MW, Scheithauer BW, Wick MR. Primary cutaneous leiomyosarcoma. A histological and immunohistochemical study of 9 cases, with ultrastructural correlation. J Cutan Pathol 1988;15:129-141.

109. DeMatteo RP, Lewis JJ, Leung D, Mudan SS, Woodruff JM, Brennan MF. Two hundred gastrointestinal stromal tumors: recurrence patterns and prognostic factors for survival. Ann Surg 2000;231:51-58.

110. Dematteo RP, Heinrich MC, El-Rifai WM, Demetri G. Clinical management of gastrointestinal stromal tumors: before and after STI-571. Hum Pathol 2002;33:466-477.

111. Weiss SW, Gnepp DR, Bratthauer GL. Palisaded myofibroblastoma. A benign mesenchymal tumor of lymph node. Am J Surg Pathol 1989;13:341-346.

112. Suster S, Rosai J. Intranodal hemorrhagic spindle-cell tumor with "amianthoid" fibers. Report of six cases of a distinctive mesenchymal neoplasm of the inguinal region that simulates Kaposi's sarcoma. Am J Surg Pathol 1989;13:347-357.

113. Smith ME, Fisher C, Weiss SW. Pleomorphic hyalinizing angiectatic tumor of soft parts. A low-grade neoplasm resembling neurilemoma. Am J Surg Pathol 1996;20:21-29.

114. Ironside JW, Moss TH, Louis DN, Lowe JS, Weller RO. Diagnostic pathology of nervous system tumors. London: Churchill Livingston; 2002.

115. Klekamp J, Samii M. Surgery of spinal nerve sheath tumors with special reference to neurofibromatosis. Neurosurgery 1998;42:279-290.

116. Beatty CW, Scheithauer BW, Katzmann JA, Roche PC, Kjeldahl KS, Ebersold MJ. Acoustic schwannoma and pregnancy: a DNA flow cytometric, steroid hormone receptor, and proliferation marker study. Laryngoscope 1995;105:693-700.

117. Chen Y, Diamond AS, Vaheesan KR, Schneider S, Valderrama E. Retroperitoneal neurofibrosarcoma in a patient with neurofibromatosis 2: a case report and review of the literature. Pediatr Pathol Mol Med 2003;22:375-381.

Cellular Schwannoma

118. Woodruff JM, Godwin TA, Erlandson RA, Susin M, Martini N. Cellular schwannoma: a variety of schwannoma sometimes mistaken for a malignant tumor. Am J Surg Pathol 1981;5:733-744.

119. Ducatman BS, Scheithauer BW, Piepgras DG, Reiman HM, Ilstrup DM. Malignant peripheral nerve sheath tumors. A clinicopathologic study of 120 cases. Cancer 1986;57:2006-2021.

120. Harkin JC, Reed RJ. Tumors of the peripheral nervous system. Atlas of tumor pathology, 2nd Series, Fascicle 3 Supplement. Washington, DC: Armed Forces Institute of Pathology; 1983.

121. Russell DS, Rubinstein LJ. Tumours of the cranial, spinal, and peripheral nerve sheaths. Pathology of tumours of the nervous system. Baltimore: William & Wilkins; 1989.

122. Woodruff JM. Cellular schwannoma and its necessary distinction from malignant peripheral nerve sheath tumors and sarcomas. Pathol Case Rev 1998; 3:118-122.

123. Casadei GP, Scheithauer BW, Hirose T, Manfrini M, Van Houton C, Wood MB. Cellular schwannoma. A clinicopathologic, DNA flow cytometric, and proliferation marker study of 70 patients. Cancer 1995;75:1109-1119.

124. Deruaz JP, Janzer RC, Costa J. Cellular schwannomas of the intracranial and intraspinal compartment: morphological and immunological characteristics compared with classical benign schwannomas. J Neuropathol Exp Neurol 1993;52:114-118.

125. Fletcher CD, Davies SE, McKee PH. Cellular schwannoma: a distinct pseudosarcomatous entity. Histopathology 1987;11:21-35.

126. Lodding P, Kindblom LG, Angervall L, Stenman G. Cellular schwannoma. A clinicopathologic study of 29 cases. Virchows Arch A Pathol Anat Histopathol 1990;416:237-248.

127. White W, Shiu MH, Rosenblum MK, Erlandson RA, Woodruff JM. Cellular schwannoma. A clinicopathologic study of 57 patients and 58 tumors. Cancer 1990;66:1266-1275.

128. Scheithauer B, Woodruff JM, Erlandson RA. Tumors of the peripheral nervous system. AFIP Atlas of Tumor Pathology, 3rd Series, Fascicle 24. Washington, DC: American Registry of Pathology; 1999.

129. White W, Shiu MH, Rosenblum MK, Erlandson RA, Woodruff JM. Cellular schwannoma. A clinicopathologic study of 57 patients and 58 tumors. Cancer 1990;66:1266-1275.

130. Nascimento AF, Fletcher CD. The controversial nosology of benign nerve sheath tumors: neurofilament protein staining demonstrates intratumoral axons in many sporadic schwannomas. Am J Surg Pathol 2007;31:1363-1370.

131. Kindblom LG, Ahlden M, Meis-Kindblom JM, Stenman G. Immunohistochemical and molecular analysis of p53, MDM2, proliferating cell nuclear antigen and Ki67 in benign and malignant peripheral nerve sheath tumours. Virchows Arch 1995;427:19-26.

132. Dickersin GR. The electron microscopic spectrum of nerve sheath tumors. Ultrastruct Pathol 1987;11:103-146.

133. Erlandson RA. Diagnostic transmission electron microscopy of tumors. New York: Raven Press; 1994.

134. Woodruff JM, Selig AM, Crowley K, Allen PW. Schwannoma (neurilemoma) with malignant transformation. A rare, distinctive peripheral nerve tumor. Am J Surg Pathol 1994;18:882-895.

135. Giangaspero F, Fratamico FC, Ceccarelli C, Brisigotti M. Malignant peripheral nerve sheath tumors and spindle cell sarcomas: an immunohistochemical analysis of multiple markers. Appl Pathol 1989;7:134-144.

136. Memoli VA, Brown EF, Gould VE. Glial fibrillary acidic protein (GFAP) immunoreactivity in peripheral nerve sheath tumors. Ultrastruct Pathol 1984;7:269-275.

137. Hirose T, Hasegawa T, Kudo E, Seki K, Sano T, Hizawa K. Malignant peripheral nerve sheath tumors: an immunohistochemical study in relation to ultrastructural features. Hum Pathol 1992;23:865-870.

138. Swanson PE, Stanley MW, Scheithauer BW, Wick MR. Primary cutaneous leiomyosarcoma. A histological and immunohistochemical study of 9 cases, with ultrastructural correlation. J Cutan Pathol 1988;15:129-141.

139. Winek RR, Scheithauer BW, Wick MR. Meningioma, meningeal hemangiopericytoma (angioblastic meningioma), peripheral hemangiopericytoma, and acoustic schwannoma. A comparative immunohistochemical study. Am J Surg Pathol 1989;13:251-261.

140. Carneiro SS, Scheithauer BW, Nascimento AG, Davis DH. Solitary fibrous tumor of the meninges: a lesion distinct from fibrous meningioma—a clinicopathologic and immunohistochemical study [Abstract]. Mod Pathol 1995;8:135A.

141. Chen Y, Diamond AS, Vaheesan KR, Schneider S, Valderrama E. Retroperitoneal neurofibrosarcoma in a patient with neurofibromatosis 2: a case report and review of the literature. Pediatr Pathol Mol Med 2003;22:375-381.

142. Casadei GP, Scheithauer BW, Hirose T, Manfrini M, Van Houton C, Wood MB. Cellular schwannoma. A clinicopathologic, DNA flow cytometric, and proliferation marker study of 70 patients. Cancer 1995;75:1109-1119.

143. Antonescu CR, Woodruff JM. Primary tumors of cranial, spinal and peripheral nerves. In: Russell and Rubinstein's pathology of tumors of the nervous systems. London: Hodder Arnold; 2006:787-835.

Plexiform Schwannoma

144. Agaram NP, Prakash S, Antonescu CR. Deep-seated plexiform schwannoma: a pathologic study of 16 cases and comparative analysis with the superficial variety. Am J Surg Pathol 2005;29:1042-1048.

145. Argenyi ZB, Goodenberger ME, Strauss JS. Congenital neural hamartoma ("fascicular schwannoma"). A light microscopic, immunohistochemical, and ultrastructural study. Am J Dermatopathol 1990;12:283-293.

146. Barbosa J, Hansen LS. Solitary multilobular schwannoma of the oral cavity. J Oral Med 1984;39:232-235.

147. Berg J, Scheithauer BW, Spinner R, Allen C, Koutlas I. Plexiform schwannoma: a clinicopathologic overview with emphasis upon the head and neck region. Hum Pathol 2008;39:633-640.

148. Fletcher CD, Davies SE. Benign plexiform (multinodular) schwannoma: a rare tumour unassociated with neurofibromatosis. Histopathology 1986;10:971-980.

149. Harkin J, Harkin JC, Arringson JH. Benign plexiform schwannoma. A lesion distinct from plexiform neurofibroma. J Neuropathol Exp Neurol 1978;37:622. (abstract)

150. Hirose T, Hasegawa T, Kudo E, Seki K, Sano T, Hizawa K. Malignant peripheral nerve sheath tumors: an immunohistochemical study in relation to ultrastructural features. Hum Pathol 1992;23:865-870.

151. Ishida T, Kuroda M, Motoi T, Oka T, Imamura T, Machinami R. Phenotypic diversity of neurofibromatosis 2: association with plexiform schwannoma. Histopathology 1998;32:264-270.

152. Iwashita T, Enjoji M. Plexiform neurilemmoma: a clinicopathological and immunohistochemical analysis of 23 tumours from 20 patients. Virchows Arch A Pathol Anat Histopathol 1987;411:305-309.

153. Kao GF, Laskin WB, Olsen TG. Solitary cutaneous plexiform neurilemmoma (schwannoma): a clinicopathologic, immunohistochemical, and ultrastructural study of 11 cases. Mod Pathol 1989;2:20-26.

154. Meis-Kindblom JM, Enzinger FM. Plexiform malignant peripheral nerve sheath tumor of infancy and childhood. Am J Surg Pathol 1994;18:479-485.

155. Woodruff JM, Marshall ML, Godwin TA, Funkhouser JW, Thompson NJ, Erlandson RA. Plexiform (multinodular) schwannoma. A tumor simulating the plexiform neurofibroma. Am J Surg Pathol 1983;7:691-697.

156. Reith JD, Goldblum JR. Multiple cutaneous plexiform schwannomas. Report of a case and review of the literature with particular reference to the association with types 1 and 2 neurofibromatosis and schwannomatosis. Arch Pathol Lab Med 1996;120:399-401.

157. Shishiba T, Niimura M, Ohtsuka F, Tsuru N. Multiple cutaneous neurilemmomas as a skin manifestation of neurilemmomatosis. J Am Acad Dermatol 1984;10:744-754.

158. Woodruff JM, Scheithauer BW, Kurtkaya-Yapicier O, et al. Congenital and childhood plexiform (multinodular) cellular schwannoma: a troublesome mimic of malignant peripheral nerve sheath tumor. Am J Surg Pathol 2003;27:1321-1329.

159. Nascimento AF, Fletcher CD. The controversial nosology of benign nerve sheath tumors: neurofilament protein staining demonstrates intratumoral axons in many sporadic schwannomas. Am J Surg Pathol 2007;31:1363-1370.

160. Casadei GP, Scheithauer BW, Hirose T, Manfrini M, Van Houton C, Wood MB. Cellular schwannoma. A clinicopathologic, DNA flow cytometric, and proliferation marker study of 70 patients. Cancer 1995;75:1109-1119.

Melanotic Schwannoma

161. Millar WG. A malignant melanocytic tumour of ganglion cells arising from a thoracic sympathetic ganglion. J Pathol 1932;35:351-357.

162. Hodson JJ. An intra-osseous tumour combination of biological importance-invasion of a melanotic schwannoma by an adamantinoma. J Pathol Bacteriol 1961;82:257-266.

163. Scheithauer B, Woodruff JM, Erlandson RA. Tumors of the peripheral nervous system. AFIP Atlas of Tumor Pathology, 3rd Series, Fascicle 24. Washington, DC: American Registry of Pathology; 1999.

164. Carney JA. Psammomatous melanotic schwannoma. A distinctive, heritable tumor with special associations, including cardiac myxoma and the Cushing syndrome. Am J Surg Pathol 1990;14:206-222.

165. Carney JA, Gordon H, Carpenter PC, Shenoy BV, Go VL. The complex of myxomas, spotty pigmentation, and endocrine overactivity. Medicine (Baltimore) 1985;64:270-283.

166. Carney JA, Hruska LS, Beauchamp GD, Gordon H. Dominant inheritance of the complex of myxomas, spotty pigmentation, and endocrine overactivity. Mayo Clin Proc 1986;61:165-172.

167. Carney JA, Stratakis CA. Epithelioid blue nevus and psammomatous melanotic schwannoma: the unusual pigmented skin tumors of the Carney complex. Semin Diagn Pathol 1998;15:216-224.

168. Carney JA, Boccon-Gibod L, Jarka DE, et al. Osteochondromyxoma of bone: a congenital tumor associated with lentigines and other unusual disorders. Am J Surg Pathol 2001;25:164-176.

169. Casey M, Mah C, Merliss AD, et al. Identification of a novel genetic locus for familial cardiac myxomas and Carney complex. Circulation 1998;98:2560-2566.

170. Stratakis CA, Carney JA, Lin JP, et al. Carney complex, a familial multiple neoplasia and lentiginosis syndrome. Analysis of 11 kindreds and linkage to the short arm of chromosome 2. J Clin Invest 1996;97:699-705.

171. Casey M, Vaughan CJ, He J, et al. Mutations in the protein kinase A R1alpha regulatory subunit cause familial cardiac myxomas and Carney complex. J Clin Invest 2000;106:R31-38.

171a. Kirschner LS, Carney JA, Pack SD, et al. Mutations of the gene encoding the protein kinase A type I-alpha regulatory subunit in patients with the Carney complex. Nat Genet 2000;26:89-92.

172. Kirschner LS, Sandrini F, Monbo J, Lin JP, Carney JA, Stratakis CA. Genetic heterogeneity and spectrum of mutations of the PRKAR1A gene in patients with the carney complex. Hum Mol Genet 2000;9:3037-3046.

173. Matyakhina L, Pack S, Kirschner LS, et al. Chromosome 2 (2p16) abnormalities in Carney complex tumours. J Med Genet 2003;40:268-277.

174. Cras P, Ceuterick-de Groote C, Van Vyve M, Vercruyssen A, Martin JJ. Malignant pigmented spinal nerve root schwannoma metastasizing in the brain and viscera. Clin Neuropathol 1990;9:290-294.

175. Gelfand ET, Taylor RF, Hendin D, Akabutu J, Callaghan JC. Melanotic malignant schwannoma of the right atrium. J Thoracic Cardiovasc Surg 1977;74:808-812.

176. Theodossiou A, Segditsas T. [Intra-abdominally situated melanotic schwannoma]. Zentralbl Allg Pathol 1971;114:168-172. [German]

177. Christensen C. Malignant melanocytic schwannoma. A case report. Acta Chir Scand 1986;152:385-386.

178. Terzakis JA, Opher E, Melamed J, Santagada E, Sloan, D. Pigmented melanocytic schwannoma of the uterine cervix. Ultrastruct Pathol 1990;14:357-366.

179. Erlandson RA. Melanotic schwannoma of spinal nerve origin. Ultrastruct Pathol 1985;9:123-129.

180. Killeen RM, Davy CL, Bauserman SC. Melanocytic schwannoma. Cancer 1988;62:174-183.

181. Antonescu CR, Woodruff JM. Primary tumors of cranial, spinal and peripheral nerves. In: Russell and Rubinstein's pathology of tumors of the nervous systems. London: Hodder Arnold; 2006:787-835.

182. Burns DK, Silva FG, Forde KA, Mount PM, Clark HB. Primary melanocytic schwannoma of the stomach. Evidence of dual melanocytic and schwannian differentiation in an extra-axial site in a patient without neurofibromatosis. Cancer 1983;52:1432-1441.

183. Sheehan D, Hrapchak B. Pigments and minerals. In: Theory and practice of histotechnology, 2nd ed. St. Louis: C.V. Mosby; 1980:214-232.

184. Vallat-Decouvelacre A, Wassef M, Lot G, et al. Spinal melanotic schwannoma: a tumor with poor prognosis. Histopathology 1999;35:558-566.

185. Jaffer S, Woodruff JM. Cytology of melanotic schwannoma in a fine needle aspirate and pleural fluid. A case report. Acta Cytol 2000;44:1095-1100.

186. Marco V, Sirvent J, Alvarez Moro J, Clavel M, Muntal MT, Bauza A. Malignant melanotic schwannoma fine-needle aspiration biopsy findings. Diagn Cytopathol 1998;18:284-286.

187. Sola-Perez J, Perez-Guillermo M, Bas-Bernal A, Gimenez-Bascunana A, Montes-Clavero C. Melanocytic schwannoma: the cytologic aspect in fine-needle aspiration cytology (FNAC): report of a case located in the spinal cord. Diagn Cytopathol 1994;11:291-296.

188. Jensen OA, Bretlau P. Melanotic schwannoma of the orbit. Immunohistochemical and ultrastructural study of a case and survey of the literature. APMIS 1990:98:713-723.

189. Miettinen M. Melanotic schwannoma coexpression of vimentin and glial fibrillary acidic protein. Ultrastruct Pathol 1987;11:39-46.

190. Myers JL, Bernreuter W, Dunham W. Melanotic schwannoma. Clinicopathologic, immunohistochemical, and ultrastructural features of a rare primary bone tumor. Am J Clin Pathol 1990;93:424-429.

191. Koch MB, Shih IM, Weiss SW, Folpe AL. Microphthalmia transcription factor and melanoma cell adhesion molecule expression distinguish desmoplastic/spindle cell melanoma from morphologic mimics. Am J Surg Pathol 2001;25:58-64.

192. Font RL, Truong LD. Melanotic schwannoma of soft tissues. Electron-microscopic observations and review of literature. Am J Surg Pathol 1984;8:129-138.

193. Janzer RC, Makek M. Intraoral malignant melanotic schwannoma. Ultrastructural evidence for melanogenesis by Schwann's cells. Arch Pathol Lab Med 1983;107:298-301.

194. Kayano H, Katayama I. Melanotic schwannoma arising in the sympathetic ganglion. Hum Pathol 1988;19:1355-1358.

195. Krausz T, Azzopardi JG, Pearse E. Malignant melanoma of the sympathetic chain: with a consideration of pigmented nerve sheath tumours. Histopathology 1984;8:881-894.

196. Mennemeyer RP, Hallman KO, Hammar SP, Raisis JE, Tytus JS, Bockus D. Melanotic schwannoma. Clinical and ultrastructural studies of three cases with evidence of intracellular melanin synthesis. Am J Surg Pathol 1979;3:3-10.

197. Fetsch JF, Michal M, Miettinen M. Pigmented (melanotic) neurofibroma: a clinicopathologic and immunohistochemical analysis of 19 lesions from 17 patients. Am J Surg Pathol 2000;24:331-343.

198. Brat DJ, Giannini C, Scheithauer BW, Burger PC. Primary melanocytic neoplasms of the central nervous systems. Am J Surg Pathol 1999;23:745-754.

199. Jellinger K, Bock F, Brenner H. Meningeal melanocytoma. Report of a case and review of the literature. Acta Neurochir (Wien) 1988;94:78-87.

200. Limas C, Tio FO. Meningeal melanocytoma ("melanotic meningioma"). Its melanocytic origin as revealed by electron microscopy. Cancer 1972;30:1286-1294.

201. Prabhu SS, Lynch PG, Keogh AJ, Parekh HC. Intracranial meningeal melanocytoma: a report of two cases and a review of the literature. Surg Neurol 1993;40:516-521.

202. Winston KR, Sotrel A, Schnitt SJ. Meningeal melanocytoma. Case report and review of the clinical and histological features. J Neurosurg 1987;66:50-57.

203. Monteagudo C, Ferrandez A, Gonzalez-Devesa M, Llombart-Bosch A. Psammomatous malignant melanoma arising in an intradermal naevus. Histopathology 2001;39:493-497.

204. DiMaio SM, Mackay B, Smith JL Jr, Dickersin GR. Neurosarcomatous transformation in malignant melanoma: an ultrastructural study. Cancer 1982;50:2345-2354.

205. Prieto VG, Woodruff JM. Expression of basement membrane antigens in spindle cell melanoma. J Cutan Pathol 1998;25:297-300.

206. Chung EB, Enzinger FM. Malignant melanoma of soft parts. A reassessment of clear cell sarcoma. Am J Surg Pathol 1983;7:405-413.

207. Enzinger FM. Clear-cell sarcoma of tendons and aponeuroses. An analysis of 21 cases. Cancer 1965;18:1163-1174.

208. Antonescu CR, Tschernyavsky SJ, Woodruff JM, Jungbluth AA, Brennan MF, Ladanyi M. Molecular diagnosis of clear cell sarcoma: detection of EWS-ATF1 and MITF-M transcripts and histopathological and ultrastructural analysis of 12 cases. J Mol Diagn 2002;4:44-52.

209. Zucman J, Delattre O, Desmaze C, et al. EWS and ATF-1 gene fusion induced by t(12;22) translocation in malignant melanoma of soft parts. Nat Genet 1993;4:341-345.

210. Dastur DK, Sinh G, Pandya SK. Melanotic tumor of the acoustic nerve. J Neurosurg 1967;27:166-170.

211. Fu YS, Kaye GI, Lattes R. Primary malignant melanocytic tumors of the sympathetic ganglia, with an ultrastructural study of one. Cancer 1975;36:2029-2041.

212. Graham DI, Paterson A, McQueen A, Milne JA, Urich H. Melanotic tumours (blue naevi) of spinal nerve roots. J Pathol 1976;118:83-89.

213. Roytta M, Elfversson J, Kalimo H. Intraspinal pigmented schwannoma with malignant progression. Acta Neurochir (Wien) 1988;95:147-154.

8 NEUROFIBROMA

Neurofibroma is a benign tumor composed of a variable admixture of Schwann, perineurial-like, perineurial, and fibroblastic cells. Residual interspersed myelinated and unmyelinated nerve fibers often are present.

GENERAL FEATURES

The term neurofibroma harkens back to the earliest attempt to classify tumors of peripheral nerves. It was the choice of Virchow and von Recklinghausen, both of whom viewed such tumors as fibroblastic in nature. Subsequent to the removal of a schwannoma subset from the all inclusive neurofibroma category, the name persisted, now comprising the tumors described in this chapter. Retention of the term neurofibroma is justified by its long-term use, historical attachment to two major clinical syndromes, and complexity of the tumor's cellular makeup. The determination of its nature, particularly its cellular composition, awaited an understanding of the exclusively Schwann cell composition of schwannoma. It is now generally agreed that neurofibroma, like schwannoma, is fundamentally a Schwann cell neoplasm. Unlike schwannoma, however, a monomorphic proliferation of readily recognized neoplastic Schwann cells, in neurofibroma the Schwann cell element is not as easily identified. Mixed with the differentiated Schwann cells are transitional forms of the cell and fibroblasts, and the resulting morphology gives neurofibroma a characteristic histologic appearance that in most instances makes distinction of the two tumors possible. This is clinically important, not only for distinguishing the two types of neurofibromatosis but, on occasion, for excluding a diagnosis of malignant peripheral nerve sheath tumor (MPNST). The principal clinicopathologic features distinguishing schwannoma from neurofibroma are summarized in Table 7-1.

Evidence that Neurofibroma is a Neoplasm Initiated by a Schwann Cell Alteration and Predominantly Schwannian in Composition.

Given its cellular heterogeneity and the association with neurofibromatosis type 1 (NF1), a disorder known for its broad spectrum of lesions, consideration had once been given to the possibility that neurofibroma was a hyperplastic process. Counter to this notion are more convincing observations supporting a neoplastic process. For NF1-associated neurofibromas, these include cellular monoclonality, as shown in an X chromosome inactivation study (1); occasional transformation to MPNST; and, most recently, other genetic aspects. Based on its identical histology, but also on recent molecular genetic findings, sporadic neurofibroma is similarly viewed as neoplastic in nature.

The prominence of Schwann cells in neurofibromas is apparent in the extensive S-100 protein expression and the ultrastructural observation of the presence of individual differentiated Schwann cells (2). Genetic evidence for the Schwann cell role in neurofibroma formation comes from the tumor's close association with NF1, a condition causally related to inactivation of the *NF1* gene. A silencing of both copies of this gene is found in inherited and sporadic neurofibromas (3–5). Within such tumors, *NF1* deletions have been traced to a cell population expressing S-100 protein (6). Studies of *NF1* gene-mutated mice show that peripheral nerve sheath tumors with the histologic features of neurofibroma do not develop in heterozygous Nf1+/- mutants (7,8), whereas they do in chimeric mice composed in part of Nf1-/- cells (9). This observation indicates that loss of the wild-type Nf1 allele is rate-limiting in tumor formation. Interestingly, although the ultrastructural features of the tumor cells in the mouse studies were consistent with Schwann cells, they generally lacked S-100 protein reactivity. In yet another study, chimeric mice with loss of Nf1 function (Nf1-/-) routinely developed neurofibromas if other cells were heterozygous (Nf1+/-) (10). In addition to indicating that Schwann cells initiate neurofibroma growth, this study suggested that mast cells may play a role in tumor formation, a critical role subsequently confirmed and detailed by others (10a).

Evidence for Morphologic Diversity of Schwann Cells in Neurofibroma and the Presence of Other Cell Types. Among the variety of cells comprising neurofibromas are perineurial–like cells (2,11,12). These, as common and sometimes more numerous than differentiated Schwann cells, possess many of the ultrastructural characteristics of perineurial cells (see fig. 8-41), but not their immunoprofile. They differ from normal perineurial cells by less uniformly thin, attenuated cell processes and a lack of tight junctions. The ultrastructure of this cell was early illustrated by Erlandson, who referred to it as a "transitional Schwann-perineurial cell" (13). The best evidence for the existence of this cell and its identity as a morphologically altered Schwann cell is found in the pseudomeissnerian body. The compact laminar component of this body, while ultrastructurally resembling perineurium, is also diffusely S-100 protein immunopositive (14) and epithelial membrane antigen (EMA) negative (see fig. 8-30D). Also present in some neurofibromas are spindle cells with the characteristics of perineurial cells, as evidenced by immunolabeling for EMA and sometimes claudin-1. These have been identified: 1) peripherally in neurofibromas; 2) in cutaneous neurofibromas, clustered around small nerves, the perineuria of which are presumed to have disintegrated during early tumor expansion (15); 3) in focal areas of localized cutaneous, subcutaneous, and plexiform neurofibromas (16,17); and 4) at the margins of pseudomeissnerian bodies (see fig. 8-30D).

Assumptions have been made that those perineurial cells found at the periphery of neurofibromas and about cutaneous nerves are remnants of nerve sheaths (18), and that the perineurial cells found at the margins of pseudomeissnerian bodies are transformed neoplastic Schwann cells (19). Although it is clear that the phenotypic perineurial cells embedded within neurofibromas are part of the neoplastic process (17,20), it remains to be determined whether they represent morphologically and immunophenotypically altered Schwann cells or proliferations of perineurial cells originating from disrupted nerve sheaths.

Fibroblasts in neurofibromas are presumed to represent either residual endoneurial fibroblasts or fibroblastic cells present in soft tissues infiltrated by tumor. As previously noted, mast cells may play a role in early neurofibroma formation (10,15).

GENETICS

NF1 and the neurofibromas in NF1 patients have a common basis in inactivating mutations of the *NF1* gene. Located at 17q11.2, it encodes the protein, neurofibromin (21–23). This protein contains a GTPase-activating protein domain that negatively regulates the proto-oncogene *p21-ras* by accelerating conversion of active ras-GTP to inactive GDP, thus functioning as a tumor suppressor (24–27). It has been postulated that neurofibroma formation is promoted by increased ras signaling resulting from a lack of neurofibromin. As currently understood, all individuals with NF1 harbor one nonfunctional *NF1* gene in every cell, the result of a germline mutation. Neurofibromas form as a result of inactivation of the remaining allele (28,29). This classic example of the "double-hit" hypothesis (30) received support from several studies (3,4,31–33). Evidence for somatic, biallelic inactivation of the *NF1* gene in sporadic neurofibromas has also been provided (34). In studies of neurofibromas, *NF1* loss of heterozygosity (LOH) is either not found or encountered in only a minority of tumors (5). One possible explanation for this is the presence of non-neoplastic cells overrun by tumor, cells that do not harbor *NF1* mutations and thereby obscure or dilute the percentage of tumor cells that do (5). Additional chromosomal losses in neurofibromas are few, but include 19p, 19q, and 22q (34a).

CLINICOPATHOLOGIC AND ANATOMIC VARIANTS

Neurofibromas develop either in patients with NF1 or, more commonly, as solitary sporadic lesions unassociated with the disorder. They are said to sometimes occur in the setting of NF2; however, each presumed example of neurofibroma in a NF2 patient (35,36) warrants close scrutiny. Some of the earlier reports may have been based on the mistaken impression that schwannomas could not present as multiple cutaneous lesions. With this possibility in mind, we reviewed the histologic slides of the tumors from one of the often cited reports (35) and found that all were schwannomas, and none neurofibromas. Neurofibromas rarely present in the newborn (37),

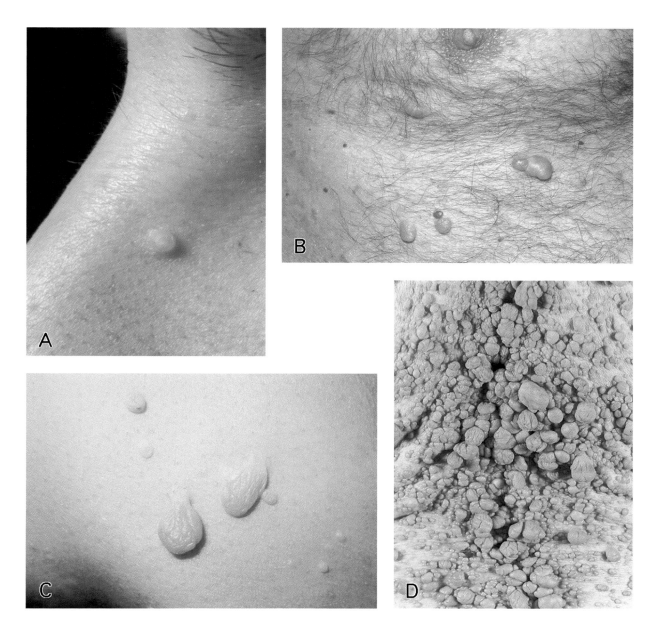

Figure 8-1

LOCALIZED CUTANEOUS NEUROFIBROMA

These tumors are solitary (A) or multiple and often neurofibromatosis type 1 (NF1) associated (B–D). The latter may be dome shaped (B) or polypoid (C). On occasion they lie densely clustered (D), as on the lower back of this markedly affected patient. (C, courtesy of Dr. H. Goebel, Mainz, Germany.)

but begin to appear in the second half of the first decade, and usually grow or multiply at puberty (38). This presentation focuses primarily upon those neurofibromas encountered in skin and soft tissues. Visceral neurofibromas and ganglioneuromatous lesions arising in the setting of NF1 are discussed in chapter 14.

Localized Cutaneous Neurofibroma. Although all neurofibromas share a common cellular makeup, a broad clinicopathologic spectrum has been described. Evidence has been provided that this most common form of neurofibroma (figs. 8-1–8-3) may not arise from nerves but from stem/progenitor cells residing

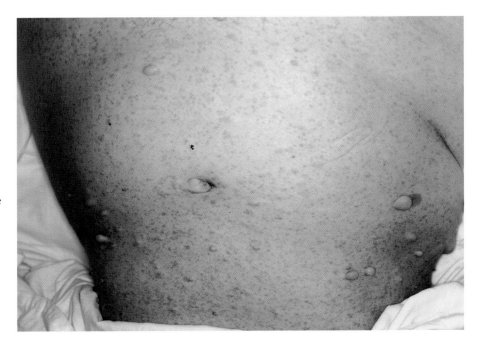

Figure 8-2

LOCALIZED CUTANEOUS NEUROFIBROMA

NF1 patient with extensive cutaneous lesions.

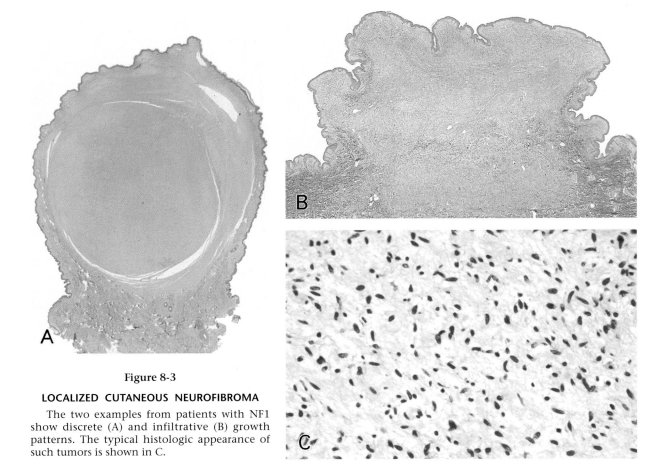

Figure 8-3

LOCALIZED CUTANEOUS NEUROFIBROMA

The two examples from patients with NF1 show discrete (A) and infiltrative (B) growth patterns. The typical histologic appearance of such tumors is shown in C.

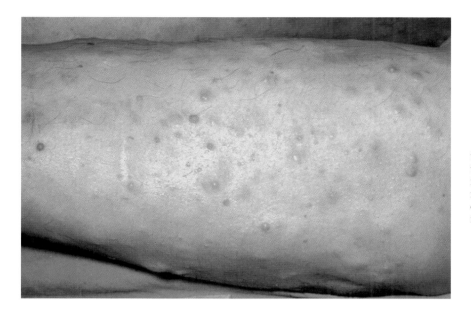

Figure 8-4

DIFFUSE CUTANEOUS NEUROFIBROMA

Such plaque-like lesions are typically larger than localized tumors. This example, occurring in a patient with NF1 features nodules much like those comprising localized neurofibromas.

in the dermis, termed skin derived precursors (SKPs) (38a). Often affecting the dermis and subcutis, there is no particular site of predilection. Soft, slightly elevated, nodular or polypoid (figs. 8-1–8-3B), such tumors are painless, slow growing, freely moveable, and usually measure more than 1 to 2 cm in maximum dimension. Most are solitary, present in young adults between age 20 and 30 years of age, and unassociated with NF1. In contrast, NF1 syndrome-associated neurofibromas are typically multiple (figs. 8-1B-D, 8-2) and may be overlain by a hyperpigmented epidermal macule, the "cafe-au-lait" spot (see fig. 15-2). Most patients with NF1 have developed cutaneous neurofibromas by the time of puberty. Thereafter, lesions simply increase in number and often in size. Only occasionally does their continued proliferation result in widespread surface involvement (fig. 8-2) to literally cover a patient with innumerable cutaneous nodules (see figs. 15-1, 15-5).

Grossly, the cut surface of localized cutaneous neurofibromas resembles that of localized intraneural examples. These are generally devoid of collagenization (see fig. 8-10C), and are homogeneously gray or gray-tan, glistening, and translucent. Their margins are often poorly delineated from surrounding dermis and underlying subcutaneous fat, and circumscribed, localized cutaneous lesions are unencapsulated (fig. 8-3A).

Whether solitary or multiple, the microscopic features of cutaneous neurofibroma consist of cells with bent or comma-shaped nuclei, similar to those of other forms of neurofibroma (fig. 8-3C). In general, no underlying nerve involvement is apparent, since the proliferation is almost entirely extraneural. We have not seen, nor are we aware of, a report of a localized cutaneous neurofibroma having undergone malignant change.

Diffuse Cutaneous Neurofibroma. The distinction between localized and diffuse cutaneous neurofibromas is usually easy, since the term diffuse is applied only to large, thick but flat lesions. Nonetheless, mixed patterns are sometimes observed, usually in individuals with NF1 (fig. 8-4). The diffuse cutaneous neurofibroma variant (figs. 8-4–8-7) is uncommon and presents primarily in children and young adults. The NF1 association is limited: only about 10 percent arise in this setting. The tumors are ill-defined, plaque-like thickenings of the dermis and subcutaneous tissue (fig. 8-5), usually of the head and neck. The content of overrun adipose tissue produces yellow patches and streaks, whereas the texture and color of the neurofibromatous tissue resembles that of localized cutaneous neurofibroma. Diffuse tumors are nondestructive of their surroundings. Instead, they permeate the dermis, entrapping cutaneous adnexa and spreading freely along connective tissue septa as well as within subcutaneous adipose tissue (fig. 8-6). Albeit a minor feature, pseudomeissnerian corpuscles may be seen. Diffuse cutaneous neurofibromas only rarely undergo malignant change.

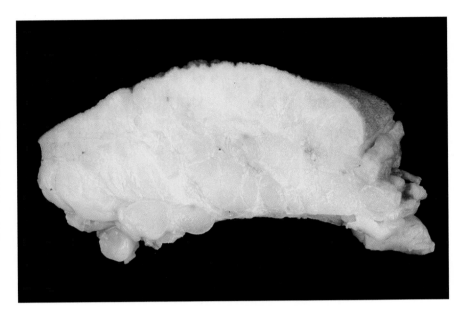

Figure 8-5

DIFFUSE CUTANEOUS NEUROFIBROMA

This NF1-associated example diffusely involves subcutaneous fat: strands of tumor separate lobules of fat. The white rather than gray-tan color is an artifact of fixation. (Fig. 3.444, left from Okazaki H, Scheithauer BW. Atlas of neuropathology. New York: Gower; 1988:190. With permission from the Mayo Foundation.)

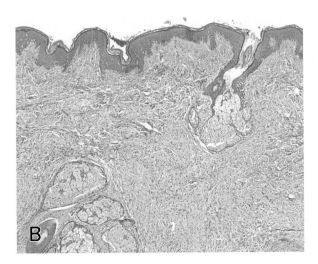

A

Figure 8-6

DIFFUSE CUTANEOUS NEUROFIBROMA

These tumors permeate dermal and subcutaneous tissues (A), surround adnexa (B), and infiltrate fat (C).

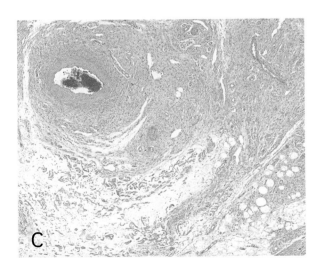

B

C

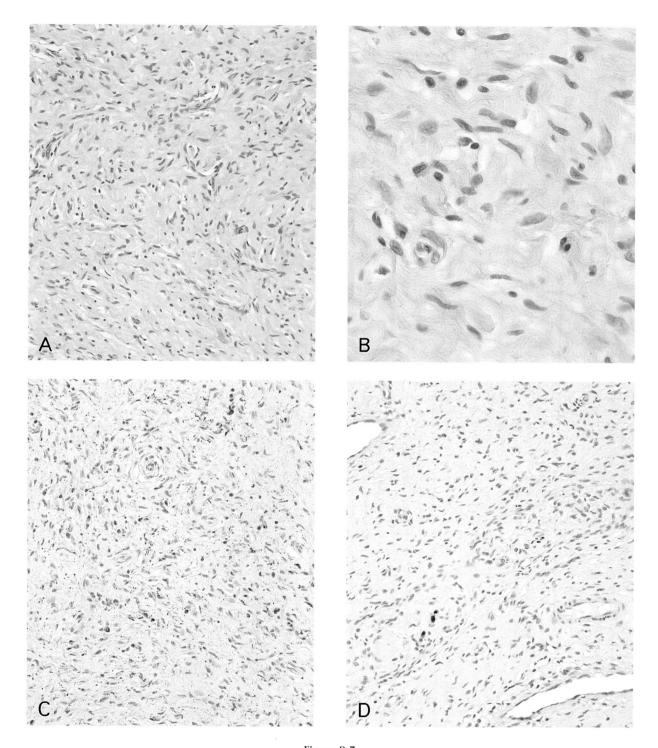

Figure 8-7

DIFFUSE CUTANEOUS NEUROFIBROMA

A: The tumor is characterized by dispersed spindled and ovoid tumor nuclei.

B: At high power, neither cell membranes nor cell processes are evident.

C: Many but not all cells are S-100 protein immunoreactive.

D: Such lesions are mainly extraneural and neuritic processes are scant (neurofilament stain).

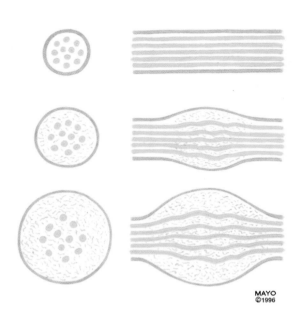

Figure 8-8

LOCALIZED INTRANEURAL NEUROFIBROMA

A schematic diagram illustrates the slow development of intraneural neurofibroma to a fusiform, mucin-rich lesion traversed by normal residual axons.

Localized Intraneural Neurofibroma. This form of neurofibroma (figs. 8-8–8-17), second in frequency to cutaneous lesions but far less common, is assumed by neurofibromas confined to a single fascicle or nerve. Its progressive, permeative intraneural growth results in segmental, fusiform nerve enlargement (figs. 8-8–8-11). The growth maintains the general contour of the uninvolved nerve. Examples range from less than one to many centimeters in greatest dimension (figs. 8-10, 8-11). Multiple lesions occur in the setting of NF1. In superficial soft tissues, localized intraneural neurofibromas come to clinical attention as a palpable lump. In deep soft tissues, they may cause tingling or pain along the course of a nerve. A number are incidental findings on imaging studies.

Localized intraneural neurofibromas may affect any nerve, spinal or cranial, from the level of the root to the smallest branches (figs. 8-12–8-17). Spinal root tumors occurring in NF1 patients preferentially affect the cervical level. Tumors arising in proximal spinal nerves may

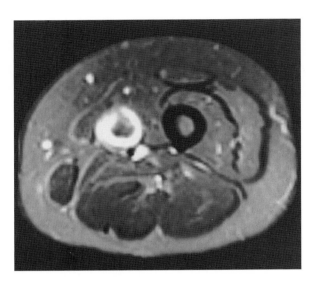

Figure 8-9

LOCALIZED INTRANEURAL NEUROFIBROMA

This axial T2-weighted magnetic resonance image (MRI) shows the target configuration often seen with this form of neurofibroma.

have both intraspinal and extraspinal components. Such "dumbbell" tumors occur both sporadically and in association with NF1. Intraneural neurofibromas also affect autonomic nerves. On gross examination, both localized and plexiform intraneural neurofibromas are covered by a thin sheath (figs. 8-10, 8-11A,B) that consists, microscopically, of perineurium and epineurium (see fig. 8-17C).

On cut section, the tumors are gray-tan to gray, and firm but translucent (figs. 8-10C, 8-11C). Color and texture variations reflect differences in collagen and mucin content. Linearly transected sections often demonstrate the centrally situated underlying residual nerve fibers (figs. 8-12, 8-14B). Compared with conventional schwannoma, intraneural neurofibromas lack the globular paraneural configuration, thick capsule, patchy bright yellow lipid accumulation, occasional foci of hemorrhage and, for the most part, cystic changes of the former. Some of these differences and the often targetoid appearance of neurofibroma as seen on cross section and on imaging scans (figs. 8-9, 8-10D) are helpful in the differentiation from MPNST (39). Localized intraneural neurofibromas undergo malignant change, but less frequently than plexiform neurofibromas.

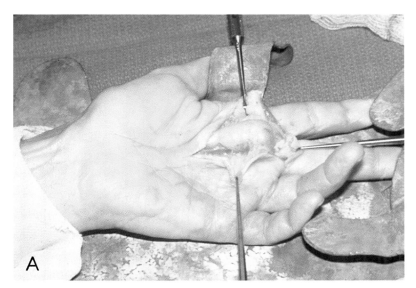

Figure 8-10

LOCALIZED INTRANEURAL NEUROFIBROMA

A: Resected neurofibroma.

B: Resection of this tumor involved its total removal, along with proximal and distal segments of the parent nerve.

C: A cross section displays the usual translucency and gray-tan color of such tumors.

D: Yet another example affecting a sensory nerve of the popliteal region in a NF1 patient shows typical T2-weighted MRI features.

E: During resection of this fusiform tumor uninvolved nerves fascicles were spared, resulting in no neurologic deficit.

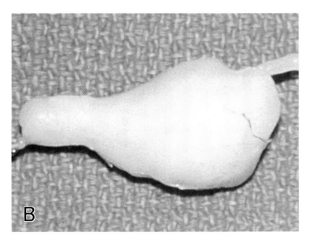

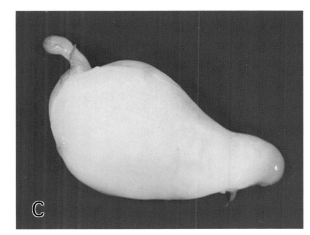

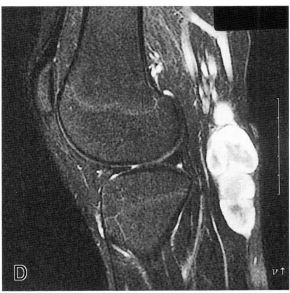

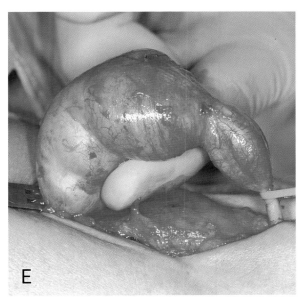

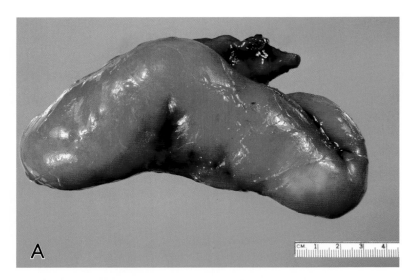

Figure 8-11

LOCALIZED INTRANEURAL NEUROFIBROMA

A: A sizable neurofibroma from the back of an 18-year-old NF1 patient. The normal nerve contour is maintained and the exterior lining of filamentous tissue seen.

B: Bulging, semi-glistening, opaque, tan cut tumor surface seen more than 3 minutes after sectioning of specimen shown in A.

C: Appearance of glistening, translucent, tan cut surface of another neurofibroma but photographed within the 3-minute time frame.

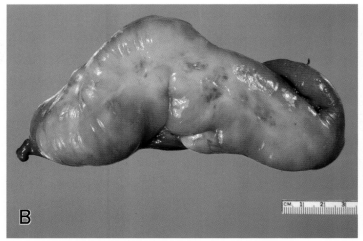

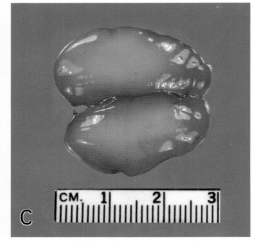

Plexiform Neurofibroma. This uncommon but highly distinctive variant of neurofibroma tends to affect sizable nerves (figs. 8-18–8-25) (2,40). Its recognition is important given its association with NF1 and the fact that it is more prone than other forms to undergo malignant change. Only rarely are plexiform tumors encountered in patients having no other features of NF1; most such lesions are small and superficially situated. The frequency of an NF1 association was investigated by MacCarron and Goldblum (41) who, using clinical records and pathology reports alone, found evidence supportive of the disorder in 85 percent of 49 patients with plexiform tumors. Any patient with a plexiform neurofibroma but no other feature of NF1 is a candidate for genetic evaluation.

The varied clinical manifestations of plexiform neurofibroma are discussed in detail in chapter 15. The process involves multiple nerve fascicles (figs. 8-19, 8-20) and is most commonly manifest as tumors of multiple branches of a nerve (figs. 8-18B; 8-19B,C; 8-21; 8-23–8-25). An affected nerve plexus, such as the brachial or sacral plexus, or other highly branching nerves, such as the trigeminal, may be altered by fusiform or ovoid masses arranged in an arbor-like pattern (fig. 8-18B,C). Less frequently, the result is a complex tangle of tumor-affected nerves likened to a "bag of worms" (figs. 8-19C; 8-21, top). Alternatively, extension of the process along the length of a nonbranching nerve may result in linear multinodularity (figs. 8-19D,E; 8-20). Such involvement of a sizable nerve, like

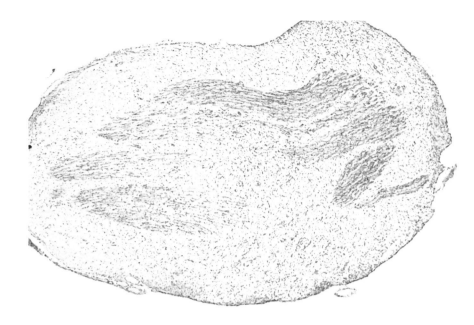

Figure 8-12

LOCALIZED INTRANEURAL NEUROFIBROMA

Residual nerve tissue is most apparent in neurofibromas of large nerves, such as this ovoid tumor involving an intradural spinal root in a patient with NF1. (Courtesy of Dr. H. Okazaki, Rochester, MN.)

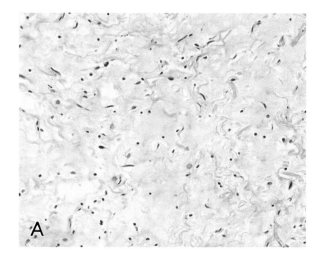

Figure 8-13

LOCALIZED INTRANEURAL NEUROFIBROMA

The proportion of stromal mucin to collagen varies in each case.

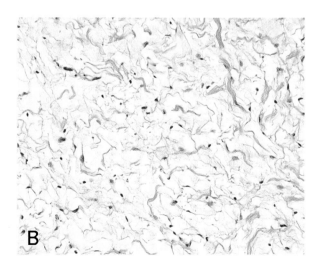

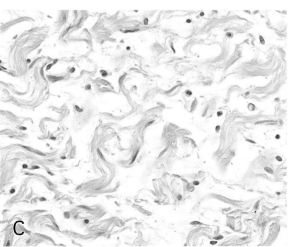

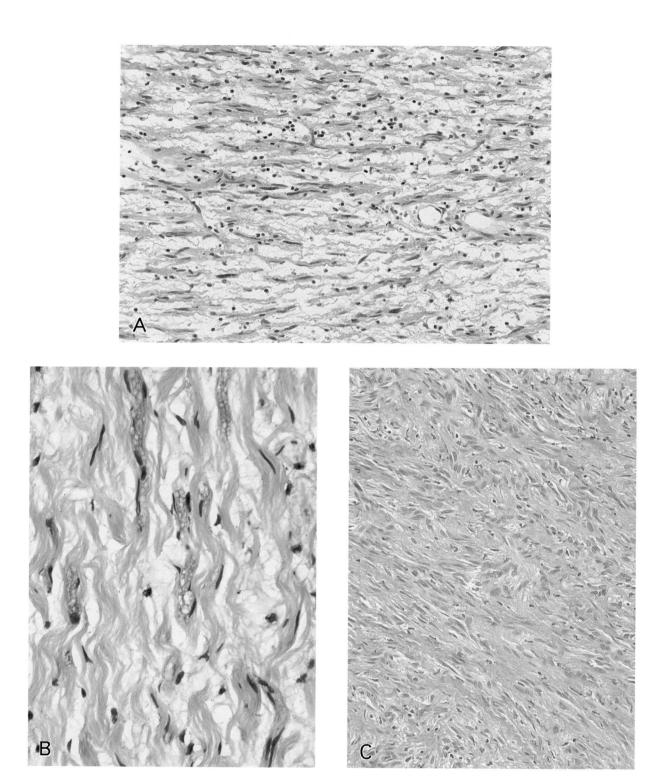

Figure 8-14

LOCALIZED INTRANEURAL NEUROFIBROMA

The cytology of such lesions varies from cells with dense, spindle-shaped curved nuclei (A,B) to ones in which nuclei are relatively plump (C). There are scattered residual myelinated nerve fibers (B).

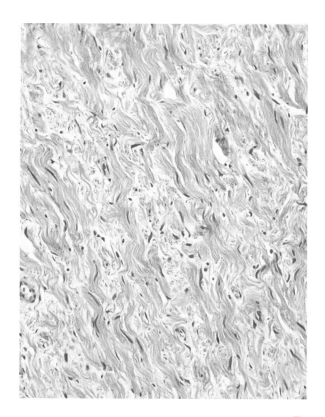 

Figure 8-15

LOCALIZED INTRANEURAL NEUROFIBROMA

Left: In longstanding tumors, there may be heavy collagen deposition.
Right: Stromal (matrical) mucin is demonstrated with the Alcian blue stain.

the sciatic, imparts the appearance of a massive, coarsely braided rope (fig. 8-21, bottom). An infrequently emphasized feature of nerves affected by plexiform neurofibromas is their marked cross-sectional enlargement compared to that of the normal nerve (fig. 8-21, bottom). Involvement of organs or viscera by plexiform neurofibromas, although grossly inconspicuous, is commonly seen at the microscopic level (see fig. 8-22). Plexiform components are also a frequent feature in massive soft tissue neurofibromas (fig. 8-27A).

The fascicles of plexiform tumors possess a mucin-rich stroma which contributes to the distension and translucency of affected nerves. This is especially the case in examples resembling a bag of worms. Most lesions have a rubbery feel but due to collagen deposition, large, often longstanding lesions may be firm and tan. Plexiform neurofibromas occasionally present as a somewhat bosselated cutaneous lesion (fig.

8-18A). Most neurofibromas affecting visceral autonomic nerves and mesentery are plexiform (fig. 8-22, see also figs. 15-14, 15-16D,H) (42). Malignant transformation of visceral examples is rare. The subject of plexiform neurofibromas affecting viscera, particularly the gastrointestinal tract (42), is discussed in chapter 15.

Massive Soft Tissue Neurofibroma. This least common form of neurofibroma (figs. 8-26, 8-27) is restricted to patients with NF1. Large and diffusely infiltrative of soft tissue, it causes extreme enlargement of the involved body region (fig. 8-26A,B). The presentation may take the form of folds of redundant soft tissue extending cape-like, as over the shoulder (see fig.15-11B), or expansive, pendulous soft tissue masses unilaterally enlarging the pelvic girdle and lower extremity (figs. 8-26B, 15-1). The tumors often infiltrate deep soft tissues, including muscle (fig. 8-26C). The now antiquated term "elephantiasis neuromatosa"

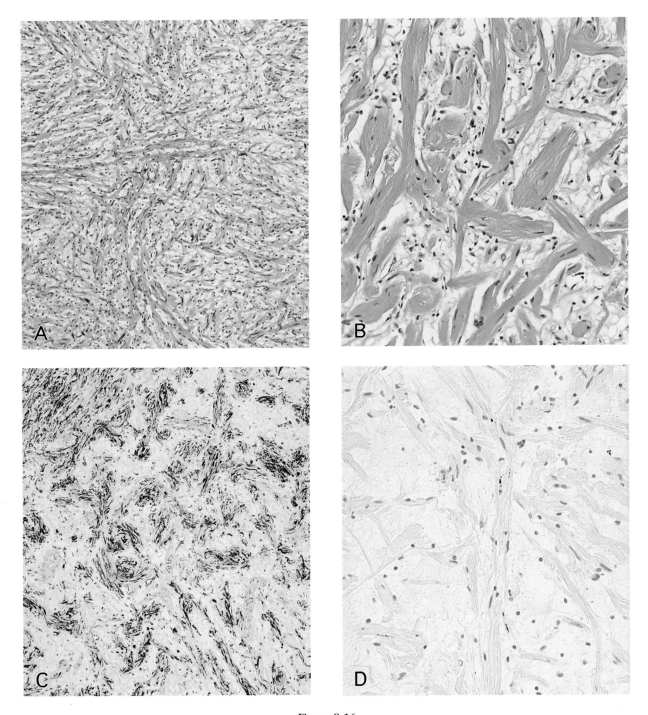

Figure 8-16

LOCALIZED INTRANEURAL NEUROFIBROMA

A,B: Collagen deposition is often progressive in neurofibroma, being laid down along the course of preexisting nerve fibers. The collagen bundles vary from long and narrow (A) to blocky in configuration (B), the latter likened to "shredded carrots."

C: Immunostains of a neurofibroma in which collagen deposition is just beginning shows abundant residual nerve fiber sheaths (S-100 protein immunostain).

D: Even after advanced collagen deposition, residual neurofilament-positive axons are present.

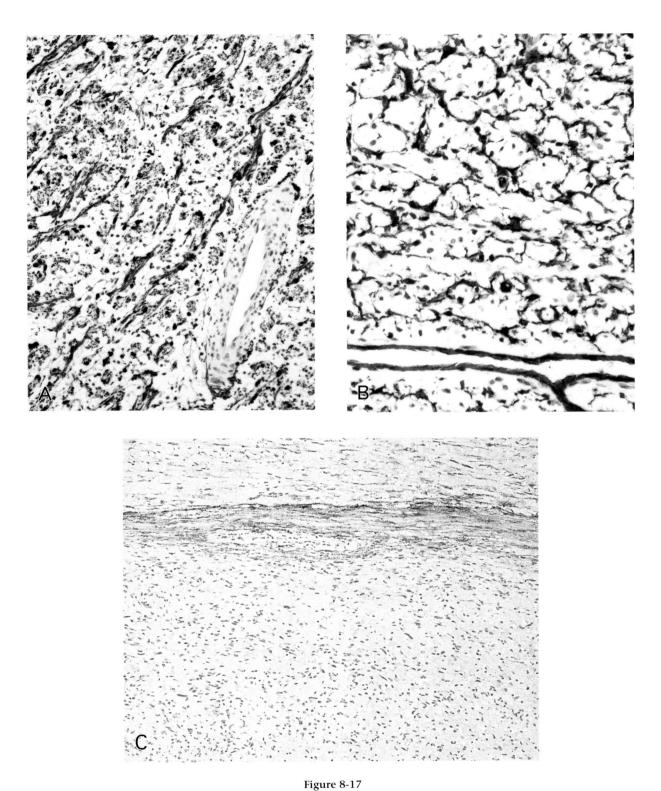

Figure 8-17

LOCALIZED INTRANEURAL NEUROFIBROMA

Immunostaining for S-100 protein (A) and CD34 (B). The grossly filamentous external covering consists in part of epithelial membrane antigen (EMA)-immunoreactive perineurium (C).

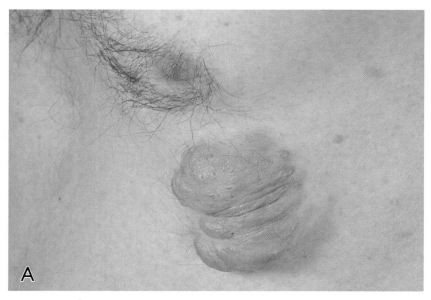

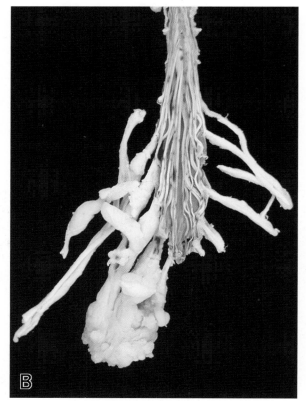

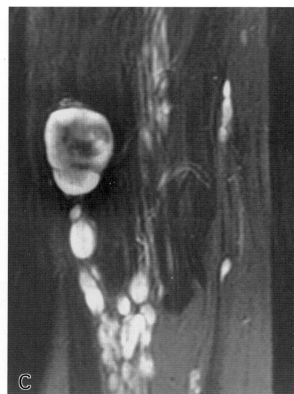

Figure 8-18

PLEXIFORM NEUROFIBROMA

A: Cutaneous and subcutaneous plexiform neurofibroma forms a protrusive lumpy mass, presumably arising from small nerves.

B: This larger example involves the lumbar plexus.

C: A coronal T2-weighted MRI of the thigh shows multiple interconnected lesions with increased signal, the largest of which has a target configuration.

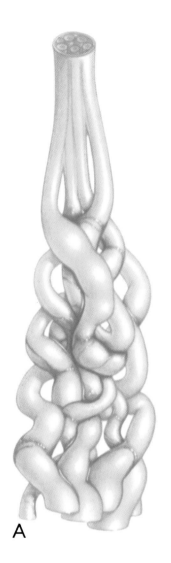
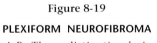
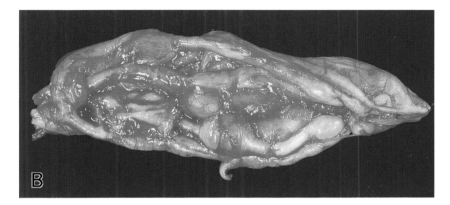
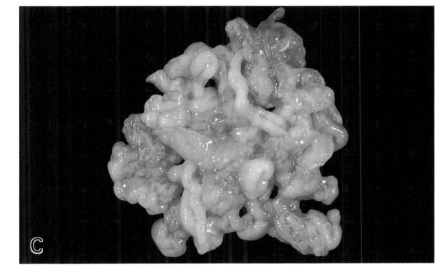
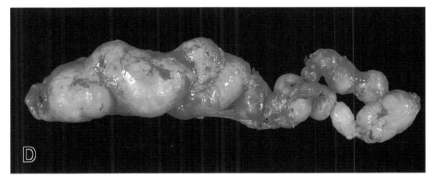
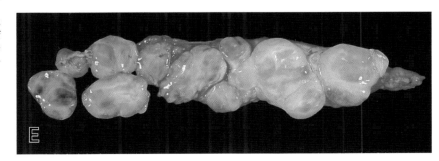

Figure 8-19

PLEXIFORM NEUROFIBROMA

A,B: These distinctive lesions consist of neurofibromatous change in multiple nerve fascicles.

C: Unfortunately, surgical specimens often consist of only fragmented nerve segments.

D,E: While occasional tumors consist of abnormal fascicles of uniform diameter, other fascicles are transformed into segmental, jelly-like expansions.

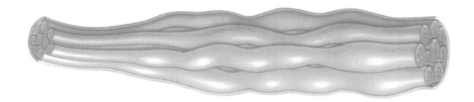

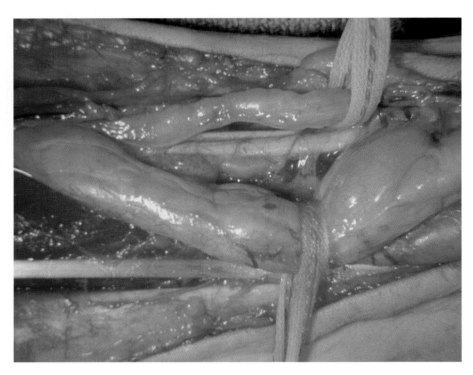

Figure 8-20

PLEXIFORM NEUROFIBROMA

Top: In large and generally nonbranching nerves, plexiform neurofibromas form a rope-like mass.

Bottom: One such tumor of the ulnar nerve involves multiple fascicles in each of two branches.

was once applied to these especially large examples. Melanin pigmentation may involve the overlying skin (fig. 8-26A,B) and appear as patchy foci within the underlying tumor (fig. 8-27E). A related form of the process is "localized gigantism," an impressive quasi-malformative process resulting in a more limited distortion of the body, such as a hand (fig. 8-26D) (43). Both forms of soft tissue neurofibroma diffusely invade soft tissue and often include a coexisting plexiform component.

Massive soft tissue neurofibromas only rarely undergo malignant change. The presence of mitoses should not prompt consideration of malignant change. Of greater concern is that their presence occasionally masks an underlying plexiform neurofibroma that is undergoing or has undergone malignant transformation.

MICROSCOPIC FINDINGS

Most neurofibroma variants share several histologic features. In their simplest form, the tumors are hypocellular and composed of widely spaced cells with ovoid to thin (fig. 8-14A,B), occasionally slightly plump (fig. 8-14C), elongated and often curved nuclei, as well as scant cytoplasm embedded in a mucocollagenous matrix (see fig. 8-3C). The majority of cells are S-100 protein immunoreactive (figs. 8-7C, 8-17A, 8-24C). Composed of mucopolysaccharides, the matrix appears watery and gray-blue on hematoxylin and eosin (H&E) stain, strongly Alcian blue positive (figs. 8-15, 8-25), weakly periodic acid–Schiff (PAS) reactive, and hyaluronidase sensitive. In lesions in which residual nerve is apparent, the neurofibroma cells are either

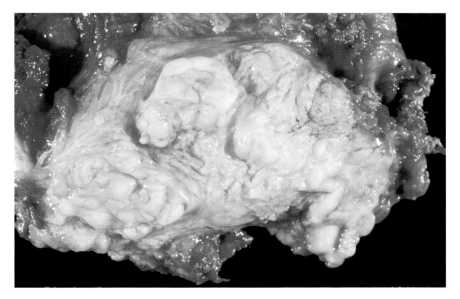

Figure 8-21

PLEXIFORM NEUROFIBROMA

Top: This example that arose in the cheek of a 7-year-old male with NF1 has a classic bag-of-worms appearance.

Bottom: Compared to the diameter of the normal adult sciatic nerve seen below, that of the above involved sciatic nerve is markedly enlarged.

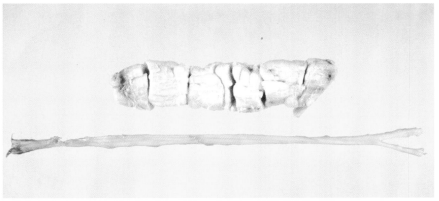

aligned along the course of its fibers (figs. 8-12, 8-14B) or lie randomly dispersed. The nuclei of neurofibroma cells are roughly one third to half the size of those of schwannoma cells and three or more times the size of lymphocyte nuclei (fig. 8-14A). In most instances, their cytoplasmic processes are indiscernible without recourse to immunohistochemistry or electron microscopy (figs. 8-3C; 8-7; 8-14A,B). Lymphocytes and histiocytes are uncommon, but mast cells are often significant in number. Far more rare are melanin-containing cells (fig. 8-27E) (44,45). These are never as numerous as in the melanotic variant of schwannoma, but when found, are most frequently seen in diffuse neurofibromas.

The proportion of stromal mucin to collagen is variable (figs. 8-13, 8-15). Plexiform tumors exhibit the most pronounced mucin formation (figs. 8-22C, 8-25A,C). The collagen fibers in localized and diffuse cutaneous neurofibromas as well as in diffuse soft tissue neurofibromas are typically delicate (figs. 8-3, 8-7A,B) and lie dispersed within variable amounts of mucin. In contrast, intraneural neurofibromas often contain coarse, refractile collagen fibers (figs. 8-13C; 8-15; 8-16A,B). Compact, aligned, and sizable bundles of collagen resembling shredded carrots are a characteristic feature of intraneural tumors, and when abundant, can cause confusion with a fibrous tumor (fig. 8-16B) (43).

The histologic features of plexiform neurofibroma are highly distinctive. Macroscopic examination (fig. 8-23A) reveals few to numerous smooth-contoured, roughly ovoid and elongated structures, identifiable as distorted enlarged nerve fascicles by their content of centrally situated dense cores of normal S-100 protein- and neurofilament protein-positive nerve fibers

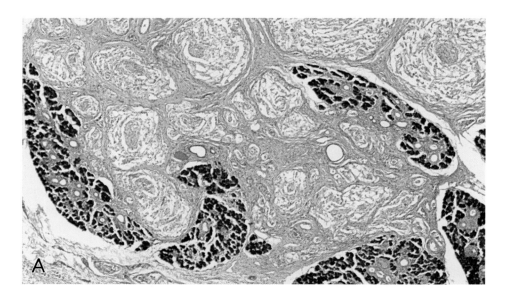

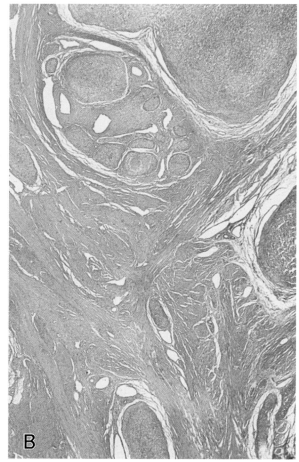

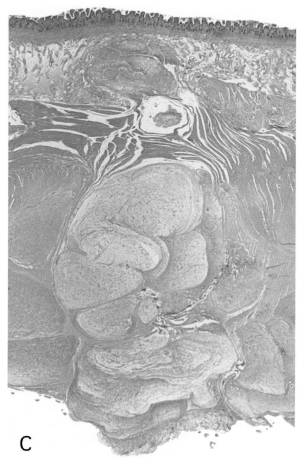

Figure 8-22

PLEXIFORM NEUROFIBROMA

Involvement of parotid gland (trigeminal nerve) (A), uterus (B), and small bowel (C) by plexiform neurofibroma.

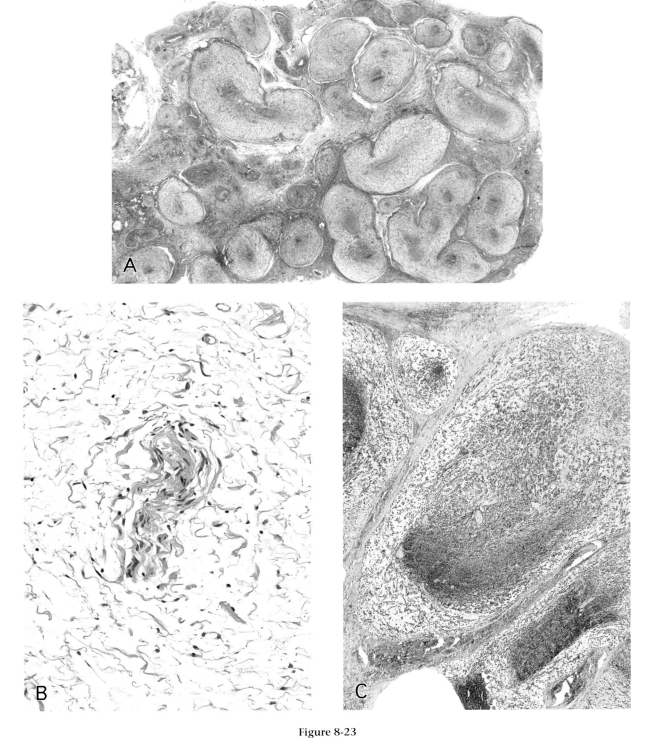

Figure 8-23

PLEXIFORM NEUROFIBROMA

A: Multiple fascicles are enlarged by neurofibroma tissue expanding out from the central core of parent nerve tissue.

B: Centrally placed nerve fibers at higher power.

C: Nerve fibers of core are readily highlighted with immunostains for S-100 protein.

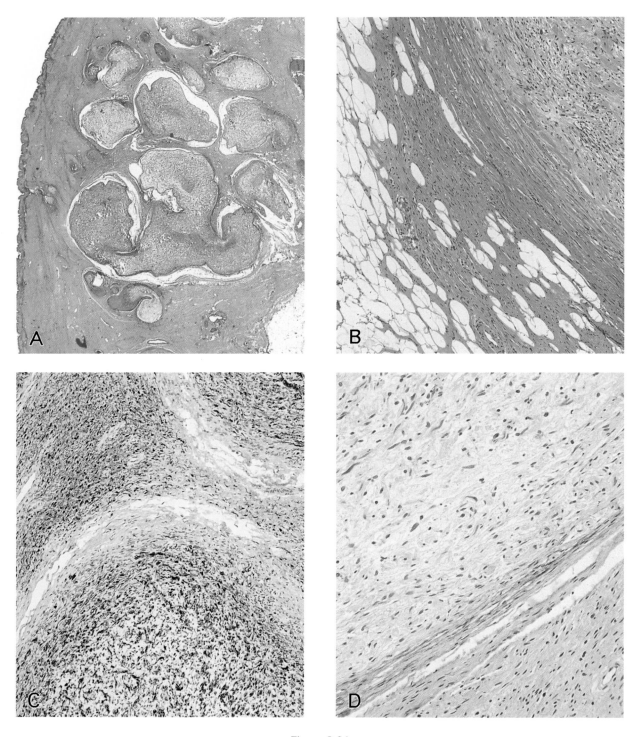

Figure 8-24

PLEXIFORM NEUROFIBROMA

A: This superficially situated example had an accompanying diffuse dermal and subcutaneous component.
B: At higher power, the extension of neurofibroma cells into the surrounding adipose tissue is well seen.
C: Immunostains for S-100 protein show reactivity in both the intraneural and extraneural components.
D: Immunoreactivity for EMA is limited to the residual perineurial sheaths surrounding affected fascicles.

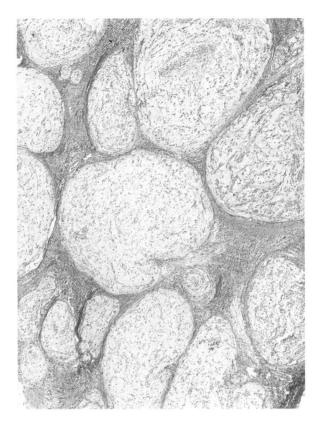
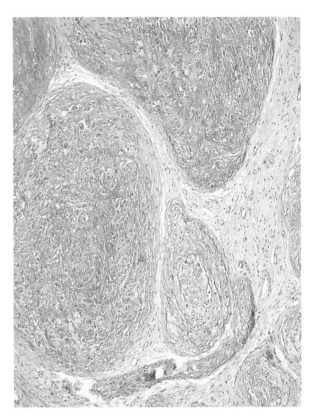

Figure 8-25

PLEXIFORM NEUROFIBROMA

Neurofibromatous tissue involving nerve fascicles is often pale and rich in mucin (left), which stains strongly with Alcian blue (right).

(fig. 8-23B,C) and their surrounding distended perineurium (fig. 8-24D). Fascicle enlargement is due to neurofibromatous tissue that insinuates between and encases the residual nerve fibers, in the process distending the perineurium. In a majority of examples there is bulk enhancement of the neurofibroma caused by the presence of a mucin-rich matrix (fig. 8-25). The grossly evident filamentous external covering of both intraneural and plexiform neurofibromas is represented microscopically by a stretched perineurium and epineurium (figs. 8-12, 8-17). In focal areas, due to oblique sectioning, this covering may appear to be thickened, thereby simulating a true capsule. Intrafascicular involvement in plexiform neurofibromas can be accompanied by tumor extension into the epineurium and surrounding soft tissues (fig. 8-24A,B). Nondestructive entrapment of cutaneous adnexa and extension into adipose tissue (figs. 8-6, 8-24B),

and permeation of both adipose tissue and skeletal muscle (figs. 8-26C; 8-27D,F) are conspicuous features of diffuse cutaneous and massive soft tissue neurofibromas, respectively.

DIAGNOSTICALLY CONFUSING MICROSCOPIC FINDINGS

Several histologic features in neurofibromas may cause diagnostic confusion. These include hypercellularity, tactile-like corpuscle formation, perineurial-like and perineurial cells, clusters of densely aggregated small nuclei, melanin-containing cells, epithelioid cell change, cellular schwannoma-like nodules, onion bulb-like changes, hyalinized laminated Schwann cell whorls, and divergent (heterologous) differentiation.

Hypercellularity with and without Epithelioid Cell Change. Infrequently, neurofibromas show a noticeable increase in cytologically nonatypical constituent cells, either as a

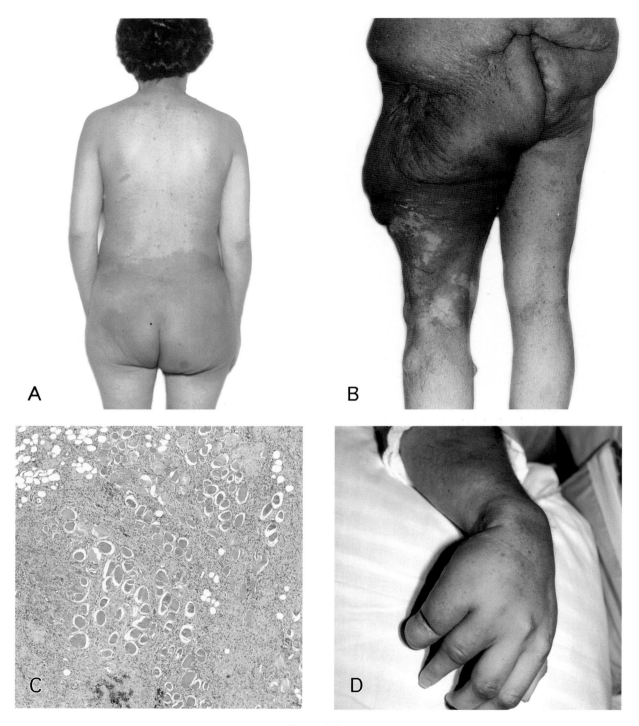

Figure 8-26

MASSIVE SOFT TISSUE NEUROFIBROMA

A: This diffuse lesion involves the buttocks and is associated with widespread cutaneous hyperpigmentation.

B: Another impressive example shows involvement not only of the hip girdle but of the leg as well ("elephantiasis neuromatosa"). The underlying lesion also included a large plexiform neurofibroma.

C: Diffuse components of such tumors freely infiltrate fat and skeletal muscle.

D: Localized gigantism of the hand of a NF1 patient is caused by a diffusely infiltrative neurofibroma.

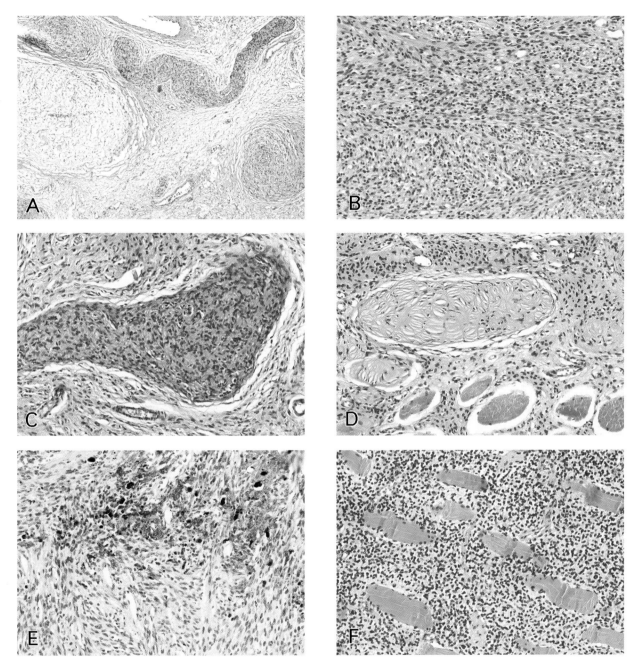

Figure 8-27

MASSIVE SOFT TISSUE NEUROFIBROMA

A: The proliferation varies from cellular to hypocellular.

B: The constituent cells vary in cytology from ones with ovoid nuclei and scant cytoplasm to others with frankly spindled cytology.

A,C: Such tumors frequently exhibit plexiform components which lie jumbled within the proliferation.

D: Pseudomeissnerian corpuscles are a common feature.

E: Less frequent is the finding of melanin pigmentation.

F: These neurofibromas typically invade surrounding soft tissues, as evidenced by extensive skeletal muscle infiltration. The increased cellularity seen here, not to be mistaken for a malignant small cell neoplasm, is explained by tumor cells having diminished cytoplasm and the lack of stromal collagen.

focal or diffuse feature. This is mostly seen in the intraneural, plexiform, and diffuse forms of neurofibroma (figs. 8-27A-C, 8-28). More rarely, an intraneural or diffuse neurofibroma contains proliferative cells that are epithelioid. The epithelioid cells, which may be few in number, are individual or arranged in nests, and multinucleated (fig. 8-29) (46). As in ordinary neurofibromas, the tumor cells have indistinct cell margins and to varying degrees a symplastic appearance. The cell cytoplasm is often dense and ranges from eosinophilic to amphophilic. Nuclei are round to ovoid, mildly to markedly pleomorphic, and devoid of large nucleoli. Mitotic activity is routinely low. The epithelioid cells express S-100 protein, typically more intensely than ordinary neurofibroma cells (fig. 8-29B,E). Stains for EMA, keratins, and HMB45 are negative. The distinction from epithelioid MPNST is primarily based on the tumor's lack of a malignant cytology (see chapter 12).

Tactile-Like Bodies, Perineurial-Like Cells, and Perineurial Cells. Cell arrangements resembling tactile corpuscles may be found in neurofibromas. These consist primarily of stacked, thin, lamellar cell processes mimicking those of Meissner corpuscles (fig. 8-30). Both the latter and the pseudomeissnerian simulators are reactive for S-100 protein. Whereas in meissnerian corpuscles this immunoreactivity is due to its composition of intricately layered nerve fibers (see fig. 2-19), their mimics consist entirely of perineurial-like cells (fig. 8-41) (14,47,48). Perineurial-like cells possess the ultrastructural features of perineurial cells but, at least in tactile-like bodies, the immunoprofile of Schwann cells. Additionally, pseudomeissnerian bodies feature a peripheral rim of EMA-positive perineurial cells (fig. 8-30D); Meissner corpuscles do not. Pseudomeissnerian bodies are most commonly found in diffuse and massive soft tissue neurofibromas (fig. 8-27D), but are also seen in the plexiform variety. Most lie, disposed singly or in clusters, within the substance of the tumor. In massive diffuse neurofibromas they form aggregates within what appears to be peritumoral fat. Pseudomeissnerian bodies are also found in large congenital nevi.

It has been suggested, although without strong support, that some tactile-like bodies in neurofibromas resemble pacinian corpuscles (48a). This is largely based upon the occasional findings of tumor cells nonspecifically disposed in a circular formations (49) and examples of pseudomeissnerian bodies rounded in shape (fig. 8-30). The view that pacinian-like corpuscles occur in neurofibromas gained early support from Weiser's demonstration (48) that their cells ultrastructurally resemble perineurial cells, the principal constituent of true pacinian corpuscles. This interpretation was revised based upon subsequent immunohistochemical studies. Even though these cellular formations closely simulate pacinian corpuscles, the suggestion that the neurofibromas harboring them should be designated "pacinian neurofibromas" (50) is unwarranted, in as much as their cells express mainly S-100 protein rather than EMA, as do true pacinian corpuscles. Some so-called pacinian neurofibromas of the hand (51) may be pacinian neuromas or perineuriomas, as reported to occur in the maxilla by Toth et al. (52). The maxilla is a known site of origin for such tumors. Others may best be interpreted as examples of nerve sheath myxoma (53,54). Cells exhibiting bona fide perineurial differentiation are occasionally found in neurofibromas. In addition to those comprising the rim of pseudomeissnerian bodies (fig. 8-30), focal collections of EMA-positive spindle cells, as mentioned above, may be part of the neoplastic process.

Densely Aggregated Small Nuclei. These crowded cell aggregates warrant attention since in the past they were sometimes considered a sign of malignant transformation in massive neurofibromas, the subset of neurofibromas in which they are usually encountered (2). In most instances, their nuclei are small, have inconspicuous cytoplasmic processes, and are separated by a mucinous and collagenous matrix. However, in some areas of massive neurofibroma as a result of diminished or absent matrix, the nuclei become densely packed (fig. 8-27F). Nuclear atypia is absent in such cells, and the finding of occasional mitotic figures is of no prognostic significance.

Melanin-Containing Cells. Melanin-pigmented cells are rarely found in neurofibromas. Such cases necessitate careful exclusion of histologic mimics including large examples of congenital neuronevus, neurocristic cutaneous hamartoma, and pigmented dermatofibrosarcoma protuberans (55). These reservations aside,

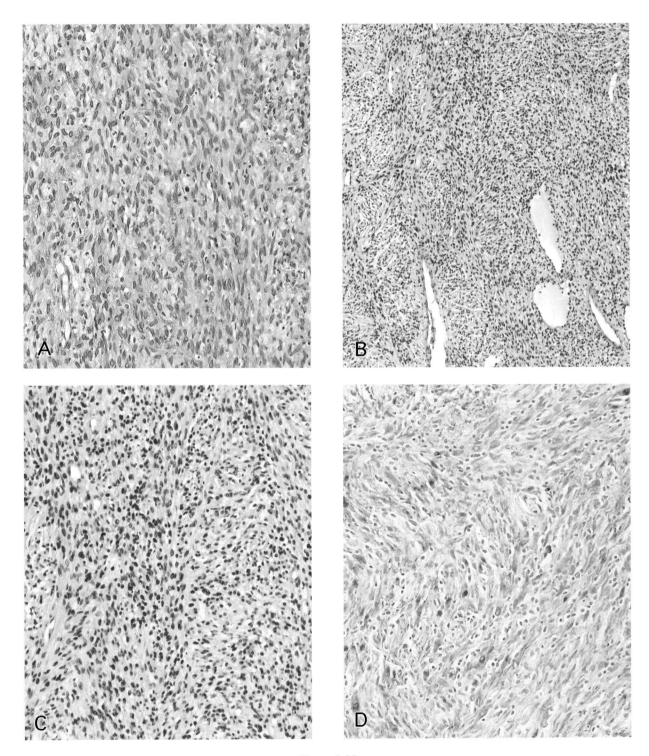

Figure 8-28

SIMPLE CELLULAR NEUROFIBROMA

Increased cellularity in a neurofibroma (A–C) is usually focal rather than diffuse. Increased nuclear size, pleomorphism, and epithelioid cell change are not features. There may be occasional mitotic figures. B and C are areas of a massive diffuse neurofibroma. As with noncellular neurofibromas, the tumors express S-100 protein (D).

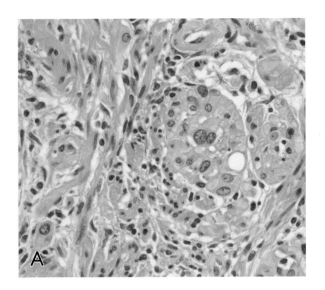

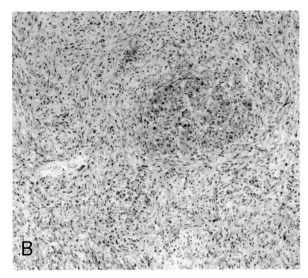

Figure 8-29

NEUROFIBROMA WITH EPITHELIOID CELL CHANGE

A: This plexiform neurofibroma has a few nests of cytologically benign epithelioid tumor cells.

B: Such nests stand out from the background neurofibroma due to their intense S-100-protein staining.

C,D: A diffuse neurofibroma involving skin and subcutaneous tissue from the back of a 64-year-old woman recurred locally 30 months after resection. The recurrence had individual and nested, enlarged round cells with abundant amphophilic cytoplasm and densely hyperchromatic, slightly pleomorphic nuclei. The nested cells were syncytially arranged.

E: The epithelioid cells were strongly positive for S-100 protein, but negative for keratins (CAM5.2 and AE1) and EMA. Followed for 153 months, the patient was alive and free of further recurrences. (Courtesy of Dr. U. Raju, Detroit, MI.)

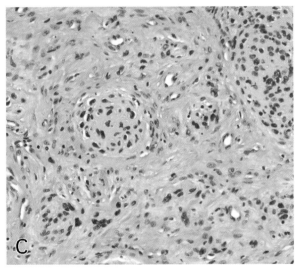

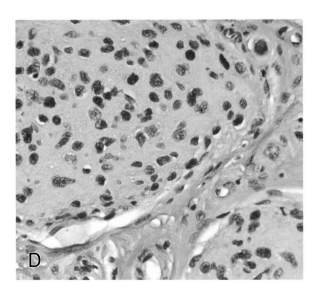

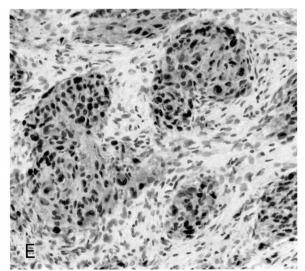

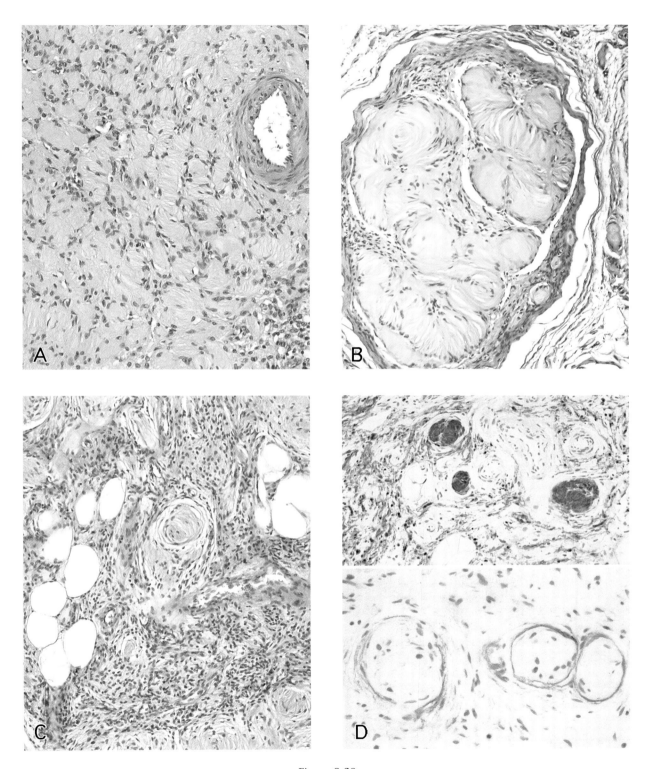

Figure 8-30

PLEXIFORM NEUROFIBROMA

Tactile-like bodies are present (A–D). These mimic Meissner corpuscles and are referred to as pseudomeissnerian bodies. Most of their constituent cells react strongly for S-100 protein, but often there is a rim of EMA-positive cells (D).

the only sizable clinicopathologic study of pigmented neurofibromas bearing such cells is that of Fetsch et al. (55) who reported 19 such tumors occurring in 17 patients; 47 percent of the affected individuals had NF1. The most common sites of involvement were the head and neck as well as the lower extremity. There was a male gender bias and a broad age range (2 to 61 years). Where data was available, 9 patients were black, 3 were Latin American/Hispanic, 1 was Asian, and 2 were white. The tumors involved primarily skin and subcutaneous tissue and varied greatly in size: 6 were greater than 10 cm and 3 were 20 cm or more. For the most part, the tumors were not grossly pigmented: only 2 exhibited small areas of brown discoloration. Histologically, the pigmented cells were arranged in irregular patches or were distributed diffusely throughout the tumors. None formed nodules. The tumors stained appropriately for melanin and melanocytic markers. The mitotic activity averaged less than 1 mitosis per 50 high-power fields. There was no nuclear atypia except for some degenerative changes. Follow-up showed that melanin-pigmented neurofibromas behaved no differently than similar nonmelanotic examples. The overwhelming predominance of dark-skinned individuals among those affected raised the question of whether the presence of intratumoral pigmented cells is the result of migration of normal melanocytes. In our own experience, the melanotic cells in some massive diffuse neurofibromas are focally distributed (figs. 8-26C, 8-27E), and sometimes seen in tumors arising in whites (fig. 8-26B). Since melanotic pigmentation is often minor and not reflected in a tumor's gross appearance or behavior, we do not think its finding warrants consideration of pigmented neurofibroma as a distinct entity.

Onion Bulb-Like Changes, Differentiated Neoplastic Schwann Cell Nodules ("Microschwannomas"), and Hyalinized Laminated Schwann Cell Whorls. These three findings represent forms of localized Schwann cell proliferation in neurofibromas. Masson (56) considered the first two to be related, viewing them as stages in a sequence of Schwann cell proliferation in neurofibroma, beginning with a concentric onion bulb-like encasement of individual nerve fibers by spindled tumor cells (fig. 8-31), and progressing to the formation of discrete Schwann cell nodules (fig. 8-32). The third finding is thought to represent partial to complete hyalinization of onion bulb-like structures not having progressed to the stage of nodule formation (fig. 8-33). The cells of all three arrangements express S-100 protein (figs. 8-31B, 8-32C), but the ultrastructural features of differentiated Schwann cells have been documented in only the first two (19,57,58).

Of these findings, the Schwann cell nodules have been the most thoroughly studied (2, 19,56–59). Feany et al. (57), reporting nine neurofibromas with such nodules, noted an adult male predilection and most frequent involvement of plexiform tumors, but no direct clinical association with NF1. Most nodules are smaller than 1 cm (57), with one illustrated example large enough (2.5 cm) to be grossly visible (19). At low magnification, they appear as a usually normochromatic, round or ovoid mass, set against a background of pale-staining neurofibroma. In some cases the nodularity is multifocal (2,57,58).

The nodules have the features of mini-schwannomas (57,58). They are identical to Antoni A tissue of schwannoma; no Antoni B tissue is found. Cell palisading has been reported (58), and occasionally a Verocay body is seen (fig. 8-32). Mitotic figures are scarce, but in one study the MIB-1 labeling index was higher on average than that reported for schwannomas in general (57). Although usually lacking encapsulation, two nodules in a multinodular example were covered by thin layers of EMA-reactive cells (58), an indication of differentiation to perineurial cells.

Neurofibroma with discrete intratumoral schwannoma has been referred to as a hybrid neurofibroma/schwannoma (57). Notable is an absence of histologic evidence, even suggestive, that the cells of either tumor cell type are undergoing transformation to those of the other. Nor is it necessary to propose such. It has been shown in genetic studies that a key step in the pathogenesis of all nonmelanotic schwannomas, including those of schwannomatosis, is a genetic or functional loss of the tumor suppressor gene product, merlin (schwannomin) (58a).

Evidence for the schwannoma arising from a clone of neoplastic cells different from that of the neurofibroma is both histologic and genetic. The schwannoma appears to arise directly from

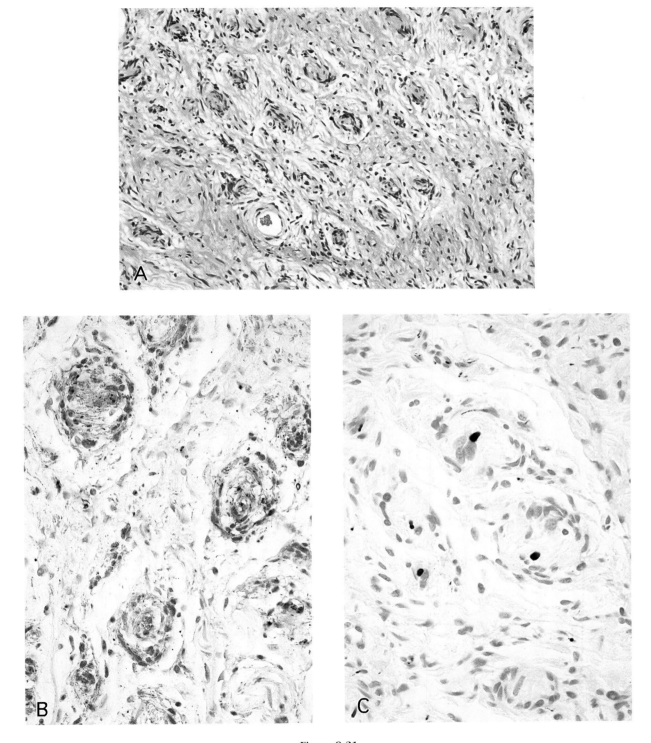

Figure 8-31

PLEXIFORM NEUROFIBROMA WITH ONION BULB-LIKE ARRANGEMENT OF NEOPLASTIC SCHWANN CELLS

A: Such arrangements of neoplastic Schwann cells are rarely seen.

B,C: The proliferative cells are arranged around individual axons (C), reactive for S-100 protein (B), and thought to be associated with the formation of minischwannomas (see fig. 8-32).

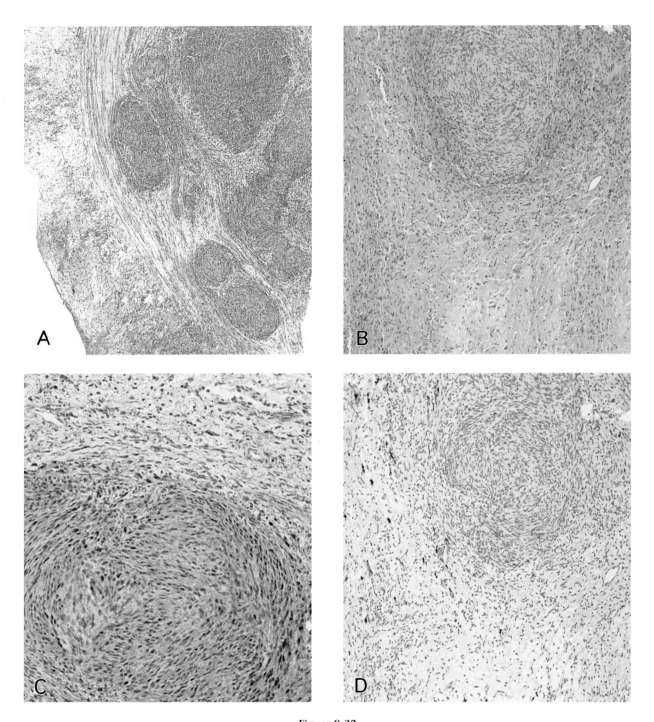

Figure 8-32

PLEXIFORM NEUROFIBROMA WITH MINISCHWANNOMAS

A: With rare exception, such schwannomas are microscopic findings.

B: They are surrounded by ordinary neurofibromatous tissue, and may stain with Alcian blue stain.

C: In contrast to the scattered S-100 protein-positive neurofibroma cells, the cells of the schwannomas are uniformly reactive for this marker.

D: In contrast to their appearance in the schwannoma, the surrounding neurofibroma contains readily identified residual nerve fibers (neurofilament protein immunostain).

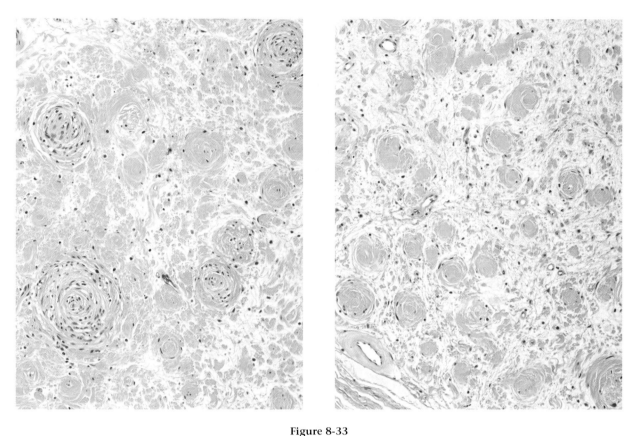

Figure 8-33

PLEXIFORM NEUROFIBROMA WITH HYALINIZED NEOPLASTIC SCHWANN CELL WHORLS

Those onion bulb-like cell formations not progressing to viable minischwannomas undergo hyalinization. In this case, cell whorls with beginning hyalinization are numerous.

individual nerve fibers in the neurofibroma, with the initial proliferative phase represented by onion-bulb cellular arrangements (fig. 8-31). Consistent with this is a nuclear size that is larger than that of the surrounding neurofibroma cells. Before reaching the nodule stage the cells coalesce, forming cell whorls (fig. 8-33). These are morphologically identical to those found in cellular schwannomas (see fig. 7-40C). Perhaps explaining why so few schwannomas are found in most cases, is the observed frequency of their hyalinization. An explanation for the development of such clones is the frequent loss of chromosome arm 22q, in some cases specifically of 22q12, the locus of the *NF2* gene, that has been reported to occur in both NF1-associated and sporadic neurofibromas (34a). Perhaps a clue why a majority of involved neurofibromas are plexiform in type is that 22q---qter is more frequently deleted in NF1-associated tumors.

The presence of a Schwann cell nodule in a neurofibroma is more than a curiosity. For pathologists unfamiliar with this tumor type it is a source of two diagnostic problems: uncertainty whether the overall tumor is a schwannoma or neurofibroma, and the distinction between an unusual neurofibroma and one that has undergone malignant transformation. If a schwannoma, the tumor would be biphasic in type, a doubtful possibility given the absence of thick-walled blood vessels in the less cellular component and of a tumor capsule. Their absence, along with the presence of numerous nerve fibers in tumor surrounding the nodule, are characteristics common to plexiform and solitary intraneural neurofibromas. Either neurofibroma variant can be focally hypercellular, but knowing they are also the principal types of neurofibroma from which MPNSTs arise, the uniformly larger size of the cells in the nodule raises concern about a malignant transformation; countering this is an absence of marked hyperchromasia or other features of anaplasia. A point useful in the distinction is that nodule formation is not a growth trait seen in early MPNST.

If the relative incidence of malignancy in schwannomas and neurofibromas serves as a reliable guide, the minischwannomas seen in this hybrid tumor are unlikely sites of malignant transformation. All neurofibromas of this type reported by Feany et al. (57) were histologically benign, as were those seen in our own laboratory (19). If such a change were to occur, one would expect the transformed cells to be epithelioid or neuroepithelial, not spindle cell in type (see chapter 12).

Divergent (Heterologous) Differentiation. This rare phenomenon is a form of mesenchymal or true epithelial differentiation. The most frequently occurring example of mesenchymal differentiation is angiosarcoma (see chapter 12). Rarer still are examples of epithelial differentiation, usually in the form of intestinal-type glands lined by both mucin-producing and endocrine-type cells (fig. 8-34). One reported glandular plexiform neurofibroma also contained an element of angiosarcoma (see fig.12-45) (19).

IMMUNOHISTOCHEMICAL FINDINGS

Although immunostains are usually unnecessary in the diagnosis of neurofibroma, all forms routinely stain for S-100 protein (figs. 8-7C, 8-16C, 8-17A, 8-23C, 8-24C, 8-28D). The proportion of immunoreactive cells varies greatly but falls short of that seen in schwannoma (60). The tactile-like bodies discussed above are also S-100 protein immunoreactive (fig. 8-30D). Staining for Leu-7 is seen in greater than half of neurofibromas (61). Despite the presence of cells with the ultrastructural features of perineurial-like cells, neurofibromas do not, as a rule, contain EMA-immunoreactive cells. When found, reactivity for this antigen is seen in residual, often compressed normal perineurium at the tumor edge, surrounding involved nerve fascicles (figs. 8-17C, 8-24D) (62), and at the periphery of some tactile-like bodies (fig. 8-30D). Only infrequently do conventional immunohistochemical methods stain collections of EMA-positive spindle cells within the

tumor cell population (18,20). Use of catalyzed signal amplification (CSA) to enhance EMA immunoreactivity results in a more frequent finding of such cells than does conventional methods (26). Neurofibromas also contain some CD34-immunoreactive cells (fig. 8-17B) (63–65). This antigen is also found in the endoneurium cells of the normal nerve, Antoni B tissue of schwannomas, and traumatic neuromas. In various mesenchymal tissues, CD34 staining occurs in the dermis (66); in dermatofibrosarcoma protuberans it is thought to be a marker of a fibroblast subset. That they are not Schwann cells has been shown by lack of double staining for CD34 and S-100 protein (67). Collagen IV staining in neurofibromas is typically pericellular and involves many cells (68). Residual axons are neurofilament protein immunoreactive (figs. 8-7D, 8-16D, 8-31C, 8-32D).

Two immunohistochemical studies of proliferation marker expression by neurofibromas have been reported (69,70). In the larger study of 26 cases (70), the MIB-1 (Ki-67) labeling indices ranged from 1 to 13 percent (mean, 4.7 percent). Atypical neurofibromas, inclusive of cellular examples, had indices one standard deviation (3.2 percent) higher than typical tumors. In comparison, 28 MPNSTs had indices of 5 to 38 percent (mean, 18.5 percent; standard deviation, 9.6 percent). A smaller study of five cutaneous and four plexiform tumors (69) found MIB-1 labeling indices of less than 1 percent in all cases; a comparison group of 26 MPNSTs showed that all but 3 tumors had values greater than 5 percent and half of all tumors had values of greater than 30 percent. Staining for p53 protein is seen in less than 5 percent of neurofibromas, including plexiform examples (42,71).

ULTRASTRUCTURAL FINDINGS

Although electron microscopy is rarely required in the diagnosis of neurofibroma, it has played an important role in the assessment of the cellular composition and the complex cell/stroma interactions that characterize these lesions. Regardless of the type of neurofibroma under consideration, individual cases and different areas of a single tumor are characterized by variations in cellular makeup (72–74).

Schwann Cells. The most numerous cells encountered ultrastructurally in neurofibromas of any form are Schwann cells (figs. 8-38, 8-39, 8-43). Often lying singly, they are primarily found among concentrations of collagen fibers (fig. 8-43), which their variously sectioned processes encircle (figs. 8-38, 8-43). Schwann cells are recognized by this latter characteristic, as well as by their thin cytoplasmic processes, content of intermediate filaments and occasional microtubules, and continuous surface basement membrane (external lamina) (figs. 8-38, 8-43). Pinocytotic vesicles are inconspicuous or absent. Scattered myelinated and unmyelinated nerve fibers are also evident (fig. 8-43), but are markedly reduced in number as compared to normal nerve.

Perineurial-Like Cells. Cells with the ultrastructural features of perineurial cells are variably distributed within neurofibromas. They lie at the periphery of unmyelinated and myelinated nerves, in the vicinity of Schwann cells (fig. 8-39), and loosely scattered within the myxocollagenous matrix (fig. 8-40). They are also found in pseudomeissnerian bodies (see below). Most perineurial-like cells feature long, straight or curved, narrow cytoplasmic processes with numerous surface pinocytotic vesicles and a discontinuous coat of basement membrane. They are referred to as perineurial-like cells since, to date, they have not been shown to express EMA immunohistochemically.

Tactile corpuscle-like formations (pseudomeissnerian bodies) in neurofibroma consist of disc-shaped packets of cells mainly represented by stacked lamellar arrays of thin, narrow processes (fig. 8-30). Their overall appearance mimics that of normal Meissner corpuscles. The latter are composed of closely packed layers of nerve fibers and thus contain S-100 protein–positive Schwann cells as well as axonal processes (see fig. 3-19). Pseudomeissnerian bodies are similarly S-100 protein immunoreactive, a finding seemingly inconsistent with the ultrastructural features of perineurial cells (fig. 8-41). The explanation for this discordance is that the bodies consist of stacked perineurial-like cells. True perineurial cell differentiation in terms of an appropriate immunostaining profile (EMA positive, S-100 protein negative) is seen at the periphery of pseudomeissnerian bodies.

Fibroblasts. Fibroblasts, characterized by an ample branching rough endoplasmic reticulum, a well-developed Golgi apparatus, sparse pino-

cytotic vesicles, and lack of basement membrane coating (fig. 8-42), are found in greatest number in cutaneous and sclerotic neurofibromas.

Transitional Cells. Cells with features of both perineurial cells and fibroblasts or of Schwann and perineurial cells are found in varying numbers within neurofibromas. Such cells are termed transitional cells and appear to be hybrid in terms of their ultrastructural features. For example, the perineurial fibroblasts are characterized by a moderately well-developed rough endoplasmic reticulum and bipolar cytoplasmic processes thicker than those of normal perineurial cells, but feature scattered pinocytotic vesicles and occasional short segments of surface basement membrane.

DNA FLOW CYTOMETRY

In one flow cytometric study of 26 neurofibromas, 66 percent were diploid and the remainder aneuploid; 1 to 8 percent of the cells were in S phase (mean 3.4 percent) (70). Of 28 MPNSTs similarly studied, 64 percent were aneuploid, and 2 to 46 percent were in S phase (mean, 12.4 percent). A smaller image analysis study of Feulgen-stained sections found that one of five neurofibromas have a hyperdiploid DNA histogram and the remainder are diploid (75).

HISTOLOGIC ATYPIA AND MALIGNANT CHANGE

Neurofibroma is remarkable both for its broad differentiation potential and biologic potential, the latter ranging from usually benign to being the source of one of the most aggressive malignant tumors of soft tissue. The relationship of specific histologic features to malignant transformation in neurofibromas has been evaluated using multiple modalities, including immunohistochemical markers of differentiation, cell proliferation and cell cycle regulators, flow cytometry, cytogenetic and molecular genetics, including microarray-based comparative genome hybridization (CGH), and clinical outcome. Hypercellularity of otherwise cytologically unremarkable neurofibroma cells (figs. 8-27B, 8-28), even if mitotically active, is not regarded as an atypical histologic change. Establishing the presence of atypical changes in a given case may require extensive tumor sampling.

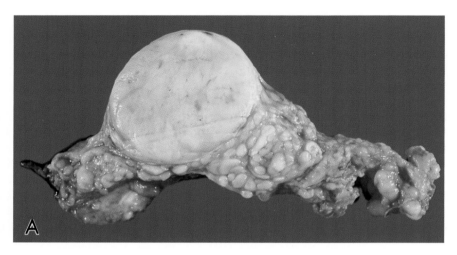

Figure 8-34

DIVERGENT DIFFERENTIATION IN A PLEXIFORM NEUROFIBROMA

This unique example from the retroperitoneum of a patient with NF1 showed the localized formation of a nodule (A) within which neurofibroma tissue was accompanied by a variety of epithelia. Microsections showed cytologically benign glands in a neurofibromatous stroma (B), mucin-producing goblet cells (C) with immunoreactivity for cytokeratin as well as carcinoembryonic antigen (D), and neuroendocrine cells (E) showing chromogranin immunoreactivity (F). The neurofibromatous stroma appeared cytologically benign throughout the gland-containing area, although early malignant transformation was noted elsewhere. (Courtesy of Dr. S. Wester, La Crosse, WI.)

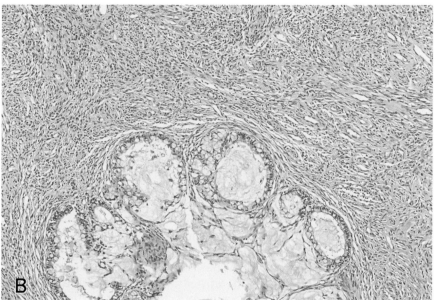

Atypical Histologic Findings Unrelated to Malignant Transformation in Neurofibromas. The most common benign atypical change in neurofibromas is "degenerative atypia." It is characterized by cells with enlarged, sometimes pleomorphic nuclei, featuring dense smudgy chromatin, inconspicuous nucleoli, and often cytoplasmic nuclear pseudoinclusions (fig. 8-35) (2,19,43). Such cells lack mitotic activity and show no appreciable MIB-1 labeling. One study of atypias in neurofibromas (76) suggested that unlike ordinary neurofibromas those with what appears to be degenerative atypia have a higher range of S-phase fractions. Similar degenerative change is seen in "ancient" and occasion-

ally in cellular schwannomas, some radiated neurofibromas (77), and normal nerve subject to incidental radiotherapy. Although affected cells typically lie scattered in a tumor lacking significant hypercellularity, we have seen a unique case in which they were abundant and arranged in sheets.

Atypical Cellular Changes Early in Malignant Transformation. There is convincing evidence for the occurrence of at least one form of atypia early in the process of malignant transformation. This is characterized by atypical, spindle-shaped neurofibroma cells interspersed among unremarkable neurofibroma cells. The nuclei of the atypical cells are enlarged, some up

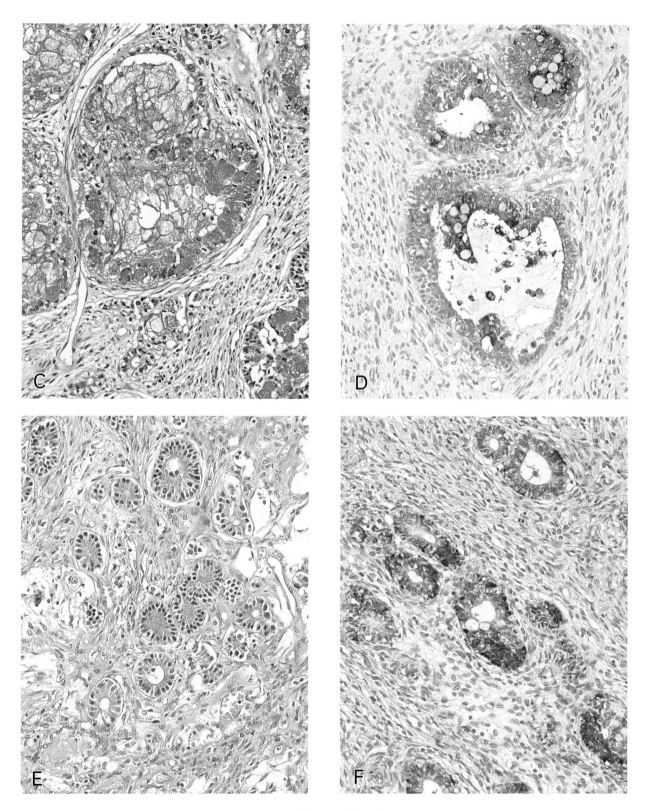

Figure 8-34, continued

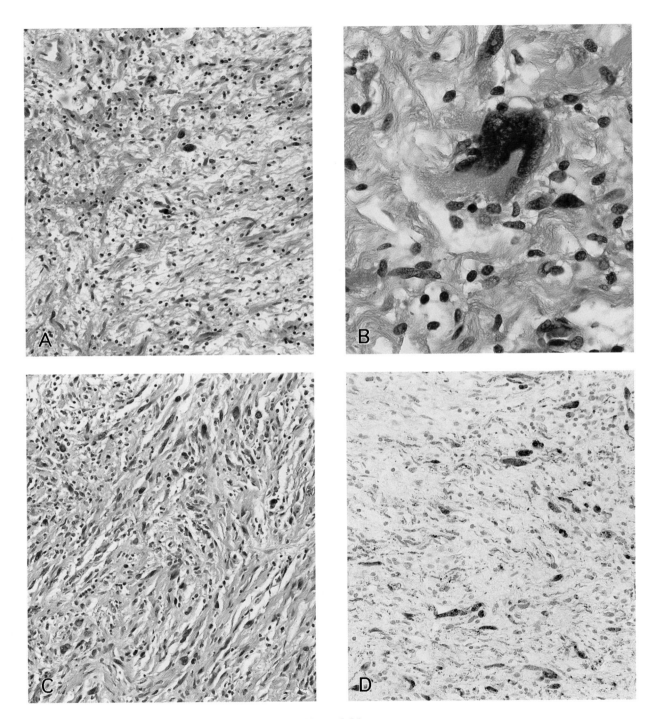

Figure 8-35

NEUROFIBROMA WITH DEGENERATIVE NUCLEAR ATYPIA (LOW-LEVEL ATYPICAL HISTOLOGIC CHANGE)

A,B: The presence of pleomorphic nuclei with smudgy chromatin and occasional nuclear inclusions is considered a degenerative change.

C: When more diffuse or involving a cellular neurofibroma, the change may raise concern about malignant transformation.

D: Such degenerative cells are S-100 protein positive but proliferation marker studies (MIB-1) show their nuclei to be unlabeled.

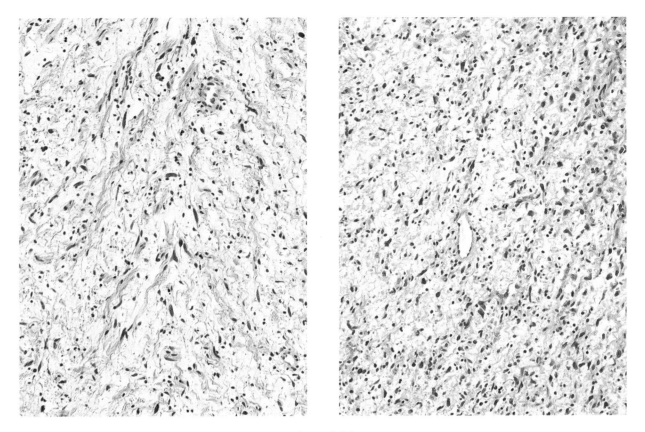

Figure 8-36

**NEUROFIBROMA WITH ATYPICAL HISTOLOGIC FINDINGS,
CONSIDERED EARLY CHANGES IN MALIGNANT TRANSFORMATION**

There is an increased number of atypical neurofibroma cells with nuclei that are enlarged to a varying degree, most less than three times the size of ordinary neurofibroma nuclei, but hyperchromatic and without smudged chromatin. Mitotic figures may be observed. The areas shown are from a plexiform neurofibroma that had undergone malignant transformation.

to three times the size of ordinary neurofibroma nuclei, and are minimally pleomorphic and uniformly hyperchromatic without smudged chromatin (fig. 8-36). Such cytologic changes are sometimes seen in proximity to areas of malignant transformation. In a recent study, 15 of 16 neurofibromas with these characteristics were found to have a deletion in chromosome band 9p21.3, a region that includes the *CDKNA/B* gene locus (78). In six tumors the deletion was homozygous. *CDKNA* is a tumor suppressor gene that encodes for p16, and its homologous deletion is found in 50 percent of conventional spindle cell MPNSTs (79,80).

Atypical Histologic Findings Considered Indicative of Malignant Transformation in Neurofibroma. Aside from the de novo appearance of cytologically malignant epithelioid or mesenchymal cells in an otherwise histologically unremarkable neurofibroma (chapter 12), we recognize two forms of malignant transformation in neurofibroma. Both typically present as localized moderate hypercellularity. The first, originally identified in neurofibromas adjacent to in-continuity MPNSTs, is characterized by sheets of uniform hyperchromatic spindle cells with at least a three-fold nuclear enlargement compared to those of ordinary neurofibromas (fig. 8-37A) (2,11,19). Mitotic figures are not expected. The second takes the form of some pleomorphic elongated and ovoid cells with ample cytoplasm and hyperchromatic, irregularly shaped nuclei (fig. 8-37B) (2,11,19). Two years after incomplete excision of the example in figure 8-37, a high-grade pleomorphic MPNST composed of similar pleomorphic cells was

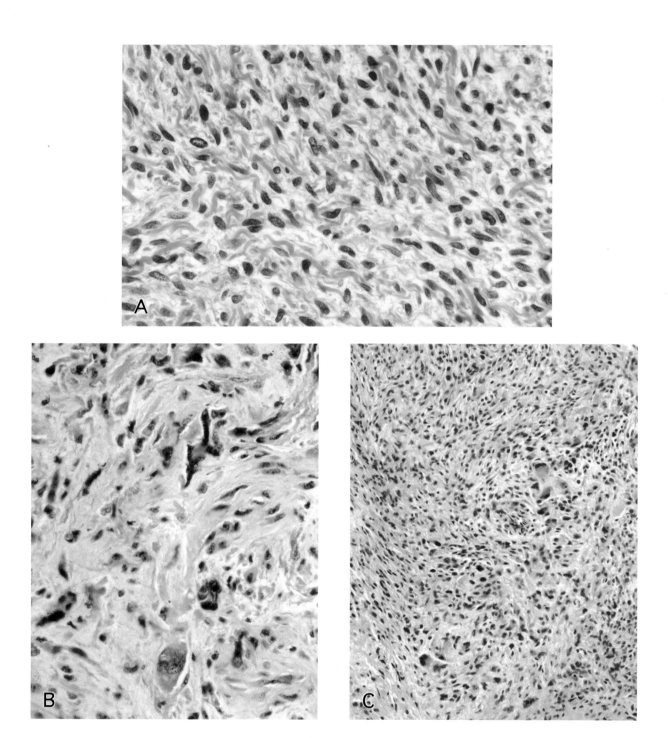

Figure 8-37

NEUROFIBROMA WITH ATYPICAL HISTOLOGIC CHANGES INDICATIVE OF MALIGNANT TRANSFORMATION

A: Type one is characterized by diffuse hypercellularity of uniformly hyperchromatic spindle cells with nuclear enlargement to at least three times the size of ordinary neurofibroma nuclei. Mitoses need not be present.

B: Type two is a microscopic group of enlarged and ovoid cells with variable, sometimes appreciable amounts of cytoplasm, and bizarre distorted hyperchromatic pleomorphic nuclei.

C: High-grade pleomorphic MPNST was found 22 months later at the site of the incompletely resected tumor illustrated in figure B.

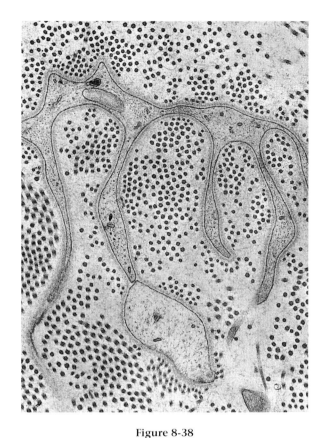

Figure 8-38

DIFFUSE NEUROFIBROMA

A Schwann cell with numerous processes appears to be enveloping collagen fibrils. The basement membrane is continuous on the cell surface.

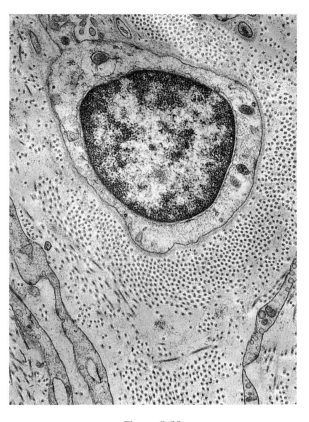

Figure 8-39

CUTANEOUS NEUROFIBROMA

A Schwann cell (top) with a continuous basement membrane is surrounded by collagen fibrils. Portions of three perineurial-like cell processes, one at the bottom right and two at the bottom left, with distinctive pinocytotic vesicles, are also evident.

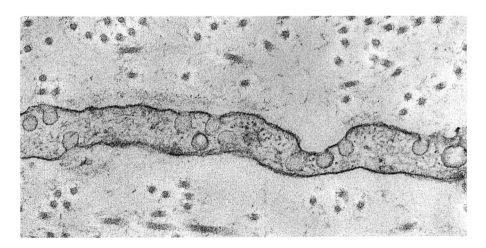

Figure 8-40

CUTANEOUS NEUROFIBROMA

A perineurial-like cell process has pinocytotic vesicles, scattered intermediate filaments, and remnants of basement membrane substance in the acellular myxocollagenous matrix.

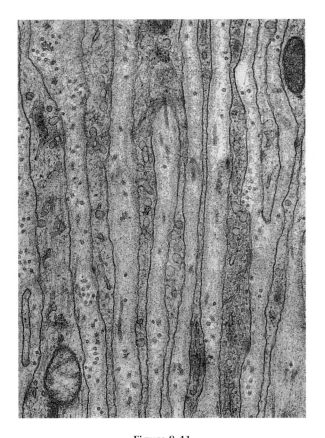

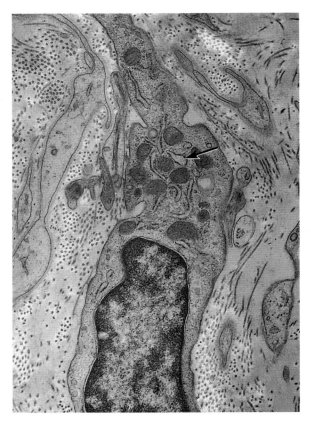

Figure 8-41

PSEUDOMEISSNERIAN BODY: ULTRASTRUCTURE

The body is composed of perineurial-like cell processes in parallel array. Pinocytotic vesicles and discontinuous basement membranes are seen.

Figure 8-42

CUTANEOUS NEUROFIBROMA IN NF1

A fibroblastic cell with a moderately well-developed rough endoplasmic reticulum (arrow), few pinocytotic vesicles, and no basement membrane, is surrounded by collagen fibrils. Schwann cell processes are coated by a continuous basement membrane.

Figure 8-43

PLEXIFORM NEUROFIBROMA

An aggregate of collagen fibrils is intermixed with two myelinated axons (top), two unmyelinated axons (arrows), and numerous complex Schwann cell processes that entrap collagen fibrils.

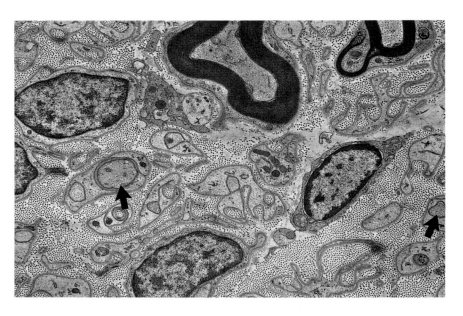

resected from the same site (fig. 8-37C). Although neither form of malignant transformation, both localized changes, were investigated for alterations of cell cycle regulation, the second corresponds to atypical cells found by Lin et al. (76) in a cellular neurofibroma that had a p53 labeling index of 5 percent.

TUMOR OF PROPOSED NEUROFIBROMATOUS NATURE BUT UNCONFIRMED

In this category is the so-called *dendritic cell neurofibroma with pseudorosettes* (DCNWPR) (81). Without gender predilection, the tumor involves mainly adults, presents as a solitary yet widely distributed skin lesion, and has yet to be reported in an individual with convincing evidence of NF1 (82). Ranging from 3 to 17 mm, the lesions are small, oval-shaped dermal growths oriented perpendicular to the epidermis. On their deep aspect they appear multifocal (fig. 8-44A).

DCNWPR consists of two types of cells: small cells possessing comma-shaped nuclei and inconspicuous cytoplasm (type I cells), among which a few larger rounded cells (type II cells) lie interspersed (fig. 8-44B). The former are histologically similar to those of cutaneous neurofibromas and some neural nevi. The latter are characterized by abundant, eosinophilic to clear cytoplasm and a round central nucleus about the same size but with less dense chromatin than type I cells. Nuclear cytoplasmic inclusions may be present. Neither cell type has a histologically defined cell membrane. Where the cell types are in close proximity, type I cells group around type II cells to form pseudorosettes. In some lesions, the same mixed cellular proliferation is found within adjacent cutaneous nerves (81,83,84), structures identified as nerves by a peripheral layer of EMA-positive cells and the presence of occasional neurofilament protein-immunopositive axons. Both cell types stain for S-100 protein: type I cells variably and type II cells intensely (fig. 8-44C). Reactivity is found not only in cell bodies, but in the long curved dendritic-appearing cell processes that give type II cells a spider-like appearance. In conventionally stained material, the small cells with comma-shaped nuclei are histologically similar to cells in cutaneous neurofibromas, and also to those of some neural nevi (85). Neither cell type reacts for

the melanocytic differentiation markers HMB45, Melan A (A103), and microphthalmia-associated transcription factor (D5) (84,85). Faint nuclear tyrosinase (T311) staining, unaccompanied by cytoplasmic reactivity, is seen in type II cells (85).

Ultrastructural studies performed on paraffin-embedded tissue show that both cells possess dendritic cell processes and rare pinocytotic vesicles, but melanosomes are lacking. A discontinuous external lamina, least evident in type II cells, has been noted (81). In one case, there were compact collagen bundles similar to those in some neurofibromas (84). In aggregate, the findings are conflicting. Unlike most neurofibromas, these lesions are multifocal, not diffuse. The cells feature dendritic processes, and no association with NF1 has been demonstrated. Unlike neural nevi, with their content of melanocytic cells, DCNWPRs show no definite evidence of melanocytic differentiation and may have an intraneural component. The absence of unequivocal immunoreactivity for melanocytic markers is similar to neurotropic melanoma (see chapter 14). The latter is associated with in situ cutaneous melanoma, the determining factor in that tumor's classification (86). In the case of DCNWPR, the confirmed presence of an intraneural component links it to tumors of peripheral nerve sheath. Whether the lesion is classifiable as a neurofibroma or represents a new form of peripheral nerve tumor remains to be determined. Further ultrastructural and genetic studies may provide clarification.

DIFFERENTIAL DIAGNOSIS

The differential diagnosis of neurofibroma includes schwannoma, low-grade MPNST, ganglioneuroma, dermatofibrosarcoma protuberans (DFSP) of both ordinary and pigmented type (Bednar tumor), nerve sheath myxoma, myxoma, and neuronevus.

A summary of the main features distinguishing localized intraneural neurofibroma from nonmelanotic schwannoma, the principal lesion in the differential diagnosis, appears in Table 7-1. Neurofibroma cells are uniformly and diffusely distributed, a pattern that contrasts sharply with the alternating dense and loose cellular arrangement characterizing conventional schwannoma, and the dense cellularity

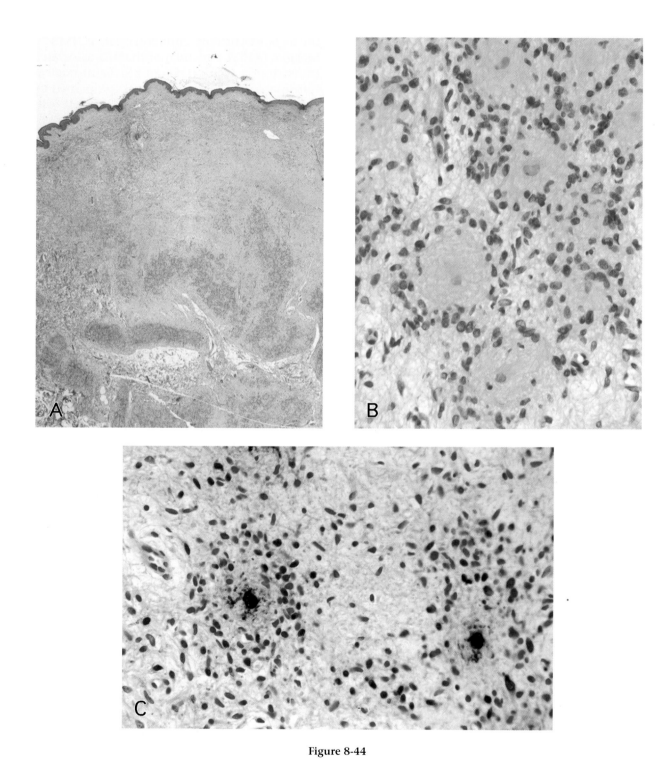

Figure 8-44

DENDRITIC CELL NEUROFIBROMA WITH PSEUDOROSETTES

A: At scanning power, multifocality of growth in skin is evident.

B: The key finding is small, comma-shaped type I cells which in areas encase large, rounded type II cells, forming rosettes.

C: S-100 protein immunoreactivity is strong in type II cells and their spider-like dendritic processes, and fainter in type I cells. (Courtesy of Dr. M. Michal, Pilsen, Czech Republic.)

that typifies cellular schwannoma. The nuclei of neurofibroma cells are approximately one third to half the size of those of schwannoma cells. Reserved to neurofibromas are broad bands of collagen simulating shredded carrots. Additionally, neurofibromas contain collagen fibers of types 1 and 3, whereas those of schwannomas are mainly of type 3 (50). Since immunoreactivity for S-100 protein is a feature of some but not all neurofibroma cells, staining is less uniform and pronounced than in schwannoma. Unlike the cellular heterogeneity that ultrastructurally characterizes neurofibromas, schwannomas consist of a uniform population of well-differentiated Schwann cells frequently associated with Luse bodies (plump aggregates of long-spacing collagen) Both tumor types may contain residual axons, but more often subcapsular and far fewer in number in schwannomas.

Distinguishing neurofibromas from low-grade MPNSTs generally poses no problem, but neurofibromas with atypical histologic features may be a challenge. Most atypical changes are degenerative. The spectrum of atypical neurofibromas and their characteristics, and our histologic criteria for a diagnosis of neurofibroma with malignant transformation, are discussed in detail elsewhere in this chapter.

The distinction of ganglioneuroma from neurofibroma rests upon the identification and the morphology of the ganglion cells, the abundance and distribution of nerve fibers, and the presence or absence of myelin sheaths. All these elements may be seen in neurofibromas overrunning dorsal root or autonomic ganglia (fig. 8-45A). In such cases, the ganglion cells are not distributed throughout the lesion, but are localized and lie among aligned nerve fiber bundles traversing normal ganglia (fig. 8-45B). Unlike the majority of dorsal root nerve fibers, those of ganglioneuroma are unmyelinated. Significantly, the nuclei of ganglion cells of ganglioneuroma are dysmorphic (see chapter 10). In contrast, those of normal dorsal root and autonomic ganglia are uninucleated, uniform in appearance, and feature central and eccentrically situated nuclei, respectively. Although normal and ganglioneuromatous ganglion cells are surrounded by satellite cells, such cells are less numerous and uniformly arranged in ganglioneuromas (fig. 8-45C).

Due to the propensity of DFSP to infiltrate dermal and adipose tissue and undergo myxoid change, it may be mistaken for diffuse neurofibroma (fig. 8-46 left). In contrast to the latter, DFSP is more cellular, consists of larger cells resembling fibroblasts, commonly shows a storiform pattern (fig. 8-46 right), and lacks both pseudomeissnerian bodies and S-100 protein immunoreactivity. Like DFSP, neurofibromas also express CD34 (64,87,88), but the pattern of CD34 staining in neurofibroma varies, never involving all the cells (65,88). In contrast, DFSPs are uniformly immunoreactive (65). Neurofibromas with pigmented cells must be distinguished from pigmented DFSP (Bednar tumor) (fig. 8-47) (89). In both tumors, the pigmented cells stain for S-100 protein, but unlike pigmented neurofibromas, the nonpigmented cells of Bednar tumor lack such immunoreactivity and ultrastructurally resemble fibroblasts (90,91). It has been suggested that the presence of pigmented cells may be due to melanocytic colonization (92).

Differing from most neurofibromas, nerve sheath myxomas (NSMs) have a distinctly lobulated architecture; hypocellularity; stringy appearing spindle cells, many of which are stellate; a subset of epithelioid cells; multinucleation; vacuolation of both nuclei and cytoplasm; and no association with nerve. Immunostaining for S-100 protein is seen in both lesions and is of no aid in the diagnosis. The lobules of NSMs are often ringed by EMA-positive cells, which are assumed to be perineurial cells.

The distinction of neurofibroma from spindle cell lipoma rests upon the frequent localization of the latter in deep soft tissue of the posterior neck in elderly patients, often conspicuous vascularity, content of fat, lack of degenerative atypia, and occasional floret cell formation. Its spindle cells are CD34 immunoreactive, and lack staining for both S-100 protein and the basement membrane markers collagen type 4 and laminin.

Due to its lack of extensive collagen fiber formation, myxoma is usually readily distinguished from myxoid neurofibromas. S-100 protein and basal lamina markers are absent in myxoma.

It may be difficult to distinguish cutaneous neurofibroma from deep portions of congenital and neuronevi (fig. 8-48). The most helpful

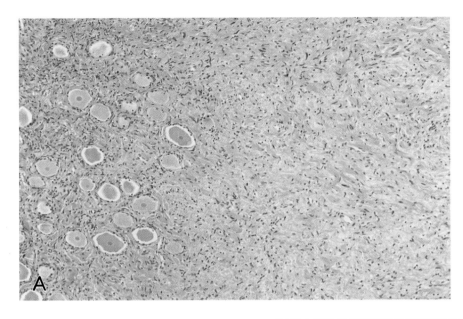

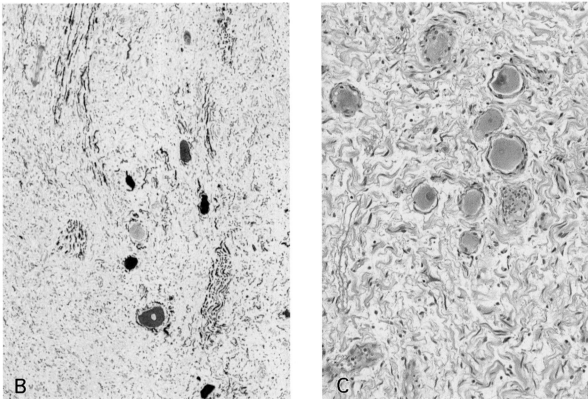

Figure 8-45

PLEXIFORM NEUROFIBROMA INVOLVING DORSAL ROOT GANGLION

A: Infiltration of dorsal root ganglion (left) by neurofibroma (right).

B: The ganglion cells are a local finding within the tumor and are accompanied by neurofilament protein-immunopositive nerve fiber bundles.

C: Unlike the ganglion cells of ganglioneuroma, here nearly all are surrounded by a uniform layer of satellite cells.

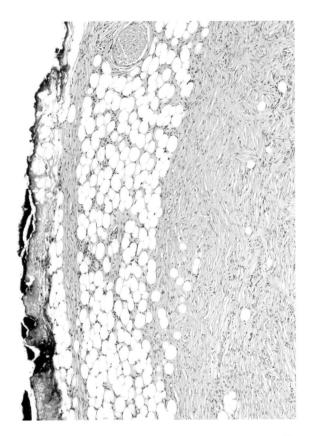 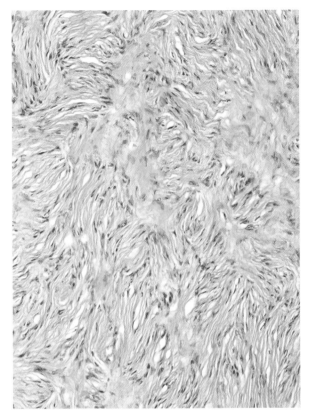

Figure 8-46

DERMATOFIBROSARCOMA PROTUBERANS

Left: This tumor commonly involves subcutaneous tissue and at low magnification is easily mistaken for a neurofibroma.

Right: Unlike in neurofibroma, these cells have a storiform growth pattern, are S-100 protein negative, but are uniformly positive for CD34.

diagnostic feature is, of course, finding classic nevus cells in the superficial portions of a neuronevus. Most neuronevus cells have conspicuous cytoplasm, whereas in neurofibromas, it is inapparent in conventionally stained material. An additional distinguishing feature is strong, diffuse S-100 protein expression in neuronevus as opposed to less uniform staining in neurofibroma.

A few lesions enter into the differential diagnosis of plexiform neurofibroma. These variously affect skin and subcutaneous and superficial soft tissue, and include primarily plexiform schwannoma and plexiform fibrohistiocytic tumor. Unlike plexiform neurofibroma, plexiform schwannoma consists of a uniform proliferation of Schwann cells sometimes forming Verocay bodies (93–96) and lacking a significant mucopolysaccharide matrix. The cells

of plexiform schwannoma are larger than those of neurofibroma and uniformly and strongly S-100 protein immunoreactive. Both lesions contain residual neurofilament protein-immunoreactive axons (usually scant and peripheral in schwannoma, numerous and central in neurofibromas), and exhibit delicate investment by EMA-positive perineurial cells. Plexiform neurofibromas are often associated with a diffuse extraneural component while the cells of plexiform schwannoma grow entirely within nerves. Plexiform schwannomas are unaccompanied by overlying cutaneous pigmentation, a feature of some plexiform neurofibromas.

Unlike plexiform neurofibroma, the dermal variant of plexiform fibrohistiocytic tumor generally measures only 1 to 2 cm and is hard in texture (97,98). This tumor is skin colored and

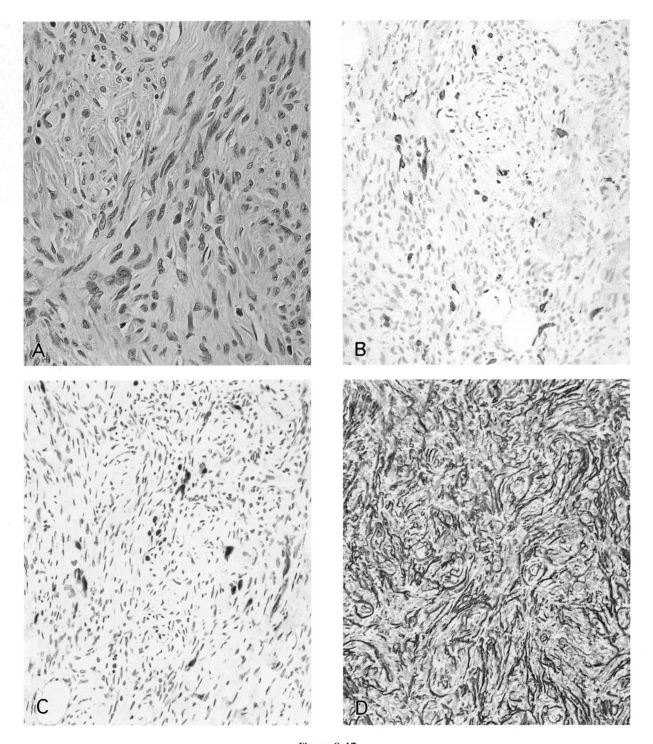

Figure 8-47

BEDNAR TUMOR

A: Unlike neurofibroma, such lesions usually are composed of S-100 protein-negative spindle cells in a storiform arrangement. Lying among them are pigmented spindle cells.

B,C: The cells are positive with a melanin stain (B, Fontana stain) and S-100 protein immunoreactive (C).

D: Bednar tumors, like ordinary dermatofibrosarcoma protuberans, show strong CD34 immunoreactivity.

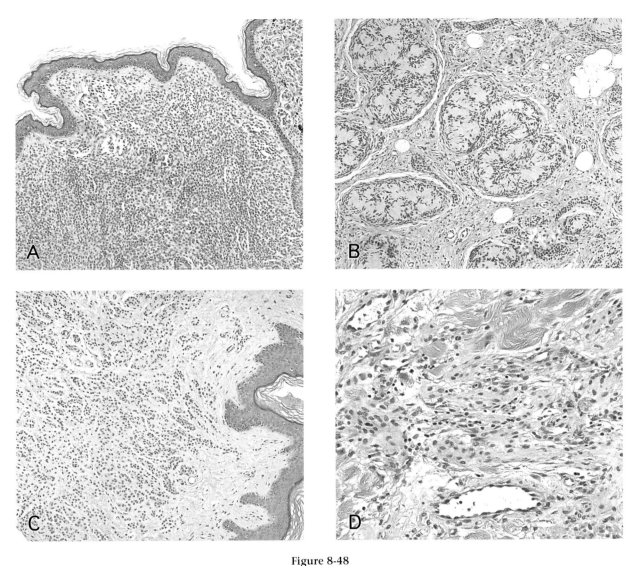

Figure 8-48

CONGENITAL NEVUS AND NEURONEVUS

Both lesions may show conspicuous schwannian differentiation. Readily recognized by its superficial component of ordinary nevus cells (A), the congenital nevus exhibits well-formed pseudomeissnerian bodies in an obviously schwannian background (B). Neuronevus similarly consists of a superficial nevus cell component (C) and a deeper portion with schwannian features (D).

unassociated with hyperpigmentation. In contrast to plexiform neurofibroma, fibrohistiocytic tumors exhibit biphasic histology, including a major component of spindle to stellate myofibroblasts with accompanying stromal collagen and lesser numbers of osteoclast-like giant cells and epithelioid mononuclear cells. The myofibroblasts are immunoreactive for HHF35 and the osteoclast-like giant cells are positive for KP-1 (CD68). Plexiform fibrohistiocytic tumors lack a nerve association and are immunonegative for S-100 protein.

TREATMENT AND PROGNOSIS

Resection of localized or diffuse cutaneous neurofibroma is curative and unassociated with neurologic deficits. Large lesions of the diffuse or massive soft tissue and extensive plexiform types may only be amenable to subtotal removal. Diffuse cutaneous neurofibromas rarely undergo malignant change. Rare examples of large, histologically unremarkable plexiform neurofibromas have been responsible for some deaths due to their anatomic location (19,37).

Although curative treatment of localized intraneural neurofibroma consists of resection, a procedure which necessarily requires sacrifice of the parent fascicle or nerve, excision of major, still functional nerves is generally unwarranted. The same is true in large examples of plexiform neurofibroma which, if entirely resected, may result in devastating neurologic loss. In addition to alleviating the mechanical disability that accompanies large neurofibromas, some are resected due to pain or rapid enlargement in size. The latter manifestations may herald malignant transformation, an uncommon occurrence in localized intraneural neurofibroma (99), but one that may occur in up to 5 percent of large plexiform tumors (100). In one recent large series of plexiform neurofibromas (41), patients whose tumors underwent such transformation were older than those with benign lesions (38 versus 22 years); the rate of tumor recurrence correspondingly differed substantially (47 versus 23 percent).

REFERENCES

1. Skuse GR, Kosciolek BA, Rowley PT. The neurofibroma in von Recklinghausen neurofibromatosis has a unicellular origin. Am J Hum Genet 1991;49:600-607.
2. Scheithauer B, Woodruff JM, Erlandson RA. Tumors of the peripheral nervous system. AFIP Atlas of Tumor Pathology, 3rd Series, Fascicle 24. Washington, DC: American Registry of Pathology; 1999.
3. Colman SD, Williams CA, Wallace MR. Benign neurofibromas in type 1 neurofibromatosis (NF1) show somatic deletions of the NF1 gene. Nat Genet 1995;11:90-92.
4. Sawada S, Florell S, Purandare SM, Ota M, Stephens K, Viskochil D. Identification of NF1 mutations in both alleles of a dermal neurofibroma. Nat Genet 1996;14:110-112.
5. Serra E, Puig S, Otero D, et al. Confirmation of a double-hit model for the NF1 gene in benign neurofibromas. Am J Hum Genet 1997;61:512-519.
6. Perry A, Roth KA, Banerjee R, Fuller CE, Gutmann DH. NF1 deletions in S-100 protein-positive and negative cells of sporadic and neurofibromatosis 1 (NF1)-associated plexiform neurofibromas and malignant peripheral nerve sheath tumors. Am J Pathol 2001;159:57-61.
7. Brannan CI, Perkins AS, Vogel KS, et al. Targeted disruption of the neurofibromatosis type-1 gene leads to developmental abnormalities in heart and various neural crest-derived tissues. Genes Dev 1994;8:1019-1029.
8. Jacks T, Shih TS, Schmitt EM, Bronson RT, Bernards A, Weinberg RA. Tumour predisposition in mice heterozygous for a targeted mutation in Nf1. Nat Genet 1994;7:353-361.
9. Cichowski K, Shih TS, Schmitt E, et al. Mouse models of tumor development in neurofibromatosis type 1. Science 1999;286:2172-2176.
10. Zhu Y, Ghosh P, Charnay P, Burns DK, Parada LF. Neurofibromas in NF1: Schwann cell origin and role of tumor environment. Science 2002;296:920-922.
10a. Yang FC, Chen S, Clegg T, et al. Nf1+/- mast cells induce neurofibroma-like phenotypes through secreted TGF-beta signaling. Genetics 2006;15;2421-2437.
11. Woodruff JM. Pathology of major peripheral nerve sheath neoplasms. In: Weiss SW. Soft tissue tumors. Baltimore: Williams & Wilkins; 1996:120-161.
12. Woodruff R, Horten BC, Erlandson RA. The peripheral nerves and paragangliomas. In: Silverberg SG, DeLellis A, Frable WJ, eds. Principles and practice of surgical pathology. New York: Lippincott; 1997:2801-2832.
13. Erlandson RA. The enigmatic perineurial cell and its participation in tumors and in tumorlike entities. Ultrastruct Pathol 1991;15:335-351.
14. Watabe K, Kumanishi T, Ikuta F, Oyake Y. Tactile-like corpuscles in neurofibromas: immunohistochemical demonstration of S-100 protein. Acta Neuropathol 1983;61:173-177.
15. Pummi KP, Aho HJ, Laato MK, Peltonen JT, Peltonen SA. Tight junction proteins and perineurial cells in neurofibromas. J Histochem Cytochem 2006;54:53-61.

16. Hirose T, Tani T, Shimada T, Ishizawa K, Shimada S, Sano T. Immunohistochemical demonstration of EMA/Glut1-positive perineurial cells and CD34-positive fibroblastic cells in peripheral nerve sheath tumors. Mod Pathol 2003;16:293-298.

17. Zamecnik M, Michal M. Perineurial cell differentiation in neurofibromas. Report of eight cases including a case with composite perineurioma-neurofibroma features. Pathol Res Pract 2001;197:537-544.

18. Perentes E, Nakagawa Y, Ross GW, Stanton C, Rubinstein LJ. Expression of epithelial membrane antigen in perineurial cells and their derivatives. An immunohistochemical study with multiple markers. Acta Neuropathol (Berl) 1987;75:160-165.

19. Antonescu CR, Woodruff JM. Primary tumors of cranial, spinal and peripheral nerves. In: Russell and Rubinstein's pathology of tumors of the nervous system. London: Hodder Arnold; 2006:787-835.

20. Kazakov DV, Pitha J, Sima R, et al. Hybrid peripheral nerve sheath tumors: schwannoma-perineuroma and neurofibroma-perineuroma. A report of three cases in extradigital locations. Ann Diagn Pathol 2005;9:16-23.

21. Cawthon RM, Weiss R, Xu GF, et al. A major segment of the neurofibromatosis type 1 gene: cDNA sequence, genomic structure, and point mutations. Cell 1990;62:193-201.

22. Viskochil D, Buchberg AM, Xu G, et al. Deletions and a translocation interrupt a cloned gene at the neurofibromatosis type 1 locus. Cell 1990;62:187-192.

23. Wallace MR, Marchuk DA, Andersen LB, et al. Type 1 neurofibromatosis gene: identification of a large transcript disrupted in three NF1 patients. Science 1990;249:181-186.

24. Ballester R, Marchuk D, Boguski M, et al. The NF1 locus encodes a protein functionally related to mammalian GAP and yeast IRA proteins. Cell 1990;63:851-859.

25. Buchberg AM, Cleveland LS, Jenkins NA, Copeland NG. Sequence homology shared by neurofibromatosis type-1 gene and IRA-1 and IRA-2 negative regulators of the RAS cyclic AMP pathway. Nature 1990;347:291-294.

26. Martin GA, Viskochil D, Bollag G, et al. The GAP-related domain of the neurofibromatosis type 1 gene product interacts with ras p21. Cell 1990;63:843-849.

27. Xu GF, Lin B, Tanaka K, et al. The catalytic domain of the neurofibromatosis type 1 gene product stimulates ras GTPase and complements ira mutants of S. cerevisiae. Cell 1990;63:835-841.

28. Gutmann DH, Collins FS. The neurofibromatosis type 1 gene and its protein product, neurofibromin. Neuron 1993;10:335-343.

29. Skuse GR, Kosciolek BA, Rowley PT. Molecular genetic analysis of tumors in von Recklinghausen neurofibromatosis: loss of heterozygosity for chromosome 17. Genes Chromosomes Cancer 1989;1:36-41.

30. Knudson AG Jr. Mutation and cancer: statistical study of retinoblastoma. Proc Natl Acad Sci U S A 1971;68:820-823.

31. Eisenbarth I, Beyer K, Krone W, Assum G. Toward a survey of somatic mutation of the NF1 gene in benign neurofibromas of patients with neurofibromatosis type 1. Am J Hum Genet 2000;66:393-401.

32. John AM, Ruggieri M, Ferner R, Upadhyaya M. A search for evidence of somatic mutations in the NF1 gene. J Med Genet 2000;37:44-49.

33. Serra E, Ars E, Ravella A, et al. Somatic NF1 mutational spectrum in benign neurofibromas: mRNA splice defects are common among point mutations. Hum Gen 2001;108:416-429.

34. Storlazzi CT, Von Steyern FV, Domanski HA, Mandahl N, Mertens F. Biallelic somatic inactivation of the NF1 gene through chromosomal translocations in a sporadic neurofibroma. Int J Cancer 2005;117:1055-1057.

34a. Koga T, Iwasaki H, Ishiguro M, Matsuzaki A, Kikuchi M. Losses in chromosomes 17, 19, and 22q in neurofibromatosis type 1 and sporadic neurofibromas: a comparative genomic hybridization analysis. Cancer Genet Cytogenet 2002;15;136:113-120.

35. Michels VV, Whisnant JP, Garrity JA, Miller GM. Neurofibromatosis type 1 with bilateral acoustic neuromas. Neurofibromatosis 1989;2:213-217.

36. Sadeh M, Martinovits G, Goldhammer Y. Occurrence of both neurofibromatoses 1 and 2 in the same individual with a rapidly progressive course. Neurology 1989;39:282-283.

37. Ralis Z, Emery JL. Congenital plexiform neurofibroma of the vagus with cardiac, pulmonary and visceral involvement. J Pathol 1972;107:55-57.

38. Riccardi VM. Von Recklinghausen neurofibromatosis. N Engl J Med 1981;305:1617-1627.

39. Bhargava R, Parham DM, Lasater OE, Chari RS, Chen G, Fletcher BD. MR imaging differentiation of benign and malignant peripheral nerve sheath tumors: use of the target sign. Pediatr Radiol 1997;27:124-129.

40. Harkin JC, Reed RJ. Tumors of the peripheral nervous system. Atlas of Tumor Pathology, 2nd Series, Fascicle 3. Washington, DC: Armed Forces Institute of Pathology; 1969.

41. McCarron KF, Goldblum JR. Plexiform neurofibroma with and without associated malignant peripheral nerve sheath tumor: a clinicopathologic and immunohistochemical analysis of 54 cases. Mod Pathol 1998;11:612-617.

42. Hochberg FH, Dasilva AB, Galdabini J, Richardson EP Jr. Gastrointestinal involvement in von Recklinghausen's neurofibromatosis. Neurology 1974;24:1144-1151.

43. Woodruff J, Horten BC, Erlandson RA. Pathology of peripheral nerves and paragangliomas. In: Silverberg SG. Principles and practice of surgical pathology. New York: Wiley; 1983.

44. Anderson B, Robertson DM. Melanin containing neurofibroma: case report with evidence of Schwann cell origin of melanin. Can J Neurol Sci 1979;6:139-143.

45. Payan MJ, Gambarelli D, Keller P, Lachard A, Garcin M, Vigouroux C, Toga M. Melanotic neurofibroma: a case report with ultrastructural study. Acta Neuropathol (Berl) 1986;69:148-152.

46. Weiss S, Goldblum J. Enzinger & Weiss's soft tissue tumors, 5th ed. Benign tumors of peripheral nerves. Philadelphia: Mosby Elsevier; 2008:838.

47. Smith TW, Bhawan J. Tactile-like structures in neurofibromas. An ultrastructural study. Acta Neuropathol (Berl) 1980;50:233-236.

48. Weiser G. An electron microscope study of "pacinian neurofibroma." Virchows Arch A Pathol Anat Histol 1975;366:331-340.

48a. Jurecka W. Tactile corpuscle-like structures in peripheral nerve sheath tumors in plastic embedded material. Am J Dermatopathol 1988;10:74-79.

49. Schochet S Jr, Barrett DA 2nd. Neurofibroma with aberrant tactile corpuscles. Acta Neuropathol (Berl) 1974;28:161-165.

50. Junqueira LC, Montes GS, Kaupert D, Shigihara KM, Bolonhani TM, Krisztan RM. Morphological and histochemical studies on the collagen in neurinomas, neurofibromas, and fibromas. J Neuropathol Exp Neurol 1981;40:123-133.

51. Levi L, Curri SB. Multiple pacinian neurofibroma and relationship with the finger-tip arterio-venous anastomoses. Br J Dermatol 1980;102:345-349.

52. Toth BB, Long WH, Pleasants JE. Central pacinian neurofibroma of the maxilla. Oral Surg Oral Med Oral Pathol 1975;39:630-634.

53. MacDonald DM, Wilson-Jones E. Pacinian neurofibroma. Histopathology 1977;1:247-255.

54. Owen DA. Pacinian neurofibroma. Arch Pathol Lab Med 1979;103:99-100.

55. Fetsch JF, Michal M, Miettinen M. Pigmented (melanotic) neurofibroma: a clinicopathologic and immunohistochemical analysis of 19 lesions from 17 patients. Am J Surg Pathol 2000;24:331-343.

56. Masson P. Tumor humaines:histologie, diagnosis et techniques, 2nd ed. Paris: Maloine; 1956:947-954.

57. Feany MB, Anthony DC, Fletcher CD. Nerve sheath tumours with hybrid features of neurofibroma and schwannoma: a conceptual challenge. Histopathology 1998;32:405-410.

58. Schober R, Reifenberger G, Kremer G, Urich H. Symmetrical neurofibroma with Schwann cell predominance and focal formation of microneurinomas. Acta Neuropathol 1993;85:227-232.

58a. Carroll SL. Molecular mechanisms promoting the pathogenesis of Schwann cell neoplasms. Acta Neuropathol 2012;123:321-348.

59. Reed R, Harkin JC. Tumors of the peripheral nervous system (supplement). Atlas of Tumor Pathology. Washington, DC: Armed Forces Institute of Pathology; 1983.

60. Hirose T, Sano T, Hizawa K. Ultrastructural localization of S-100 protein in neurofibroma. Acta Neuropathol (Berl) 1986;69:103-110.

61. Perentes E, Rubinstein LJ. Immunohistochemical recognition of human neuroepithelial tumors by anti-Leu 7 (HNK-1) monoclonal antibody. Acta Neuropathol 1986;69:227-233.

62. Ariza A, Bilbao JM, Rosai J. Immunohistochemical detection of epithelial membrane antigen in normal perineurial cells and perineurioma. Am J Surg Pathol 1988;12:678-683.

63. Chaubal A, Paetau A, Zoltic K, Miettinen M. CD34 immunoreactivity in nervous system tumors. Acta Neuropathol 1994;88:454-458.

64. Ramani P, Bradley NJ, Fletcher CD. QBEND/10, a new monoclonal antibody to endothelium: assessment of its diagnostic utility in paraffin sections. Histopathology 1990;17:237-242.

65. Weiss SW, Nickoloff BJ. CD-34 is expressed by a distinctive cell population in peripheral nerve, nerve sheath tumors, and related lesions. Am J Surg Pathol 1993;17:1039-1045.

66. Miettinen M, Lindenmayer AE, Chaubal A. Endothelial cell markers CD31, CD34, and BNH9 antibody to H- and Y-antigens—evaluation of their specificity and sensitivity in the diagnosis of vascular tumors and comparison with von Willebrand factor. Mod Pathol 1994;7:82-90.

67. Khalifa MA, Montgomery EA, Ismiil N, Azumi N. What are the CD34+ cells in benign peripheral nerve sheath tumors? Double immunostaining study of CD34 and S-100 protein. Am J Clin Pathol 2000;114:123-126.

68. Chanoki M, Ishii M, Fukai K, et al. Immunohistochemical localization of type I, III, IV, V, and VI collagens and laminin in neurofibroma and neurofibrosarcoma. Am J Dermatopathol 1991;13:365-373.

69. Kindblom LG, Ahlden M, Meis-Kindblom JM, Stenman G. Immunohistochemical and molecular analysis of p53, MDM2, proliferating cell nuclear antigen and Ki67 in benign and malignant peripheral nerve sheath tumours. Virchows Arch 1995;427:19-26.

70. Scheithauer BW, Halling KC, Nascimento AG, Hill EM, Sim FH, Katzmann JA. Neurofibroma and malignant peripheral nerve sheath tumor: a proliferation index and DNA ploidy study [Abstract]. Pathol Res Pract 1995;19:771.

71. Halling KC, Scheithauer BW, Halling AC, et al. p53 expression in neurofibroma and malignant peripheral nerve sheath tumor. An immunohistochemical study of sporadic and NF1-associated tumors. Am J Clin Pathol 1996;106:282-288.

72. Erlandson RA. Diagnostic transmission electron microscopy of tumors. New York: Raven Press; 1994.

73. Kimura K, Kihara I, Kitamura S. The fine structure of glomerular epithelial cells in experimental renal amyloidosis. Acta Pathol Jpn 1974;24:779-796.

74. Ushigome S, Takakuwa T, Hyuga M, Tadokoro M, Shinagawa T. Perineurial cell tumor and the significance of the perineurial cells in neurofibroma. Acta Pathol Jpn 1986;36:973-987.

75. Salmon I, Kiss R, Segers V, et al. Characterization of nuclear size, ploidy, DNA histogram type and proliferation index in 79 nerve sheath tumors. Anticancer Res 1992;12:2277-2283.

76. Lin BT, Weiss LM, Medeiros LJ. Neurofibroma and cellular neurofibroma with atypia: a report of 14 tumors. Am J Surg Pathol 1997;21:1443-1449.

77. Foley KM, Woodruff JM, Ellis FT, Posner JB. Radiation-induced malignant and atypical peripheral nerve sheath tumors. Ann Neurol 1980;7:311-318.

78. Beert E, Brems H, Daniels B, et al. Atypical neurofibromas in neurofibromatosis type 1 are premalignant tumors. Genes Chromosomes Cancer 2011;50:1021-1032.

79. Kourea HP, Orlow I, Scheithauer BW, Cordon-Cardo C, Woodruff JM. Deletions of the INK4A gene occur in malignant peripheral nerve sheath tumors but not in neurofibromas. Am J Pathol 1999;155:1855-1860.

80. Nielsen GP, Stemmer-Rachamimov AO, Ino Y, Moller MB, Rosenberg AE, Louis DN. Malignant transformation of neurofibromas in neurofibromatosis 1 is associated with CDKN2A/p16 inactivation. Am J Pathol 1999;155:1879-1884.

81. Michal M, Fanburg-Smith JC, Mentzel T, et al. Dendritic cell neurofibroma with pseudorosettes: a report of 18 cases of a distinct and hitherto unrecognized neurofibroma variant. Am J Surg Pathol 2001;25:587-594.

82. Simpson R, Seymour MJ. Dendritic cell neurofibroma with pseudorosettes: two tumors in a patient with evidence of neurofibromatosis. Am J Surg Pathol 2001;25:1458-1459.

83. Kazakov DV, Mukensnabl P, Zamecnik M, Michal M. Intraneural dendritic cell neurofibroma with pseudorosettes. Am J Dermatopathol 2004;26:72-75.

84. Michal M, Zamecnik M, Fanburg-Smith JC, et al. Histologically benign cutaneous dendritic cell tumor with pseudorosettes.[Letter]. Am J Surg Pathol 2002;26:1644-1648.

85. Woodruff JM, Busam KJ. Histologically benign cutaneous dendritic cell tumor with pseudorosettes. Am J Surg Pathol 2002;26:1644-1645; author reply 1645-1648.

86. Reed RJ, Leonard DD. Neurotropic melanoma. A variant of desmoplastic melanoma. Am J Surg Pathol 1979;3:301-311.

87. Aiba S, Tabata N, Ishii H, Ootani H, Tagami H. Dermatofibrosarcoma protuberans is a unique fibrohistiocytic tumour expressing CD34. Br J Dermatol 1992;127:79-84.

88. Cohen PR, Rapini RP, Farhood AI. Expression of the human hematopoietic progenitor cell antigen CD34 in vascular and spindle cell tumors. J Cutan Pathol 1993;20:15-20.

89. Bednar B. Storiform neurofibromas of the skin, pigmented and nonpigmented. Cancer 1957;10:368-376.

90. Dupree WB, Langloss JM, Weiss SW. Pigmented dermatofibrosarcoma protuberans (Bednar tumor). A pathologic, ultrastructural, and immunohistochemical study. Am J Surg Pathol 1985;9:630-639.

91. Lautier R, Wolff HH, Jones RE. An immunohistochemical study of dermatofibrosarcoma protuberans supports its fibroblastic character and contradicts neuroectodermal or histiocytic components. Am J Dermatopathol 1990;12:25-30.

92. Fletcher CD, Theaker JM, Flanagan A, Krausz T. Pigmented dermatofibrosarcoma protuberans (Bednar tumour): melanocytic colonization or neuroectodermal differentiation? A clinicopathological and immunohistochemical study. Histopathology 1988;13:631-643.

93. Woodruff JM, Marshall ML, Godwin TA, Funkhouser JW, Thompson NJ, Erlandson RA. Plexiform (multinodular) schwannoma. A tumor simulating the plexiform neurofibroma. Am J Surg Pathol 1983;7:691-697.

94. Agaram NP, Prakash S, Antonescu CR. Deep-seated plexiform schwannoma: a pathologic study of 16 cases and comparative analysis with the superficial variety. Am J Surg Pathol 2005;29:1042-1048.

95. Berg JC, Scheithauer BW, Spinner RS, Allen C, Koutlas IG. Plexiform schwannoma: clinicopathologic overview with emphasis upon the head and neck region. Hum Pathol 2008;39:633-640.

96. Harkin J, Arrington JH, Reed RJ. Benign plexiform schwannoma: a lesion distinct from plexiform neurofibroma. J Neuropathol Exp Neurol 1978;37:622 [abstract].

97. Enzinger FM, Zhang RY. Plexiform fibrohistiocytic tumor presenting in children and young adults. An analysis of 65 cases. Am J Surg Pathol 1988;12:818-826.

98. Hollowood K, Holley MP, Fletcher CD. Plexiform fibrohistiocytic tumour: clinicopathological, immunohistochemical and ultrastructural analysis in favour of a myofibroblastic lesion. Histopathology 1991;19;503-513.

99. Sorensen SA, Mulvihill JJ, Nielsen A. Long-term follow-up of von Recklinghausen neurofibromatosis. Survival and malignant neoplasms. N Engl J Med 1986;314:1010-1015.

100. Ducatman BS, Scheithauer BW, Piepgras DG, Reiman HM, Ilstrup DM. Malignant peripheral nerve sheath tumors. A clinicopathologic study of 120 cases. Cancer 1986;57:2006-2021.

9 PERINEURIAL CELL TUMORS

Aside from the Schwann cell, the perineurial cell is the other principal supportive cell of the peripheral nerve sheath. Its histologic, immunohistochemical, and ultrastructural features are discussed in chapter 2. The nature of the cell was considered by Bunge and associates (1) to be a modified fibroblast, but histopathologic findings suggest an origin from neural crest progenitors of the Schwann cells, and/or embryonic Schwann cells. Alone or with other nerve sheath elements, perineurial cells contribute to the formation of a variety of lesions (2). Among these are reactive processes (traumatic, plantar, pacinian, and palisaded encapsulated neuromas) and a variety of benign nerve sheath tumors, including nerve sheath myxoma. The term perineurioma, however, is reserved for peripheral nerve sheath tumors (PNSTs) composed purely of neoplastic perineurial cells. Their incidence is far lower than that of schwannomas and neurofibromas. Nearly all are benign, although rare malignant examples have been reported. Also included in this chapter is a discussion of hybrid PNSTs with a perineuriomatous component.

PERINEURIOMA

Perineurioma is a tumor composed exclusively of neoplastic perineurial cells. In 1978, Lazarus and Trombetta (3) first suggested the existence of a purely perineurial cell tumor. When unassociated with the perineurium of normal nerve fascicles, perineurial cells cannot be identified with certainty with routine histochemical stains. The evidence provided by Lazarus and Trombetta for a perineurioma was ultrastructural. They described a tumor consisting of cells having the characteristics of normal perineurial cells unaccompanied by any with the features of Schwann cells. Immunohistochemical confirmation of their finding was later provided by observations of immunoreactivity for epithelial membrane antigen (EMA) in both normal perineurial cells (4–6) and those of the tumor (7). With routine histochemical stains, perineurial cells closely resemble fibroblasts; thus, providing immunohistochemical evidence of EMA expression is a required diagnostic step. Unfortunately, since perineurial tumor cell processes are extremely thin and often widely separated by collagen, the presence of EMA reactivity may only be apparent if higher titers of antisera or long incubation times are employed (8,9). If doubt persists, recourse can be made to the gold standard in establishing the diagnosis: a tumor of cells with the ultrastructural features of perineurial cells in the absence of S-100 protein immunoreactivity. This immunohistochemical qualification is necessary since perineurial cells are indistinguishable in fine structural terms from the perineurial-like cells of neurofibroma (see chapter 8). Additional markers helpful in establishing the diagnosis of perineurioma are claudin-1 (10) and Glut-1 (11). The former is a transmembrane protein present in the tight junctions of perineurial cells, and the latter a human erythrocyte glucose transporter protein-1 in the perineurial cells of perineuriomas (12), in the capsule of schwannomas, and as occasional elements of neurofibromas (11).

Perineuriomas have a wide anatomic distribution, ranging from intraneural, to soft tissue, intraosseous, and intestinal. The characteristics of individual perineurial tumor cells are the same at each site, but clinical presentations and histologic appearances differ. These variations are delineated below.

The most common genetic abnormalities of perineuriomas involve chromosome 22 (8,13,14), specifically the *NF2* (neurofibromatosis type 2) gene (15–17). First identified was monosomy of the long arm of chromosome 22 in intraneural perineuriomas (13), an aberration also found in schwannoma and meningioma. Its demonstration is key to classifying intraneural perineuriomas as neoplasms rather than reactive lesions (9). A conventional soft tissue perineurioma arose in a patient with NF2 (18). Chromosomal rearrangements and/or deletions of 10q may be a recurrent feature of sclerosing perineurioma (14).

Intraneural Perineurioma

General Features. The term *intraneural perineurioma* was coined in 1995 by Emory et al. (13). Of all perineurioma variants, it is the most difficult to diagnose and treat. The 2007 work of Boyanton et al. (19) indicates that approximately 50 cases have been reported in the English language literature. Some were reported under the nonspecific umbrella term "localized hypertrophic neuropathy" (20), a designation we now reserve for discrete localized, nonhereditary Schwann cell proliferations characterized by true (Schwann cell) onion bulb formation and apparently reactive in nature (see chapter 5).

Clinical Features. Intraneural perineuriomas typically present in adolescence or early adulthood, and males and females are equally affected (19). An antecedent history of trauma is exceptional (21). The lesions are typically slowly growing and painless. The most common presenting symptom is muscle weakness progressive over months to many years. Sensory disturbances are less often noted. On physical examination, localized muscle atrophy may be apparent. Electromyography demonstrates denervation. Although the affected nerve is only occasionally palpable, magnetic resonance imaging (MRI) generally shows segmental, cylindrical nerve enlargement. In their review, Boyanton et al. (19) found the ulnar, median, peroneal, and posterior interosseous nerves to be most frequently affected. Cranial nerve involvement is rare (22). With the exception of two cases, one with involvement of two adjacent spinal nerve roots (13) and the other of both ulnar nerves (23), all other reported tumors have been solitary.

Gross Findings. Intraneural perineuriomas produce a segmental, firm, sausage-shaped enlargement of an often but not always (15,24) sizeable nerve; the nerve diameter is increased several fold (fig. 9-1A). When the epineurium is stripped, the process is seen to involve individual, distinctly enlarged nerve fascicles (fig. 9-1B). Most examples measure 2 to 10 cm in length, although one lesion exceeded 30 cm (fig. 9-1C) (13).

Microscopic Findings. Cross sections of affected nerves show the histologic process to advantage. The recognition of intraneural perineurioma is based upon finding perineurial cells circumferentially enwrapping nerve fibers (fig. 9-2). These distinctive cellular arrangements have been termed pseudo-onion bulbs, given their superficial resemblance to the true Schwann cell–derived onion bulbs that typify hypertrophic neuropathies (see chapter 5). In contrast, perineurial cells in a circumferential arrangement, but not surrounding Schwann cells or a nerve fiber, are referred to as a perineurial cell whorls. Whereas the telltale pseudo-onion bulbs of intraneural perineurioma are obvious in cross sections, longitudinal sections show only ill-defined, parallel, rope-like bundles of perineurial cells accompanying nearly indiscernible nerve fibers (fig. 9-3A,B). Most, if not all, fascicles are affected and thus enlarged. On occasion, some fascicles of an otherwise markedly involved nerve appear spared (fig. 9-4A). The perineuria of affected fascicles may also be thickened by proliferative perineurial cells (fig. 9-4B,C). Although these may extend from the perineurium into the endoneurium, they do not invade epineurial tissue.

Compared to normal nerve fascicles, those of perineuriomas are hypercellular due to the abundance of overlapping perineurial cells arrayed concentrically around axons (fig. 9-2). Despite their number, arrangement, and occasional enlarged or hyperchromatic examples (fig. 9-4D), most tumor cells appear cytologically normal. The nuclei are elongated and chromatin is delicate (fig. 9-3A). Mitoses are absent or rare (fig. 9-4D). The cell layers surrounding the nerve fibers vary considerably in number, but five or six lamellae are often seen. In addition, cells at the periphery of a whorl occasionally sweep toward and contribute to the structure of an adjacent whorl (fig. 9-2B,C). Particularly large whorls may enclose several or even numerous nerve fibers (fig. 9-5). Endoneurial capillaries may also be enshrouded by perineurial whorls (fig. 9-2C). In well-established or chronic lesions, stains for axons and myelin show them to be reduced, scant, or even absent (fig. 9-3C,D) despite the persistence of Schwann cells at the centers of most whorls (fig. 9-6, left). Collagenization characterizes chronic lesions (fig. 9-6, right).

Immunohistochemical Findings. Like normal perineurial cells, those of intraneural perineuriomas forming pseudo-onion bulbs exhibit immunoreactivity for EMA (figs. 9-7A, 9-3B). The EMA staining pattern is membranous and widespread. Reactivity is limited to pseudo-onion bulbs, perineurial cells involving septa, and residual

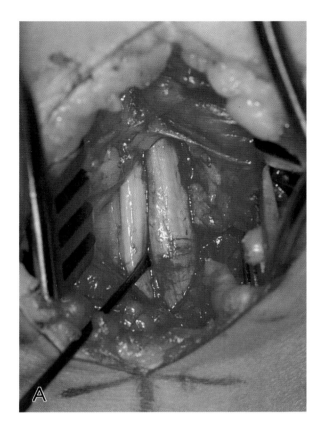

Figure 9-1

INTRANEURAL PERINEURIOMA

A: This operative photograph of a peroneal nerve lesion shows the normal tibial (left) beside the affected peroneal (right) nerve.

B: Enlargement of individual fascicles of an affected nerve is readily apparent in this tibial example.

C: One remarkably extensive tumor involved a sciatic nerve from the level of the sciatic notch to the knee. The epineurium has been opened to demonstrate the enlarged fascicles.

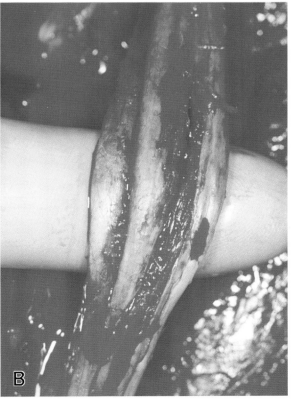

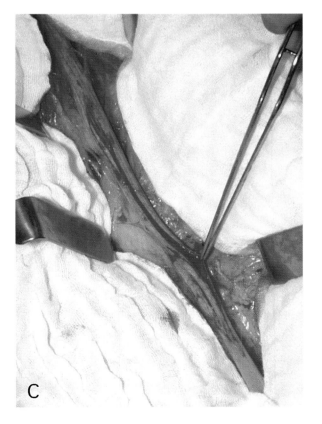

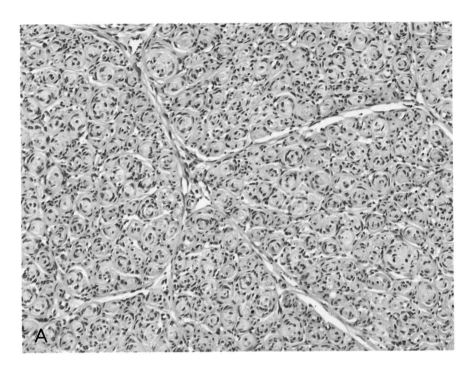

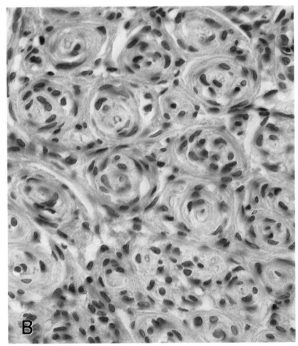
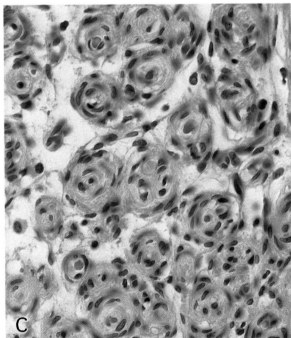

Figure 9-2

INTRANEURAL PERINEURIOMA

A: Making a correct diagnosis requires examination of cross sections of the affected nerve to discern the reason for the enlargement of fascicles, four of which appear in this field.

B: At higher power, individual nerve fibers are surrounded by whorls of cells that should express epithelial membrane antigen (EMA) (see fig. 9-3A). Such structures are referred to as pseudo-onion bulbs.

B,C: There is occasional "spinning off" of perineurial cells from one pseudo-onion bulb to another.

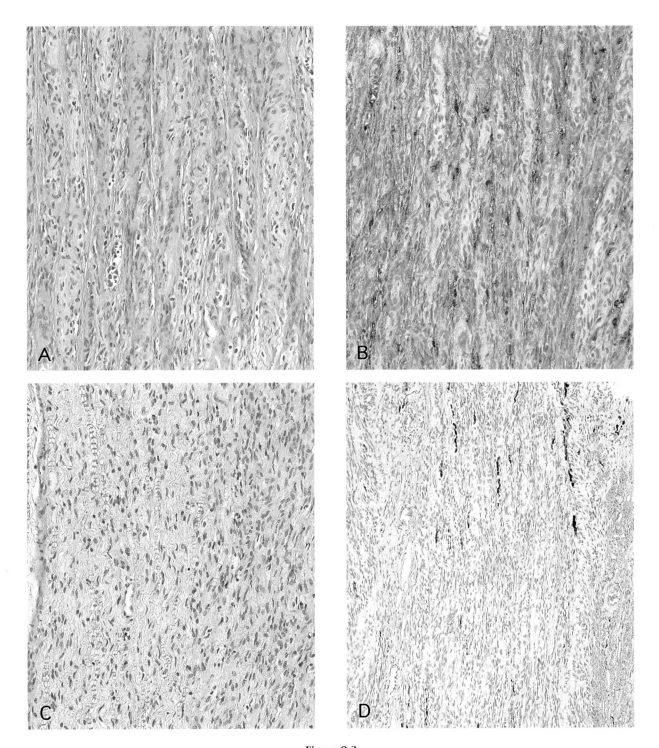

Figure 9-3

INTRANEURAL PERINEURIOMA

A,B: Although assessment of longitudinal sections makes the diagnosis more difficult, perineurial wrapping of fibers imparts a characteristic ropy appearance (A) which is accentuated on EMA stain (B).

C: Luxol-fast blue-periodic acid–Schiff (PAS) preparation of a variably affected fascicle shows graduation of myelin loss.

D: Axonal loss is seen well with neurofilament protein immunostains.

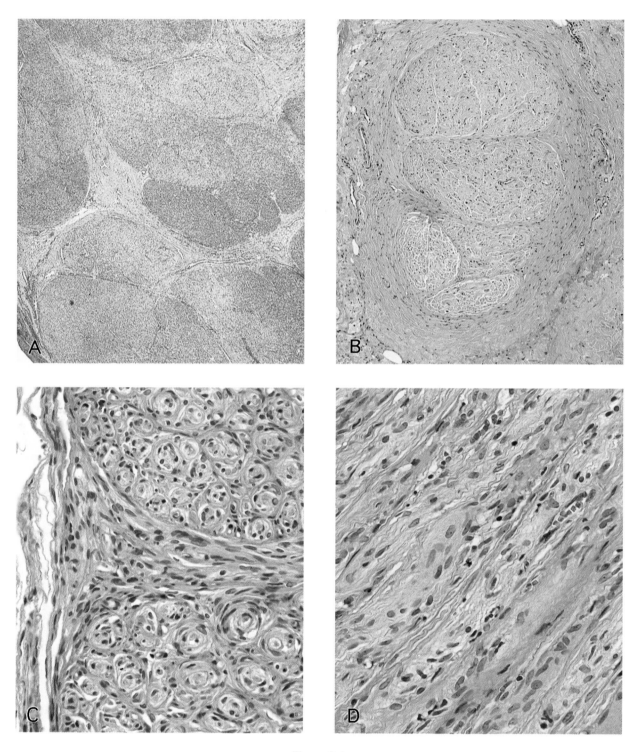

Figure 9-4

INTRANEURAL PERINEURIOMA

Although the gross appearance of such tumors does not suggest malignancy, some microscopic features may be misleading. These include marked variation in endoneurial cellularity (A), conspicuous involvement of the perineurium (B,C), and the occurrence of occasional mitoses, particularly when seen in longitudinal sections (D).

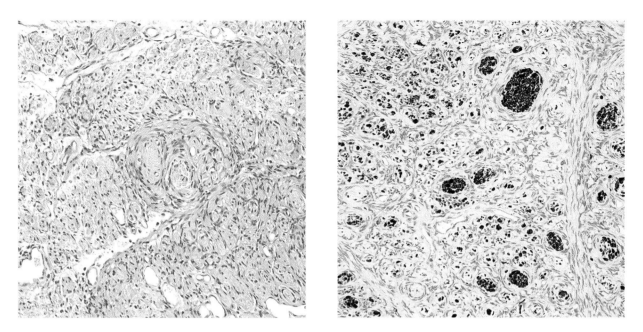

Figure 9-5

INTRANEURAL PERINEURIOMA

Microscopic variations include partial involvement of nerve fascicles, with some fibers unaffected and others showing only scant perineurial cell ensheathment (left). In some instances, large pseudo-onion bulbs surround bundles of nerve fibers (left), a finding best seen on neurofilament stain (right).

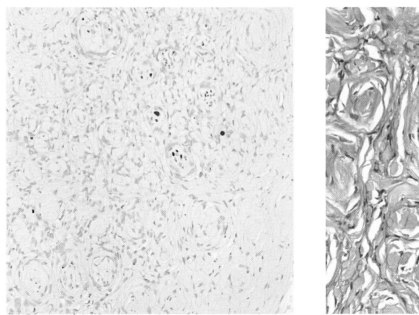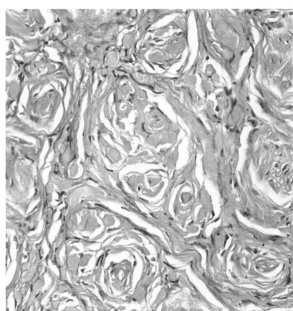

Figure 9-6

INTRANEURAL PERINEURIOMA

In longitudinal sections, extensive collagen deposition is associated with near-total loss of nerve fibers and myelin, here illustrated with a neurofilament protein preparation (left) and a Luxol-fast blue-PAS stain for myelin (right). Blue myelin sheaths are seen.

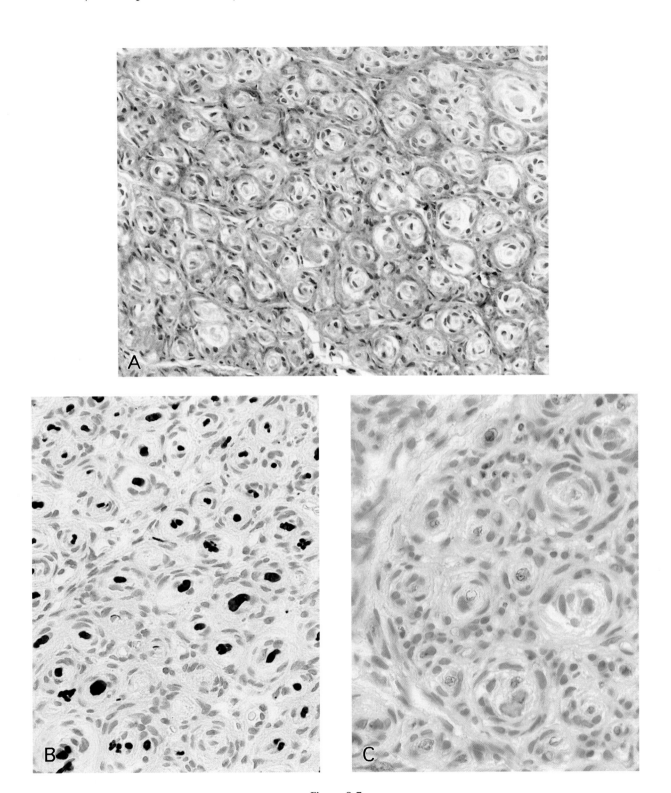

Figure 9-7

INTRANEURAL PERINEURIOMA

Pseudo-onion bulbs consist of multilayer wrappings of EMA-positive perineurial cells (A) around neurofilament-reactive axons (B) and their S-100 protein-positive Schwann sheaths (C).

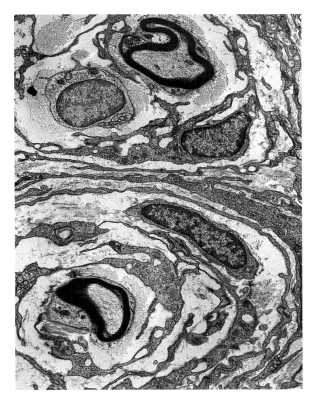

Figure 9-8

INTRANEURAL PERINEURIOMA

Ultrastructure of pseudo-onion bulbs shows myelinated nerve fibers circumferentially surrounded by layers of perineurial cells.

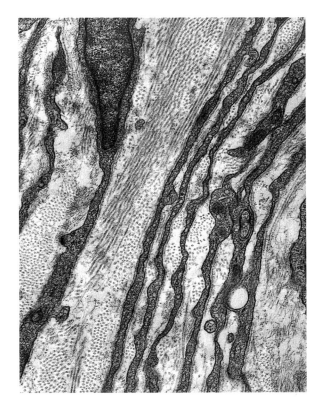

Figure 9-9

INTRANEURAL PERINEURIOMA

High magnification of a pseudo-onion bulb shows nine thin perineurial cell cytoplasmic processes and part of a nucleus. Numerous pinocytotic vesicles, surface basal lamina, and abundant stromal collagen fibrils are evident.

normal perineurium. Lack of S-100 protein expression in the concentrically layered cells clearly distinguishes the pseudo-onion bulbs of perineurioma from lesions featuring Schwann cell–derived true onion bulbs. Axons and Schwann cells (residual nerve fibers), whether myelinated or not, are immunoreactive for neurofilament protein (figs. 9-5, right; 9-7B) and S-100 protein (fig. 9-7C), respectively. Also supportive of the diagnosis is immunoreactivity for claudin-1 and Glut-1. Collagen 4 and laminin staining is also seen (19), but does not distinguish the lesion from the equally reactive Schwann cell processes. One study reported significant nuclear immunoreactivity for the proliferation marker MIB-1, with the labeling index ranging from 5 to 15 percent (13).

Ultrastructural Findings. The fine structure of intraneural perineuriomas reveals two essential components: one or more myelinated or un-

myelinated axons and non-neoplastic Schwann sheaths surrounded by concentric layers of neoplastic, rather normal-appearing perineurial cells (fig. 9-8) (2). The latter are separated by an often discontinuous basal lamina substance and varying numbers of collagen fibrils (fig. 9-9). The ultrastructural features of normal perineurium are described in chapter 1.

Molecular Findings. The early study of three cases provided evidence of chromosome 22 abnormalities (13). The authors identified a monosomy of the long arm of chromosome 22 in two tumors. A subsequent fluorescence in situ hybridization (FISH) analysis of one tumor by Huguet et al. (15) found a deletion of the *bcr* locus (22q11) in 75 of 100 nuclei. Cytogenetic studies of two tumors displayed mostly simple karyotypes with some numerical changes (13). Unusual associations include one patient who had Beckwith-Wiedemann syndrome (25), another with NF1 as well as a family history for the disorder (26), and two patients with café au lait spots (27).

Differential Diagnosis. The differential diagnosis of intraneural perineurioma is limited since the pseudo-onion bulb formation is mimicked only by the Schwann cell–derived, true onion bulbs occurring in hypertrophic neuropathies. Such disorders are either inherited and generalized (hereditary sensorimotor neuropathies) or, on rare occasion, sporadic and focal in occurrence (see chapter 4). The schwannian nature of these more discrete and uniform-sized onion bulbs is readily confirmed by S-100 protein immunostaining and lack of EMA staining.

Even infrequently occurring, cylindrically shaped neurofibromas involving a segment of nerve pose no differential diagnostic problem. Their less cellular appearance and large Schwann cell component, and the way in which residual axons, unaccompanied by encircling perineurial cells, appear to float in an Alcian blue–positive, mucopolysaccharide-rich matrix, is very different from perineurioma. Admittedly, neurofibromas occasionally show onion bulb-like structures superficially resembling those of perineurioma, but their cells are S-100 protein rather than EMA reactive. In comparison, the neoplastic cells of intraneural perineuriomas encircle nerve fibers and are EMA reactive, while S-100 protein expression is strictly limited to encircled Schwann cells.

Intraneural perineurioma must not be mistaken for malignant peripheral nerve sheath tumor (MPNST). In view of the former's uniform cylindrical shape, small diameter, and generally limited nerve involvement, confusion is unlikely. Nonetheless, the cellularity of intraneural perineurioma in some cross sections (fig. 9-4A,B), and particularly in some longitudinal sections (fig. 9-3A), and the occasional finding of a mitotic figure (fig. 9-4D), may cause concern. Should the differential arise, especially with a frozen section, the simplest solution is to examine a cross section of the lesion: MPNSTs lack pseudo-onion bulb formation. The positive reaction of pseudo-onion bulbs for EMA confirms the diagnosis of perineurioma; perineurial cell MPNSTs occur, but they are rare and their cells may whorl but do not form pseudo-onion bulbs.

Treatment and Prognosis. In a review of reported cases, Boyanton et al. (19) found that the most common treatment approaches are resection with nerve grafting, simple resection, and excisional biopsy. Among the 35 cases with available follow-up information, 16 patients had been treated by surgical resection. Of these, 15 underwent nerve grafting and 1 had a primary anastomosis. Five patients (31 percent) reported no improvement and 11 (69 percent) reported some improvement in motor function. Our experience indicates that biopsy alone is sufficient for diagnosis; fascicles confirmed to be nonfunctional by direct nerve stimulation should be selected for biopsy. Even if only partially functional, affected nerves should be preserved. Excision and nerve graft reconstruction should only be considered in the setting of a totally nonfunctional nerve. The margins of these well-localized lesions must be microscopically examined to assure their normalcy. Even after reconstruction, recovery of nerve function may not be obtained. Long-term follow-up has confirmed the benign nature of intraneural perineurioma by showing no risk of recurrence or metastasis (13,19).

Soft Tissue Perineurioma

General Features. The first description of an extraneural soft tissue tumor composed solely of perineurial cells is attributed to Lazarus and Trombetta (3). Given the difficulty in distinguishing perineurial cells from fibroblasts in conventionally stained tissue, it is no surprise that before their paper appeared such tumors had been classified as storiform perineurial fibromas (28). Perineurial cells have characteristic immunohistochemical and ultrastructural features (see above). Applying these criteria, over 100 *soft tissue perineuriomas* have been reported to date. Unlike intraneural examples, this form of perineurioma preferentially affects adults. Three histologic growth patterns have been identified, leading to the classification of soft tissue perineuriomas into *conventional* and the less frequently occurring *reticular (retiform)* and *sclerosing* variants. A recently described subset of soft tissue perineuriomas occurring in the intestines is sufficiently clinicopathologically unique to warrant a separate discussion (see below). Like intraneural perineurioma, the soft tissue variety exhibits an abnormality of chromosome 22 (fig. 9-10).

Clinical Features. Soft tissue perineuriomas occur over a wide age range (9 to 79 years) (29,30) and, although widely distributed, most often affect the limbs and trunk (30). Most are situated in the subcutis, and most of the remainder reside in deep soft tissue. Infrequently affected sites include the retroperitoneum (30), paratesticular region (30), kidney (31,32), soft tissues of the breast (33), nasal cavity and maxillary sinus (8), intraosseous sites such as the mandible (34), and choroid plexus (35). In the hand (36), where the majority are dermal and subcutaneous, the tumors involve the fingers and palm and are of the sclerosing variety (36–39). A majority (8 of 11) of reticular tumors (40–42) arose in an upper extremity, half involving a hand. Based on a sample of 100 cases collected from multiple reports, including one literature review (8,30,43), conventional soft tissue perineuriomas show a slight female bias in patients ranging from 10 to 79 years of age (mean, 43 years). A female prevalence (8 of 11), with a narrower age range (31 to 61 years; mean, 42 years), is seen in individuals with reticular tumors (40–42). In contrast, sclerosing tumors show a striking predilection for males and affect mainly young adults (age range 9 to 55 years; mean, 23 years) (37–39). There has been a one report of a soft tissue perineurioma arising in a patient with NF2 (18) and another in a patient with NF1 (44).

Gross Findings. There is no apparent nerve association. One exception was an example associated with a mandibular nerve (34); although initially considered a meningioma, retrospective study confirmed its perineurial nature. The tumors, usually solitary, are nodular and ovoid (fig. 9-11A), and rarely polypoid (45). They are grossly well circumscribed but not encapsulated (fig. 9-11A) (9). Multinodular examples of conventional soft tissue perineuriomas also occur (fig. 9-11B,C) (46–49). Sclerosing soft tissue perineuriomas are also typically ovoid and well marginated (fig. 9-11D) (37). Conventional tumors vary greatly in size (range, 0.3 to 20.0 cm; mean, 4.1 cm) (30). Reticular examples range from 1.5 to 10.0 cm (mean, 3.9 cm) (40–42). With a size range of 0.7 to 4.0 cm (mean, 1.7 cm) (37–39), sclerosing soft tissue perineuriomas are considerably smaller.

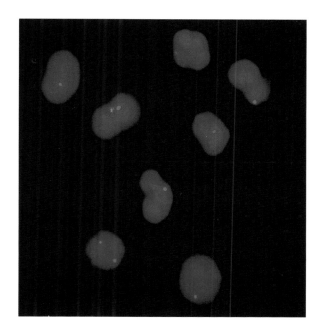

Figure 9-10

SOFT TISSUE PERINEURIOMA

The fluorescence in situ hybridization (FISH) preparation of isolated nuclei is shown. Six of the nuclei show only one signal for M-BCR, a chromosome 22 marker, thus indicating monosomy.

The cut surfaces of conventional perineuriomas are most often white-tan (fig. 9-11A), rubbery to firm, and infrequently soft, gelatinous, or mucoid. One very large example, in addition to being focally necrotic, exhibited cyst formation (50). Of reticular tumors, some are described as yellow-white; cystic change is exceptional (40). Sclerosing tumors are typically firm and homogeneously off-white (37). One massive, hypocellular perineurial cell tumor consisted primarily of dense collagen and showed degenerative nuclear atypia as well as dystrophic calcification (51). The tumor presented as a 12-cm extrapelvic and intrapelvic dumbbell-shaped mass that had passed through the sciatic notch and was apposed to the sciatic nerve. The tumor was classified as a sclerosing perineurioma. Dystrophic calcification and osseous metaplasia are rare in such tumors (52), and it is possible that this tumor was a sclerosed conventional soft tissue perineurioma.

Microscopic Findings. Although usually well circumscribed, in the series of 81 conventional soft tissue perineuriomas reported by Hornick

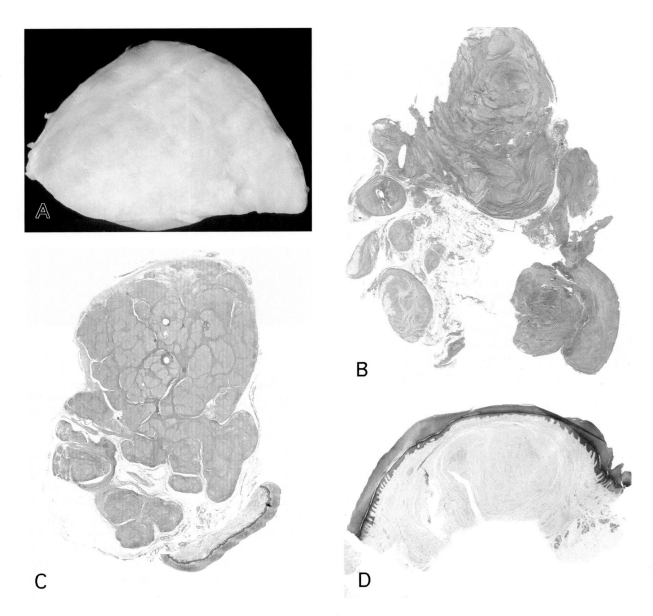

Figure 9-11

SOFT TISSUE PERINEURIOMA

A: Cross section of half of a gross specimen shows a rounded contour, circumscription, uniform texture, and white-tan appearance.

B,C: Multinodular examples are uncommon.

D: On macrosections, circumscription of dermal tumors is less evident.

and Fletcher (30), 1 in 7 showed focal entrapment or infiltration of surrounding fat or skeletal muscle. The lower-power histologic appearance of conventional tumors is variable. The tumor cells often have a layered or lamellar appearance (fig. 9-12A), but sometimes the pattern is vaguely fascicular (fig. 9-12B), bundled (fig.

9-12C), or storiform (47). Often, the cell layers are wrinkled (fig. 9-12A). Whorl formation may be seen (fig. 9-12D). A myxoid matrix is often conspicuous (fig. 9-13, left) (30,43,46). Hornick and Fletcher found at least 40 percent of their tumors to be focally myxoid, and 20 percent to be almost exclusively so. Collagen fibers are a

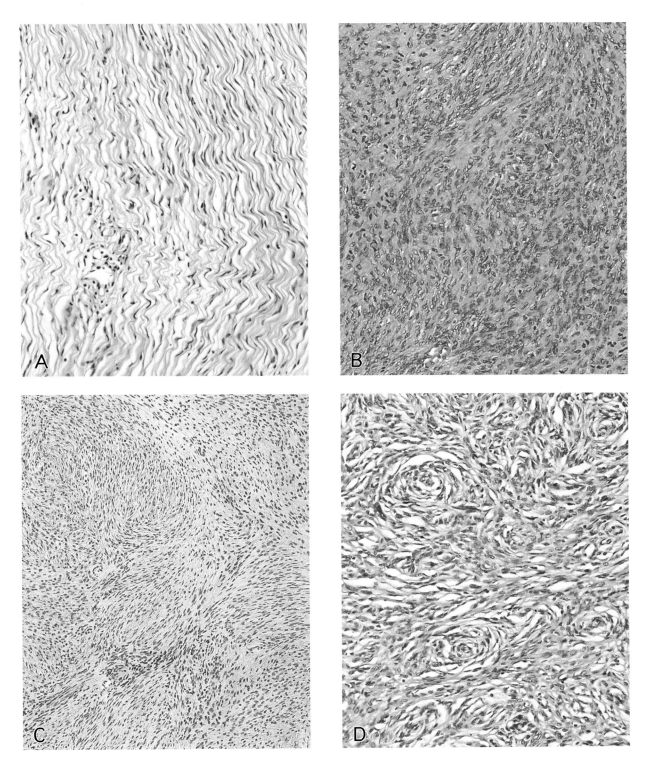

Figure 9-12

SOFT TISSUE PERINEURIOMA

The most common growth patterns seen histologically are lamellar (A), vague fasciculation (B), bundles (C), and cell whorls (D).

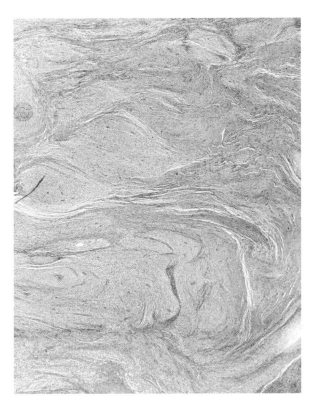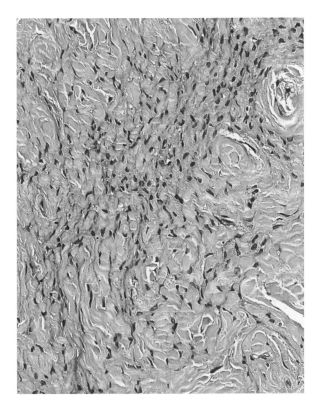

Figure 9-13

SOFT TISSUE PERINEURIOMA

Left: Less than half of the tumors are focally or mostly myxoid. In some examples, the myxoid change has a mosaic appearance.

Right: In heavily collagenized tumors the collagen fibers may be arrayed in micronodules.

constant component of perineuriomas, and may be arranged in bundles or micronodules (fig. 9-13, right). Cellularity varies considerably among the tumors. Of those reported by Hornick and Fletcher, nearly half were hypocellular, and about 20 percent markedly hypercellular. Individual tumor cells are usually spindle shaped, with thin, elongated and bipolar cytoplasmic processes (fig. 9-14A,B). Nuclei are most often fusiform, tapered, and bent (fig. 9-14A), but may be ovoid or disc shaped (fig. 9-14C). Silver impregnations for axons are negative, as are myelin stains. Although cell crowding and hyperchromasia may be seen (30), nuclear pleomorphism and the degenerative changes of the kind seen in ancient schwannoma and atypical neurofibroma (fig. 9-14D) are uncommon (51). The designation *atypical cellular perineurioma* has been suggested for cellular perineuriomas featuring scattered nuclear atypia or infiltrative

growth (53). In most conventional perineuriomas, mitoses are absent or infrequent. In addition, necrosis is usually lacking. Blood vessels, although inconspicuous, are often numerous. A distinctive feature of the collagenous zones of some tumors is dissection of collagen by tumor cells with resultant encirclement of collagen bundles and nodules (fig. 9-13, right). Psammoma body formation is rare (16).

The defining histology of the reticular (retiform) perineurioma is a predominantly net-like or lace-like pattern of tumor growth (fig. 9-16A–C) (40–42). The cells are fusiform and arranged in anastomosing cords, and feature bipolar cytoplasmic processes, palely eosinophilic cytoplasm, and centrally situated fusiform or ovoid nuclei (fig. 9-16B) (40). The cell cords often encircle islands of fibromyxoid stroma (40), which sometimes give way to globular collagen deposits (42). Additional features are

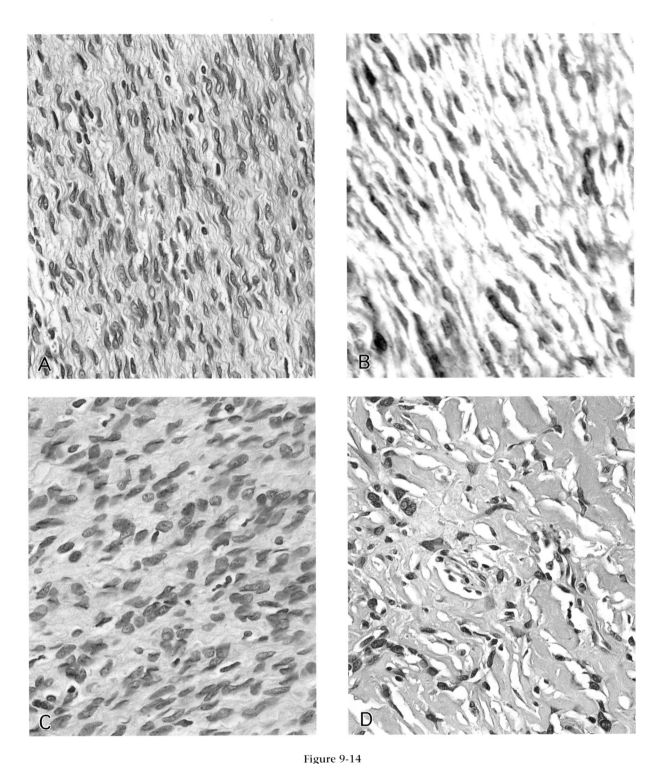

Figure 9-14

SOFT TISSUE PERINEURIOMA

A,B: At high power, the tumor cells most often are thin with wrinkled elongated nuclei from which extend bipolar cytoplasmic processes that are more evident in EMA-stained sections (B).

C: Less frequent are tumor cells with plump or coin-shaped nuclei.

D: Pleomorphic nuclei represent degenerative changes.

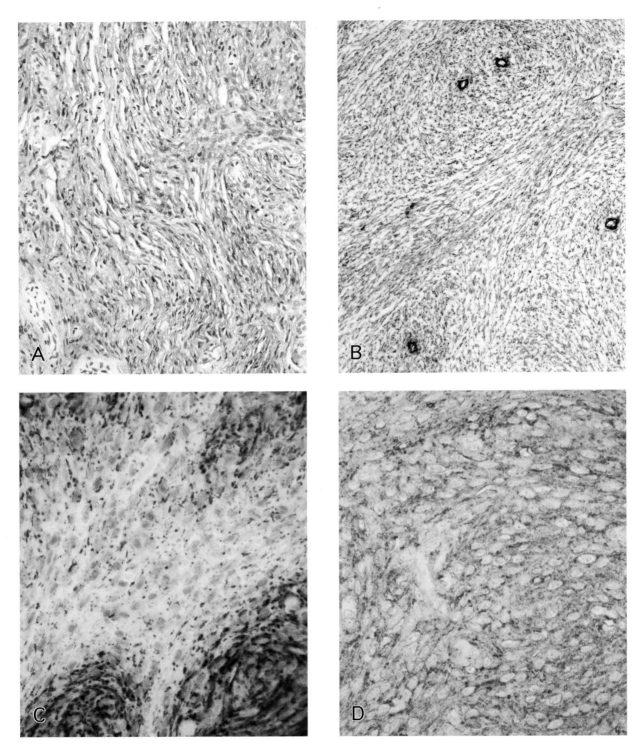

Figure 9-15

SOFT TISSUE PERINEURIOMA

A: Reactivity for EMA is requisite to the diagnosis.
B: Diffuse collagen 4 immunostaining is attributed to the presence of pericellular basal lamina.
C,D: Frequent findings are expression of claudin-1 (C) and Glut-1 (D).

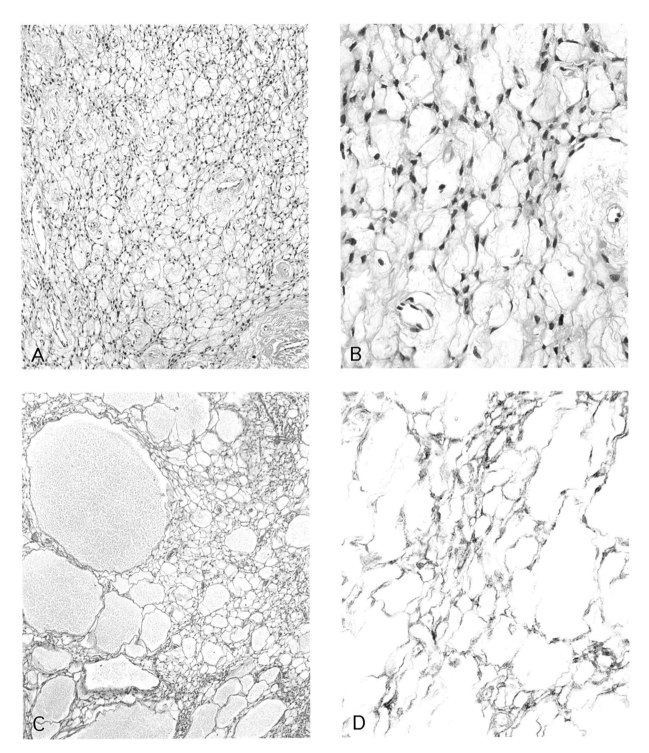

Figure 9-16

RETICULAR VARIANT OF SOFT TISSUE PERINEURIOMA

A,B: The defining histology is a predominantly net-like growth, seen here at medium (A) and high power (B).

C: Prominent cystic changes are sometimes observed.

D: Like conventional soft tissue perineuriomas, the tumor cells express EMA. (Courtesy of Dr. C. D. Fletcher, Boston, MA.)

linear arrays of tumor cells separated by matrix (42) and cystic spaces, which may be prominent (fig. 9-16C) (40). Most reticular tumors also exhibit zones of conventional perineurioma (40,41). Infrequent features include enlarged hyperchromatic nuclei, presumably degenerative in nature, and partial tumor hyalinization (40). Mitoses are generally absent.

The sclerosing perineurioma is characterized by a variable number of epithelioid and spindle cells with small nuclei growing in cords, arcades, and whorls. These are embedded in a dense collagenous matrix (fig. 9-17A-C). Only rarely is a centrally located nerve twig identified (38,46).

Immunohistochemical Findings. The immunoprofile of soft tissue perineuriomas, established initially by work on conventional tumors, is immunoreactivity for EMA (figs. 9-15A, 9-16D, 9-17D), collagen type 4 (fig. 9-15B), laminin, and vimentin, but lack of S-100 protein staining. Expression of claudin-1 (fig. 9-15C) (10) and Glut-1 (fig. 9-15D) (11,39,41) are also seen. Claudin-1 has been reported in 29 percent (30) to 92 percent (10) of tumors. In the latter study, claudin-1 expression was occasionally stronger and more diffuse than EMA expression, while in the former study staining for Glut-1 was more intense than that for EMA. As mentioned earlier, a prolonged incubation or a higher antibody titer than is used to label carcinomas may be required to obtain a positive EMA reaction in perineuriomas. The difference in reported claudin-1 expression may also be due to the use of different immunohistochemical methods (30). CD34 staining was evident in 64 percent of 78 conventional perineuriomas in one report (30), and in 2 of 5 reticular tumors in another (40). Pertinent negative reactions include those for glial fibrillary acidic protein (GFAP) (30), desmin (30), and desmoplakin. One study of conventional soft tissue perineuriomas found immunopositivity for smooth muscle actin in 21 percent of 77 tumors (30), while another study found it in 6 of 14 sclerosing tumors (37). Although soft tissue perineuriomas are usually keratin immunonegative, focal keratin expression was noted in two reticular tumors (40) and in a small number of cells in 4 of 14 sclerosing tumors (37).

Ultrastructural Findings. Given the variation in the sensitivity of EMA immunoreactivity among various laboratories, electron microscopy continues to play a useful role in the diagnosis of soft tissue perineurioma. Such tumors are composed of normal-appearing perineurial cells, usually loosely organized in a collagenous or myxocollagenous stroma (fig. 9-18). Viewed in cross section, circular aggregates of stromal collagen fibrils are surrounded by perineurial cell processes (fig. 9-19). Diagnostically helpful attributes of neoplastic perineurial cells include an elongated nucleus with variably clumped, marginated chromatin; an inconspicuous nucleolus; long, thin cytoplasmic processes; cytoplasm containing few organelles and scant filaments; prominent pinocytotic vesicles distributed along the cell membrane and occasionally in the cytoplasm; an often discontinuous basal lamina thinner than that lining normal perineurial cells; and scattered rudimentary intercellular tight junctions (figs. 9-18, 9-19) (2,8,40,54). Ribosome-lamella complexes were a prominent feature of one reported tumor (55).

Molecular Findings. Genetic studies have shown a pathogenetic relationship to loss of *NF2* gene function in soft tissue perineuriomas. Studies focusing on the region 22q11-q13.1, including the *NF2* gene (22q12.2), first found a monosomy of chromosome 22 by FISH analysis, consistent with a loss of genetic material from chromosome band 22q11 (fig. 9-10) (8). Molecular methods have also demonstrated a cryptic deletion (38) and point mutations (17) at the *NF2* locus. The above genetic aberrations were identified in 8 of 16 tumors, all 8 of which were either of the conventional or sclerosing variety. In cytogenetic studies, perineuriomas display mostly simple karyotypes, characterized by one or a few chromosomal rearrangements or numerical changes (13,14,38,56). Included in these studies were one conventional and three sclerosing lesions. Rearrangements and/or deletions of 10q were a consistent finding in the latter (14).

Differential Diagnosis. The differential diagnosis for soft tissue perineurioma is broad, and varies according to the morphologic form and the location. The single nodule lesions most easily confused with conventional tumors are listed in Table 9-1. If multinodular, a plexiform schwannoma (see chapter 7) should be ruled out. In contrast to perineurioma, plexiform neurofibroma is extensively immunoreactive for S-100 protein. Not mentioned in the table

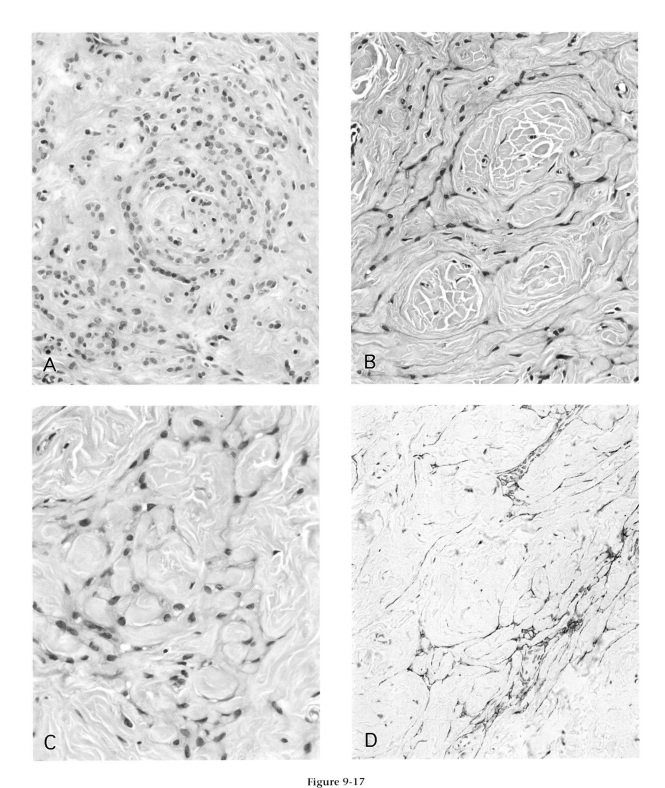

Figure 9-17

SCLEROSING VARIANT OF SOFT TISSUE PERINEURIOMA

The tumor cells are small, round to ovoid, and arrayed in vaguely circular (A,B) and irregular (C) cords among sclerotic fibrous tissue. Staining for EMA confirms the diagnosis (D). (Courtesy of Dr. J. F. Fetsch, Washington, DC.)

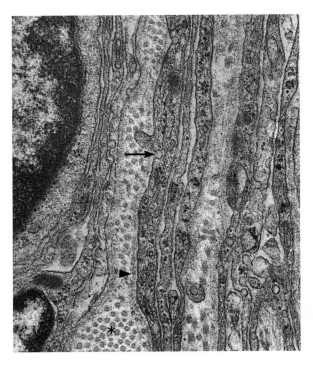

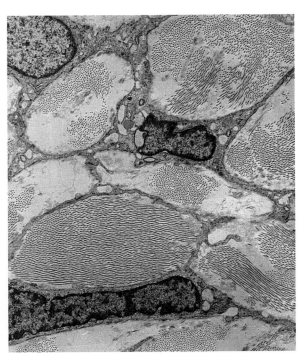

Figure 9-18

**SOFT TISSUE PERINEURIOMA:
PERINEURIAL CELL PROCESSES**

Seen are pinocytotic vesicles (arrow), remnants of basal lamina (arrowhead), and cross-sectioned collagen fibrils. A portion of a nucleus is also seen.

Figure 9-19

SOFT TISSUE PERINEURIOMA

Encirclement of collagen bundles by the long processes of perineurial cells is a common feature of this tumor.

Table 9-1

DIFFERENTIAL DIAGNOSIS OF CONVENTIONAL SOFT TISSUE PERINEURIOMA (STP)

Location	Distinguishing Features of Resembling Lesions
Dermal and Subcutaneous Tumors (8,47,76,81)	DFSP[a] – typically infiltrative, hypercellular, uniformly storiform, and CD34 positive, but EMA[b] negative
	Extracranial fibrous meningioma (82) – frequent psammoma body formation, 80% S-100 protein positive, ultrastructurally lacks basal lamina and pinocytotic vesicles
Subcutaneous and Deep Tumors (8,47,76,81)	Solitary fibrous tumor – commonly circumscribed with ovoid to spindle cells in patternless, nonstoriform arrangement, and usually CD34 and sometimes EMA positive; pericytoma-like branching blood vessels
	Fibromatosis – infiltrative, less cellular tumor with cells having shorter, straighter nuclei that are embedded in a dense collagenous matrix; sometimes immunostains for myoid markers
	Low-grade fibromyxoid sarcoma (59,60) – the closest histologic mimic of STP, this usually presents in the proximal extremities of young adults; histologically bland spindle cells with variously collagenous/hyalinized and myxoid areas, arcades of small blood vessels, and occasional giant collagen rosettes
	Low-grade myxofibrosarcoma (58,83) – fibroblastic tumor with elongated, thin-walled, curvilinear blood vessels, occasional vacuolated cells simulating lipoblasts (pseudo-lipoblasts), and atypical hyperchromatic cells; EMA negative
	Cellular myxoma (40) – features of intramuscular myxoma but with increased cellularity; no storiform growth or cell whorls; EMA negative

[a]DFSP = dermatofibrosarcoma protuberans.
[b]EMA = epithelial membrane antigen.

Table 9-2

DIFFERENTIAL DIAGNOSIS OF SOFT TISSUE PERINEURIOMA VARIANTS

Variant Type	Distinguishing Features of Resembling Lesions
Reticular/Retiform STP[a] (40–42,81)	Myoepithelial tumors of soft tissue (84) – have an identifiable acinar or ductal component, and are variably positive for S-100 protein, cytokeratins, GFAP[b], and SMA
	Ossifying fibromyxoid tumor of soft parts (devoid of ossification) (85) – a more nested tumor with more rounded cells with eosinophilic cytoplasm; often S-100 protein and desmin positive, but EMA[c] negative
	Extraskeletal myxoid chondrosarcoma (86,87) – grossly distinctive with fleshy, firm, tan tissue interrupted by irregular deposits of gray myxoid material; histologically, there may be a lace-like cellular arrangement, rarely microcysts, and cells that are larger with more obvious eosinophilic cytoplasm; infrequently EMA positive; associated with a t(9;22) (q22-31;q11-12) translocation
	Myxoid synovial sarcoma (88) – grossly myxoid areas may be prominent, but cream-tan, firm and fleshy tumor typically dominates; histologically, solid fascicular spindle cell areas are present, the cells are more plump and atypical, and are occasionally EMA positive; there usually is a t(x;18)(p11.2;q11.2) translocation and either SYT-SSX1 or SYT-SSX2 transcripts
Sclerosing STP	Sclerosing adnexal tumor – perhaps the closest histologic simulator of STP; in contrast the lesion may show ductal structures, a demonstrable myoepithelial layer, and is consistently positive for keratins as well as other epithelial markers
	Fibroma of tendon sheath – deeper lesion involving tendon sheath and composed of myofibroblastic cells that lack EMA reactivity
	Sclerotic fibromas of dermis – solitary or multiple lesions (Cowden disease); hypocellular, hyalinized lesions not shown to be EMA positive
	Regressing glomus tumor – often painful and predominantly affecting young adult females; tumor cells cluster around blood vessels, have more cytoplasm, are muscle specific and smooth muscle actin positive, but EMA negative
	Epithelioid neurofibroma and schwannoma – both are composed at least in part (epithelioid neurofibroma) by rounded cells and are diffusely or extensively S-100 protein positive
	Epithelioid hemangioendothelioma – can show cord-like growth, which may also be nested; cells uniformly epithelioid, with a vacuolated cytoplasm; CD31, CD34, and factor VIII antigen positive
	Epithelioid sarcoma – (a crucial distinction because its aggressive growth results in a frequently fatal outcome); epithelioid cells are larger than those of STP, have eosinophilic cytoplasm, have well-formed cell membranes, are cytologically malignant, and are keratin positive

[a]STP = soft tissue perineurioma.
[b]GFAP = glial fibrillary acidic protein; SMA = smooth muscle actin.
[c]EMA = epithelial membrane antigen.

are simulators of atypical perineurioma: the closest are dermatofibrosarcoma protuberans with fibrosarcomatous areas (57), low-grade myxofibrosarcoma with some pleomorphic nuclei (so-called malignant fibrous histiocytoma) (58), low-grade fibromyxoid sarcoma (59,60), MPNST with perineurial cell differentiation (61,62), and follicular dendritic cell tumor (53). The first two are EMA negative. Specific criteria for a diagnosis of perineurial cell MPNST are still to be determined, but at present their distinction from atypical cellular perineurioma is thought to rest with the finding of numerous rather than few mitoses, marked rather than mild nuclear atypia, and the presence of necrosis in the former (see chapter 12) (53,61). The

overlapping microscopic features of follicular dendritic cell tumor, a malignant neoplasm (63,64), are tumor circumscription, storiform growth, and staining for EMA (see section on intestinal perineuriomas).

Tumors that mimic the reticular and sclerosing perineurioma variants are listed in Table 9-2. One lesion mentioned in the literature (36) but not warranting consideration as a simulator of soft tissue perineurioma is localized interdigital neuritis (Morton neuroma; chapter 3), a reactive change confined to the foot, a site not involved by perineurioma.

Treatment and Prognosis. The preferred treatment of soft tissue perineurioma is gross total excision. The prognosis is excellent. To date, no examples have recurred or metastasized following such treatment. Even in instances in which total excision is difficult, as in the nasal cavity-maxillary sinus example referred to above (8), we advocate careful observation rather than aggressive adjuvant therapy.

Intestinal Perineurioma

General Features. A significant recent finding concerning soft tissue perineuriomas is the identification by Hornick and Fletcher (65) and by Agaimy and Wuensch (65a) of the intestine as a site of involvement. The finding clarifies the nature of a small group of intestinal spindle cell tumors that were previously unclassified or misclassified.

Clinical Features. Nine of 10 patients with intestinal perineuriomas reported by Hornick and Fletcher (65) had large bowel tumors, 4 of which affected the sigmoid colon; the remaining tumor involved the jejunum. Eight of the patients were female ranging from 35 to 59 years (mean, 51 years). Six of the patients with large bowel tumors were asymptomatic and undergoing routine colorectal cancer screening; another presented because of abdominal pain and gastrointestinal bleeding. Of the last 2, 1 was admitted with a mass lesion. The patient with the jejunal lesion had a 2-year history consistent with small bowel obstruction. The case report of Agaimy and Wuensch (65a) documented a 30-year-old woman with a gastric lesion evaluated for recurrent upper gastrointestinal bleeding.

Gross Findings. Eight of the large bowel lesions consisted of small polyps ranging in size from 0.2 to 0.6 cm. Two were nonpolypoid lesions, 1 in the colon and another jejunal which measured 3.0 cm and 4.5 cm, respectively. The latter was myxoid. The single gastric tumor measured 1.5 cm and was firm to soft with a vaguely whorled, tan-white cut surface.

Microscopic Findings. The polypoid lesions described above were intramucosal, whereas the nonpolypoid tumors were submucosal (65). The former were nonulcerated, expanded the lamina propria, uniformly entrapped crypts, and often had irregular borders (fig. 9-20A). Hyperplastic epithelial changes were present in nearby colonic epithelium for a majority of the lesions. In addition to the polypoid perineuriomas, 5 patients in this group had varying numbers of hyperplastic

polyps and tubular adenomas. Of the 2 submucosal tumors, the colonic mass was circumscribed and the jejunal mass (fig. 9-21) focally infiltrative of the muscularis propria and subserosa. The gastric lesion was entirely submucosal in location.

In this study (65), all forms of gastrointestinal perineurioma were nonencapsulated and comprised of cells typical of perineurioma, i.e., uniform bland, pale eosinophilic spindle cells with ovoid to elongated and tapered nuclei, as well as bipolar cytoplasmic processes (figs. 9-20B, 9-21). The latter were more apparent in the submucosal masses. Mitoses were rare or absent. The cells generally showed a diffuse arrangement, but in the gastric tumor formed distinct whorls. The stroma of the jejunal mass was myxoid (fig. 9-21). No lesion showed necrosis.

Immunohistochemical Findings. Nine of the 10 tumors were EMA immunopositive (fig. 9-20C) (65). Staining was weak in 4, requiring assessment at high magnification. In one case the diagnosis was based on ultrastructural evidence (30). There was immunoreactivity for claudin-1 in 4 cases (fig. 9-20D) and for CD34 in 2. All were immunonegative for S-100 protein and most for an assortment of markers, including GFAP, neurofilament protein, smooth muscle markers, h-caldesmon, c-kit, and keratin. The gastric tumor was nonreactive for CD117, CD21, and CD35.

Ultrastructural Findings. In the single jejunal tumor studied (65), the features were identical to those of their soft tissue counterparts, and included spindle cells with long bipolar cytoplasmic processes featuring numerous pinocytotic vesicles, basal lamina, and a collagenous matrix (fig. 9-22).

Differential Diagnosis. The differential diagnosis varies according to the location of the tumor within the bowel wall (65). Polypoid lesions are distinguished from other peripheral nerve tumors (solitary polypoid intestinal ganglioneuroma, neuroma, neurofibroma, schwannoma) by the lack of S-100 protein expression, and from leiomyoma of the muscularis mucosae by the latter's immunoreactivity for smooth muscle actin (66). The recently described benign colonic fibrous polyp, which in its growth pushes aside intestinal crypts and may be associated with hyperplastic polyposis (67), is also a close simulator. Examples described thus far have been found to be nonreactive for EMA, but

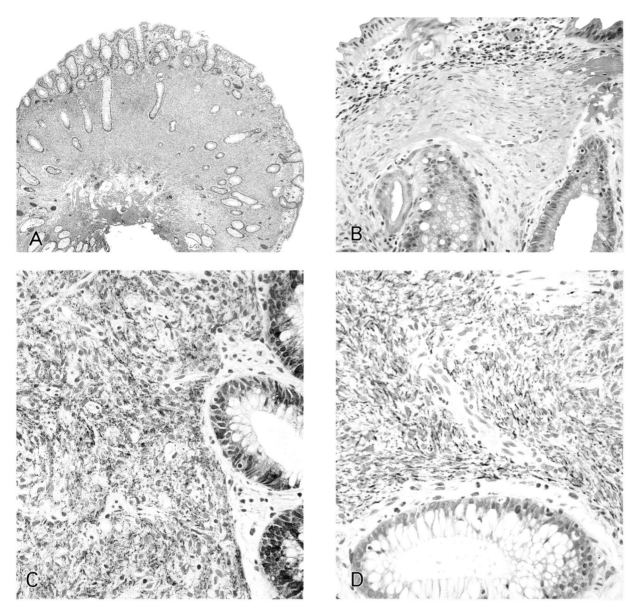

Figure 9-20

INTRAMUCOSAL INTESTINAL PERINEURIOMA

A: Polypoid colonic perineurioma expands the mucosal lamina propria and enwraps crypts.

B: The spindle cell process seen at medium power.

C,D: Diagnostic confirmation usually rests with immunoreactivity of tumor cells for EMA (C) and claudin-1 (D). (Courtesy of Drs. J. L. Hornick and C. D. Fletcher, Boston, MA.)

Hornick and Fletcher (65) suggest that further investigation of such lesions should include immunostains for claudin-1.

For submucosal intestinal perineurioma, of greatest concern is the distinction from the gastrointestinal stromal tumor (GIST). Other considerations include schwannoma, neurofibroma, and follicular dendritic cell tumor. GIST, an interstitial cell of Cajal tumor that is frequently clinically malignant (see chapter 13), most commonly arises in the stomach and less often in the small intestine. Most are composed

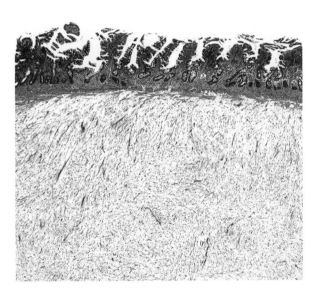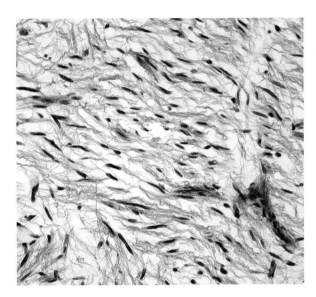

Figure 9-21

INTRAINTESTINAL PERINEURIOMA

Left: A myxoid tumor involves the jejunal submucosa.

Right: At high power, the tumor is composed of loosely arrayed, uniform, bland pale eosinophilic spindle cells with ovoid, elongated nuclei and bipolar cytoplasmic processes. (Courtesy of Drs. J. L. Hornick and C. D. Fletcher, Boston, MA.)

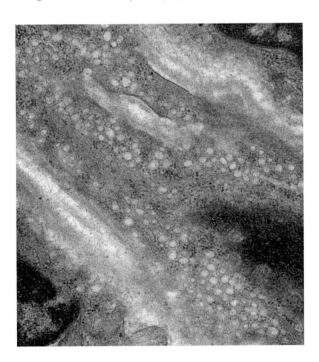

Figure 9-22

INTESTINAL PERINEURIOMA: ULTRASTRUCTURE

The tumor seen in figure 9-21 has cells with processes replete with pinocytotic vesicles and continuous external lamina, consistent with perineurial cells. (Courtesy of Drs. J. L. Hornick and C. D. Fletcher, Boston, MA.)

of uniform spindle cells with pale eosinophilic cytoplasm and a syncytial appearance, and arranged in short fascicles or whorls. In a minority of cases the cells may be palisaded or epithelioid, in part or totally. Commonly, tumor nuclei are abutted by vacuoles. Elongated eosinophilic bodies, termed skeinoid fibers, may be present. Most GISTs express KIT (CD117) (68) and h-caldesmon (69); intestinal perineuriomas, in contrast, are negative for both (65).

Intestinal schwannomas may be mistaken for perineurioma, because at this site the schwannomas typically are nonencapsulated, devoid of Antoni A tissue and Verocay bodies, and commonly have a peripheral cuff of lymphoid cells, with or without germinal center formation. If a neurofibroma is mistaken for an intestinal perineurioma, it would be one arising below the submucosa in the bowel wall or in a paraserosal location. As indicated above, both schwannoma and neurofibroma express S-100 protein. Follicular dendritic cell tumor (70) sometimes has a vaguely storiform pattern and EMA immunoreactivity (70,71). The tumor has a dispersed small lymphocytic component and cells expressing CD21 and CD35, all lacking in perineurioma.

HYBRID BENIGN PERIPHERAL NERVE SHEATH TUMORS

Hybrid PNSTs, defined as those of the three major benign PNSTs found to contain a histologic component typical of another (72), are discussed in this chapter because the large majority have partial perineuriomatous features. Of these, schwannoma with perineurioma is the combination most often observed (73–75). In contrast, reported examples of neurofibroma with perineurioma are few in number (74,76). In both variants the different histologic elements are intimately admixed. Contrary to this, is the arrangement assumed by the different elements in the hybrid neurofibroma/schwannoma, discussed by Feany et al. (72). Here the schwannoma takes the form of a discrete microscopic nodule or nodules embedded in an otherwise histologically unremarkable neurofibroma (see fig. 8-32). Given the form assumed by the schwannomatous component in this tumor, and knowing that deletions in the region of the *NF2* gene occur with some frequency in neurofibroma (77), it is logical to conclude that the miniature schwannomas represent a clone of neoplastic Schwann cells different from those giving rise to the neurofibroma (see chapter 8).

Hybrid Schwannoma/Perineurioma

The largest group of reported hybrid PNSTs is from a study of 42 patients (75) who ranged in age from 2 to 85 years (mean, 38 years) and were of equal gender (74). The most common symptom was a painless nodule. The tumors, all solitary, usually involved the superficial subcutis or dermis. Although widely distributed, about three fourths of the cases were sited in a lower or upper limb girdle. Seventy-seven percent of the tumors were 3.5 cm or smaller. None of the tumors grossly had a nerve of origin. Almost all were well circumscribed (fig. 9-23A), unencapsulated, and composed of bland spindle cells (fig. 9-23B–D). These had a mostly storiform pattern (fig. 9-23B) but sometimes were arranged in whorls or lamellae (fig. 9-24B). There were two unequal-sized tumor cell populations. The larger consisted of spindle cells with plump tapered nuclei, paley eosinophilic cytoplasm, and indistinct cell borders (fig. 9-23C). The nuclei of the cells in the smaller population were generally slender (fig. 9-23D). There was staining for EMA (fig. 9-24A,B) and S-100 protein (fig. 9-24C) in both populations, with lesser staining for CD34 (98 percent), GFAP (84 percent), and claudin-1 (80 percent). Double staining revealed alternating parallel layers of S-100 protein- and EMA-positive cells. No co-expression of the markers was seen in the cells. In most cases, the neoplastic Schwann cells were about twice as numerous as the neoplastic perineurial cells. About one third of the tumors contained rare neurofilament protein-positive axons. Although showing predominantly schwannomatous growth, the tumors were devoid of other common features of conventional schwannoma, and while there was a lesser growth of perineuriomatous cells, the general impression on initial examination was of a soft tissue perineurioma.

Hybrid Reticular (Retiform) Schwannoma/Perineurioma

This subset of hybrid tumor is based on two reports (74,78) representing seven patients (five females and two males) ranging in age from 28 to 52 years. Most lesions involved the hands (finger, 5; thenar eminence, 1; knee, 1). Histologically, the tumors were characterized by the multilobular growth of spindle and sometimes epithelioid cells embedded in a loose myxoid matrix. Surrounding the lobules were compact spindle cells, the two differing areas separated by variably thickened dense, sclerotic collagenous septa. The compact cells resembled Antoni A tissue by often possessing eosinophilic cytoplasm and tapered spindled nuclei. Well-formed Verocay bodies were not seen. The cells within the myxoid lobules were usually reactive for EMA and negative for S-100 protein. The reverse held for the surrounding compact cell population. Areas with the immunophenotype of perineurial cells usually dominated. Unlike the above pattern, the knee lesion was characterized by whorled, pale cells with the immunophenotype of Schwann cells, separated by sheets of deeply eosinophilic cells with the staining pattern of perineurial cells (74).

Significance of Hybrid Benign PNSTs with Intimately Admixed Phenotypically Different Tumor Cell Types

The presence of different tumor cell types in this group of hybrid PNSTs is traced to the neoplastic Schwann cell and its convertibility

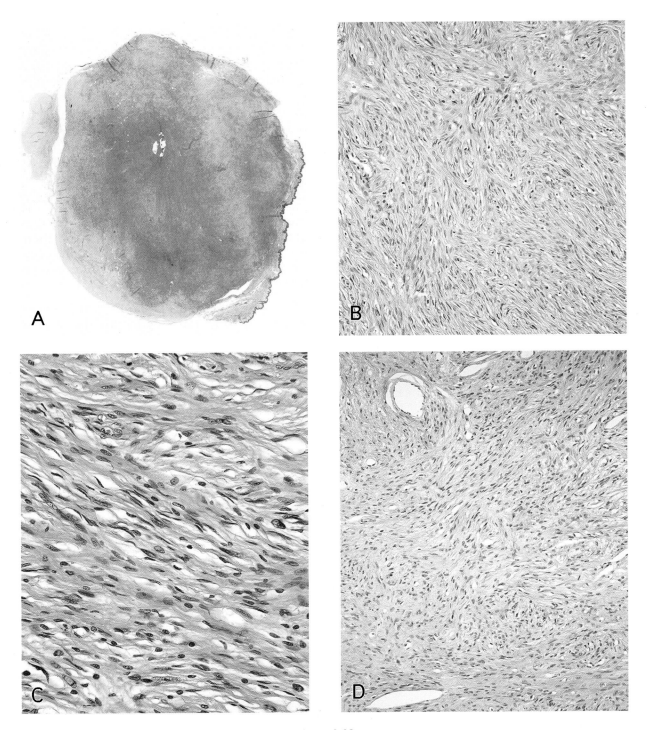

Figure 9-23

HYBRID SCHWANNOMA/PERINEURIOMA

A: Such tumors mainly arise in soft tissue of the trunk and proximal extremities, and are typically well circumscribed and unencapsulated.

B–D: Microscopically they consist of closely packed eosinophilic spindle cells showing either plump (B,C) or thin (D) nuclei, and most often growing in a storiform arrangement (B).

D: Vessels of the tumor are thin walled. (Courtesy of Drs. J. L. Hornick and C. D. Fletcher, Boston, MA.)

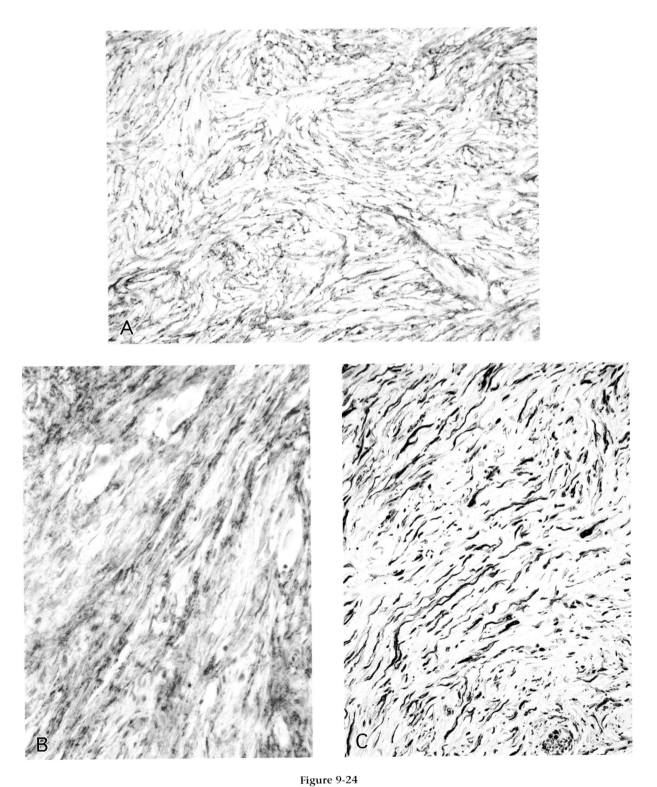

Figure 9-24

HYBRID SCHWANNOMA/PERINEURIOMA

Immunostaining of the tumor for both EMA (A,B) and S-100 protein (C) is required for the diagnosis. A lamellar growth pattern is evident in B. (A,C, Courtesy of Drs. J. L. Hornick and C. D. Fletcher, Boston, MA.)

to a perineurial cell. The evidence for this is found in neurofibromas, tumors of known Schwann cell origin (see chapter 8). In addition to differentiated Schwann cells, a major neurofibroma component is the perineurial-like cell, a morphologic form of Schwann cell possessing ultrastructural features resembling those of the perineurial cell (see figs. 8-40, 8-41). Aggregates of these cells form S-100 protein expressive pseudomeissnerian bodies (see fig. 8-41). Cells at their rim may also express EMA (see fig. 8-30D), thereby acquiring the immunophenotype of perineurial cells. The same phenotypic change is seen in cells at the margins of minischwannomas found in the type of hybrid neurofibroma/schwannoma not displaying an intimate admixture of different tumor cell types (79). The molecular mechanism for such a change is unknown, but the close proximity of numerous nerve fibers in both tumors suggests their role. Normally, some perineurial cells are found in neurofibromas, but occasional examples designated perineurioma/neurofibroma, or the reverse (74,76), show a larger than usual population. We presume the additional perineurial cells are similarly formed.

An explanation for the formation of the hybrid schwannoma/perineurioma (75), with its sizeable population of both schwannoma and perineurioma cells, is more complex. Characterized by a main location in the dermis and subcutis of a limb or limb girdle, no apparent nerve association, a dominant storiform growth pattern, and the presence of thin, not thick-walled, vessels, in balance, the tumor has more features of perineurioma than schwannoma. Countering findings are an overall predominance of schwannoma cells and an absence of credible reports of perineurial cells developing a Schwann cell immunophenotype. Based on the latter findings, it is logical to conclude that the perineuriomatous component of these tumors arise from neoplastic Schwann cells. But how?

The answer may lie in their common location, the dermis and subcutis, sites rich in small nerves and microenvironmental cues. In a study using genetic mouse models, in which NF1-deficient stem/progenitor skin-derived precursor (SKP) cells gave rise to cutaneous neurofibromas, it was shown that the tumor microenvironment played an essential role in their formation. Similarily located, the hybrid schwannoma/perineurioma likely arises from small nerves or nerve twigs. A possible origin from from NF2-deficient SKP cells must also be considered.

Likely, the neoplastic Schwann cells initially produced are in such small number as to facilitate their conversion to perineurial cells. The result is a tumor early acquiring the features of a perineurioma. However, microenviromental signals in the dermis and subcutis are subject to fluctuation. Signal variation may lead to irregular accretion of differentiated neoplastic Schwann cells. The tumors would be unencapsulated because perineurial (capsular) cells are spread throughout the mass rather than peripherally distributed.

Regardless of the pathway taken in the tumor's formation, a combination of schwannoma and perineurioma, both known to arise in the context of a *NF2* deletion, is evidence that at least some perineuriomas have a Schwann cell lineage. A shared Schwann cell lineage would explain the architectural similarity of the microcystic/reticular schwannoma (see fig. 7-16D,E), and the reticular variant of soft tissue perineurioma (see fig. 9-16), tumors differing by specific features reflective of phenotypes that may have been induced by microenvironmental factors.

Differential Diagnosis

The differential diagnosis for hybrid perineurioma-schwannoma differs with tumor location. Those presenting in the trunk and proximal extremities, given their lack of classic features of schwannoma but presence of bland spindle cells arranged in a storiform and sometimes in a focally lamellar pattern, may initially be regarded as soft tissue perineuriomas. The entity in the differential diagnosis of tumors involving the hand is nerve sheath myxoma. EMA-reactive cells in nerve sheath myxomas are far fewer in number, and when found, are peripherally rather than centrally situated within lobules. Also, the interlobular cells of nerve sheath myxoma are immunonegative for S-100 protein.

REFERENCES

Perineurioma

1. Bunge MB, Wood PM, Tynan LB, Bates ML, Sanes JR. Perineurium originates from fibroblasts: Demonstration in vitro with a retroviral marker. Science 1989;243:229-231.

2. Erlandson RA. The enigmatic perineurial cell and its participation in tumors and in tumorlike entities. Ultrastruct Pathol 1991;15:335-351.

3. Lazarus SS, Trombetta LD. Ultrastructural identification of a benign perineurial cell tumor. Cancer 1978;41:1823-1829.

4. Pinkus GS, Kurtin PJ. Epithelial membrane antigen—a diagnostic discriminant in surgical pathology: Immunohistochemical profile in epithelial, mesenchymal, and hematopoietic neoplasms using paraffin sections and monoclonal antibodies. Hum Pathol 1985;16:929-940.

5. Perentes E, Nakagawa Y, Ross GW, Stanton C, Rubinstein LJ. Expression of epithelial membrane antigen in perineurial cells and their derivatives. An immunohistochemical study with multiple markers. Acta Neuropathol 1987;75:160-165.

6. Theaker JM, Gatter K, Puddle J. Epithelial membrane antigen expression by the perineurium of peripheral nerve and in peripheral nerve tumors. Histopathology 1988;13:171-179.

7. Ariza A, Bilbao JM, Rosai J. Immunohistochemical detection of epithelial membrane antigen in normal perineurial cells and perineurioma. Am J Surg Pathol 1988;12:678-683.

8. Giannini C, Scheithauer BW, Jenkins RB, et al. Soft-tissue perineurioma. Evidence for an abnormality of chromosome 22, criteria for diagnosis, and review of the literature. Am J Surg Pathol 1997;21:164-173.

9. Scheithauer BW, Woodruff JM, Erlandson RA. Tumors of the peripheral nervous system. AFIP Atlas of Tumor Pathology, 3rd Series, Fascicle 24. Washington, DC: American Registry of Pathology; 1999.

10. Folpe AL, Billings SD, McKenney JK, Walsh SV, Nusrat A, Weiss SW. Expression of claudin-1, a recently described tight junction-associated protein, distinguishes soft tissue perineurioma from potential mimics. Am J Surg Pathol 2002;26:1620-1626.

11. Hirose T, Tani T, Shimada T, Ishizawa K, Shimada S, Sano T. Immunohistochemical demonstration of EMA/Glut1-positive perineurial cells and cd34-positive fibroblastic cells in peripheral nerve sheath tumors. Mod Pathol 2003;16:293-298.

12. Fogt F, Capodieci P, Loda M. Assessment of perineurial invasion by GLUT-1 immunohisto-chemistry. Appl Immunohistochem 1995;3:194-197.

13. Emory TS, Scheithauer BW, Hirose T, Wood M, Onofrio BM, Jenkins RB. Intraneural perineurioma. A clonal neoplasm associated with abnormalities of chromosome 22. Am J Clin Pathol 1995;103:696-704.

14. Brock J, Perez-Atayde A, Kozakewich HP, Richkind KE, Fletcher JA, Vargas SO. Cytogenetic aberrations in perineurioma. Variation with subtype. Am J Surg Pathol 2005;29:1164-1169.

15. Huguet P, de la Torre J, Pallares J, et al. Intraosseous intraneural perineurioma: Report of a case with morphological, immunohistochemical and FISH study. Med Oral 2004;9:64-68.

16. Tsang WY, Chan JK, Chow LT, Tse CC. Perineurioma: an uncommon soft tissue neoplasm distinct from localized hypertrophic neuropathy and neurofibroma. Am J Surg Pathol 1992;16:756-763.

17. Lasota J, Fetsch JF, Wozniak A, Wasag B, Sciot R, Miettinen M. The neurofibromatosis type 2 gene is mutated in perineurial cell tumors: A molecular genetic study of eight cases. Am J Pathol 2001;158:1223-1229.

18. Pitchford C, Schwartz H, Atkinson J, Cates J. Soft tissue perineurioma in a patient with neurofibromatosis type 2: a tumor not previously associated with the nf2 syndrome. Am J Surg Pathol 2006;30:1624-1629.

19. Boyanton BL Jr, Jones JK, Shenaq SM, Hicks MJ, Bhattacharjee MB. Intraneural perineurioma. A systematic review with illustrative cases. Arch Pathol Lab Med 2007;131:1382-1392.

20. Bilbao JM, Khoury N, Hudson A, Briggs SJ. Perineurioma (localized hypertrophic neuropathy). Arch Pathol Lab Med 1984;108:557-560.

21. Peckham NH, O'Boynick PL, Meneses A, Kepes JJ. Hypertrophic mononeuropathy. A report of two cases and review of the literature. Arch Pathol Lab Med 1982;106:534-537.

22. Li D, Schauble B, Moll C, Fisch U. Intratemporal facial nerve perineurioma. Laryngoscope 1996;106:328-333.

23. Beekman R, Slooff W, Van Oosterhout MF, Lammens M, Van Den Berg LH. Bilateral intraneural perineurioma presenting as ulnar neuropathy at the elbow. Muscle Nerve 2004;30:239-243.

24. Damm DD, White DK, Merrell JD. Intraneural perineurioma- not restricted to major nerves. Med Oral Pathol Oral Radiol Endo 2003;96:192-196.

25. Chen L, Li Y, Lin J. Intraneural perineurioma in a child with beckwith-wiedemann syndrome. J Pediatr Surg 2005;40:E12-E14.

26. Mitsumoto H, Wilbourn A, Goren H. Perineurioma as the cause of localized hypertrophic neuropathy. Muscle Nerve 1980;3:403-412.

27. Stanton C, Perentes E, Phillips L, VandenBerg SR. The immunohistochemical demonstration of early perineurial change in the development of localized hypertrophic neuropathy. Hum Pathol 1988;19:1455-1457.

28. Harkin JC, Reed RJ. Tumors of the peripheral nervous system. Atlas of Tumor Pathology, 2nd Series, Fascicle 3 (supplement). Washington, DC: Armed Forces Institute of Pathology; 1983.

29. Balarezo FS, Muller RC, Weiss RG, Brown T, Knibbs D, Joshi VV. Soft tissue perineuriomas in children: Report of three cases and review of the literature. Pediatr Dev Pathol 2003;6:137-141

30. Hornick JL, Fletcher CD. Soft tissue perineurioma: clinicopathologic analysis of 81 cases including those with atypical histologic features. Am J Surg Pathol 2005;29:845-858.

31. Kahn DG, Duckett T, Bhuta SM. Perineurioma of the kidney. Report of a case with histologic, immunohistochemical, and ultrastructural studies. Arch Pathol Lab Med 1993;117:654-657.

32. Val-Bernal JF, Hernando M, Garijo MF, Villa P. Renal perineurioma in childhood. Gen Diagn Pathol 1997;143:75-81.

33. Carneiro F, Brandao O, Correia AC, Sobrinho-Simoes M. Spindle cell tumor of the breast. Ultrastruct Pathol 1989;13:593-598.

34. Landini G, Kitano M. Meningioma of the mandible. Cancer 1992;69:2917-2920.

35. Giannini C, Scheithauer BW, Steinberg J, Cosgrove TJ. Intraventricular perineurioma. Neurosurgery 1998;43:1478-1481.

36. Burgues O, Monteagudo C, Noguera R, Revert A, Molina I, Llombarg-Bosch A. Cutaneous sclerosing Pacinian-like perineurioma. Histopathology 2001;39:498-502.

37. Fetsch JF, Miettinen M. Sclerosing perineurioma: A clinicopathologic study of 19 cases of a distinctive soft tissue lesion with a predilection for the fingers and palms of young adults. Am J Surg Pathol 1997;21:1433-1442.

38. Sciot R, Cin PD, Hagemeijer A, et al. Cutaneous sclerosing perineurioma with cryptic NF2 gene deletion. Am J Surg Pathol 1999;23:849-853.

39. Yamaguchi U, Hasegawa T, Hirose T, et al. Sclerosing perineurioma: a clinicopathological study of five cases and diagnostic utility of immunohistochemical staining for glut1. Virchows Arch 2003;443:159-163.

40. Graadt van Roggen JF, McMenamin ME, Belchis DA, Nielsen GP, Rosenberg AC, Fletcher CD. Reticular perineurioma. A distinctive variant of soft tissue perineurioma. Am J Surg Pathol 2001;25:485-493.

41. Mentzel T, Kutzner H. Reticular and plexiform perineurioma: clinicopathological and immunohistochemical analysis of two cases and review of perineurial neoplasms of the skin and soft tissues. Virchows Arch 2005;447:677-682.

42. Michal M. Extraneural retiform perineuriomas. A report of four cases. Pathol Res Pract 1999;195:759-763.

43. Rankine AJ, Filion PR, Platten MA, Spagnolo DV. Perineurioma: A clinicopathological study of eight cases. Pathology 2004;36:309-315.

44. Ausmus GG, Piliang MP, Bergfeld WF, Goldblum JR. Soft-tissue perineurioma in a 20-year-old patient with neurofibromatosis type 1 (NF1): Report of a case and review of the literature. J Cutan Pathol 2007;34:726-730.

45. Donnellan R, Rughubar K, Govender D, Chetty R. Perineurioma: an unusual cause of an external auditory canal polyp. ORL J Otorhinolaryngol Relat Spec 1997;59:336-338.

46. Antonescu CR, Woodruff JM. Primary tumors of cranial, spinal and peripheral nerves. In: Russell and Rubinstein's pathology of tumors of the nervous systems. London: Hodder Arnold; 2006:787-835.

47. Mentzel T, Dei Tos AP, Fletcher CD. Perineurioma (storiform perineurial fibroma): Clinico-pathological analysis of four cases. Histopathology 1994;25:261-267.

48. Weidner N, Nasr A, Johnston J. Plexiform soft tissue tumor composed of perineurial fibroblasts (perineurioma). Ultrastruct Pathol 1993;17:251-262.

49. Zelger B, Weinlich L, Zelger B. Perineurioma. A frequently unrecognized entity with emphasis on a plexiform variant. Adv Clin Pathol 2000;4:25-33.

50. Aoki T, Hisaoka M, Hashimoto H, Nakata H, Sakai A, Okabe S. Giant degenerative perineurial cell tumor. Skeletal Radiol 1996;25:757-761.

51. Hirose T, Scheithauer BW. "Sclerosing" perineurioma: a tumor variant? Int J Surg Pathol 1999;7:133-140.

52. Rank J, Rostad S. Perineurioma with ossification: a case report with immunohistochemical and ultrastructural studies. Arch Pathol Lab Med 1998;122:366-370.

53. Zamecnik M, Koys F, Gomolcak P. Atypical cellular perineurioma. Histopathology 2002;40:296-299.

54. Weidenheim KM, Campbell WJ. Perineurial cell tumor. Immunocytochemical and ultrastructural characterization. Relationship to other peripheral nerve tumors with a review of the literature. Virchows Arch A Pathol Anat Histopathol 1986;408:375-383.

55. Dhimes P, Martinez-Gonzalez MA, Carabias E, Perez-Espejo G. Ultrastructural study of a perineurioma with ribosome-lamella complexes. Ultrastruct Pathol 1996;20:167-172.

56. Mertens F, Dal Cin P, De Wever I, et al. Cytogenetic characterization of peripheral nerve sheath tumours: a report of the CHAMP study group. J Pathol 2000;190:31-38.

57. Connelly JH, Evans HL. Dermatofibrosarcoma protuberans. A clinicopathologic review with emphasis on fibrosarcomatous areas. Am J Surg Pathol 1992;16:921-925.

58. Mentzel T, Calonje E, Wadden C, et al. Myxofibrosarcoma: clinicopathologic analysis of 75 cases with emphasis on the low-grade variant. Am J Surg Pathol 1996;20:391-405.

59. Evans HL. Low-grade fibromyxoid sarcoma. A report of 12 cases. Am J Surg Pathol 1993;17:595-600.

60. Folpe AL, Lane K, Paull G, Weiss SW. Low-grade fibromyxoid sarcoma and hyalinizing spindle cell tumor with giant rosettes: a clinicopathologic study of 73 cases supporting their identity and assessing the impact of high-grade areas. Am J Surg Pathol 2000;24:1353-1360.

61. Hirose T, Sumitomo M, Kudo E, et al. Malignant peripheral nerve sheath tumor (MPNST) showing perineurial cell differentiation. Am J Surg Pathol 1989;13:613-620.

62. Hirose T, Scheithauer BW, Sano T. Perineurial malignant peripheral nerve sheath tumor (MPNST): a clinicopathologic, immunohistochemical, and ultrastructural study of seven cases. Am J Surg Pathol 1998;22:1368-1378.

63. Andriko JW, Kaldjian EP, Abbondanzo SL, Jaffe ES. Reticulum cell neoplasms of lymph nodes: a clinicopathologic study of 11 cases with recognition of a new subtype derived from fibroblastic reticular cells. Am J Surg Pathol 1998;22:1048-1058.

64. Monda L, Warnke R, Rosai JA. Primary lymph node malignancy with features suggestive of dendritic reticulum cell differentiation. A report of 4 cases. Am J Pathol 1986;122:S62-72.

65. Hornick J, Fletcher CD. Intestinal perineuriomas: clinicopathologic definition of a new anatomic subset in a series of 10 cases. Am J Surg Pathol 2005;29:859-865.

65a. Agaimy A, Wuensch P. Perineurioma of the stomach. A rare spindle cell neoplasm that should be distinguished from gastrointestinal stromal tumor. Pathol Res Pract 2005;201:463-467.

66. Miettinen M, Shekitka KM, Sobin LH. Schwannomas in the colon and rectum: A clinicopathologic and immunohistochemical study of 20 cases. Am J Surg Pathol 2001;25:846-855.

67. Eslami-Varzaneh F, Washington K, Robert ME, Kashgarian M, Goldblum JR, Jain D. Benign fibroblastic polyps of the colon: a histologic, immunohistochemical, and ultrastructural study. Am J Surg Pathol 2004;28:374-378.

68. Sarlomo-Rikala M, Kovatich AJ, Barusevicius A, Miettinen M. CD117: A sensitive marker for gastrointestinal stromal tumors that is more specific than CD34. Mod Pathol 1998;11:728-734.

69. Miettinen MM, Sarlomo-Rikala M, Kovatich AJ, Lasota J. Calponin and h-caldesmon in soft tissue tumors: consistent h-caldesmon immunoreactivity in gastrointestinal stromal tumors indicates traits of smooth muscle differentiation. Mod Pathol 1999;12:756-762.

70. Chang K, Jin YT, Chen FF, Su IJ. Follicular dendritic cell sarcoma of the colon mimicking stromal tumor. Histopathology 2001;38:25-29.

71. Pileri SA, Grogan TM, Harris NL, et al. Tumours of histiocytes and accessory dendritic cells: an immunohistochemical approach to classification from the international lymphoma study group based on 61 cases. Histopathology 2002;41:1-29.

Hybrid Peripheral Nerve Sheath Tumors

72. Feany M, Anthony DC, Fletcher DM. Nerve sheath tumours with hybrid features of neurofibroma and schwannoma: a conceptual challenge. Histopathology 1998;32:495-410.

73. Bundock E, Fletcher C. Nerve sheath tumors with hybrid features of perineurioma and schwannoma. Mod Pathol 2004;17:12A.

74. Kazakov DV, Pitha J, Sima R, et al. Hybrid peripheral nerve sheath tumors: Schwannoma-perineurioma and neurofibroma-perineurioma. A report of three cases in extradigital locations. Ann Diagn Pathol 2005;9:16-23.

75. Hornick JL, Bundock EA, Fletcher CD. Hybrid schwannoma/perineurioma: clinicalpathologic analysis of 42 distinctive benign nerve sheath tumors. Am J Surg Pathol 2009;33:1534-1561.

76. Zamecnik M, Michal M. Perineurial cell differentiation in neurofibromas. Report of eight cases including a case with composite perineurioma-neurofibroma features. Pathol Res Pract 2001;197:537-544.

77. Koga T, Iwasaki H, Ishiguro M, Matsuzaki A, Kikucki M. Losses in chromosomes 17, 19, and 22q in neurofibromatosis type 1 and sporadic neurofibromas: a comparative genomic hybridization analysis. Cancer Genet Cytogenet 2002;136:113-120.

78. Michal M, Kazakov DV, Belousova I, Bisceglia M, Zamecnik M, Mukenshabe P. A benign neoplasm with histopathological features of both schwannoma and retiform perineurioma (benign schwannoma-perineurioma): a report of six cases of a distinctive soft tissue tumor with a predilection for the fingers. Virchows Arch 2004;445:347-353.

79. Schrober R, Reifenberger G, Kremer G, Urich H. Symmetrical neurofibroma with Schwann cell predominance and focal formation of microneurinomas. Acta Neuropathol 1993;85:227-232.

80. Le LQ, Shipman T, Burns DK, Parada LF. Cell of origin and microenvironmental contribution for NF-1 associated dermal neurofibromas. Cell Stemm Cell 2009;4:453-463.

81. Macarenco RS, Ellinger F, Oliveira AM. Perineurioma: a distinctive and underrecognized peripheral nerve sheath neoplasm. Arch Pathol Lab Med 2007;131:625-636.

82. Carneiro SS, Scheithauer BW, Nascimento AG, Hirose T, Davis DH. Solitary fibrous tumor of the meninges: a lesion distinct from fibrous meningioma. A clinicopathologic and immunohistochemical study. Am J Clin Pathol 1996;106:217-224.

83. Merck C, Angervall L, Kindblom LG, Oden A. Myofibrosarcoma: A malignant soft tissue tumor of fibroblastic-histiocytic origin. A clinicopathologic and prognostic study of 110 cases using multivariate analysis. Acta Pathol Microbiol Immunol Scand Suppl 1983;282:1-40.

84. Kilpatrick SE, Hitchcock MG, Kraus MD, Calonje E, Fletcher CD. Mixed tumors and myoepitheliomas of soft tissue: a clinicopathologic study of 19 cases with a unifying concept. Am J Surg Pathol 1997;21:12-22.

85. Enzinger FM, Weiss SW, Liang CY. Ossifying fibromyxoid tumor of soft parts. A clinicopathological analysis of 59 cases. Am J Surg Pathol 1989;13:817-827.

86. Antonescu CR, Argani P, Erlandson RA, Healey JH, Ladanyi M, Huvos AG. Skeletal and extraskeletal myxoid chondrosarcoma; a comparative clinicopathologic, ultrastructural and molecular study. Cancer 1998;83:1504-1521.

87. Meis-Kindblom JM, Bergh P, Gunterberg B, Kindblom LG. Extraskeletal myxoid chondrosarcoma: a reappraisal of its morphologic spectrum and prognostic factors based on 117 cases. Am J Surg Pathol 1999;23:636-650.

88. Krane JF, Bertoni F, Fletcher CD. Myxoid synovial sarcoma: an underappreciated morphologic subset. Mod Pathol 1999;12:456-462.

MISCELLANEOUS BENIGN NEUROGENIC TUMORS

NERVE SHEATH MYXOMA

Definition. *Nerve sheath myxoma* is a benign, usually cutaneous, multilobulated and predominantly myxoid neoplasm with Schwann cell differentiation, but lacking features warranting classification as a conventional schwannoma.

General Features. The nerve sheath myxoma, a tumor rich in mucinous matrix, composed of cells consistently S-100 protein immunoreactive, and featuring basement membrane formation, was originally described by Harkin and Reed in their 1969 Armed Forces Institute of Pathology (AFIP) Fascicle *Tumors of the Peripheral Nervous System* (1). A subsequent study (2) comparing this tumor with neurothekeoma, a cutaneous neoplasm reported in 1980 by Gallagher and Helwig (3), suggested that both were myxoid and cellular forms of the same neoplastic process. This conceptual linkage was fostered by a common origin in skin; a micronodular, lobular, or nested growth pattern; an entire or partial composition of spindle and epithelioid cells; and a variable content of stromal mucin. Nonetheless, clinical, histologic, immunohistochemical, and ultrastructural findings accumulated over time (Table 10-1) have led to the conclusion that nerve sheath myxoma is a Schwann cell tumor, whereas neurothekeoma is not.

Clinical Features. Nerve sheath myxoma occurs over a broad age range (8 to 72 years) but affects mainly young and middle-aged adults (mean age, 36 years) (4). Fetsch et al. (4) mention only one possible congenital example. Males and females are nearly equally represented (4). The tumor shows a predilection for the distal extremities, notably the hands and fingers, followed by the knees and pretibial region, ankle, and foot. Involvement of the trunk or the head and neck is infrequent (4). A few lesions have arisen in the oral mucosa (5). Typical examples present as solitary, mobile, flesh-colored to translucent nodules undergoing slow, painless growth (4).

Gross Findings. The largest study of nerve sheath myxoma (4) found the tumors to range from 0.4 to 4.5 cm in greatest dimension, with one consisting of two separate nodules measuring 3.0 and 4.0 cm. Eighty-five percent were smaller than 2.5 cm. All had a rubbery to firm consistency and on sectioning were well-

Table 10-1

DIFFERENCES BETWEEN NERVE SHEATH MYXOMA (NSM)[a] AND NEUROTHEKEOMA[b]

Feature	NSM	Neurothekeoma
Main Age Group	Young and middle-aged adults	Children and young adults
Gender	Ratio approximately equal	2:1 female/male
Main Location	Distal extremities	Face, shoulder, upper arms
Histology	Multiple nodules/lobules with fibrous borders; spindled, stellate, and epithelioid cells in cords, rings, syncytial-like arrangements; routinely abundant myxoid matrix	Multiple nodules/lobules without fibrous borders; epithelioid and spindle cells; stroma often collagenous in 1/3 of cases variably myxoid
Key Immunoreactivity	S-100 protein and GFAP[c] positive	S-100 protein always and GFAP usually negative
Local Recurrence	Common	Uncommon
Classification	A probable Schwann cell tumor	Tumor of unknown cellular differentiation

[a]Data from reference 4.
[b]Data from reference 15.
[c]GFAP = glial fibrillary acidic protein.

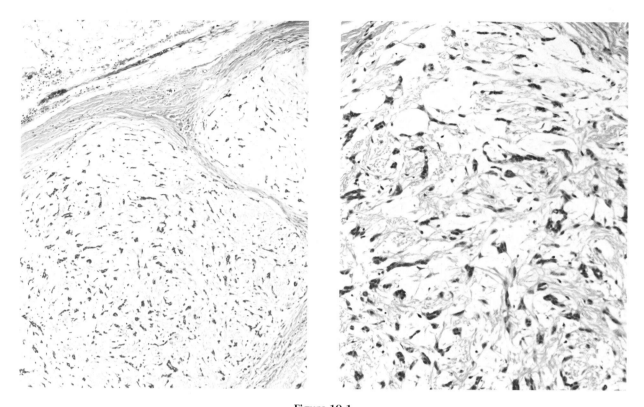

Figure 10-1

NERVE SHEATH MYXOMA

Left: The tumor is characterized by distinct lobularity, septation, and a high mucin content. At medium power, the cells most often are spindled.

Right: At higher power, such cells have pale pink cytoplasm and small dark nuclei, and are arranged in cords and syncytial-like aggregates. (Courtesy of Dr. J. Fetsch, Washington, DC.)

demarcated, translucent to white, glistening, and mucoid. The overlying epidermis was intact and devoid of hyperpigmentation.

Microscopic Findings. Nerve sheath myxoma forms a highly myxoid, multilobular, nonencapsulated mass within dermal and subcutaneous tissue. Varying in size and shape, the lobules usually exhibit rounded contours and are sharply demarcated by fibrous rims. The cells within the lobules are variously spindled, stellate, epithelioid, and ring shaped. Most often they are dispersed as stringy cells in an abundant, myxoid matrix (fig. 10-1). Intercellular collagen is scant. Most cells possess thin, bipolar or multipolar processes that merge with scant eosinophilic cytoplasm surrounding small, round or ovoid nuclei (fig. 10-1, right). As previously noted, epithelioid, ring cell forms having vacuolated cytoplasm are occasionally encountered (fig. 10-2) (4). Cellular interconnec-

tions are common, thus cords of cells or syncytial arrangements develop (fig. 10-1). The tumor cell nuclei feature faintly granular chromatin and sometimes cytoplasmic-nuclear pseudoinclusions. Cytologic atypia is rare and mitoses are infrequent (4,6,7). The intratumoral mucin stains strongly with Alcian blue preparations (fig. 10-3A) and consists of hyaluronic acid and perhaps chondroitin sulfates 4 and 6 (8,9).

Immunohistochemical Findings. The intralobular cells comprising nerve sheath myxomas are diffusely immunoreactive for S-100 protein (fig. 10-3B) (4,8,10,11), and often very immunoreactive for glial fibrillary acidic protein (GFAP) (fig. 10-3C) (4). Staining for CD57 (Leu-7) and neuron-specific enolase is seen in a majority of cases (4). Strong pericellular expression for collagen 4 is also a feature (fig. 10-3D) (4). Epithelial membrane antigen (EMA) positivity, usually limited to the perineurial cells comprising the

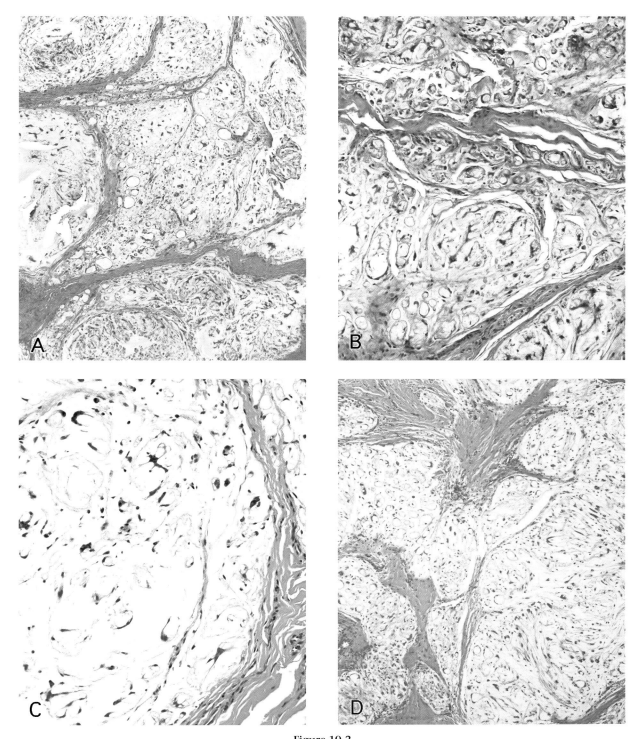

Figure 10-2

NERVE SHEATH MYXOMA

A,B: Aggregates of ringed tumor cells, which may histologically simulate a chondroid tumor, are uncommon.

C: The nuclei of the ring cells are distorted, and at higher power the cells may be mistaken for adipose cells.

D: Clarification of the diagnosis is usually provided by finding adjacent areas of stringy spindle tumor cells. (Courtesy of Dr. J. Fetsch, Washington, DC.)

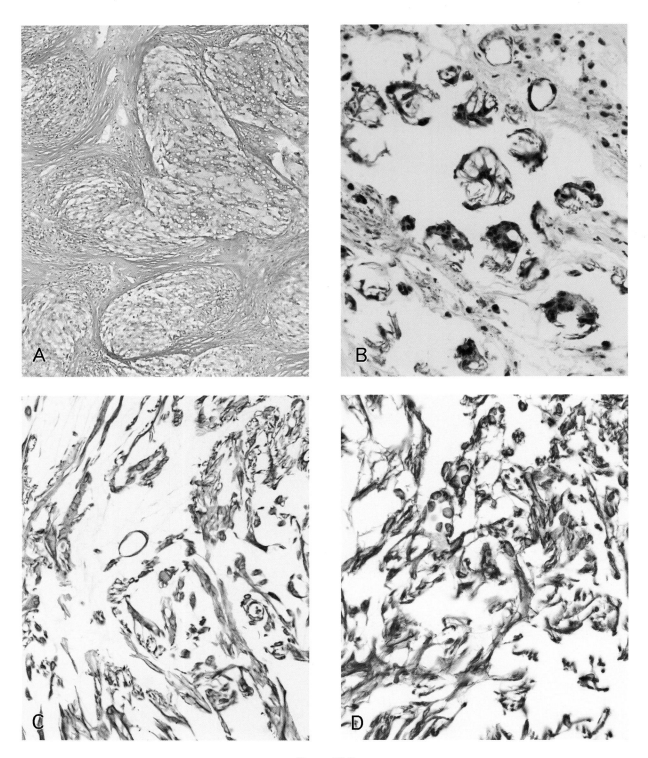

Figure 10-3

NERVE SHEATH MYXOMA

The presence of abundant myxoid matrix is highlighted with the Alcian blue stain (A). The tumor cells are immunopositive for S-100 protein (B), glial fibrillary acidic protein (GFAP) (C), and collagen 4 (D). (C and D courtesy of Dr. J. Fetsch, Washington, DC.)

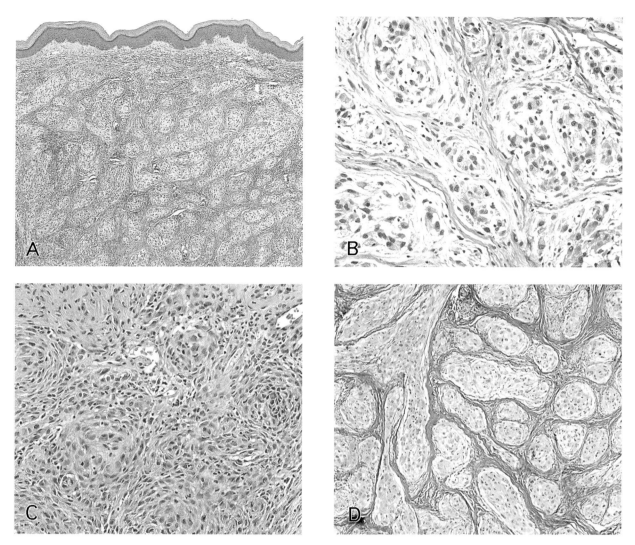

Figure 10-4

NEUROTHEKEOMA

This cutaneous tumor is most commonly moderately cellular (A) and less commonly mildly cellular (B) or hypercellular (C). The cell nests are usually round to ovoid in configuration (A,B), sometimes elongated (D), and often encircled by fibrous tracts. Some cell nests form tight whorls (C).

compacted rim of the lobules, is seen in over half the cases (4). Importantly, the tumor cells are nonreactive for both HMB45 and CD10 (4).

Ultrastructural Findings. The features of nerve sheath differentiation are present in typical nerve sheath myxomas (6,8,12,13). Although the findings are variously interpreted as evidence of Schwann or perineurial cell differentiation, a critical review of published illustrations and reported immunoreactivities indicates that the constituent cells are mainly schwannian.

Differential Diagnosis. The tumor most often histologically mistaken for nerve sheath myxoma is neurothekeoma with myxoid stroma (14,15). Neurothekeoma comprises a group of cutaneous, mainly cellular, multilobular or micronodular tumors (fig. 10-4A,D) composed of spindle and epithelioid cells that are generally more plump than those of nerve sheath myxoma (figs. 10-4B,C; 10-5). Their immunoprofile is nonspecific, but all are reactive for NKI-C3 (fig. 10-6) (15) and negative for S-100 protein (11,15).

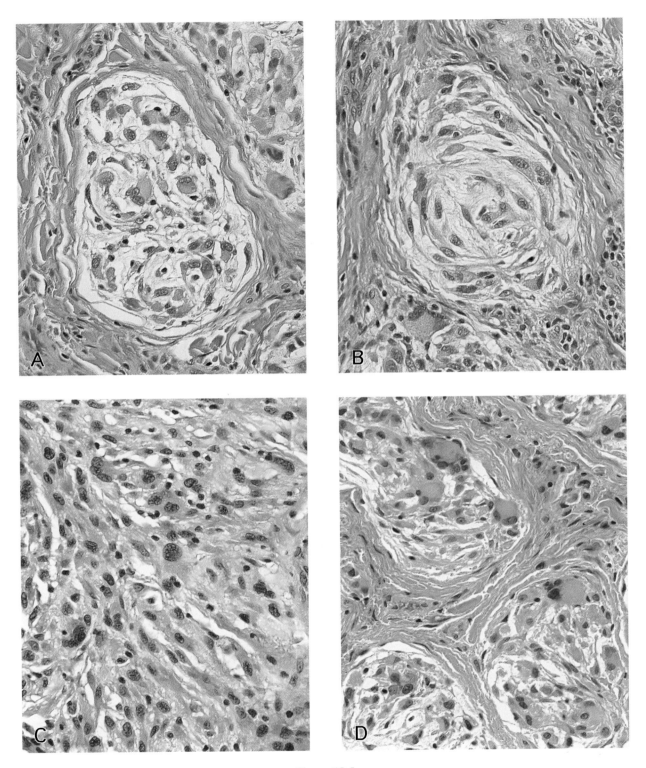

Figure 10-5

NEUROTHEKEOMA

The tumor cells are epithelioid (A), spindled (B), mixed epithelioid and spindled (C), and occasionally multinucleated (D).

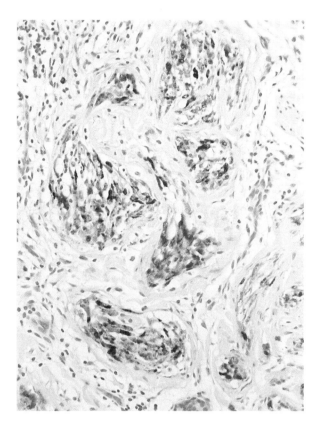

Figure 10-6

NEUROTHEKEOMA

Unlike nerve sheath myxoma, neurothekeomas are consistently S-100 protein immunonegative, but NK1-C3 immunopositive.

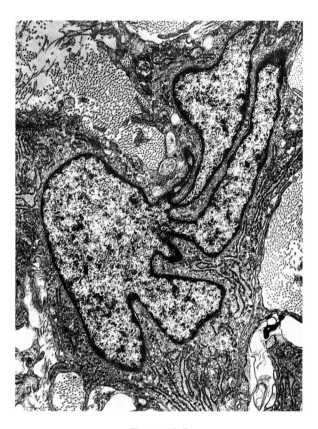

Figure 10-7

CELLULAR NEUROTHEKEOMA: ULTRASTRUCTURE

The tumor cells have fibroblastic features including prominent rough endoplasmic reticulum and lack of basal lamina.

The fact that 89 percent of neurothekeomas are reactive for neuron-specific enolase (15) is no proof of a neuroectodermal derivation. They feature no expression for GFAP (4,16), collagen type 4, or laminin, and are almost never reactive for EMA (14,17). Interestingly, consistent expression for CD10, a marker found to be present by Fetsch et al. (14) stands in contrast to its absence in nerve sheath myxomas. In summary, the cellular constituents of neurothekeoma exhibit neither the features of intrinsic nerve sheath cells (Schwann or perineurial cells) nor of melanocytes. Instead, their immunohistochemical and ultrastructural attributes suggest that at least some are myofibroblastic in nature. From 38 (14) to 60 percent (15) of neurothekeomas show at least focal staining for smooth muscle actin, whereas desmin preparations are always negative (14,15). Ultrastructurally, well-developed, often dilated rough endoplasmic reticulum and lack of basement membranes (fig. 10-7) are features in keeping with fibroblastic differentiation (5,18). The comparative clinicopathologic characteristics of nerve sheath myxoma and neurothekeoma are summarized in Table 10-1. Confusion with nerve sheath myxoma occurs in 33 percent and 10 percent of neurothekeomas that are focally or diffusely myxoid, respectively (fig. 10-8) (15).

Additional lesions, not all neoplastic, also enter into the differential diagnosis of nerve sheath myxoma. Focal mucinosis (19), a nonneoplastic process occasionally associated with hyperthyroidism, lacks not only the circumscription and lobulation typical of nerve sheath myxoma, but its cellularity as well. Cutaneous myxoma (superficial angiomyxoma) is also multinodular, highly myxoid, involves both

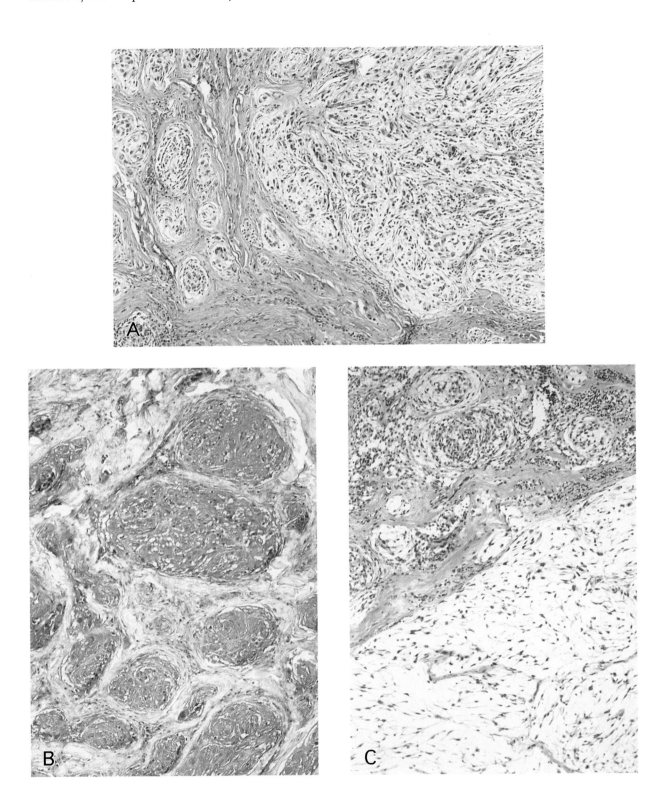

Figure 10-8

NEUROTHEKEOMA

Approximately one third of these tumors have partial myxoid features (A), as emphasized by an Alcian blue stain (B), and about 10 percent are extensively myxoid (C). It is this last group of tumors that may be mistaken for nerve sheath myxoma.

dermis and subcutis (20,21), and is one of the several tumors encountered in Carney complex (22,23). It contains mononucleated and multinucleated, stellate- and spindle-shaped tumor cells. The lesions typically lack peripheral fibrous circumscription, often contain scattered acute and chronic inflammatory cells, and on immunohistochemical evaluation, often stain for CD34, sometimes for actin, but generally not at all or only weakly for S-100 protein (14).

Rarely, conventional schwannomas focally exhibit such an abundance of myxoid stroma as to resemble a primary myxoid tumor. In contrast to nerve sheath myxoma, such tumors are usually encapsulated. If it arises in the skin and subcutaneous tissue, its identification as a schwannoma rests upon finding any classic histologic feature of conventional schwannoma, particularly islands of Antoni A tissue, perhaps with Verocay body formation. In contrast to nerve sheath myxoma, a partly myxoid, superficial plexiform neurofibroma would unlikely contain stellate and epithelioid cells. Also, a few aligned neurofilament protein-immunoreactive axons are present.

A partial Schwann cell tumor that may be misinterpreted as a nerve sheath myxoma is the reticular, or "retiform," variant of the perineurioma hybrid, perineurioma-schwannoma, a tumor that involves the hand (24). In contrast to nerve sheath myxoma, the intralobular cells of reticular perineurioma are immunoreactive for EMA rather than S-100 protein. Reticular schwannomas (25) affect viscera and are not in the differential diagnosis.

Treatment and Prognosis. Nerve sheath myxomas are clinically benign. The largest series to date reports a recurrence rate of 47 percent, all following simple excision (4). For this reason complete local excision with attention to margins is recommended.

BENIGN GRANULAR CELL TUMOR

Definition. *Granular cell tumor* (GCT) is a neoplasm composed of lysosome-rich granular cells that are generally considered neurogenic in nature.

General Features. GCT is an uncommon, usually benign lesion which, in contrast to other benign superficially situated lesions resembling granular cell tumors (26,27), is almost always immunoreactive for S-100 protein (28). Initially thought to be myogenic (29), and long referred to as a granular cell myoblastoma, GCT has been found to have features consistent with a neurogenic tumor. Supporting this view is the involvement of small to medium-sized nerves (30). This includes cranial nerves, either within the cranium (31–33) or in their extracranial course (34,35), as well as peripheral nerves (36–38). The neurogenic nature of GCTs is further suggested by features associated with Schwann cells, including immunoreactivity for S-100 protein (28,39) and Leu-7, as well as the ultrastructural finding of basement membrane typically surrounding tumor cell clusters (see fig. 10-20) (40,41). Immunoreactivity for markers of muscle differentiation is lacking. The continued use of the descriptive designation GCT reflects the lack of a better understanding of the nature of these tumors. Clinically malignant GCTs, some histologically indistinguishable from benign GCT, are discussed in chapter 12.

Clinical Features. GCTs affect all age groups. Their peak incidence is in the fourth through the sixth decades. Uncommon in the first decade, they become more frequent in the second (42). Rare examples occurring in neonates must be distinguished from congenital gingival granular cell tumor, or epulis, a clinically similar lesion presenting in this age group and typically affecting the mucosa of the alveolar ridge (see Differential Diagnosis) (43,44). GCTs show a two-fold predilection for females and a proclivity for blacks over other racial groups (45). In a review of 325 reported cases, Peterson (45) found that 40 percent of patients in which race was indicated were black. Most GCTs are solitary masses, but up to 10 percent are multifocal (46,47). We know of only two reports of an association with neurofibromatosis type 1 (NF1) (46,48). Only rarely is a diagnosis of GCT clinically suspected.

GCTs arise at a wide variety of sites. Most affect the deep dermis and subcutaneous tissue (fig. 10-9C), particularly of the head, neck, trunk, and extremities (45). The single most common site is the tongue, representing 25 percent of cases (fig. 10-9A) (45). Its lateral borders, tip, and dorsum are most often affected (fig. 10-10) (49,50). Breast lesions represent 5 to 15 percent of all GCTs (45,51); the lower figure corresponds to tumors of breast parenchyma and

305

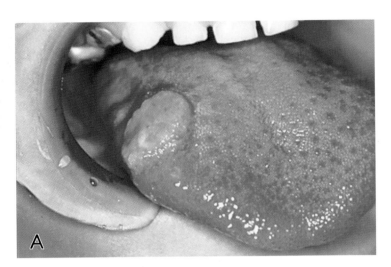

Figure 10-9

GRANULAR CELL TUMOR

A,B: The tongue is the most common site of origin for this tumor.

C: This example involving the vulva shows overlying marked pseudoepitheliomatous hyperplasia.

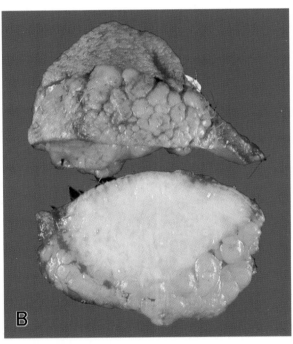

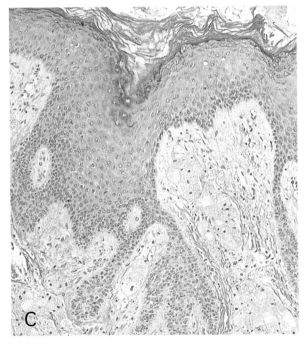

the higher figure represents examples affecting subcutaneous tissue and skin.

In the respiratory system (45), the larynx and bronchi are preferentially affected, representing 7.0 percent and 3.4 percent of all cases, respectively. The majority of laryngeal GCTs originate in the posterior aspect of a true vocal cord. Subglottic examples are rare and occur mainly in childhood (52). The trachea is rarely involved.

From 5 to 11 percent of GCTs affect the gastrointestinal tract (45,53). While the esophagus, large bowel, and perianal region account for the majority of cases (54,55), examples occur at all levels, including stomach and small bowel. Most esophageal tumors affect its distal portion, while tumors involving the large bowel arise throughout its length (55). Although most gastrointestinal tumors are solitary and involve the lamina propria or submucosa (fig. 10-11), multiplicity also occurs. The greatest number of multiple GCTs reported to date includes two cases featuring 26 and 52 lesions. In both instances, the colon was the affected site (56,57). GCTs also involve the gallbladder and bile ducts (55).

Genital GCTs are rare, and usually affect the vulva (58,59) and penis (60) as superficial

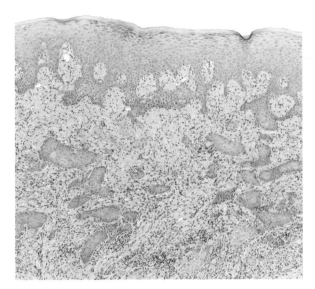 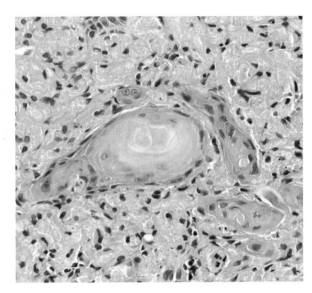

Figure 10-10

GRANULAR CELL TUMOR

Low-power magnification shows that the lesion, situated on the lateral border of the tongue (left), is covered by proliferative squamous epithelium mimicking invasive carcinoma (pseudo-epitheliomatous hyperplasia) (right). (Courtesy of Dr. I.G. Koutlas, Minneapolis, MN.)

lesions. Vulvar lesions are frequently multifocal are found in a somewhat younger patient population (59).

Gross Findings. Most GCTs are solitary, nodular lesions seldom measuring more than 3 cm in maximum dimension. Circumscribed tumors are more common than ones poorly demarcated or grossly infiltrative. Surface irregularity of overlying skin or squamous mucosa is often seen and is due to pseudoepitheliomatous hyperplasia (fig. 10-9C). On cross section, the generally firm tumors appear gray-white to faintly yellow (fig. 10-9B). In one reported example, as well as in a case of our own (fig. 10-12), cutaneous plaques or multinodularity perhaps reflected a plexiform pattern of growth (37).

Microscopic Findings. GCTs are poorly marginated and consist of cells disposed in sheets, nests, lobules, or ribbons (figs. 10-13, left; 10-14) within a variably dense fibrous stroma. Limited infiltration of surrounding adipose tissue may be seen. The tumor cells are monotonous, plump, polyhedral to somewhat elongated, with distinct cell borders. Their abundant eosinophilic cytoplasm is granular in appearance (figs. 10-14A,C). The nuclei are typically eccentrically placed, small and regular, and somewhat hyperchromat-

ic, and generally contain inconspicuous nucleoli (fig. 10-14A,B). Occasional tumors feature degenerative nuclear changes (fig.10-14C).

In addition to uniform granularity, a reportedly constant feature of GCT is the presence in scattered cells of one or several eosinophilic cytoplasmic globules, once referred to as "pustule-ovoid bodies of Milian" (fig. 10-15A) (61). Demystified, they simply represent aggregates of secondary lysosomes spatially separated from the surrounding cytoplasm by a halo (61). A typical but less common feature is refractile eosinophilic lysosomes that are ovoid to elongated in shape. Termed angulate bodies, they lie within stromal histiocytes (fig. 10-15C) (62).

Both these features and the abundant cytoplasmic granularity (lysosomes) are moderately periodic acid–Schiff (PAS)-positive (figs. 10-14B; 10-15B,D) and diastase resistant. In addition, the tumor cells stain with Sudan black B and are magenta with trichrome preparations. These various cellular features of GCT are constant and are readily evident in cytologic preparations (fig. 10-16) (63,64). Multinucleation, nuclear pleomorphism, readily identifiable nucleoli, and mitotic figures are uncommon features. The pattern of reticulin staining varies considerably,

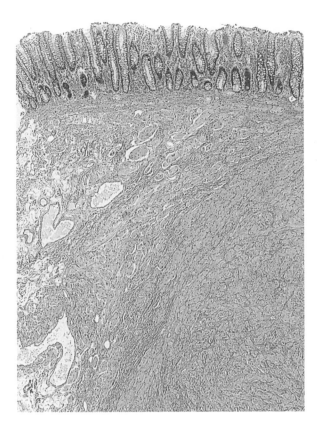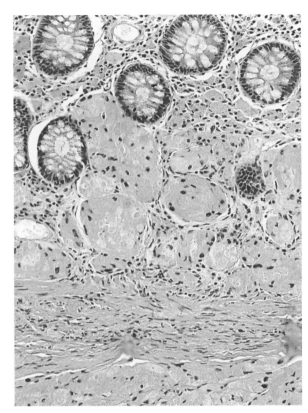

Figure 10-11

GRANULAR CELL TUMOR

Left: This tumor in the colon involves the submucosa.
Right: Both the lamina propria and submucosa are involved.

surrounding either individual or clustered granular cells. Reactive changes are often evident in the forms of extensive collagenization (fig.10-13, right), aggregation of lymphoid cells at the periphery of most lesions, and proliferation of overlying squamous epithelium sufficient to mimic squamous cell carcinoma (pseudoepitheliomatous hyperplasia) (fig. 10-10, left).

Although most GCTs are superficial, affecting dermal and subcutaneous tissues, some involve deep soft tissues, including muscle. Gastrointestinal GCTs primarily involve the lamina propria and submucosa (fig. 10-11). A notable feature, given its bearing upon the assumed line of differentiation of GCTs, is common involvement of the small nerves in or around the tumor (fig. 10-17); large nerves are less often affected (fig. 10-18). In other instances, the neural derivation of GCT is suggested simply by the finding of residual axons within a tumor.

Rare, superficially situated examples exhibit a plexiform pattern of growth suggestive of nerve involvement (fig. 10-11) (37).

Immunohistochemical Findings. A variety of markers are exhibited by GCTs. Numerous reports support the possibility of a neurogenic nature. For example, the tumors are routinely reactive for S-100 protein (figs. 10-18C, 10-19A,B) (28,65–67), and, as more recently demonstrated, most are reactive for the primarily neural marker, calretinin (68). CD57 (Leu-7) is evident in about one third of cases (39). Staining for myelin-associated protein has produced erratic results, but reactivity for the integral myelin protein PO and the peripheral myelin protein P2 has been reported (69). Nonetheless, stains for myelin basic protein are inconclusive (39,70,71). As expected, given their high content of secondary lysosomes, GCTs show strong reactivity for CD68 (KP-1) (fig. 10-19C) (65,66),

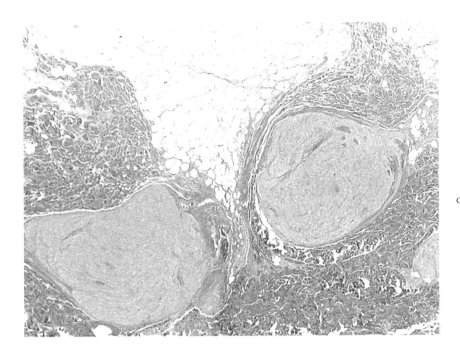

Figure 10-12
GRANULAR CELL TUMOR
Rare tumors have a multinodular or plexiform-like growth pattern.

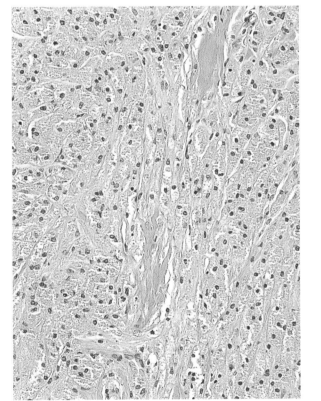
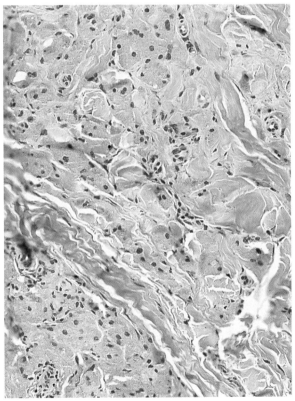

Figure 10-13

GRANULAR CELL TUMOR

Left: These tumors are most often disposed in sheets with uniform cells grouped between delicate fibrovascular septa.
Right: Occasional examples are fibrotic.

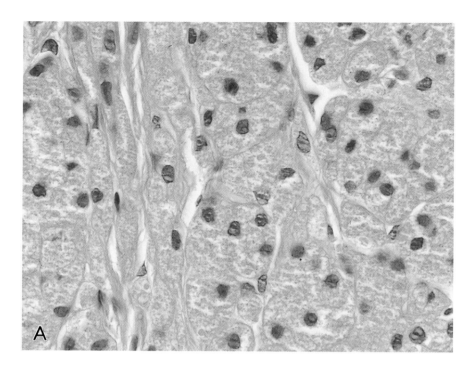

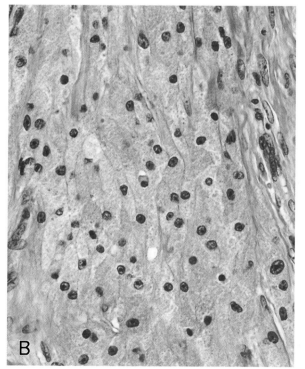

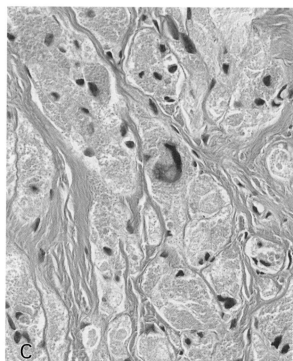

Figure 10-14

GRANULAR CELL TUMOR

Due to the accumulation of secondary lysosomes, the cells appear coarsely granular (A), a feature highlighted with the periodic acid–Schiff (PAS) stain (B). The nuclei are small and range from showing slightly open chromatin with discernible nucleoli (A) to having dense chromatin (B). Degenerative nuclear atypia is uncommon (C).

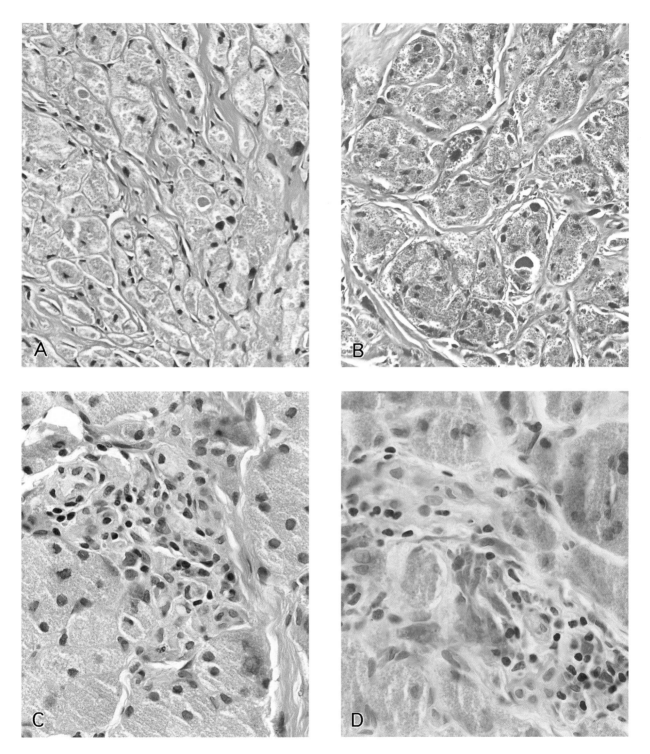

Figure 10-15

GRANULAR CELL TUMOR

Two cytologic features typical of GCT are globules representing collections of secondary lysosomal material that presumably detach from the surrounding cytoplasm (A, center), and angulate bodies (C), collections of membrane-bound angulate lysosomes in stromal fibrohistiocytic cells. Both are accentuated with the PAS stain (B and D).

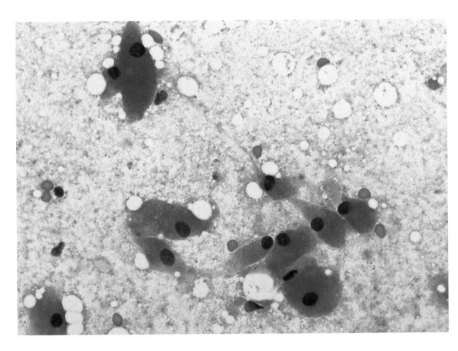

Figure 10-16

GRANULAR CELL TUMOR: CYTOLOGY

On smear preparations, the cells appear polygonal or angular in configuration and possess dense granular cytoplasm and dense round nuclei.

alpha-1-antitrypsin, and alpha-1-antichymotrypsin (66). Nonspecific but consistent findings are positivity for gene product 9.5 (65), inhibin alpha-subunit (65,68,72), and neuron-specific enolase (66). A number of studies have reported lack of both neurofilament protein and GFAP (67,73). Immunostains for laminin are positive (67) as well as for collagen 4 (fig. 10-19D), which stain around groups of tumor cells. Angulate bodies containing histiocytes are CD68 immunoreactive and S-100 protein negative (74).

Ultrastructural Findings. The fine structural features of GCTs are distinctive. The light microscopic granularity of their polygonal to spindle-shaped cells is due to the presence of numerous large pleomorphic secondary lysosomes. Varying in type, these include autophagosomes, residual bodies, multivesicular bodies, and material resembling ceroid lipofuscin (figs. 10-20, 10-21) (32,47,67,75–78). Ultrastructurally, the lysosomes consist of membrane-bound aggregates of microgranules and irregularly shaped, variably electron-dense masses containing assorted inclusions, among them remnants of organelles and concentric lamellae likened to myelin debris (figs. 10-20, 10-21). Stromal fibrohistiocytic cells intimately associated with the granular tumor cells frequently contain membrane-bound structures featuring parallel arrays of microtubules, termed angulate bodies, and

scattered dense lipid bodies (62). The terms angulate lysosomes (79) and "Gaucher-like bodies" (fig. 10-22) have also been applied to angulate bodies. Interestingly, these bodies are only rarely found in the cytoplasm of the granular tumor cells. A peripheral nerve origin of most GCTs is supported by the finding of a distinct basement membrane often surrounding granular cell clusters (fig. 10-20), the occasional presence of similarly disposed extracellular long-spacing collagen, and the presence among tumor cells of arrays of neuronal processes (32,47,75).

As is further discussed below, ultrastructural studies also are useful for excluding such mimics of GCT as granular cell leiomyoma (75,80) and leiomyosarcoma (81).

Hybrid Granular Cell and Perineurial Cell Tumors. Biphenotypic benign peripheral nerve sheath tumors composed of cells with features of Schwann and perineurial cells, the two principal nerve sheath elements, are commonly referred to as *hybrid peripheral nerve sheath tumors.* Hybrid perineurial and Schwann cell tumors are discussed in chapter 9. The term hybrid PNST tumor is used here because GCTs are generally considered to be Schwann cell tumors.

One patient had five such hybrid tumors, which were removed (82). This 47-year-old man had at least 20 extremity-based, cutaneous lesions present since childhood, but no history of

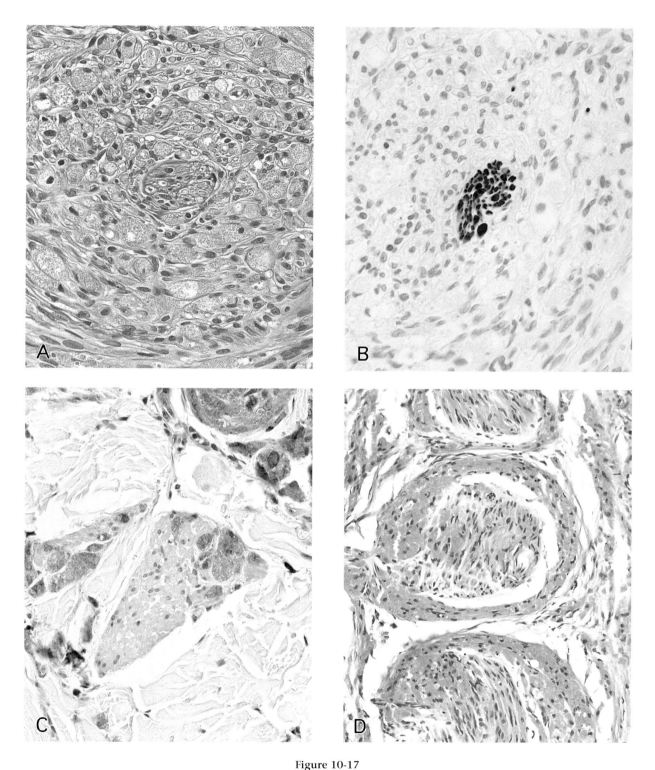

Figure 10-17

GRANULAR CELL TUMOR

Careful sampling sometimes reveals GCTs to involve minute nerves (A), a feature highlighted by neurofilament protein immunostaining (B; same case as fig. 10-12). Although perineurial growth is the rule, in some cases granular cells actually lie within the nerve (C; S-100 protein immunostain). On rare occasion, there is also perineurial extension (D).

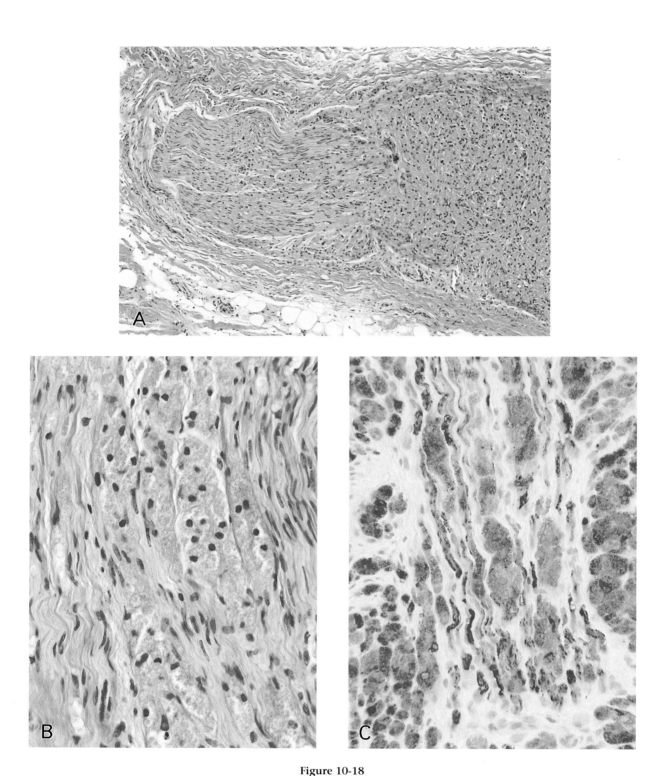

Figure 10-18

GRANULAR CELL TUMOR

This lesion arose in a grossly recognizable nerve. At low power (A), the contours of the affected nerve are still apparent (left). In addition to a solid growth phase (A, right), permeation of the nerve by GCT is readily evident at higher power (B). The granular cells are most apparent with an S-100 protein immunostain (C). This stain permits comparison of the neoplastic cells to aligned Schwann cells of the underlying nerve.

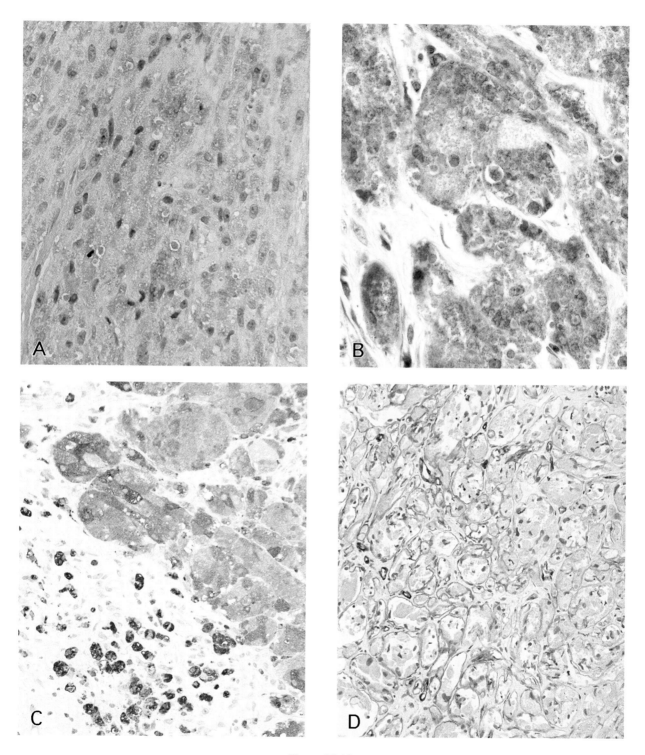

Figure 10-19

GRANULAR CELL TUMOR

A,B: Immunoreactivity for S-100 protein varies considerably from one tumor to the next.

C: Staining for CD68 is also a typical feature of GCT. The stromal histiocytes stain more than the tumor cells.

D: Collagen 4 staining highlights the basement membrane around granular cell clusters.

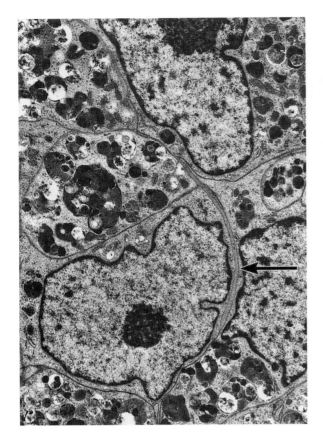

Figure 10-20

GRANULAR CELL TUMOR

Some cells have cytoplasm filled with pleomorphic secondary lysosomes. Basement membrane (arrow) separates cell clusters.

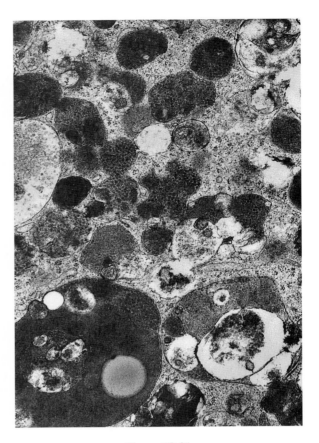

Figure 10-21

GRANULAR CELL TUMOR

High magnification of the secondary lysosomes present in granular cells tumors.

Figure 10-22

ANGULATE BODY IN A GRANULAR CELL TUMOR

Membrane-limited angulate bodies (angulate lysosomes) contain numerous aligned microtubules and are a common feature of histocytes found in GCTs.

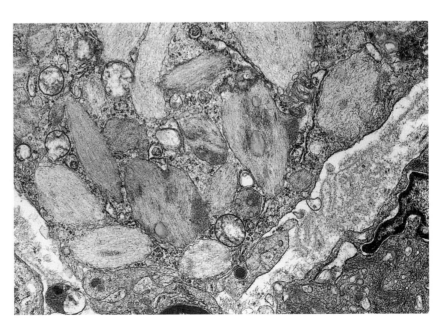

a genetic disorder, specifically neurofibromatosis. Ranging from 0.4 to 3.0 cm in greatest dimension, each lesion was well circumscribed, unencapsulated, and involved mainly dermis. All were composed of bland spindle cells, possessed tapered nuclei as well as indistinct cytoplasm, and assumed a storiform arrangement. Scattered among them were large granular cells. The nongranular spindle cells expressed EMA but not S-100 protein, an immunostaining pattern of perineurial cells rather than of Schwann or granular cells.

An earlier report described two circumscribed cutaneous tumors, possibly examples of this same hybrid tumor, that were histologically unique given their superficial resemblance to intraneural perineurioma (83). Both were solitary lesions of the hand. One each occurred in an adult woman and a man, and were small (0.8 and 1.4 cm, respectively). The published diagnosis was perineurioma with granular cells.

Differential Diagnosis. Although granular cells are present in some schwannomas (84), neurofibromas, and possibly traumatic neuromas (85), the distinctive, basic features of these three lesions are readily apparent. Despite their frequent expression of CD68 (see fig. 6-25D) (65,66), we have not encountered a schwannoma with widespread granular change. Nonetheless, lesions to be considered in the differential diagnosis of GCT include neurogenic as well as mesenchymal and ectodermal lesions. With the exception of carcinoma, these generally pose little diagnostic challenge.

Due to their firmness on palpation and section as well as infiltrative margins, GCTs of the breast are notoriously difficult to distinguish from mammary adenocarcinoma. This is also true at the microscopic level, particularly at frozen section (86). Confusion with squamous carcinomas may also arise due to misinterpretation of the often associated pseudoepitheliomatous hyperplasia overlying cutaneous or mucosal GCTs, particularly of the vulva (see fig. 10-9C). The distinction from carcinoma may necessitate immunohistochemistry. Unlike carcinoma, GCTs are CD68 (KP-1) positive (65) and lack both keratin and EMA staining. Since some carcinomas, including those of mammary origin, may be S-100 protein immunoreactive, use of this determinant alone cannot be relied upon for the diagnosis.

Granular cells may be seen in a wide array of non-neurogenic tumors (87). The ones bearing the closest histologic resemblance to GCT include malignant GCT, congenital GCT or epulis (44,88,89), primitive non-neural GCT of skin (26,87,90), and granular cell leiomyoma. Most clinically malignant GCTs are histologically indistinguishable from benign GCTs; only a minority show cellular pleomorphism, marked hyperchromasia, mitotic activity, and focal necrosis, all features lacking in benign examples (see chapter 12). Although congenital GCT, or epulis, shares many histologic similarities with benign GCT, important differences exist. The congenital GCT occurs exclusively in newborns, affects the alveolar ridge (fig. 10-23A), and histologically demonstrates a plexiform capillary pattern not present in GCT (fig. 10-23B). Their cells possess uniformly granular cytoplasm similar to that of GCT but without the presence of globular inclusions or angulate body-containing histiocytes (fig. 10-23C). Although immunoexpressive of the lysosomal markers CD68 and alpha-1-antitrypsin (88), they do not stain for S-100 protein. On balance, the congenital GCT exhibits aspects of a reactive process, reinforced by its nonrecurrence and the fact that most undergo spontaneous regression, even if incompletely excised.

The so-called primitive non-neural GCT is a nodular cutaneous lesion residing primarily in the papillary, and less often the reticular, dermis or superficial subcutaneous tissue. Based upon combined data from the two largest series of cases (87,90), these tumors affect younger individuals (mean and median ages, 23 and 28 years, respectively) than do GCTs and show no gender predilection. They are similar in size but, in contrast to GCT, are well circumscribed and usually encircled by an epithelial collarette. Their cells, arranged in sheets without nesting, exhibit mainly vesicular rather than hyperchromatic nuclei and exhibit more in the way of atypia and mitotic activity. They immunostain for the melanoma marker NKI-C3. Most stain for CD68, a reflection of their content of secondary lysosomes at the ultrastructural level (91), but no S-100 protein reactivity is seen. One example reportedly metastasized to local lymph nodes, but the patient was disease free 70 months following lymphadenectomy (87). Occurring after a tooth

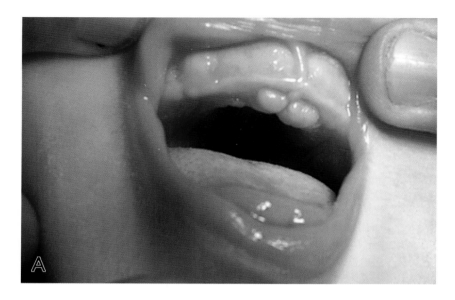

Figure 10-23

CONGENITAL GRANULAR CELL TUMOR (EPULIS)

A: Two symmetric protrusions are present on the upper gum.

B: Microscopically, the lesion is covered by intact epithelium and features a somewhat plexiform vascular pattern.

C: At higher power, cytoplasmic angulate bodies are lacking. Such lesions are typically S-100 protein immunonegative. (Courtesy of Dr. I.G. Koutlas, Minneapolis, MN.)

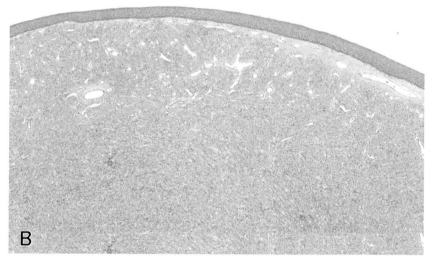

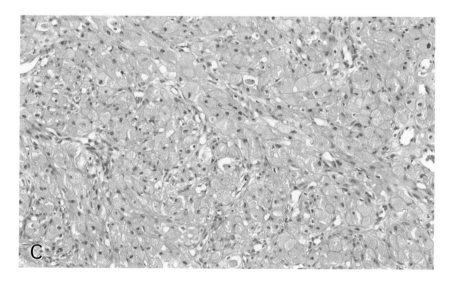

extraction, the sole oral example of a presumed non-neural GCT (92) consisted of variably granular to clear spindle cells and had the appearance of a robust granulomatous reaction.

The distinction of GCT from granular cell leiomyoma may require either immunohistochemical staining for muscle markers, such as HHF-35 and smooth muscle actin, or recourse to electron microscopy (75,80). Granular cell change in smooth muscle tumors may be associated with immunoreactivity for neuron-specific enolase and NKI-C3 (93).

Less easily confused with GCT are melanoma, rhabdomyoma, hibernoma, and astrocytoma with granular cells. In contrast to GCTs, HMB45 is usually expressed in melanomas (28). Unlike rhabdomyoma, GCTs lack cytoplasmic cross striations as well as immunohistochemical and ultrastructural features of myogenic differentiation. The cells of GCTs differ from those of hibernomas in that they do not have vacuolated cytoplasm. Finally, intracerebral granular cell astrocytomas are distinguished from benign GCT by the lack of GFAP staining in the latter (94).

Treatment and Prognosis. The recommended treatment of benign GCT is local excision, preferably with negative margins. The recurrence rate is estimated at 2 to 8 percent when margins of resection are deemed free of involvement, whereas the rates are 21 to 50 percent after incomplete excision (49).

GANGLIONEUROMA

Definition. *Ganglioneuroma* is a benign neoplasm consisting of mature autonomic ganglion cells, satellite cells, and numerous unmyelinated axons, associated with Schwann cells in a somewhat collagenous background.

General Features. Many years after the original 1870 description of Loritz (95), Stout (96) summarized the clinical and pathologic features of ganglioneuromatous neoplasms. His study found a minority of tumors to be composite in nature, containing either a diffuse admixture or localized collections of neuroblastoma cells; such lesions metastasized at rates of 18 or 65 percent, respectively. On the other hand, tumors lacking neuroblastic cells did not metastasize. These "fully differentiated" examples he called ganglioneuromas. They had a benign clinical outcome, but a postoperative mortality rate of 10 percent when resection was aggressive. Thus, Stout underscored the need to distinguish between pure ganglioneuroma and similar tumors containing less-differentiated elements.

The origin of ganglioneuroma and its relationship to neuroblastic tumors remains unsettled. No doubt the ganglion cells of ganglioneuromas have their origin in neuroblasts. Perhaps most ganglioneuromas, unlike the cells of neuroblastoma, mature at a pace approximating that of normal development. Maturation of neuroblastoma or ganglioneuroblastoma to ganglioneuroma is also known to occur, either spontaneously or after therapy, as well as in metastases (97–102). These occurrences suggest that patient age and tumor distribution aside (see below), ganglioneuromas represent fully differentiated neuroblastomas.

Ganglioneuromas are associated with, or arise in, transition from other neuroectodermal tumors. Examples of the first include the concurrence of ganglioneuroma and schwannoma of the vagus nerve (103) and mediastinal ganglioneuroma with retroperitoneal pheochromocytoma (104). Examples of the second, referred to as "composite tumors," include ganglioneuroma in transition from pheochromocytoma (105) and of ganglioneuromatous components in extra-adrenal paragangliomas, such as of the cauda equina region (106,107) and duodenum (108). Synchronous mediastinal ganglioneuroma and retroperitoneal pheochromocytoma has also been reported (104). Ganglioneuromatous differentiation of rhabdomyosarcoma (110) as well as of olfactory neuroblastoma (109) have been reported after therapy.

Although uncommon, the association of ganglioneuroma with multiple endocrine neoplasia (MEN) 2B as well as with NF1 (112) is well established. A Turner syndrome (113) or Beckwith-Wiedemann syndrome (114) association is infrequent. Only a single example has been associated with Cowden syndrome (115). Familial ganglioneuromas unassociated with a specific syndrome have also been described (116). In any case, whether heritable or sporadic in occurrence, ganglioneuromas are far less common than are schwannomas and neurofibromas.

Ganglioneuromas rarely affect animals but have been noted in association with C-cell hyperplasia of the thyroid gland in the rat (117).

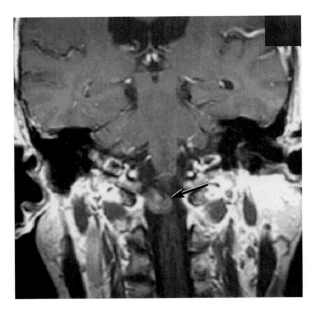 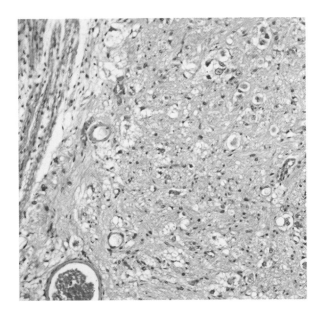

Figure 10-24

SPINAL INTRADURAL GANGLIONEUROMA

Left: As seen on magnetic resonance imaging (MRI), the spinal root tumor (arrow) compresses the spinal cord.
Right: The intimate association of tumor with spinal nerve is readily evident.

Clinical Features. Ganglioneuromas most often arise where sympathetic ganglia are found, particularly in the mediastinum, retroperitoneum, and pelvis. They represent 5 percent of all mediastinal tumors, most being paraspinal. Also often involved are retroperitoneal ganglia and the adrenal medulla. Most pelvic examples are presacral (118) or coccygeal. Less common sites include the skull base, parapharyngeal region, and cranial nerve ganglia (103). Aware of examples affecting odd sites, such as the uterus, ovary, kidney, breast, and vulva, Stout (96) anticipated the finding of ganglioneuromas at still more sites. Subsequent reports of visceral (see below), ocular choroidal (119), orbital (120), posterior cranial fossa (121), spinal intradural (fig. 10-24) (115,122), mandibular (123), and even internal auditory canal ganglioneuromas (124) have proven him right. Although ganglioneuromatous tumors occur in skin, their morphology varies from conventional to consisting of dermal ganglion cells alone, both associated with overlying seborrheic keratosis-like changes (fig. 10-25) (125–129). Oral mucosal examples are rare (fig. 10-26).

A few ganglioneuromas originate in viscera and presumably represent their parasympa-

thetic counterparts. Their anatomic distribution and morphology varies, and they are broadly divided into diffuse and localized varieties. Diffuse examples occur in viscera in the setting of MEN 2B and NF1 (130). Such lesions, also occasionally sporadic (131) or unassociated with the classic features of MEN 2B (132), are discussed in chapter 5. Localized, polypoid visceral ganglioneuromas unassociated with a heritable syndrome are rare (133). Unlike neurofibromas occurring in patients with NF1, most of which arise in the stomach and small bowel, visceral ganglioneuromas affect primarily the colon and rectum (134). These tumors have also been observed in the appendix (135), lung (136), urinary bladder (137,138), and prostate gland (139). The two latter tumors occurred in the setting of NF1. Visceral ganglioneuromas are generally smaller than their soft tissue counterparts and show no neuroblastoma association.

The general clinical features of ganglioneuromas are well known (111). They usually affect older children and young adults, presenting between ages 10 and 20, and show a distinct female predilection. Most patients come to attention due to mass effects, but some tumors are incidental findings on physical examination or

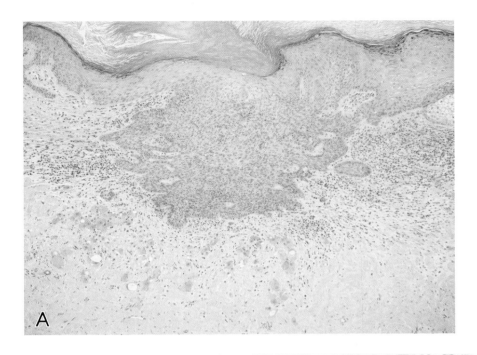

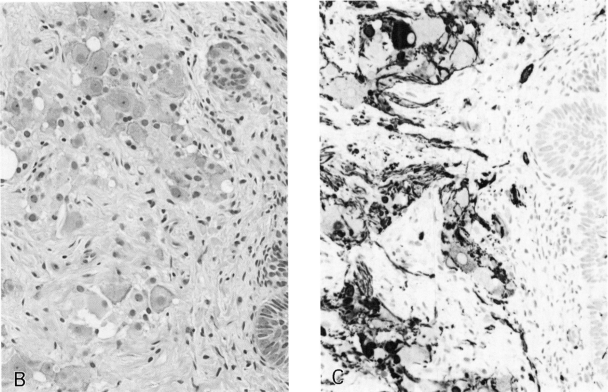

Figure 10-25

CUTANEOUS GANGLIONEUROMA

A,B: This rare lesion consists of mature ganglion cells within the dermis.
C: The lesional cells are highlighted by a neurofilament stain.

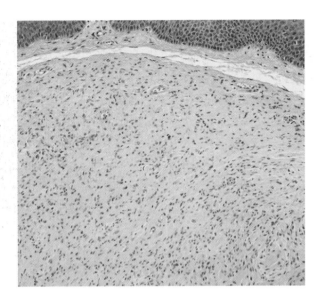 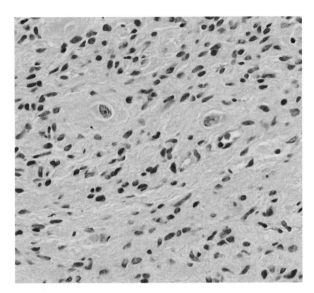

Figure 10-26

ORAL MUCOSAL GANGLIONEUROMA

Left: The tumor lies immediately beneath squamous mucosa.
Right: On hematoxylin and eosin (H&E) stain, scattered ganglion cells are associated with abundant nerve fibers.

imaging studies. Occasional examples are first noted at autopsy.

Endocrine Effects. Some ganglioneuromas are endocrine active. An association with the "watery diarrhea syndrome" (Verner-Morrison syndrome), a condition mediated by tumoral production of vasoactive intestinal polypeptide (VIP), is best known. VIP may be expressed by differentiating and mature ganglion cells in ganglioneuroma and ganglioneuroblastoma, as well as in those of composite ganglioneuroma-pheochromocytoma (140,141). Not surprisingly, the composite tumor may also be associated with hypertension (105). Elevation of urinary catecholamine metabolites, including vanillylmandelic acid and homovanillic acid, may be associated with pure ganglioneuromas as well as composite ganglioneuroma-pheochromocytoma (142). The blood levels found are related to the tumor size (143). Significant elevations, more than three times normal, should prompt a careful search for a neuroblastoma component. Virilization is rarely seen (144). One ganglioneuroma was reportedly associated with myasthenia gravis (145).

Radiologic Features. Regardless of the method used, ganglioneuromas appear as solitary, smooth-contoured masses. Paraspinal tumors are often associated with expansion of one or occasionally more spinal foramina and occasionally with intraspinal extension. Intradural extension is rare (146,147). On computerized tomography (CT), ganglioneuromas are sharply defined masses that show soft tissue attenuation; delicate or amorphous calcification is sometimes seen, but is far less frequent than in neuroblastoma. Contrast enhancement is most pronounced on magnetic resonance imaging (MRI), which also shows cyst formation to greater advantage. An uncommon feature, although well recognized by radiologists (148), is intratumoral accumulation of adipose tissue (149). On ultrasound examination, ganglioneuromas appear hypoechoic and hypovascular.

Gross Findings. Often large, ganglioneuromas are typically circumscribed, smooth-contoured masses either ovoid, somewhat flattened, or intimately conforming to their surroundings (figs. 10-27–10-30). Most are smaller than 15 cm, but rare tumors measure 50 cm and weigh up to 6 kg. Although most appear grossly encapsulated, at the microscopic level, ganglioneuromas possess only a thin pseudo-capsule (fig. 10-27). Occasional tumors focally exhibit an irregular interface with adjacent soft tissue (fig. 10-30, right). As a result, adherence to surrounding tissue may complicate complete

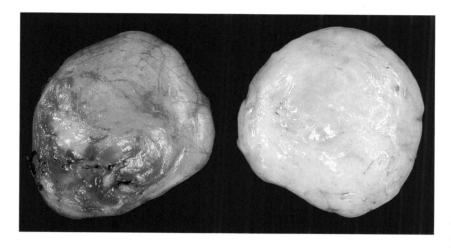

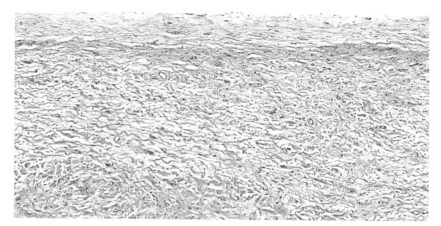

Figure 10-27

GANGLIONEUROMA

Top: Grossly, most ganglioneuromas are ovoid in shape, but unlike schwannomas, are often flattened rather than globoid. A thick pancake shape is common. Occasional examples are multilobate.

Bottom: Microsections show them to be enveloped by a thin fibrous pseudocapsule.

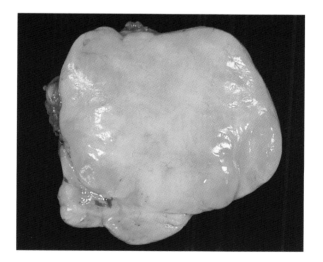

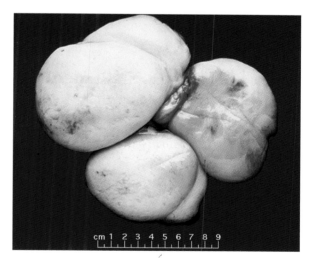

Figure 10-28

GANGLIONEUROMA

The cut surfaces of these posterior mediastinal examples vary from soft, pale, glistening, and mucin-rich (left) to firm and somewhat fibrous (right). The range closely resembles that exhibited by neurofibroma, and is a reflection of the uniform cellularity of the lesion.

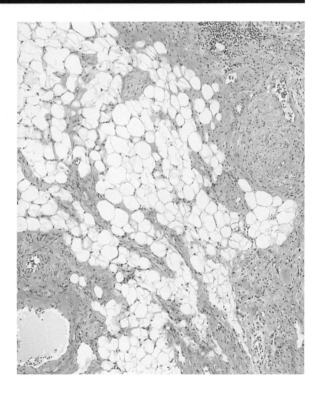

Figure 10-29

GANGLIONEUROMA

Some tumors, such as this intercostal example, are macrocystic.

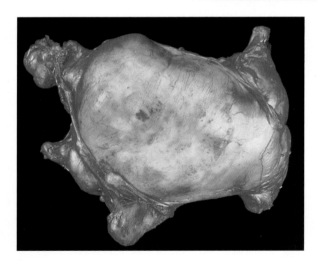

Figure 10-30

GANGLIONEUROMA

Above: Irregular in contour, with peripheral lobulation, this posterior mediastinal lesion was adherent to surrounding structures.

Right: Occasional tumors lack complete encapsulation and irregularly spread into surrounding soft tissue.

resection. The same is true of tumors with irregular contours that surround vital structures (fig. 10-30). Ganglioneuromas grossly resemble neurofibromas in all but their shape, being globular to lobulated rather than fusiform.

Nearly all ganglioneuromas are solitary. Only rare examples have been multiple, as in one case in which several tumors involved an entire segment of the sympathetic chain (150), and others in which bilateral spinal foramina and epidural spaces were affected (146,147). The latter tumors only rarely extended intradurally to involve dorsal and ventral roots (146). Intradural ganglioneuromas limited to spinal nerve root are rare (115).

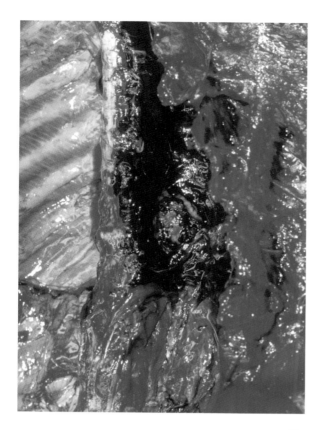 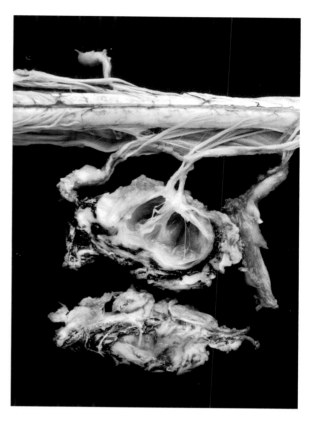

Figure 10-31

HEMORRHAGE IN PARASPINOUS GANGLIONEUROMA

Left: An autopsy photograph demonstrates peritumoral hemorrhage that extended into soft tissue.
Right: The discrete tumor is bivalved to demonstrate lesional hemorrhage.

Most ganglioneuromas are solid, but cyst formation may be seen (fig. 10-29). Only a few exhibit grossly apparent calcification. On cut surface, most are firm, homogeneously light tan, and often somewhat translucent (figs. 10-27, 10-28). Adipose-rich examples appear, in part, bright yellow. Massive spontaneous hemorrhage of ganglioneuromas is rarely seen (fig. 10-31) (151).

Paragangliomas, including duodenal and cauda equina region tumors which more often affect the filum terminale than a spinal nerve root, are known to rarely undergo ganglioneuromatous maturation (152). Such maturation also occurs in pheochromocytoma. Occasionally, the two components are grossly evident: the ganglioneuroma element is tan and distinct from the pheochromocytoma, which is red-brown (fig. 10-32A,B). The distinction is highlighted by fixation in Zenker solution which shows the chromaffin-positive pheochromocytoma to be dark brown. Microscopically, the two tumor elements are spatially distinct (fig. 10-32C). With the exception of one example occurring in the region of the organ of Zuckerkandl (153), reported examples of composite tumors have all occurred in the adrenal gland. In one reported instance, the process was bilateral (154).

Microscopic Findings. The essential morphologic features of ganglioneuroma include ganglion cells with long axonal processes and Schwann cells forming both axonal and satellite cells encompassing the ganglion cells (fig. 10-33). The presence of neuroblasts must be sought by thorough sampling so as to exclude a diagnosis of ganglioneuroblastoma. The distribution of ganglion cells within ganglioneuromas varies. They are either localized (fig. 10-33B) or widely scattered (fig. 10-33C). As a result, occasional microsections lack ganglion cells entirely and consist only

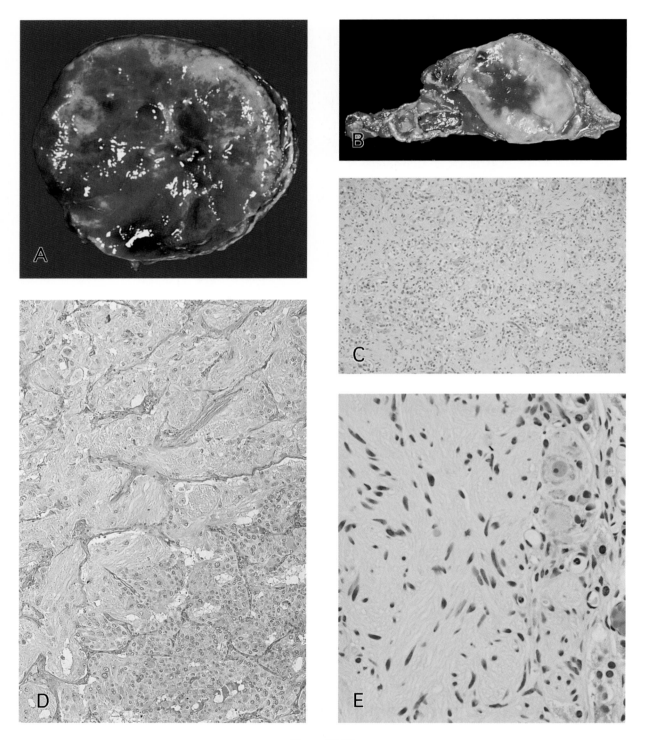

Figure 10-32

**GANGLIONEUROMATOUS MATURATION OF PHEOCHROMOCYTOMA
(COMPOSITE PHEOCHROMOCYTOMA-GANGLIONEUROMA)**

The process may be grossly evident and varies in extent. Firm and cream colored, such foci of maturation may be limited, as beneath the capsule (A), or may comprise the majority of the tumor (B). Microscopically, the two components are typically distinct (C–E). (A,B, courtesy of Dr. J.A.Carney, Rochester, MN.)

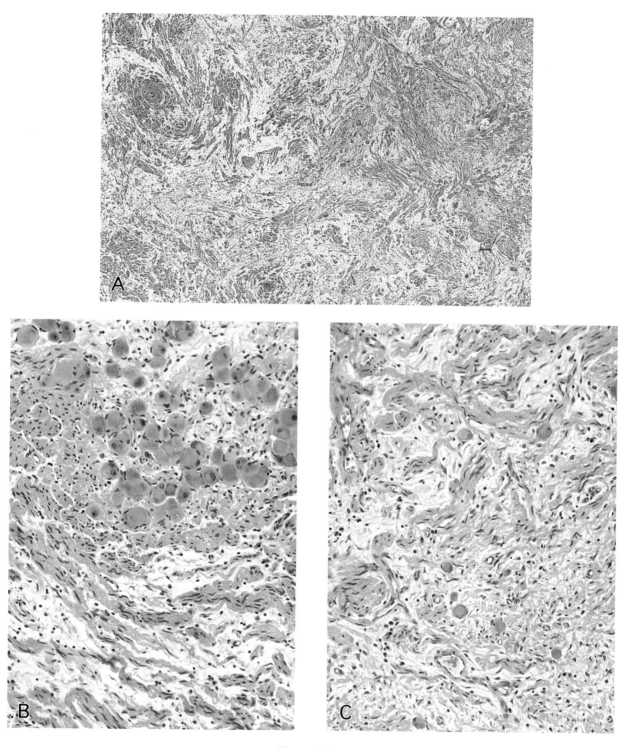

Figure 10-33

GANGLIONEUROMA

The essential components of this tumor include ganglion cells, their processes, and ensheathing Schwann cells (A). These vary in proportion and in their distribution. This example exhibited areas with numerous, concentrated ganglion cells (B) and other areas in which they were dispersed (C).

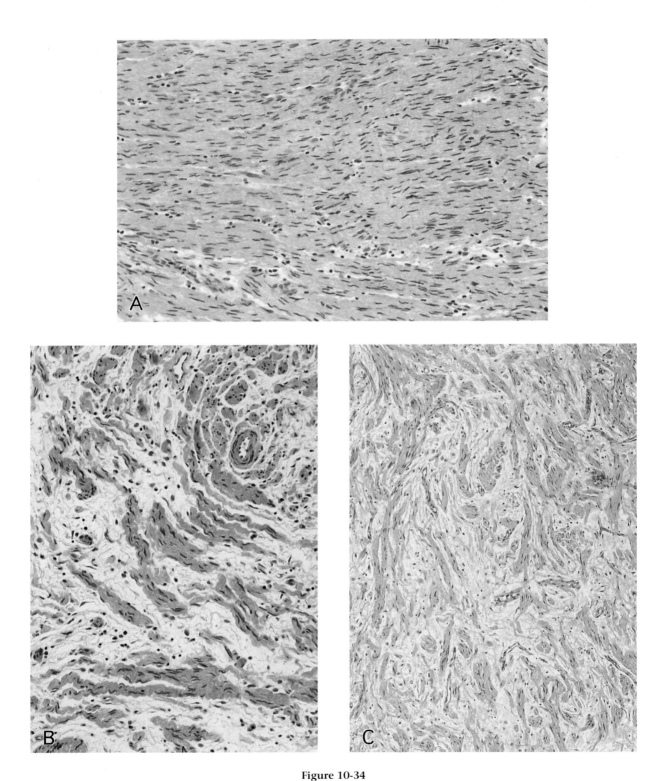

Figure 10-34

GANGLIONEUROMA

A,B: The arrangement of nerve fibers varies from compact and aligned bundles, the appearance of which mimics that of schwannoma (A), to fields in which nerve fiber bundles of varying size are dispersed (B).

C: Despite finding scattered ganglion cells, the jumbled bundles may mimic the pattern of a neurofibroma.

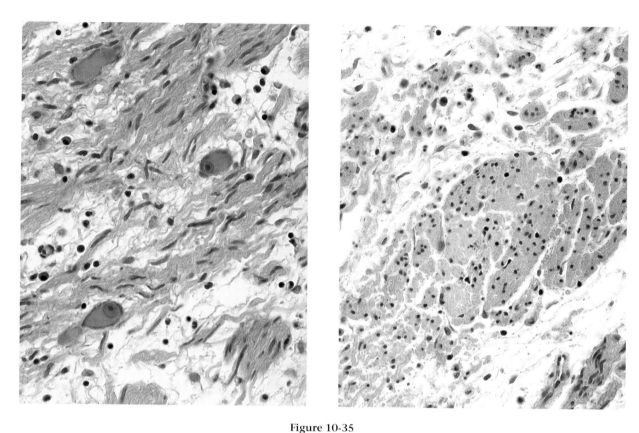

Figure 10-35

GANGLIONEUROMA

Whether longitudinally (left) or cross cut (right), nerve fiber bundles vary markedly in appearance.

of fields of neuritic processes with ensheathing Schwann cells (fig. 10-34C). Thus, the number of neuritic processes in ganglioneuromas often appears out of proportion to the ganglion cells. Either compactly arrayed or loose textured, the processes typically form aligned, entangled bundles (fig. 10-34A,B), the appearance of which depends upon their orientation (fig. 10-35).

Despite the variation in cytology (fig. 10-36), the ganglion cells are well differentiated and easily recognized on the basis of: 1) size, which is generally greater than 20 µm due to varying amounts of abundant eosinophilic to amphophilic cytoplasm; 2) the presence of single or multiple vesicular nuclei, often eccentrically situated and possessing single, prominent nucleoli; and 3) the finding of Nissl substance, which varies from scant to relatively abundant (fig. 10-37A). Cytologic abnormalities include cellular and nuclear pleomorphism, cytoplasmic vacuolation, and large, often pale and

spherical cytoplasmic inclusions (fig. 10-36C,D), some of which resemble the Lewy bodies seen in Parkinson disease. Secretory granules may be evident with the argyrophil (Grimelius) stain, but these are not always seen (fig. 10-37B). Varying numbers of satellite cells, modified Schwann cells with often flattened nuclei, surround the ganglion cells. Their number and uniformity of distribution fall short of that seen in normal ganglia. Axons are abundant. Although their small diameter makes them inapparent with the hematoxylin and eosin (H&E) stain, silver impregnation (Bodian or Bielschowsky preparations) shows them to advantage (fig. 10-37C). Peanut agglutinin, a marker of advanced neuronal differentiation, labels both ganglion cells and their processes (155). Although Schwann cell cytoplasm surrounds axons, myelination is usually limited to entrapped normal nerve fibers (fig. 10-38). Thus, myelin stains such as Luxolfast blue are generally negative (fig. 10-37D). If

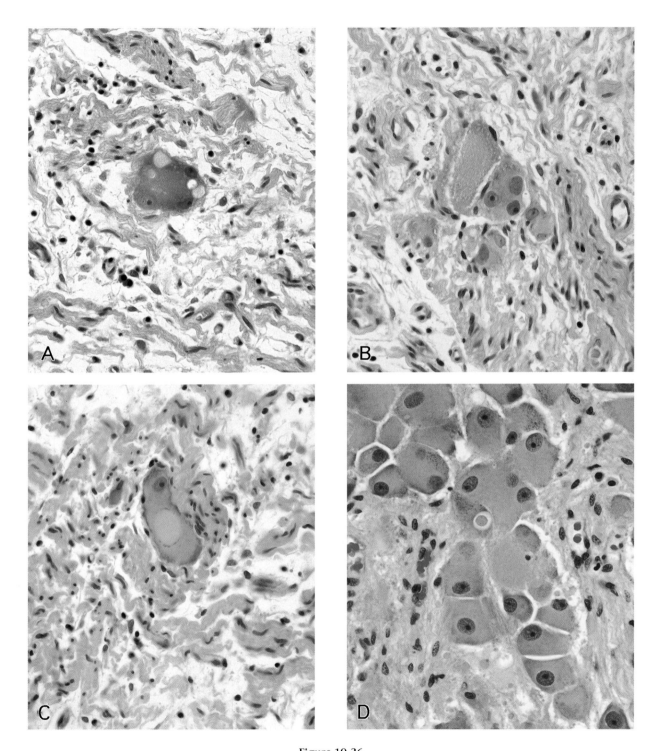

Figure 10-36

GANGLIONEUROMA

Even at high power, the distribution of ganglion cells varies: some are isolated (A), others clustered (B). Many contain abundant Nissl substance. The large vesicular nuclei and prominent nucleoli are hallmarks of ganglion cells. Cytologic abnormalities are common and include multinucleation (B,D), vacuolation (A), and spherical, eosinophilic cytoplasmic masses (C,D), some closely resembling Lewy bodies (D; see also fig. 10-41). (D courtesy of Dr. J. Wilson, New York, NY.)

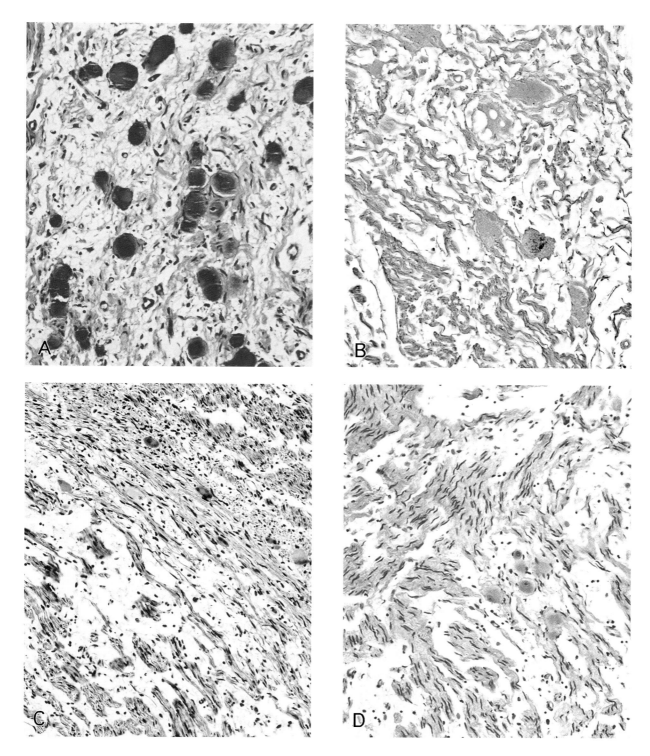

Figure 10-37

GANGLIONEUROMA

Ganglion cells vary in their content of Nissl substance (A) and argyrophilic granules (B). Their processes are readily visualized with silver impregnations (C), but myelin stains are typically negative (D). (A, cresyl violet; B, Grimelius; C, Bielschowsky; D, Luxol-fast blue-PAS stains).

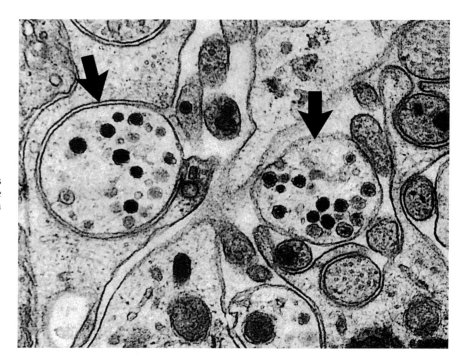

Figure 10-38

GANGLIONEUROMA

Two cross-sectioned axons (arrows) contain dense-core neurosecretory granules with an average diameter of 100 nm.

present, residual normal sympathetic ganglion tissue is recognized by its characteristic anatomic features, including clustered ganglion cells and traversing nerve fiber bundles (see fig. 2-17).

Ganglioneuromas often undergo degenerative changes, including the accumulation within ganglion cells of brown cytoplasmic pigment termed neuromelanin (fig. 10-39A). Unlike true melanin, it consists of pigmented lysosomes (156). Both argyrophil and argentaffin positive, it also differs from lipofuscin by lacking PAS and acid-fast reactivity as well as autofluorescence (157). Degenerative changes affecting the stroma are also common, particularly in sizable tumors. They include mainly fibrosis or some degree of mucin accumulation as seen in neurofibroma (fig. 10-39B). As a result, trichrome stains may show impressive collagen deposition and Alcian blue positivity may be evident. Adipose tissue is occasionally encountered in ganglioneuromas and takes the form of ill-defined lobules at the tumor periphery (fig. 10-40). Marked adipose deposition is uncommon (fig. 10-40) (149). Vascular hyalinization may also be seen and is the presumed basis of focal hemorrhage with resultant cystic change. Massive hemorrhage sufficient to produce hemothorax is rare (151). Lymphocytic infiltrates, when present,

are usually centered about vessels (fig. 10-39C) and must not be mistaken for neuroblasts. The distinction is readily made with the leukocyte common antigen (LCA) immunostain. Small numbers of mast cells may be seen. Whereas coarse, patchy calcification is common, psammoma bodies are rare (154).

In most instances of composite ganglioneuroma-pheochromocytoma, the two components are minimally admixed (fig. 10-32C) (140,141,153,154,158). Nonetheless, in one example of nodular and diffuse adrenal medullary hyperplasia of MEN 2B, clear transition of pheochromocytes to intermediate and ganglion cells was observed (159). Although all three cell types exhibited tyrosine hydroxylase activity, the process of transition was accompanied by loss of phenylethanolamine-N-methyltransferase, the enzyme that synthesizes epinephrine. One morphologically unique, testosterone-secreting adrenal ganglioneuroma consisted in part of nodules of Leydig cells containing both lipochrome pigment and Reinke crystalloids (144).

Immunohistochemical Findings. Ganglion cells and their axonal processes are immunopositive for synaptophysin (fig. 10-41A), neurofilament protein (fig. 10-41B), tubulin, cathepsin-D (160), and neuron-specific enolase. The latter,

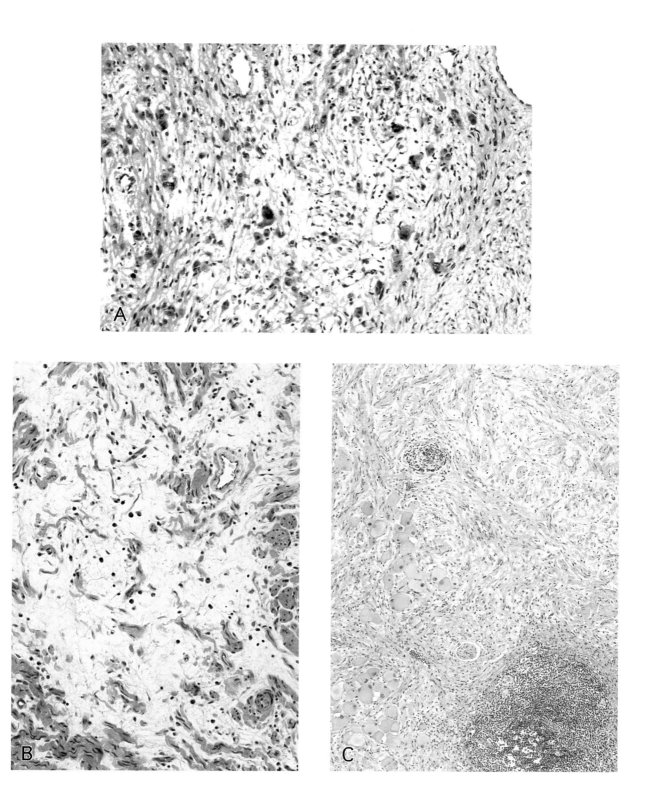

Figure 10-39

GANGLIONEUROMA

A: Neuromelanin deposition is commonly seen and is considered a degenerative feature.

B,C: The same is true of stromal mucin accumulation (B) and fibrosis and chronic inflammation (C).

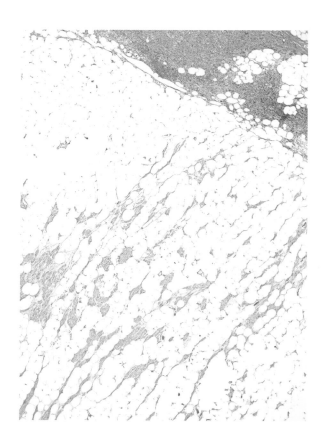
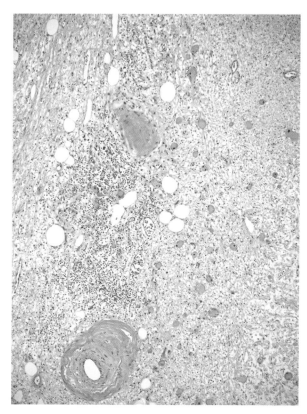

Figure 10-40

ADIPOSE-RICH GANGLIONEUROMA

Abundant adipose tissue is noted in this adrenal ganglioneuroma of a 15-year-old male.

although reliably present, is not a specific marker of neuronal differentiation (161,162). Reactivity for neurofilament protein is mainly for the high molecular weight phosphorylated epitope (163,164). The Schwann cell element of ganglioneuroma exhibits strong staining for S-100 protein (fig. 10-41C) and often for GFAP. Despite the lack of obvious myelination, staining for myelin basic protein has been reported (164). Collagen 4 reactivity highlights the basal lamina surrounding the Schwann cells.

Chromogranin A staining within the ganglion cell cytoplasm is said to be a regular finding (164), but we have found it to vary (fig. 10-42, left). Of the various hormones elaborated by ganglioneuroma, VIP is the best known (fig. 10-42, right) (140,141) and is often seen in differentiating and mature ganglion cells. It may also be found in tumors unassociated with the watery diarrhea syndrome (fig. 10-42, right). Calcitonin immunoreactivity has also been reported (140).

Ultrastructural Findings. The fine structural features of ganglioneuroma cells resemble those of mature sympathetic ganglion cells. These include: 1) large, round to oval, electron-lucent nuclei with prominent nucleoli; 2) abundant cytoplasm containing well-developed, often dilated rough endoplasmic reticulum; 3) prominent Golgi complexes; 4) numerous pleomorphic secondary lysosomes; 5) bundles of intermediate filaments (neurofilaments) which extend into proximal processes; 6) scattered microtubules; and 7) dense-core secretory granules ranging in size from 90 to 130 nm (figs. 10-38, 10-43). In one reported tumor, 125-nm granules were thought to correlate with the presence of calcitonin and coexisting 350-nm granules with VIP (140). Rarely seen presynaptic terminations of axons reportedly contain 40- to 60-nm vesicles. Cytoplasmic tubular inclusions (165) and Pick-like bodies (166) also have been identified in ganglion cells. While the axons of ganglioneuromas are

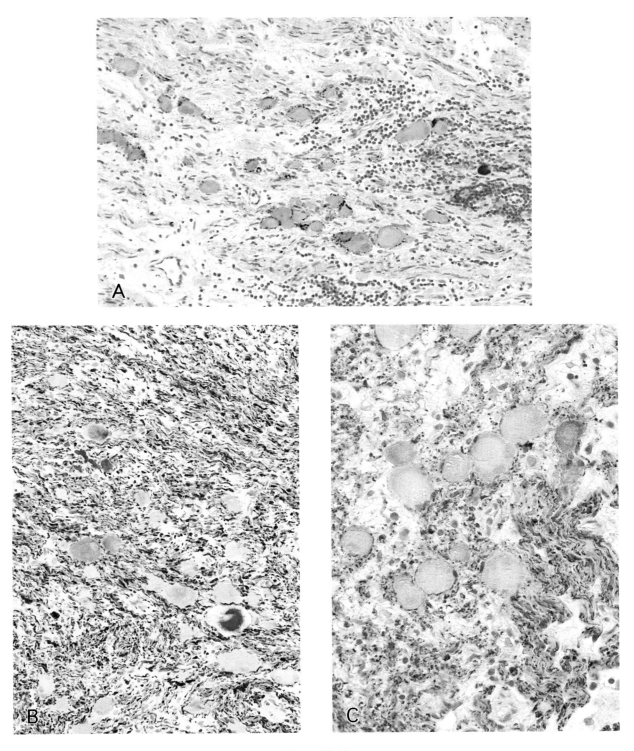

Figure 10-41

GANGLIONEUROMA

Ganglion cells show reactivity for synaptophysin (A) and neurofilament protein (B). The latter also stains spherical cytoplasmic neurofilament accumulations and ganglion cell processes. The ensheathing Schwann cells are S-100 protein reactive (C).

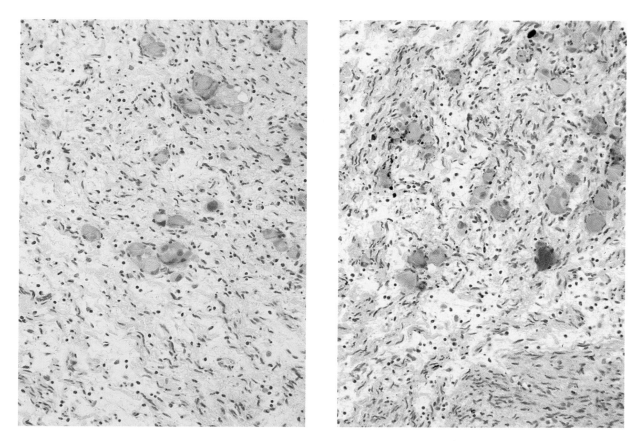

Figure 10-42

GANGLIONEUROMA

Chromogranin staining of ganglion cells (left) reflects their content of hormones and neurotransmitter substances, in this case, vasoactive intestinal polypeptide (right).

Figure 10-43

GANGLIONEUROMA

A portion of a ganglion cell (top) is bordered by an elongated satellite cell (center). Numerous lysosomal inclusions are found in the cytoplasm of the ganglion cell. The outer cell membrane of the satellite cell is separated from the stroma by a thin basement membrane (arrow).

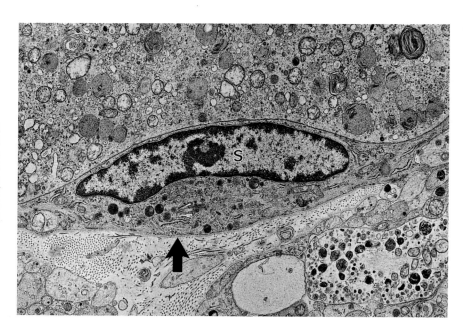

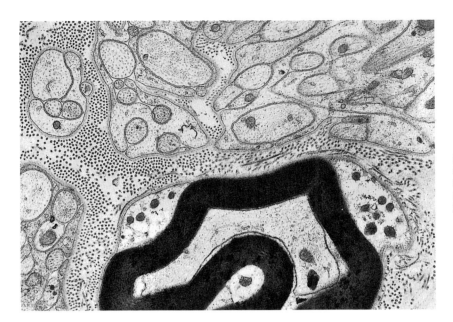

Figure 10-44

GANGLIONEUROMA

Prominent unmyelinated axons (bottom) are much smaller than a normal, apparently entrapped myelinated axon (top). The stroma consists of numerous collagen fibrils, here seen in cross section.

typically unmyelinated, scattered myelinated axons, presumably overrun normal nerve fibers, are occasionally encountered (fig. 10-44). Basal lamina surrounds the outer surface of the flattened satellite cells encompassing the ganglion cells (fig. 10-43). The interstitium of ganglioneuromas contain not only varying quantities of collagen fibrils but scattered Luse bodies (long-spacing collagen) as well. Ultrastructural studies, while delineating the architecture and cellular makeup of ganglioneuroma, are not diagnostically necessary.

Molecular Findings. Unlike neuroblastoma and occasional ganglioneuroblastomas, ganglioneuromas do not show *N-MYC* amplification, a marker of aggressive behavior in neuroblastic tumors (167).

Differential Diagnosis. Ganglioneuroma is usually readily distinguished from both neurofibroma and schwannoma, since these tumors lack both a ganglion cell component and abundant unmyelinated nerve fibers. Confusion only arises at surgery, on gross examination, and at microscopy in instances where these nerve sheath tumors overrun dorsal root sympathetic ganglia (fig. 10-45). Residual normal ganglion tissue is characterized by the orderly arrangement and uniform cytology of clustered ganglion cells as well as by separation of the clusters by organized bundles of myelinated or unmyelinated nerve fibers. Intraneural neuro-

fibromas lack the high density of nerve fibers that characterizes ganglioneuroma; instead, nerve fibers in neurofibromas are few in number, often myelinated, and either widely separated by intervening neurofibroma tissue or lie bundled at the center of affected nerve fascicles. The latter pattern is best seen in plexiform neurofibromas. Another distinguishing feature is the presence of more extensive stromal mucin (mucopolysaccharide) accumulation in neurofibromas. Unlike schwannomas, ganglioneuromas are grossly somewhat flattened and lack a thick capsule, an often peripherally displaced or partly intracapsular myelinated nerve, hyalinized blood vessels, Antoni A and B patterns, palisading of cells, and Verocay bodies. Localized mucosal neuromas, such as of the pharynx (168), may feature overrun ganglion cells and thus enter into the differential diagnosis. The finding of any ganglion cells in cutaneous lesions excludes consideration of neurofibroma or schwannoma.

Ganglioneuromatous transformation is known to occur in both pheochromocytoma (see fig. 10-32A–C), paraganglioma (106–108), and the spectrum of neuroblastic tumors, including a rare example of olfactory neuroblastoma (109). Composite ganglioneuroma-pheochromocytoma was discussed above. Thorough tissue sampling is the key to establishing the correct diagnosis. Neuroblastoma occurs at a younger age and its primary sites

Figure 10-45

GANGLIONEUROMA

A: Mimicry of ganglioneuroma results when schwannomas involve dorsal root ganglia.

B: Unlike ganglioneuroma, the schwannoma component is devoid of nerve fibers and well-formed Schwann sheaths (neurofilament protein immunostain).

C: In a similar manner, neurofibromas may also mimic ganglioneuromas.

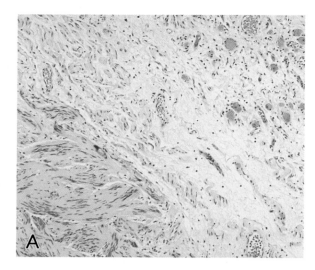

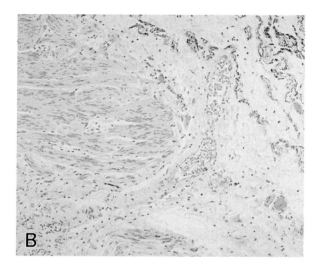

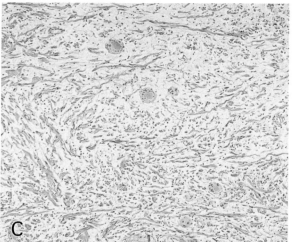

differ from those of ganglioneuroma. Most are infradiaphragmatic, whereas ganglioneuromas are supradiaphragmatic.

Two neuronal neoplasms often mistaken for ganglioneuroma are immature ganglioneuroma and ganglioneuroblastoma. Immature ganglioneuroma features a broad range of ganglion cell maturation, absence of or only rare neuroblasts, and abundant axonal processes unassociated with ensheathing Schwann cells (fig. 10-46). Ganglioneuroblastoma (fig. 10-47), particularly of the stroma-rich type (169), enters into the differential diagnosis when a nonrepresentative biopsy contains only the mature ganglionic element. Adequate tissue sampling resolves the issue. The finding of immature neurons lacking ample Nissl-containing cytoplasm, vesicular nuclei, and conspicuous nucleoli should

prompt a search for neuroblasts. As previously noted, by expressing neuron-specific enolase and synaptophysin reactivity, neuroblasts are readily distinguished from the scattered, LCA-positive lymphocytes, a common feature of ganglioneuroma. Metastatic neuroblastoma or ganglioneuroblastoma that has matured may also mimic ganglioneuroma (fig. 10-48).

Ganglioneuroma is a common component of the rare, histologically malignant and cytologically heterogenous tumor variously referred to as ectomesenchymoma (170) or gangliorhabdomyosarcoma (171). It is discussed in chapter 12.

Treatment and Prognosis. Ganglioneuromas are benign tumors that cause symptoms of mass effect or, far less often, of endocrine activity; resection is curative, even in instances in which intimate adherence to or growth around nearby

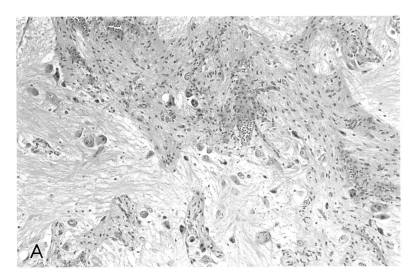

Figure 10-46

IMMATURE GANGLIONEUROMA

This neuronal neoplasm mimics mature ganglioneuroma and consists of both mature ganglion cells and small forms with less cytoplasm and smaller nucleoli (A,B). Atypia as well as rare neuroblasts may be seen (B). Neuronal processes unassociated with Schwann cells are a common feature (A,B) and readily evident with the H&E (A,B) and S-100 protein (C) stains.

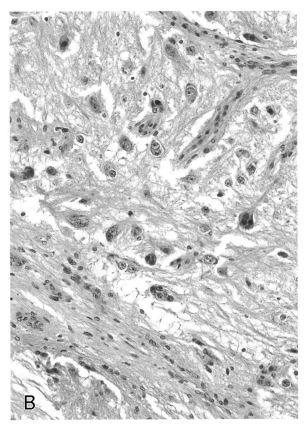

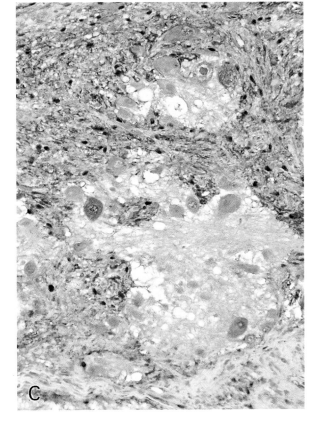

structures complicates the resection (111). The occasional finding of ganglioneuromatous tissue in regional lymph nodes or at sites remote from that of the primary indicates that maturation of metastatic neuroblastoma has taken place. The prognosis in such instances is also excellent. Nonetheless, at least one example of recurrence of neuroblastoma 15 years after conversion to ganglioneuroma has been reported (172). On rare occasion, ganglioneuroma may give rise to malignant peripheral nerve sheath tumor (see chapter 12).

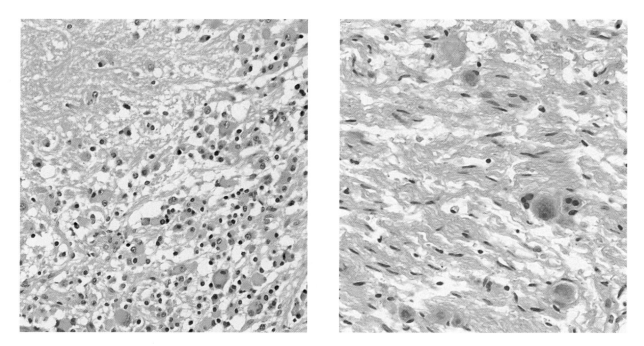

Figure 10-47

GANGLIONEUROBLASTOMA

This neuronal neoplasm consists of both a neuroblastic (left) and a variably mature ganglioneuromatous (right) component. Careful sampling of such tumors is required to avoid an erroneous diagnosis of ganglioneuroma.

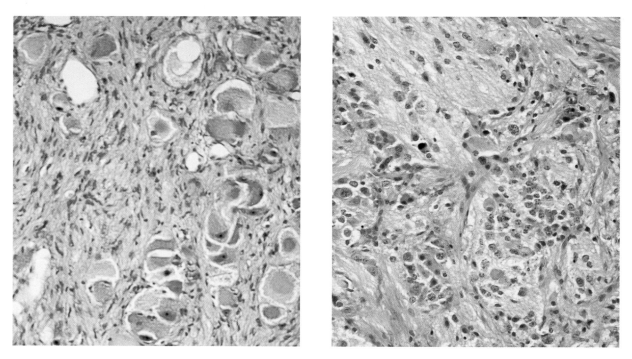

Figure 10-48

NEUROBLASTOMA WITH GANGLIONEUROMATOUS MATURATION OF METASTASIS

The orbital metastasis (left) of an adrenal gland primary (right).

REFERENCES

Nerve Sheath Myxoma

1. Harkins J, Reed RJ. Tumors of the peripheral nervous system. Atlas of Tumor Pathology, 2nd Series, Fascicle 3. Washington, DC: Armed Forces Institute of Pathology; 1969.
2. Pulitzer DR, Reed RJ. Nerve-sheath myxoma (perineurial myxoma). Am J Dermatopathol 1985;7:409-421.
3. Gallager RL, Helwig EB. Neurothekeoma—a benign cutaneous tumor of neural origin. Am J Clin Pathol 1980;74:759-764.
4. Fetsch JF, Laskin WB, Miettinen M. Nerve sheath myxoma: a clinicopathologic and immunohisto-chemical analysis of 57 morphologically distinctive, S-100 protein- and GFAP-positive, myxoid peripheral nerve sheath tumors with a predilection for the extremities and a high local recurrence rate. Am J Surg Pathol 2005;29:1615-1624.
5. Scheithauer BW, Woodruff JM, Erlandson RA. Tumors of the peripheral nervous system. AFIP Atlas of Tumor Pathology, 3rd Series, Fascicle 24. Washington, DC: American Registry of Pathology; 1999.
6. Goldstein J, Lifshitz T. Myxoma of the nerve sheath. Report of three cases, observations by light and electron microscopy and histochemical analysis. Am J Dermatopathol 1985;7:423-429.
7. Holden CA, Wilson-Jones E, MacDonald DM. Cutaneous lobular neuromyxoma. Br J Dermatol 1982;106:211-215.
8. Angervall L, Kindblom LG, Haglid K. Dermal nerve sheath myxoma. A light and electron microscopic, histochemical and immunohisto-chemical study. Cancer 1984;53:1752-1759.
9. Blumberg AK, Kay S, Adelaar RS. Nerve sheath myxoma of digital nerve. Cancer 1989;63:1215-1218.
10. Argenyi ZB, LeBoit PE, Santa Cruz D, Swanson PE, Kutzner H. Nerve sheath myxoma (neurothekeoma) of the skin: light microscopic and immunohistochemical reappraisal of the cellular variant. J Cutan Pathol 1993;20:294-303.
11. Laskin WB, Fetsch JF, Miettinen M. The "neurothekeoma": immunohistochemical analysis distinguishes the true nerve sheath myxoma from its mimics. Hum Pathol 2000;31:1230-1241.
12. Argenyi ZB, Kutzner H, Seaba MM. Ultrastruc-tural spectrum of cutaneous nerve sheath myxoma/cellular neurothekeoma. J Cutan Pathol 1995;22:137-145.
13. Webb JN. The histogenesis of nerve sheath myxoma: report of a case with electron microscopy. J Pathol 1979;127:35-37.
14. Fetsch JF, Laskin WB, Hallman JR, Lupton GP, Miettinen M. Neurothekeoma: an analysis of 178 tumors with detailed immunohistochemical data and long-term patient follow-up information. Am J Surg Pathol 2007;31:1103-1114.
15. Hornick JL, Fletcher CD. Cellular neurothekeoma: detailed characterization in a series of 133 cases. Am J Surg Pathol 2007;31:329-340.
16. Barnhill RL, Mihm MC Jr. Cellular neurothekeoma. A distinctive variant of neurothekeoma mimicking nevomelanocytic tumors. Am J Surg Pathol 1990;14:113-120.
17. Kao GF, Penneys NS. Immunohistochemical findings of 34 neurothekeomas (benign peripheral nerve sheath tumor) [Abstract]. J Cutan Pathol 1990;17:304.
18. Barnhill RL, Dickersin GR, Nickeleit V, et al. Studies on the cellular origin of neurothekeoma: clinical, light microscopic, immunohistochemical, and ultrastructural observations. J Am Acad Dermatol 1991;25(1 Pt 1):80-88.
19. Kerns MJ, Mutasim DF. Focal cutaneous mucinosis in Graves disease: relation to pretibial myxedema. Am J Dermatopathol 2010;32:196-197.
20. Allen PW, Dymock RB, MacCormac LB. Superficial angiomyxomas with and without epithelial components. Report of 30 tumors in 28 patients. Am J Surg Pathol 1988;12:519-530.
21. Calonje E, Guerin D, McCormick D, Fletcher CD. Superficial angiomyxoma: clinicopathologic analysis of a series of distinctive but poorly recognized cutaneous tumors with tendency for recurrence. Am J Surg Pathol 1999;23:910-917.
22. Carney JA, Hruska LS, Beauchamp GD, Gordon H. Dominant inheritance of the complex of myxomas, spotty pigmentation, and endocrine overactivity. Mayo Clin Proc 1986;61:165-172.
23. Carney JA. The Carney complex (myxomas, spotty pigmentation, endocrine overactivity, and schwannomas). Dermatol Clin 1995;13:19-26.
24. Michal M, Kazakov DV, Belousova I, Bisceglia M, Zamecnik M, Mukensnabl P. A benign neoplasm with histopathological features of both schwannoma and retiform perineurioma (benign schwannoma-perineurioma): a report of six cases of a distinctive soft tissue tumor with a predilection for the fingers. Virchows Arch 2004;445:347-353.
25. Liegl B, Bennett MW, Fletcher CD. Microcystic/reticular schwannoma: a distinct variant with predilection for visceral locations. Am J Surg Pathol 2008;32:1080-1087.

341

Benign Granular Cell Tumor

26. LeBoit PE, Barr RJ, Burall S, Metcalf JS, Yen TS, Wick MR. Primitive polypoid granular-cell tumor and other cutaneous granular-cell neoplasms of apparent nonneural origin. Am J Surg Pathol 1991;15:48-58.

27. Zaenglein AL, Meehan SA, Orlow SJ. Congenital granular cell tumors localized to the arm. Pediatr Dermatol 2001;18:234-237.

28. Gleason BC, Nascimento AF. HMB-45 and Melan-A are useful in the differential diagnosis between granular cell tumor and malignant melanoma. Am J DermatoPathol 2007;29:22-27.

29. Abrikossoff A. [Myomas originating from transversely striated voluntary musculature.] Virchows Arch A Pathol Anat Histol 1926;260:215-233. [German]

30. Fust JA, Custer RP. On the neurogenesis of so-called granular cell myoblastoma. Am J Clin Pathol 1949;19:522-535.

31. Carvalho GA, Lindeke A, Tatagiba M, Ostertag H, Samii M. Cranial granular-cell tumor of the trigeminal nerve. Case report. J Neurosurg 1994;81:795-798.

32. Chimelli L, Symon L, Scaravilli F. Granular cell tumor of the fifth cranial nerve: further evidence for Schwann cell origin. J Neuropathol Exp Neurol 1984;43:634-642.

33. May M, Beckford NS, Bedetti CD. Granular cell tumor of facial nerve diagnosed at surgery for idiopathic facial nerve paralysis. Otolaryngol Head Neck Surg 1985;93:122-126.

34. Bangle R Jr. An early granular-cell myoblastoma confined within a small peripheral myelinated nerve. Cancer 1953;6:790-793.

35. Budzilovich GN. Granular cell "myoblastoma" of vagus nerve. Acta Neuropathol 1968;10:162-165.

36. Dahlin LB, Lorentzen M, Besjakov J, Lundborg G. Granular cell tumour of the ulnar nerve in a young adult. Scand J Plast Reconstr Surg Hand Surg 2002;36:46-49.

37. Lee J, Bhawan J, Wax F, Farber J. Plexiform granular cell tumor. A report of two cases. Am J DermatoPathol 1994;16:537-541.

38. Yasutomi T, Koike H, Nakatsuchi Y. Granular cell tumour of the ulnar nerve. J Hand Surg Br 1999;24:122-124.

39. Mazur MT, Shultz JJ, Myers JL. Granular cell tumor. Immunohistochemical analysis of 21 benign tumors and one malignant tumor. Arch Pathol Lab Med 1990;114:692-696.

40. Lack EE, Worsham GF, Callihan MD, et al. Granular cell tumor: a clinicopathologic study of 110 patients. J Surg Oncol 1980;13:301-316.

41. Ordonez NG. Granular cell tumor: a review and update. Adv Anat Pathol 1999;6:186-203.

42. Brannon RB, Anand PM. Oral granular cell tumors: an analysis of 10 new pediatric and adolescent cases and a review of the literature. J Clin Pediatr Dent 2004;29:69-74.

43. Reinshagen K, Wessel LM, Roth H, Waag KL. Congenital epulis: a rare diagnosis in paediatric surgery. Eur J Pediatr Surg 2002;12:124-126.

44. Tucker MC, Rusnock EJ, Azumi N, Hoy GR, Lack EE. Gingival granular cell tumors of the newborn. An ultrastructural and immunohistochemical study. Arch Pathol Lab Med 1990;114(8):895-898.

45. Peterson LJ. Granular-cell tumor. Review of the literature and report of a case. Oral Surg Oral Med Oral Pathol 1974;37:728-735.

46. Martin RW 3rd, Neldner KH, Boyd AS, Coates PW. Multiple cutaneous granular cell tumors and neurofibromatosis in childhood. A case report and review of the literature. Arch Dermatol 1990;126:1051-1056.

47. Seo IS, Azzarelli B, Warner TF, Goheen MP, Senteney GE. Multiple visceral and cutaneous granular cell tumors. Ultrastructural and immunocytochemical evidence of Schwann cell origin. Cancer 1984;53:2104-2110.

48. Kontani K, Okaneya T, Takezaki T. Recurrent granular cell tumour of the bladder in a patient with von Recklinghausen's disease. BJU Int 1999;84:871-872.

49. Alessi DM, Zimmerman MC. Granular cell tumors of the head and neck. Laryngoscope 1988;98(Pt 1):810-814.

50. Miller AS, Leifer C, Chen SY, Harwick RD. Oral granular-cell tumors. Report of twenty-five cases with electron microscopy. Oral Surg Oral Med Oral Pathol 1977;44:227-237.

51. DeMay RM, Kay S. Granular cell tumor of the breast. Pathol Annu 1984;19(Pt 2):121-148.

52. Compagno J, Hyams VJ, Ste-Marie P. Benign granular cell tumors of the larynx: a review of 36 cases with clinicopathologic data. Ann Otol Rhinol Laryngol 1975;84(Pt 1):308-314.

53. Szumilo J, Skomra D, Zinkiewicz K, Zgodzinski W. Multiple synchronous granular cell tumours of the esophagus: a case report. Ann Univ Mariae Curie Sklodowska Med 2001;56:253-256.

54. Goldblum JR, Rice TW, Zuccaro G, Richter JE. Granular cell tumors of the esophagus: a clinical and pathologic study of 13 cases. Ann Thorac Surg 1996;62:860-865.

55. Johnston J, Helwig EB. Granular cell tumors of the gastrointestinal tract and perianal region: a study of 74 cases. Dig Dis Sci 1981;26:807-816.

56. Bodic O, Couderc JP, Cuilliere P, et al. [Multiple granular cell tumor of the colon]. Ann Pathol 1992;12:130-134. [French]

57. Melo CR, Melo IS, Schmitt FC, Fagundes R, Amendola D. Multicentric granular cell tumor of the colon: report of a patient with 52 tumors. Am J Gastroenterol 1993;88:1785-1787.

58. Ashokkumar O, Rodin A. Granular cell tumour of the vulva: very rare neoplasm of female genitalia. J Obstet Gynaecol 2004;24:830.

59. Papalas JA, Shaco-Levy R, Robboy SJ, Selim MA. Isolated and synchronous vulvar granular cell tumors: a clinicopathologic study of 17 cases in 13 patients. Int J Gynecol Pathol 2010;29:173-180.

60. Laskin WB, Fetsch JF, Davis CJ Jr, Sesterhenn IA. Granular cell tumor of the penis: clinico-pathologic evaluation of 9 cases. Hum Pathol 2005;36:291-298.

61. Epstein DS, Pashaei S, Hunt E Jr, Fitzpatrick JE, Golitz LE. Pustulo-ovoid bodies of Milian in granular cell tumors. J Cutan Pathol 2007;34:405-409.

62. Shintaku M, Sasaki M. Angulate body cell: an immunohistochemical and ultrastructural study. Brain Tumor Pathol 1992;9:41-47.

63. Frable MA, Fischer RA. Granular cell myoblastomas. Laryngoscope 1976;86:36-42.

64. Lowhagen T, Rubio CA. The cytology of the granular cell myoblastoma of the breast. Report of a case. Acta Cytologica 1977;21:314-315.

65. Le BH, Boyer PJ, Lewis JE, Kapadia SB. Granular cell tumor: immunohistochemical assessment of inhibin-alpha, protein gene product 9.5, S100 protein, CD68, and Ki-67 proliferative index with clinical correlation. Arch Pathol Lab Med 2004;128:771-775.

66. Maiorano E, Favia G, Napoli A, et al. Cellular heterogeneity of granular cell tumours: a clue to their nature? J Oral Pathol Med 2000;29:284-290.

67. Miettinen M, Lehtonen E, Lehtola H, Ekblom P, Lehto VP, Virtanen I. Histogenesis of granular cell tumour--an immunohistochemical and ultrastructural study. J Pathol 1984;142:221-229.

68. Fine SW, Li M. Expression of calretinin and the alpha-subunit of inhibin in granular cell tumors. Am J Clin Pathol 2003;119:259-264.

69. Mukai M. Immunohistochemical localization of S-100 protein and peripheral nerve myelin proteins (P2 protein, P0 protein) in granular cell tumors. Am J Pathol 1983;112:139-146.

70. Clark HB, Minesky JJ, Agrawal D, Agrawal HC. Myelin basic protein and P2 protein are not immunohistochemical markers for Schwann cell neoplasms. A comparative study using antisera to S-100, P2, and myelin basic proteins. Am J Pathol 1985;121:96-101.

71. Penneys NS, Adachi K, Ziegels-Weissman J, Nadji M. Granular cell tumors of the skin contain myelin basic protein. Arch Pathol Lab Med 1983;107:302-303.

72. Murakata LA, Ishak KG. Expression of inhibin-alpha by granular cell tumors of the gallbladder and extrahepatic bile ducts. Am J Surg Pathol 2001;25:1200-1203.

73. Ulrich J, Heitz PU, Fischer T, Obrist E, Gullotta F. Granular cell tumors: evidence for heterogeneous tumor cell differentiation. An immunocytochemical study. Virchows Arch B Cell Pathol Incl Mol Pathol 1987;53:52-57.

74. Sobel HJ, Marquet E. Granular cells and granular cell lesions. Pathol Annu 1974;9:43-79.

75. Abenoza P, Sibley RK. Granular cell myoma and schwannoma: fine structural and immunohistochemical study. Ultrastruct Pathol 1987;11:19-28.

76. Alvarez-Fernandez E, Carretero-Albinana L. Bronchial granular cell tumor. Presentation of three cases with tissue culture and ultrastructural study. Arch Pathol Lab Med 1987;111:1065-1069.

77. Buley ID, Gatter KC, Kelly PM, Heryet A, Millard PR. Granular cell tumours revisited. An immunohistological and ultrastructural study. Histopathology 1988;12:263-274.

78. Damiani S, Koerner FC, Dickersin GR, Cook MG, Eusebi V. Granular cell tumour of the breast. Virchows Arch A Pathol Anat Histopathol 1992;420:219-226.

79. Dingemans KP, Mooi WJ, van den Bergh Weerman MA. Angulate lysosomes. Ultrastruct Pathol 1983;5:113-122.

80. Christ ML, Ozzello L. Myogenous origin of a granular cell tumor of the urinary bladder. Am J Clin Pathol 1971;56:736-749.

81. Suster S, Rosen LB, Sanchez JL. Granular cell leiomyosarcoma of the skin. Am J Dermatopathol 1988;10:234-239.

82. Zarineh A, Costa ME, Rabkin MS. Multiple hybrid granular cell tumor-perineuriomas. Am J Surg Pathol 2008;32:1572-1577.

83. Diaz-Flores L, Alvarez-Arguelles H, Madrid JF, Varela H, Gonzalez MP, Gutierrez R. Perineurial cell tumor (perineurioma) with granular cells. J Cutan Pathol 1997;24:575-579.

84. Carpenter PM, Grafe MR, Varki NM. Granular cells in a cellular neurilemmoma. Arch Pathol Lab Med 1992;116:1083-1085.

85. Rosso R, Scelsi M, Carnevali L. Granular cell traumatic neuroma: a lesion occurring in mastectomy scars. Arch Pathol Lab Med 2000;124:709-711.

86. Townsend MC, Stellato TA. Granular cell myoblastoma of the breast: a report of five cases and a review. Breast 1985;11:12-21.

87. Lazar AJ, Fletcher CD. Primitive nonneural granular cell tumors of skin: clinicopathologic analysis of 13 cases. Am J Surg Pathol 2005;29:927-934.

88. Filie AC, Lage JM, Azumi N. Immunoreactivity of S100 protein, alpha-1-antitrypsin, and CD68 in adult and congenital granular cell tumors. Mod Pathol 1996;9:888-892.

89. Torsiglieri AJ Jr, Handler SD, Uri AK. Granular cell tumors of the head and neck in children: the experience at the Children's Hospital of Philadelphia. Int J Pediatr Otorhinolaryngol 1991;21:249-258.

90. Chaudhry IH, Calonje E. Dermal non-neural granular cell tumour (so-called primitive polypoid granular cell tumour): a distinctive entity further delineated in a clinicopathological study of 11 cases. Histopathology 2005;47:179-185.

91. Habeeb AA, Salama S. Primitive nonneural granular cell tumor (so-called atypical polypoid granular cell tumor). Report of 2 cases with immunohistochemical and ultrastructural correlation. Am J Dermatopathol 2008;30:156-159.

92. Lerman M, Freedman PD. Nonneural granular cell tumor of the oral cavity: a case report and review of the literature. Oral Surg Oral Med Oral Pathol Oral Radiol Endod 2007;103:382-384.

93. Mentzel T, Wadden C, Fletcher CD. Granular cell change in smooth muscle tumours of skin and soft tissue. Histopathology 1994;24:223-231.

94. Nakamura T, Hirato J, Hotchi M, Kyoshima K, Nakamura Y. Astrocytoma with granular cell tumor-like changes. Report of a case with histochemical and ultrastructural characterization of granular cells. Acta Pathol Jpn 1990;40:206-211.

Ganglioneuroma

95. Loritz W. Ein Fall von gangliosen Neurom (Ganglion). Virchows Arch Pathol Anat 1870;49:435-441.

96. Stout AP. Ganglioneuroma of the sympathetic nervous system. Surg Gynecol Obstet 1947;84:101-110.

97. Cushing H, Wolbach SB. The transformation of a malignant paravertebral sympathicoblastoma into a benign ganglioneuroma. Am J Pathol 1927;3:203-216.7.

98. Fox F, Davidson J, Thomas LB. Maturation of sympathicoblastoma into ganglioneuroma; report of 2 patients with 20-and 46-year survivals respectively. Cancer 1959;12:108-116.

99. Garvin JH Jr, Lack EE, Berenberg W, Frantz CN. Ganglioneuroma presenting with differentiated skeletal metastases. Report of a case. Cancer 1984;54:357-360.

100. Hayes FA, Green AA, Rao BN. Clinical manifestations of ganglioneuroma. Cancer 1989;63:1211-1214.

101. MacMillan RW, Blanc WB, Santulli TV. Maturation of neuroblastoma to ganglioneuroma in lymph nodes. J Pediatr Surg 1976;11:461-462.

102. Sitarz AL, Santulli TV, Wigger HJ, Berdon WE. Complete maturation of neuroblastoma with bone metastases in documented stages. J Pediatr Surg 1975;10:533-536.

103. Johnson DC, Teleg M, Eberle RC. Simultaneous occurrence of a ganglioneuroma and a neurilemmoma of the vagus nerve: a case report. Otolaryngol Head Neck Surg 1981;89:75-76.

104. Takeda S, Minami M, Inoue Y, Matsuda H. Synchronous mediastinal ganglioneuroma and retroperitoneal pheochromocytoma. Ann Thorac Surg 2005;80:1525-1527.

105. Moore PJ, Biggs PJ. Compound adrenal medullary tumor. South Med J 1995;88:475-478.

106. Schmitt HP, Wurster K, Bauer M, Parsch K. Mixed chemodectoma-ganglioneuroma of the conus medullaris region. Acta Neuropathol 1982;57:275-281.

107. Sonneland PR, Scheithauer BW, LeChago J, Crawford BG, Onofrio BM. Paraganglioma of the cauda equina region. Clinicopathologic study of 31 cases with special reference to immunocytology and ultrastructure. Cancer 1986;58:1720-1735.

108. Scheithauer BW, Nora FE, LeChago J, et al. Duodenal gangliocytic paraganglioma. Clinicopathologic and immunocytochemical study of 11 cases. Am J Clin Pathol 1986;86:559-565.

109. Miura K, Mineta H, Yokota N, Tsutsui Y. Olfactory neuroblastoma with epithelial and endocrine differentiation transformed into ganglioneuroma after chemoradiotherapy. Pathol Int 2001;51:942-947.

110. Sebire NJ, Ramsay AD, Malone M, Risdon RA. Extensive posttreatment ganglioneuromatous differentiation of rhabdomyosarcoma: malignant ectomesenchymoma in an infant. Pediatr Dev Pathol 2003;6:94-96.

111. Geoerger B, Hero B, Harms D, Grebe J, Scheidhauer K, Berthold F. Metabolic activity and clinical features of primary ganglioneuromas. Cancer 2001;91:1905-1913.

112. Jansson S, Dahlstrom A, Hansson G, Tisell LE, Ahlman H. Concomitant occurrence of an adrenal ganglioneuroma and a contralateral pheochromocytoma in a patient with von Recklinghausen's neurofibromatosis. An immunocytochemical study. Cancer 1989;63:324-329.

113. Sasaki Y, Nakayama H, Ikeda M. Turner syndrome and ganglioneuroma. J Pediatr Hematol Oncol 2000;22:89-90.

114. Thornburg CD, Shulkin BL, Castle VP, McAllister-Lucas LM. Thoracic neural crest tumors in Beckwith-Wiedemann syndrome. Med Pediatr Oncol 2003;41:468-469.

115. Tei R, Morimoto T, Miyamoto K, et al. Intradural extramedullary ganglioneuroma associated with multiple hamartoma syndrome. Neurol Med Chir (Tokyo) 2007;47:513-515.

116. Robertson CM, Tyrrell JC, Pritchard J. Familial neural crest tumours. Eur J Pediatr 1991;150:789-792.

117. Crissman JW, Valerio MG, Asiedu SA, Evangelista-Sobel I. Ganglioneuromas of the thyroid gland in a colony of Sprague-Dawley rats. Vet Pathol 1991;28:354-362.

118. Cerullo G, Marrelli D, Rampone B, et al. Presacral ganglioneuroma: a case report and review of literature. World J Gastroenterol 2007;13:2129-2131.

119. Woog JJ, Albert DM, Craft J, Silberman N, Horns D. Choroidal ganglioneuroma in neurofibromatosis. Graefes Arch Clin Exp Ophthalmol 1983;220:25-31.

120. Cannon TC, Brown HH, Hughes BM, Wenger AN, Flynn SB, Westfall CT. Orbital ganglioneuroma in a patient with chronic progressive proptosis. Arch Ophthalmol 2004;122:1712-1714.

121. Keefe JF, Kobrine AI, Kempe LG. Primary ganglioneuroma of the posterior cranial fossa: case report. Mil Med 1976;141:115-116.

122. Levy DI, Bucci MN, Weatherbee L, Chandler WF. Intradural extramedullary ganglioneuroma: case report and review of the literature. Surg Neurol 1992;37:216-218.

123. Young WG. Histopathologic study of ganglioneuroma in the mandible. J Oral Surg 1967;25:327-335.

124. Ozluoglu LN, Yilmaz I, Cagici CA, Bal N, Erdogan B. Ganglioneuroma of the internal auditory canal: a case report. Audiol Neurootol 2007;12:160-164.

125. Hammond RR, Walton JC. Cutaneous ganglioneuromas: a case report and review of the literature. Hum Pathol 1996;27:735-738.

126. Lee JY, Martinez AJ, Abell E. Ganglioneuromatous tumor of the skin: a combined heterotopia of ganglion cells and hamartomatous neuroma: report of a case. J Cutan Pathol 1988;15:58-61.

127. Murphy JG, Barnett NP, Goldstein AL, Colby SM. Gender moderates the relationship between substance-free activity enjoyment and alcohol use. Psychol Addict Behav 2007;21:261-265.

128. Rios JJ, Diaz-Cano SJ, Rivera-Hueto F, Villar JL. Cutaneous ganglion cell choristoma. Report of a case. J Cutan Pathol 1991;18:469-473.

129. Wallace CA, Hallman JR, Sangueza OP. Primary cutaneous ganglioneuroma: a report of two cases and literature review. Am J Dermatopathol 2003;25:239-242.

130. Thway K, Fisher C. Diffuse ganglioneuromatosis in small intestine associated with neurofibromatosis type 1. Ann Diagn Pathol 2009;13:50-54.

131. Ledwidge SF, Moorghen M, Longman RJ, Thomas MG. Adult transmural intestinal ganglioneuromatosis is not always associated with multiple endocrine neoplasia or neurofibromatosis: a case report. J Clin Pathol 2007;60:222-223.

132. Nguyen AT, Zacharin MR, Smith M, Hardikar W. Isolated intestinal ganglioneuromatosis with a new mutation of RET proto-oncogene. Eur J Gastroenterol Hepatol 2006;18:803-805.

133. Al-Daraji WI, Abdellaoui A, Salman WD. Solitary polypoidal rectal ganglioneuroma: a rare presentation of a rare tumor. J Gastroenterol Hepatol 2005;20:961-963.

134. Beer TW. Solitary ganglioneuroma of the rectum: report of two cases. J Clin Pathol 1992;45:353-355.

135. Zarabi M, LaBach JP. Ganglioneuroma causing acute appendicitis. Hum Pathol 1982;13:1143-1146.

136. Markaki S, Edwards C. Intrapulmonary ganglioneuroma. A case report. Arch Anat Cytol Pathol 1987;35:183-184.

137. Scheithauer BW, Santi M, Richter ER, Belman B, Rushing EJ. Diffuse ganglioneuromatosis and plexiform neurofibroma of the urinary bladder: report of a pediatric example and literature review. Hum Pathol 2008;39:1708-1712.

138. Wyman HE, Chappell BS, Jones WR Jr. Ganglioneuroma of bladder: report of a case. J Urol 1950;63:526-532.

139. Nassiri M, Ghazi C, Stivers JR, Nadji M. Ganglioneuroma of the prostate. A novel finding in neurofibromatosis. Arch Pathol Lab Med 1994;118:938-939.

140. Mendelsohn G, Eggleston JC, Olson JL, Said SI, Baylin SB. Vasoactive intestinal peptide and its relationship to ganglion cell differentiation in neuroblastic tumors. Lab Invest 1979;41:144-149.

141. Trump DL, Livingston JN, Baylin SB. Watery diarrhea syndrome in an adult with ganglioneuroma-pheochromocytoma: identification of vasoactive intestinal peptide, calcitonin, and catecholamines and assessment of their biologic activity. Cancer 1977;40:1526-1532.

142. Usuda H, Emura I. Composite paraganglioma-ganglioneuroma of the urinary bladder. Pathol Int 2005;55:596-601.

143. Lucas K, Gula MJ, Knisely AS, Virgi MA, Wollman M, Blatt J. Catecholamine metabolites in ganglioneuroma. Med Pediatr Oncol 1994;22:240-243.

144. Aguirre P, Scully RE. Testosterone-secreting adrenal ganglioneuroma containing Leydig cells. Am J Surg Pathol 1983;7:699-705.

145. Nagashima F, Hayashi J, Araki Y, et al. Silent mixed ganglioneuroma/pheochromocytoma which produces a vasoactive intestinal polypeptide. Intern Med 1993;32:63-66.

146. Kyoshima K, Sakai K, Kanaji M, et al. Symmetric dumbbell ganglioneuromas of bilateral C2 and C3 roots with intradural extension associated with von Recklinghausen's disease: case report. Surg Neurol 2004;61:468-473; discussion 473.

147. Ugarriza LF, Cabezudo JM, Ramirez JM, Lorenzana LM, Porras LF. Bilateral and symmetric C1-C2 dumbbell ganglioneuromas producing severe spinal cord compression. Surg Neurol 2001;55:228-231.

148. Duffy S, Jhaveri M, Scudierre J, Cochran E, Huckman M. MR imaging of a posterior mediastinal ganglioneuroma: fat as a useful diagnostic sign. AJNR Am J Neuroradiol 2005;26:2658-2662.

149. Adachi S, Kawamura N, Hatano K, et al. Lipomatous ganglioneuroma of the retroperitoneum. Pathol Int 2008;58:183-186.

150. Shotton JC, Milton CM, Allen JP. Multiple ganglioneuroma of the neck. J Laryngol Otol 1992;106:277-278.

151. Vaziri M, Mehrazma M. Massive spontaneous hemothorax associated with Von Recklinghausen's disease. Ann Thorac Surg 2006;82:1500-1501.

152. de Montpreville VT, Mussot S, Gharbi N, Dartevelle P, Dulmet E. Paraganglioma with ganglioneuromatous component located in the posterior mediastinum. Ann Diagn Pathol 2005;9:110-114.

153. Yoshimi N, Tanaka T, Hara A, Bunai Y, Kato K, Mori H. Extra-adrenal pheochromocytoma-ganglioneuroma. A case report. Pathol Res Pract 1992;188:1098-1100; discussion 1101-1103.

154. Chetty R, Duhig JD. Bilateral pheochromocytoma-ganglioneuroma of the adrenal in type 1 neurofibromatosis. Am J Surg Pathol 1993;17:837-841.

155. Kahn HJ, Baumal R, Thorner PS, Chan H. Binding of peanut agglutinin to neuroblastomas and ganglioneuromas: a marker for differentiation of neuroblasts into ganglion cells. Pediatr Pathol 1988;8:83-93.

156. Graham DG. On the origin and significance of neuromelanin. Arch Pathol Lab Med 1979;103:359-362.

157. Mullins JD. A pigmented differentiating neuroblastoma: a light and ultrastructural study. Cancer 1980;46:522-528.

158. Salmi J, Pelto-Huikko M, Auvinen O, et al. Adrenal pheochromocytoma-ganglioneuroma producing catecholamines and various neuropeptides. Acta Med Scand 1988;224:403-408.

159. Brady S, Lechan RM, Schwaitzberg SD, Dayal Y, Ziar J, Tischler AS. Composite pheochromocytoma/ganglioneuroma of the adrenal gland associated with multiple endocrine neoplasia 2A: case report with immunohistochemical analysis. Am J Surg Pathol 1997;21:102-108.

160. Magro G, Ruggieri M, Fraggetta F, Grasso S, Viale G. Cathepsin D is a marker of ganglion cell differentiation in the developing and neoplastic human peripheral sympathetic nervous tissues. Virchows Arch 2000;437:406-412.

161. Becker H, Wirnsberger G, Ziervogel K, Hofler H. Immunohistochemical markers in (ganglio)neuroblastomas. Acta Histochem Suppl 1990;38:107-114.

162. Sasaki A, Ogawa A, Nakazato Y, Ishida Y. Distribution of neurofilament protein and neuron-specific enolase in peripheral neuronal tumours. Virchows Arch A Pathol Anat Histopathol 1985;407:33-41.

163. Molenaar WM, Baker DL, Pleasure D, Lee VM, Trojanowski JQ. The neuroendocrine and neural profiles of neuroblastomas, ganglioneuroblastomas, and ganglioneuromas. Am J Pathol 1990;136:375-382.

164. Trojanowski JQ, Molenaar WM, Baker DL, Pleasure D, Lee VM. Neural and neuroendocrine phenotype of neuroblastomas, ganglioneuroblastomas, ganglioneuromas and mature versus embryonic human adrenal medullary cells. Prog Clin Biol Res 1991;366:335-341.

165. Matsuda M, Nagashima K. Cytoplasmic tubular inclusion in ganglioneuroma. Acta Neuropathol 1984;64:81-84.

166. Bender BL, Ghatak NR. Light and electron microscopic observations on a ganglioneuroma. Acta Neuropathol 1978;42:7-10.

167. Goto S, Umehara S, Gerbing RB, et al. Histopathology (International Neuroblastoma Pathology Classification) and MYCN status in patients with peripheral neuroblastic tumors: a report from the Children's Cancer Group. Cancer 2001;92:2699-2708.

168. Daneshvar A. Pharyngeal traumatic neuromas and traumatic neuromas with mature ganglion cells (pseudoganglioneuromas). Am J Surg Pathol 1990;14:565-570.

169. Shimada H, Chatten J, Newton WA Jr, et al. Histopathologic prognostic factors in neuroblastic tumors: definition of subtypes of ganglioneuroblastoma and an age-linked classification of neuroblastomas. J Natl Cancer Inst 1984;73:405-416.

170. Karcioglu Z, Someren A, Mathes SJ. Ectomesenchymoma. A malignant tumor of migratory neural crest (ectomesenchyme) remnants showing ganglionic, schwannian, melanocytic and rhabdomyoblastic differentiation. Cancer 1977;39:2486-2496.

171. Kodet R, Kasthuri N, Marsden HB, Coad NA, Raafat F. Gangliorhabdomyosarcoma: a histopathological and immunohistochemical study of three cases. Histopathology 1986;10:181-193.

172. Goldman RL, Winterling AN, Winterling CC. Maturation of tumors of the sympathetic nervous system. Report of long-term survival in 2 patients, one with disseminated osseous metastases, and review of cases from the literature. Cancer 1965;18:1510-1516.

11 BENIGN AND MALIGNANT NON-NEUROGENIC TUMORS

BENIGN NON-NEUROGENIC TUMORS

Lipoma

Soft tissue lipomas secondarily compressing peripheral nerves are uncommon (1,2). They are well circumscribed by a delicate capsule, arise in subfacial tissue or in intermuscular planes, and are composed entirely of mature adipose tissue. In the upper extremity, the posterior interosseous nerve is most often affected by compression (3).

Lipoma of nerve sheath, defined by Terzis et al. (2), is rare and is a discrete, delicately encapsulated epineurial lesion (see chapter 6, fig. 6-8B) (4–6). Such tumors presumably arise in those portions of peripheral nerves having an appreciable content of epineurial adipose tissue (7). Such tumors usually affect the median or sciatic nerves or the brachial plexus and are typically painless. Most patients are adult females. Lesion duration is often less than 5 years, but the presentation may be in childhood.

Computerized tomography (CT) and magnetic resonance imaging (MRI) studies show that the circumscribed, solid lesions have the signal characteristics of fat. Open resection results in relief of symptoms without recurrence. Excision of both soft tissue and nerve sheath lipomas is curative and unassociated with neurologic deficits. Neither is accompanied by macrodactyly. For a discussion of lipomatosis of nerve, the reader is referred to chapter 6.

Cranial nerve lipomas, also termed *lipochoristomas*, are rare. Comprising less than 1 percent of cerebellopontine angle and acoustic meatus tumors, they present in adulthood and favor males. Most affect the 8th nerve, but occasionally, other cranial nerves are involved, including the trigeminal or facial (8–11). Up to 5 percent are bilateral (12). Although clinically confused with acoustic schwannoma, due to hearing loss, dizziness, or unilateral tinnitus, the neuroimaging characteristics of adipose tissue permit a preoperative diagnosis in nearly all instances (fig. 11-1, top). Microscopically, they consist of mature adipose tissue, fibrous tissue and tortuous vessels intimately associated with nerve fibers and fascicles, and neurons of Scarpa ganglion (fig. 11-1, bottom). As is the case in lipomas affecting other central nervous system (CNS) sites, the occasional presence of heterologous elements, particularly skeletal or smooth muscle (see figs. 6-15, 6-16) (13), suggests that lipomas of the 8th nerve may be malformative rather than neoplastic in nature. This view is supported by the recent molecular genetic finding that *HMGA2* rearrangements, although common in true lipomas, are rare in lipomatous lesions of the nervous system including such "lipomas" and lipofibromatous hamartomas (14). The relationship of muscle-containing lesions to intracranial neuromuscular choristoma (15), a rhabdomyomatous lesion with scant adipose tissue content (16) or none at all (17), remains unsettled (see Neuromuscular Choristoma, chapter 6). Although surgery leads to improvement in 50 percent of patients, new neurologic deficits are produced in most instances; preservation of hearing is possible in only 20 percent (12).

Spinal epidural lipomatosis, a rare disorder often associated with the administration of exogenous corticosteroids or with endogenous steroid excess (Cushing syndrome), may produce radiculopathy (18). It affects primarily the thoracolumbar region and occurs mainly in obese males. Surgical decompression is the treatment of choice.

Paraganglioma

General Features. Fully 90 percent of *paragangliomas* arise in the adrenal gland (pheochromocytoma). Of extra-adrenal paragangliomas, a similar proportion affects the carotid body, glomus jugulare, glomus tympanicum, and ganglia of the autonomic nervous system. Syndrome associations include von Hippel-Lindau disease and multiple

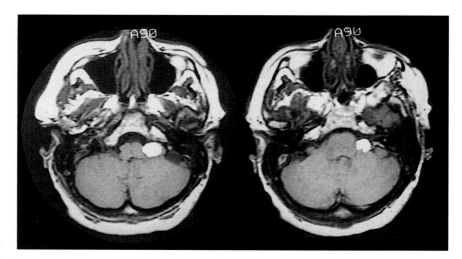

Figure 11-1

LIPOMA OF 8TH NERVE

Top: The magnetic resonance imaging (MRI) appearance of this lesion, here seen as a bright signal on a T1-weighted sequence, is diagnostic. (Courtesy of Dr. G.M. Miller, Rochester, MN.)

Bottom: Nerve fascicles and accompanying ganglion cells are entrapped by benign adipose tissue. (Courtesy of Dr. P.C. Burger, Baltimore, MD.)

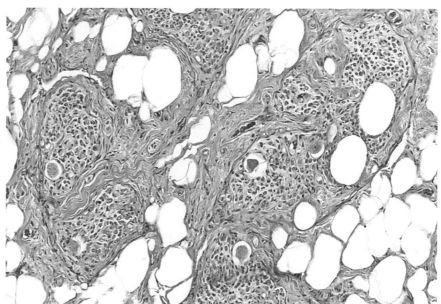

endocrine neoplasia type 2 (MEN 2). Mutations in the succinate dehydrogenase genes play a role in the tumorigenesis of paragangliomas (19).

Clinical Features. On occasion, extra-adrenal paragangliomas arise at sites lacking paraganglia, including the duodenum (20,21), filum terminale (22), pituitary gland, and pineal region (23). Cranial nerve examples also include paragangliomas of facial (24), hypoglossal (25), and vagal (26) nerves.

Sizable large nerves are occasionally affected by paraganglioma. These include nerve roots of the cauda equina (22,27–29) or other spinal levels (30). With few exceptions, paragangliomas of the cauda equina occur in adults, with a 2 to 1 male predilection. They cause low back pain, sensorimotor deficits, and bowel and bladder dysfunction. CT and MRI scans show contrast-enhancing, sausage-shaped masses. Most measure several centimeters in size, but one massive, 13-cm example has been reported (29). Their delicate fibrous capsules occasionally undergo calcification or ossification (fig. 11-2D) (31).

Microscopic Findings. Histologic patterns vary considerably. Most tumors show the zellballen formation typical of paragangliomas at other sites. Others feature a ribbon or pseudorosette pattern like that of carcinoid

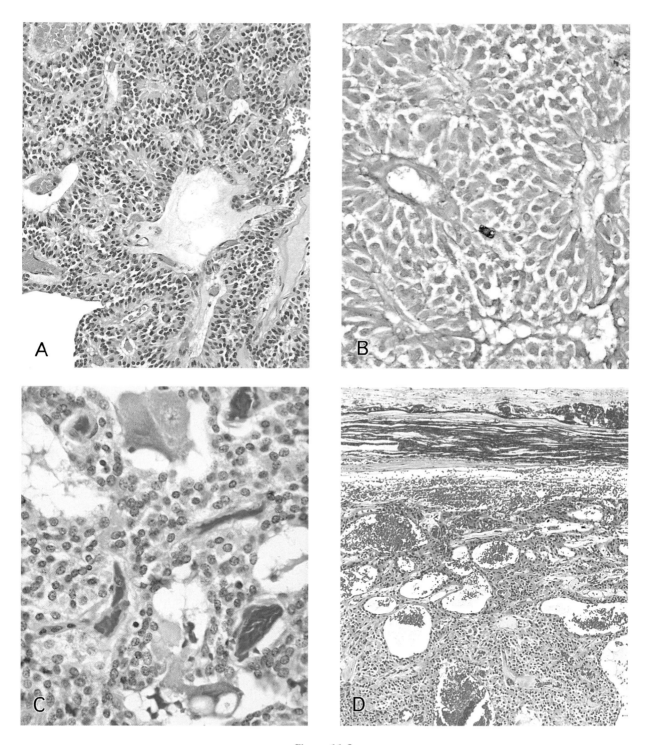

Figure 11-2

PARAGANGLIOMA OF NERVE ROOT

A,B: Although the occurrence of perivascular pseudorosettes and mucin accumulation may simulate myxopapillary ependymoma (A), argyrophilia (Grimelius stain) readily permits the correct diagnosis (B).

C: Half of cauda equina lesions show ganglionic differentiation.

D: Occasional examples have capsular calcifications. (D, courtesy of Dr. N. Karpinski, San Diego, CA.)

tumor (fig. 11-2A). Ganglionic differentiation (fig. 11-2C) is seen in up to half of cauda equina region paragangliomas (22). Oncocytic paraganglioma is rare (32). The neuroendocrine nature of the chief cells is confirmed by argyrophilia (fig. 11-2B), occasional argentaffin staining, and immunoreactivity for synaptophysin, chromogranin, and such neuropeptides as somatostatin, serotonin, or metenkephalin (22,33,34). Cytokeratin expression by chief cells is a frequent feature of paragangliomas of the cauda equina region (35). Clusters of chief cells are encircled by sustentacular cells, modified Schwann cells immunoreactive for S-100 protein and/or glial fibrillary acidic protein (GFAP).

Ultrastructural Findings. The ultrastructural findings are those of paragangliomas occurring at other sites (36) and include the presence within chief cells of 100- to 400-nm secretory granules, occasionally numerous or atypical mitochondria, moderately developed Golgi complexes, small stacks of rough endoplasmic reticulum, lysosomes in small number, occasional arrays of intermediate filaments and process formation, and rudimentary junctions. Sustentacular cells vary in number and may be absent, particularly in malignant examples.

Differential Diagnosis. Spinal intradural paragangliomas must be distinguished from myxopapillary ependymoma. In contrast to paraganglioma, ependymomas far more often break through their capsules to involve surrounding leptomeninges and nerve roots, exhibit widespread GFAP positivity, and lack both neuronal differentiation and immunoreactivity for neuroendocrine markers (6). Concurrence of paraganglioma and myxopapillary ependymoma has been described (39).

Treatment and Prognosis. While most nerve root paragangliomas lend themselves to gross total resection, some are locally invasive. This is particularly true of recurrent tumors. Of subtotally resected lesions, approximately 10 percent recur at 1 year (28). The aggressive potential of both adrenal and extra-adrenal paragangliomas is related to the anaplastic changes, which include diminution of or lack of neuropeptide immunoreactivity (34,37) and sustentacular cells (34), as well as the occurrence of metastases. The latter is rare in paraganglioma of nerve (30,38).

Angiomas of Nerve

General Features. Benign vascular lesions rarely affect nerve. They vary in type from *hemangioma* to *venous angioma* and *arteriovenous malformation* (40).

Clinical Features. The clinicopathologic features of the approximately 15 reported hemangiomas were recently summarized (41–43), as were those affecting the sciatic nerve (40). Half of the patients are of pediatric age, with a female sex predilection. There is also no association with prior trauma. Involved nerves include the median, ulnar, digital, sciatic, peroneal, and tibial; cranial nerves are rarely affected (44). Pain is the most common symptom, although early lesions may present as asymptomatic lumps. On MRI, flow voids are usually apparent. Angiography shows a tumor blush.

Microscopic Findings. Most hemangiomas are soft, globular lesions resembling nerve sheath tumor but with vessels infiltrating between nerve fascicles. Multiple tumors are rare, as is extensive "hemangiomatosis" of nerve (45). Affecting primarily epineurium, the hemangiomas are of *capillary* (figs. 11-3, 11-4), *venous* (figs. 11-5, 11-6), or *cavernous* (figs. 11-7, 11-8A) type (46).

A curious case of "angiomatosis of nerve" (fig. 11-9) associated with multiple soft tissue tumors (fig. 11-10) in the setting of progressive peripheral neuropathy has been reported (47). It featured a massive proliferation of small vessels with abnormally thick walls, extensively replacing both the endoneurium and perineurium of multiple peripheral nerves (fig. 11-9A,B). That the cells comprising the vessels were either pericytes or smooth muscle cells was suggested by intense immunoreactivity for actin and smooth muscle actin (fig. 11-9C), as well as by the ultrastructural features. The patient also exhibited multiple, often partially calcified soft tissue tumors. Histologically, these resembled infantile myofibromatosis (fig. 11-9D) and showed immunohistochemical and ultrastructural features of either smooth muscle or myofibroblastic differentiation. At surgery, a peripheral nerve branch appeared to course directly into one such tumor. This association of a diffuse polyneuropathy with widespread angiomatosis and multifocal soft tissue tumors (fig. 11-10) may well be a manifestation of a previously

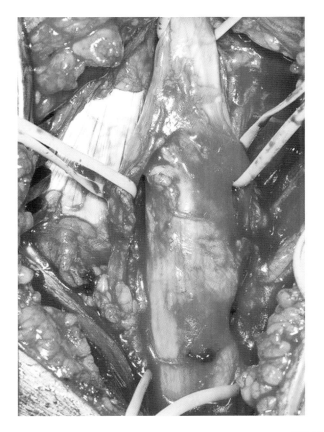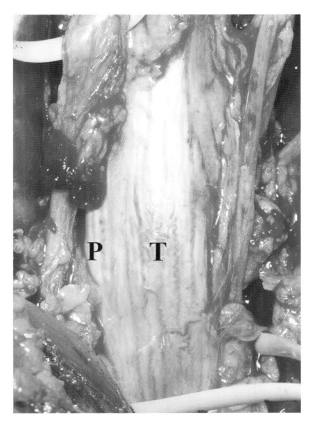

Figure 11-3

CAPILLARY HEMANGIOMA OF TIBIAL DIVISION OF THE SCIATIC NERVE

Left: The sciatic nerve proximal to the bifurcation shows no obvious abnormality.

Right: Upon opening the epineurium, red streaking corresponding to the hemangioma is well seen. P = peroneal division; T = tibial division. (Fig. 11 from Van Gompel JJ, Griessenauer CJ, Scheithauer BW, Amrami KK, Spinner RJ. Vascular malformations, rare causes of sciatic neuropathy: a case series. Neurosurgery 2010;67:1141.)

unrecognized syndrome. Soft tissue angiomatosis with involvement of small peripheral nerve fascicles has also been described (48).

Differential Diagnosis. Hemangiomas with a compact pattern of growth, particularly ones featuring mitotic activity, should not be mistaken for angiosarcoma (fig. 11-8B) (see below). An occasional feature of capillary hemangiomas is extramedullary erythropoiesis.

Treatment and Prognosis. Treatment has varied from intraneural dissection with gross total or partial tumor resection to excision of the affected nerve. With the exception of one case in which two partial resections failed to alleviate pain and necessitated amputation (45), all patients have experienced symptomatic improvement without tumor recurrence. A conservative, nerve-sparing approach is therefore recommended.

Glomus Tumor Variants

Glomus tumors are benign vascular neoplasms comprising about 1 percent of soft tissue tumors. They rarely affect nerve. Only 10 cases have been reported; the affected nerves included the radial nerve in the axillary region (fig. 11-11) (49), a dermal nerve in the shoulder (50), and digital nerves (51,52). All tumors occurred in adults, only two involving sizable, grossly apparent nerves. In the dermal example, a nerve association was evident only at the histologic level where nerve fiber bundles traversed the lesion and perilesional epineurium was observed (50). The various tumors ranged in size from several millimeters to 2.5 cm and appeared discrete. The largest resembled a schwannoma and "shelled out" with preservation of adjacent nerve fascicles (49). A nerve-sparing

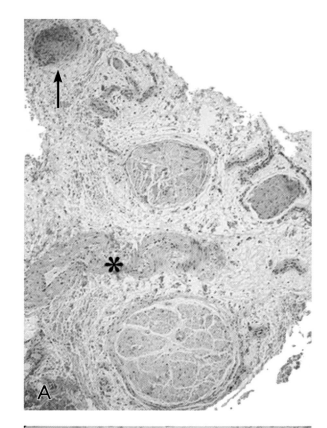

Figure 11-4

CAPILLARY HEMANGIOMA OF TIBIAL NERVE

A: The hemangioma, present as tufts of densely compacted capillaries (arrowhead), is associated with a sizeable vein (*).

B,C: The capillary tufts are well seen at higher power (B) and on CD31 stain (arrowheads) (C). (Fig. 12 from Van Gompel JJ, Griessenauer CJ, Scheithauer BW, Amrami KK, Spinner RJ. Vascular malformations, rare causes of sciatic neuropathy: a case series. Neurosurgery 2010;67:1141.)

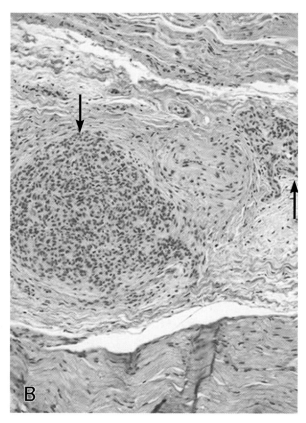

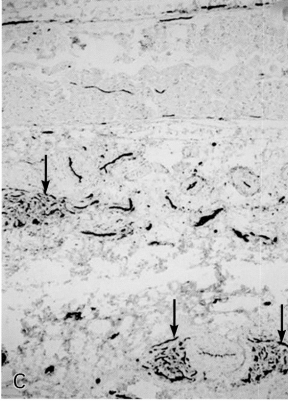

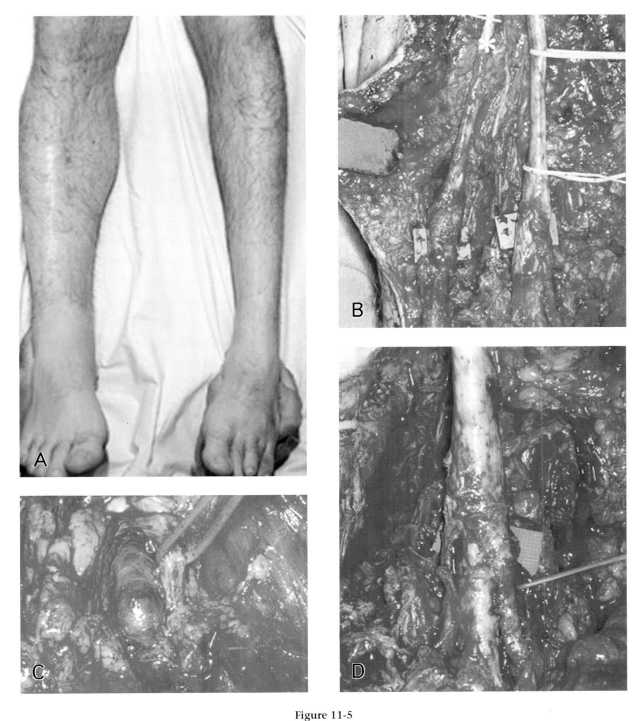

Figure 11-5

VENOUS ANGIOMA OF SCIATIC BIFURCATION IN KLIPPEL-TRENAUNAY SYNDROME

A: There is atrophy of the left lower limb.

B: Intraoperatively, the tibial and peroneal nerves appear abnormal (* = peroneal).

C: At high magnification red tape surrounds the vein of the tibial nerve.

D: The tibial nerve features a large vein within its perineurium. (Fig. 8 from Van Gompel JJ, Griessenauer CJ, Scheithauer BW, Amrami KK, Spinner RJ. Vascular malformations, rare causes of sciatic neuropathy: a case series. Neurosurgery 2010;67:1139.)

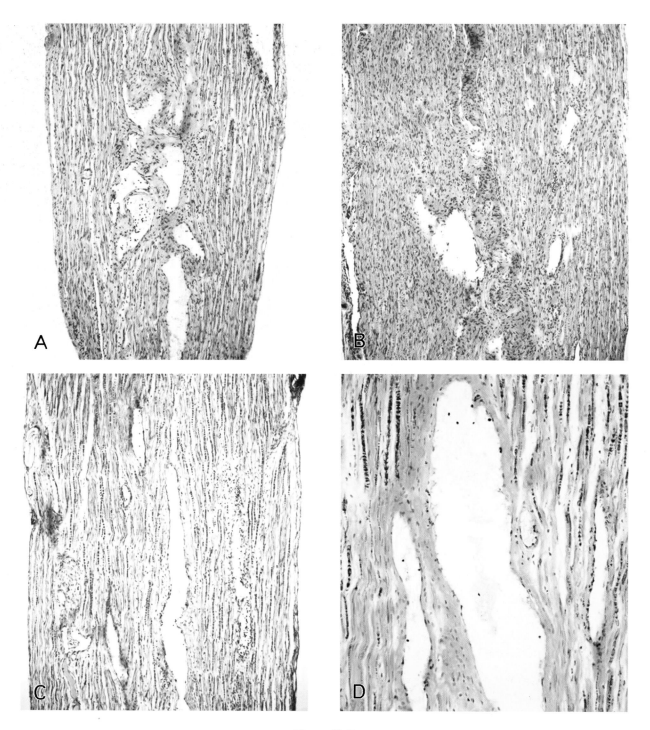

Figure 11-6

VENOUS MALFORMATION OF SCIATIC BIFURCATION IN KLIPPEL-TRENAUNAY SYNDROME

A,B: The biopsy reveals numerous thin-walled but media-containing veins within the endoneurium (hematoxylin and eosin [H&E] stain).

C,D: Veins are further highlighted on Luxol fast blue (C) and Masson trichrome stain (D). (Fig. 9 from Van Gompel JJ, Griessenauer CJ, Scheithauer BW, Amrami KK, Spinner RJ. Vascular malformations, rare causes of sciatic neuropathy: a case series. Neurosurgery 2010;67:1140.)

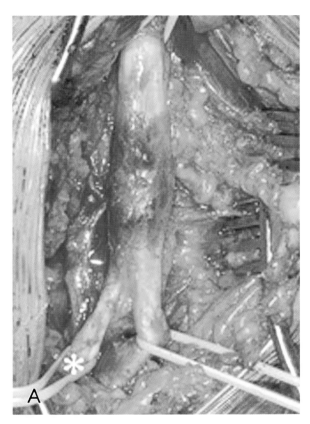

Figure 11-7

**CAVERNOUS AND VENOUS
HEMANGIOMA OF SCIATIC BIFURCATION**

A: The asterisk indicates the peroneal nerve.

A,B: Blue discoloration of the sciatic nerve is seen just proximal to the bifurcation.

C: On dissection, vessels interdigitate between the nerves. (Fig. 2 from Van Gompel JJ, Griessenauer CJ, Scheithauer BW, Amrami KK, Spinner RJ. Vascular malformations, rare causes of sciatic neuropathy: a case series. Neurosurgery 2010;67:1135.)

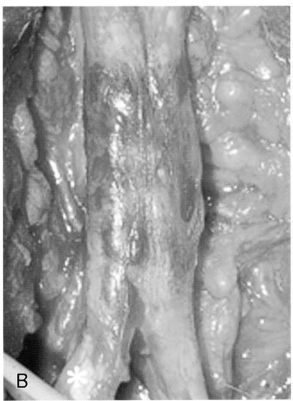

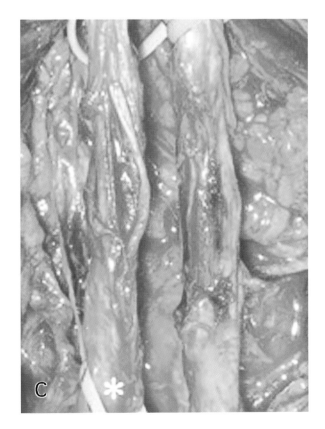

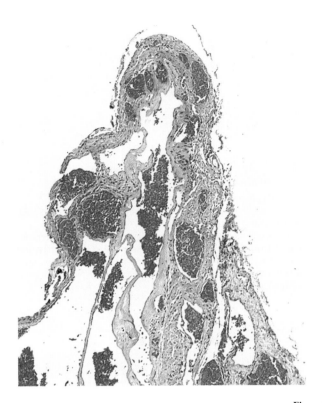 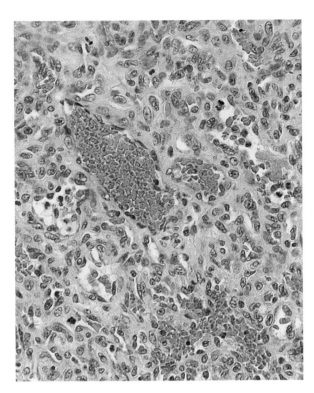

Figure 11-8

VASCULAR TUMORS OF NERVE

Left: Cavernous angiomas, such as this facial nerve lesion, consist of large vascular spaces composed of hyaline vessels. (Courtesy of Dr. D. Horoupian, Stanford, CA.)

Right: Whereas most capillary hemangiomas feature lobular architecture, with obvious lumen formation, occasional examples are cellular and mitotically active.

surgical approach is recommended. The occurrence of glomus tumors within nerve remains to be explained since glomus bodies are not normally encountered there.

Glomangiomas are less common than glomus tumors; most involve the distal upper extremity. Nerve-based examples are rare (fig. 11-12A–C) (53). Histologically, the tumors superficially resemble cavernous angiomas but with glomus cells in the interstices (fig. 11-12D).

Hemangioblastoma

General Features. Principally involving the CNS, *hemangioblastomas* are tumors of adulthood that most commonly arise in the cerebellum. Depending upon the site(s) in brain or spinal cord, one third to nearly all are associated with von Hippel-Lindau disease, an autosomal dominant disorder characterized by retinal, cerebellar, and/or spinal hemangioblastomas; renal

cell carcinoma; cysts or cystic neoplasms of the pancreas, liver, or epididymis; pheochromocytoma; and extra-adrenal paragangliomas (54). The 5 percent that arise in the spinal cord, often from its dorsal aspect, lie in close proximity to spinal nerve roots which may, on occasion, be directly involved (55,56).

Hemangioblastomas limited to nerve are rare. With the exception of two reported examples (57,58), all have been intradural, arising either from a sensory nerve root (55–60) or from a ganglion (61). Some are dumbbell shaped with intradural and extradural components (62). In one instance, multiple lesions of the filum terminale presented in pregnancy (63). In another case (55), multiple cervical, thoracic, and lumbar spinal cord hemangioblastomas of microscopic dimension were an incidental autopsy finding. Only one presumed cranial nerve example has been reported (64).

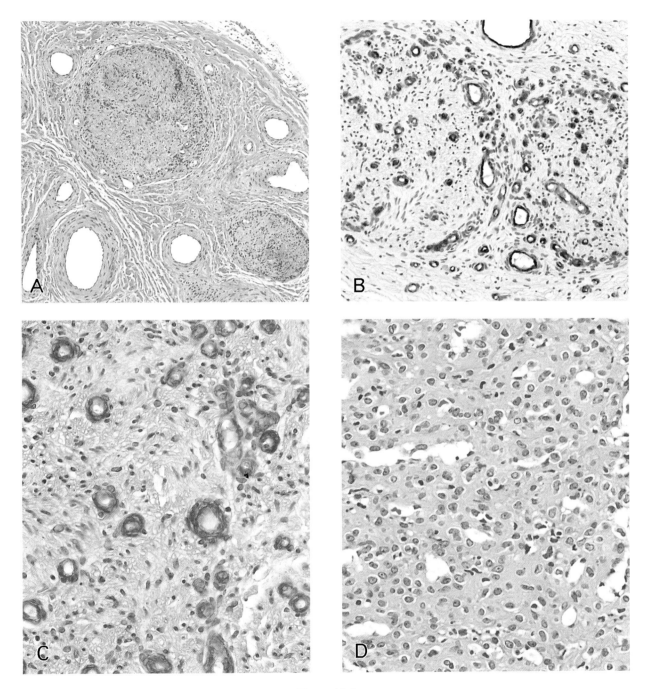

Figure 11-9

ANGIOMATOSIS OF PERIPHERAL NERVE

A: Sections of the sural nerve show that the architecture of the perineurium and endoneurium is retained. Myelinated fibers are severely and diffusely decreased. A striking proliferation of small vessels with thickened walls is present in the perineurium and extends into the endoneurium, partially replacing it.

B: These vessels are accentuated on immunostains for factor VIII-related antigen.

C: The cells present in the wall of the numerous, thickened perineurial and endoneurial vessels show intense immunoreactivity for alpha-smooth muscle actin.

D: The soft tissue nodules, this one from the lateral neck, show infantile myofibromatosis or hemangiopericytoma-like features. (All figures courtesy of Drs. C. Giannini, Treviso, Italy and P. J. Dyck, Rochester, MN.)

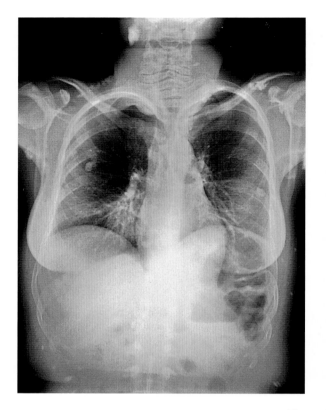
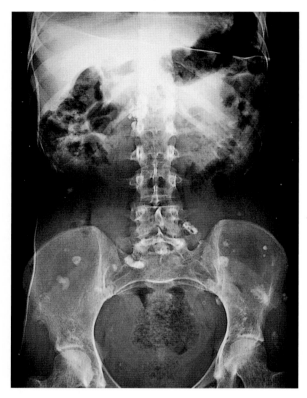

Figure 11-10

ANGIOMATOSIS OF PERIPHERAL NERVE WITH SOFT TISSUE TUMOR ASSOCIATION

Multiple, calcified, subcutaneous and deep soft tissue nodules ranging in size from 0.5 to 3.0 cm are present in the lateral neck, axilla, chest (left), and abdomen (right). (Left is fig. 1 from Giannini C, Wright A, Dyck PJ. Polyneuropathy associated with nerve angiomatosis and multiple soft tissue tumors. A newly recognized syndrome. Am J Surg Pathol 1995;19:1326.)

Figure 11-11

GLOMUS TUMOR OF NERVE

A,B: This well-demarcated brachial plexus example (A) arose in the epineurium of the radial nerve, displaced fascicles, and showed the typical histologic features of glomus tumor (B).

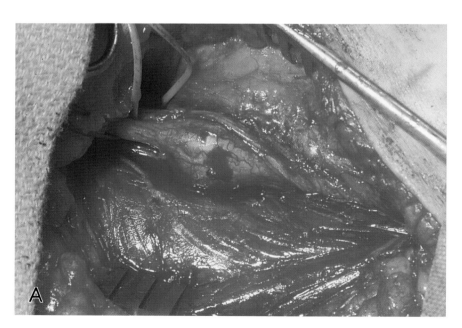

358

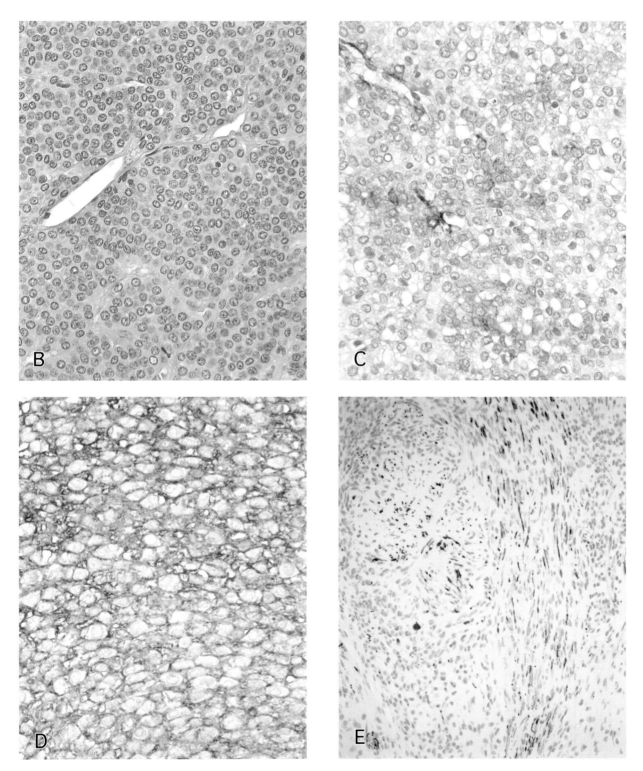

Figure 11-11, continued

C,D: The lesions show immunoreactivity for smooth muscle actin (C) and collagen 4 (D).

E: Infiltration of the nerve is evidenced by neurofilament protein immunoreactive axons within its substance. (Courtesy of Dr. S. E. MacKennan, St.Louis, MO.)

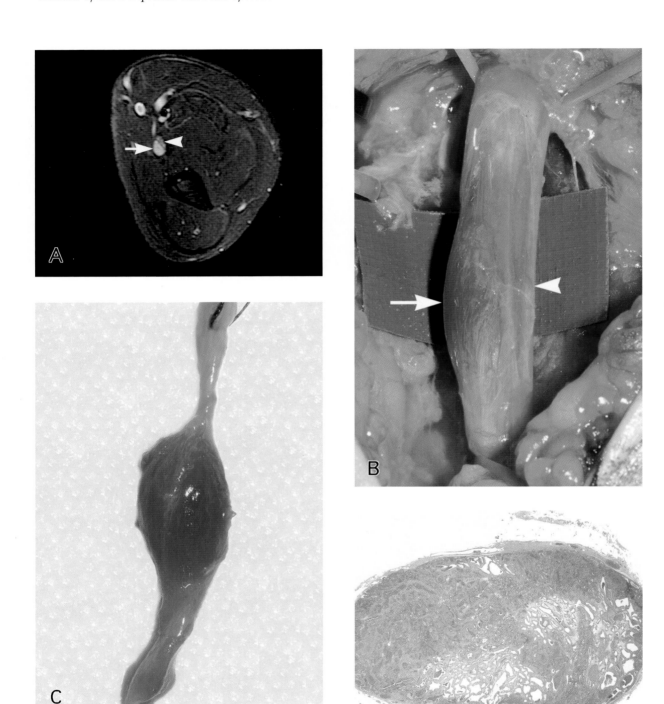

Figure 11-12

GLOMANGIOMA OF MEDIAN NERVE

A: Axial T2-weighted fast spin echo MRI with fat suppression shows focal enlargement of the nerve (arrow) and hyperintense fascicles (arrowhead).

B: The operative photo shows fusiform enlargement of the nerve affecting a fascicular group.

C: The tumor was totally resected.

D: Low-power micrograph shows the abundance of vasculature.

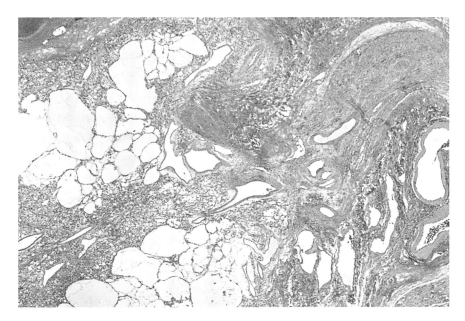

Clinical Features. Patient ages range from 17 to 79 years, with no sex predilection. Sensory symptoms predominate, due to the high frequency of posterior nerve root involvement in intradural tumors. With increase in tumor size, one lesion measuring up to 6.8 cm (60), spinal cord or anterior root compression produces motor symptoms.

Gross and Microscopic Findings. Grossly, the tumors are demarcated and yellow-red, and associated with prominent feeder vessels. Microscopically, they are often multinodular and show microcystic degeneration. They lie within epineurium, frequently abutting feeder vessels of varying size (fig. 11-13). At higher magnification, the stromal cells of hemangioblastoma, with their round nuclei and vacuolated, lipid-rich cytoplasm, fill the interstices between innumerable capillaries (fig. 11-14A). They are uniformly S-100 protein and inhibin immunopositive (fig. 11-14B,C). Unlike hemangioblastomas involving brain or spinal cord, which on occasion show unexplained GFAP reactivity, reported peripheral nerve examples are nonreactive for this antigen (57,58). Where fascicles are involved, the tumor cells lie among nerve fibers (fig. 11-14D). Hemangioblastomas have been reported to occur in soft tissue (65,66); however, their frequent lack of inhibin immunoreactivity (65) brings some of these diagnoses into question.

Differential Diagnosis. The principal entity in the differential diagnosis of hemangioblastoma of nerve or any other site is metastatic renal cell carcinoma, a lesion often associated with von Hippel-Lindau disease. Renal cell carcinomas stain for keratin and epithelial membrane antigen (EMA); however, 15 to 20 percent of primary and 50 percent of metastatic renal cell carcinomas are S-100 protein positive.

Treatment and Prognosis. The prognosis of patients with hemangioblastoma is excellent. No reported examples have recurred. Although invasion of nerve fascicles may necessitate sacrifice of the parent nerve, sparing it by microsurgical resection of the lesion appears to be the treatment of choice (58). Whereas radiotherapy plays a limited role in the treatment of cerebellar and spinal cord hemangioblastomas (67), adjuvant treatment has not been employed in peripheral nerve lesions.

Meningioma

Definition. *Peripheral nerve* and *ectopic meningiomas* are defined as meningiomas without a dural association that involve soft tissue, including peripheral nerve, skin, or viscera.

General Features. These are rare tumors, representing less than 1 percent of all meningiomas. Nearly all are sporadic in occurrence. In most instances, the finding of a meningioma outside the CNS is due to direct peripheral extension

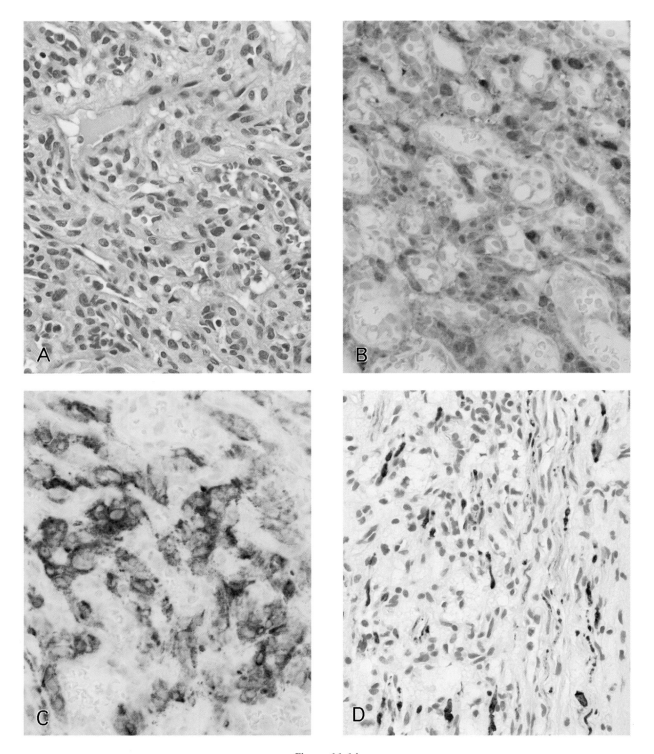

Figure 11-14

HEMANGIOBLASTOMA OF LUMBAR NERVE ROOT

A: Tumor stromal cells are vacuolated due to an abundance of cytoplasmic lipid.
B,C: Expected immunoreactivities include staining for S-100 protein (B) and inhibin (C).
D: Axons within these tumors are identified by their neurofilament protein immunoreactivity.

of cranial (68–70) or spinal nerve (71) meningiomas via osseous foramina. This is expected given the intimate association of the arachnoid membrane with proximal, intradural segments of cranial and spinal peripheral nerves. In one large study of meningiomas (72), 90 percent of which involved cranial dura, extension outside the CNS was noted in 20 percent. In decreasing order of frequency, secondarily affected sites included the orbit, skull and scalp, paranasal sinuses and nose, and the parotid and parapharyngeal regions.

Meningiomas rarely appear to be primarily in peripheral nerve. A review found that of approximately 75 meningiomas reported to arise outside the CNS, only 2 arose in a major peripheral nerve (69,73,74). One additional case has recently been described (75). Several other examples, variously quoted as originating in nerve, did not in fact do so (76,77).

Arachnoidal cells normally reside in the leptomeninges (arachnoid membrane), not in peripheral nerve. Similarly, meningiomas arise in the leptomeninges, and only secondarily involve dura. To the extent that cranial and proximal spinal nerve roots are ensheathed by arachnoid membrane, the growth of meningiomas may, to a significant extent, be along nerve. Thus, some meningiomas exit the CNS, even without a dural attachment (78,79), and follow the course of a nerve (71). Just how meningiomas arise in extradural portions of peripheral nerves is unclear, however. Proposed mechanisms underlying the occurrence of meningiomas outside the CNS include: 1) extradural trapping of arachnoidal cells during development; 2) migration of arachnoidal cells along developing peripheral nerves; and 3) metaplasia of soft tissue or peripheral nerve sheath cells to arachnoidal cells (80,81).

The distinction between lesions resulting from entrapment as opposed to migration is often difficult, since a parent nerve may not be found. Presumed examples of trapping include meningiomas involving calvarial diploe (82,83) and skin overlying the skull or spine (84,85). Rare examples of post-traumatic extracranial meningioma may also be viewed as a form of arachnoidal cell entrapment (86).

Peripheral meningiomas, perhaps arising by migration of arachnoidal cells along nerve, include those affecting the soft tissues of the head and neck (87), parotid and parapharyngeal regions (88), maxilla and oral cavity (89,90), nasopharynx (91), orbit, and temporal bone (87). Meningiomas of proximal nerve plexuses may also fall into this group (73–75). The fact that the leptomeninges are continuous with the perineurium may explain the occurrence of proximal examples (92), but the occasional finding of arachnoidal cell nests around otherwise normal peripheral nerves (74) suggests that the migration of these cells may also play a role.

The metaplasia concept perhaps better explains the finding of meningiomas at sites truly remote from the CNS. Experiments showing not only nerve sheath but a portion of the leptomeninges to be neuroectodermal in derivation (93) make this a plausible mechanism. A likely candidate to undergo arachnoidal metaplasia is the perineurial cell. Arachnoidal and perineurial cells share some similarities, both being vimentin and EMA reactive (94). There are differences, however. Electron microscopic studies show that meningothelial cells contain intermediate filaments and are interconnected by well-formed desmosomes, whereas perineurial cells are joined by tight junctions and possess a discontinuous pericellular basement membrane and pinocytotic vesicles, features alien to arachnoidal cells. Nonetheless, since some heterotopic meningiomas feature an intimate association with nerve, particularly cutaneous examples (85), arachnoidal metaplasia of nerve sheath or mesenchymal cells may explain the occurrence of meningiomas at remote sites (95), including finger (77), muscle of the thigh (96), and viscera, particularly the lung (97–99).

Only two peripheral nerve meningiomas have been reported to date. Both arose in adult females and involved the brachial plexus (73,74). A possible third example, a psammomatous meningioma, arose in the left neck of a 15-year-old male; firmly attached to the left accessory nerve, it also featured a fibrous string-like attachment to the vertebral column (100). One mandibular nerve tumor considered a meningioma (75) has since been found to be a perineurioma.

Microscopic Findings. Both peripheral nerve meningiomas reported to date were centered upon or accompanied medium sized or large

Table 11-1

FEATURES DIFFERENTIATING MENINGIOMA, SCHWANNOMA, AND SOFT TISSUE PERINEURIOMA

Features	Meningioma	Soft Tissue Schwannoma	Perineurioma
Antoni A and/or B pattern	(–)	Frequent	(–)
Verocay bodies	(–)	Frequent	(–)
Whorls	Frequent, tight	Rare, vague	Occasional, loose
Psammoma bodies	20%	Rare	(–)
Reticulin pattern	Variable	Intercellular	Intercellular
S-100 protein	18-80%	100%	(–)
EMA[a]	70-95%	(–)	100%
Cytokeratin	5%	(–)	(–)
Progesterone receptor	(+)	(–)	(–)
Glut-1	Weakly (+)	(–)	(+)
Claudin	Variable	(–)	(+)
Interdigitating cell membranes	Yes	No	No
Entangled cell processes	No	Yes	No
Junctions	Well-formed desmosomes	Rudimentary	Rudimentary and tight
Basement membranes	Absent	Continuous	Discontinuous

[a]EMA = epithelial membrane antigen.

nerves and were located in the epineurium (fig. 11-15A,B). As in the CNS, their morphologic spectrum includes a meningothelial (73) as well as a transitional example replete with psammoma bodies (74). Both were World Health Organization (WHO) grade I lesions. Immunohistochemistry, performed in one case, showed reactivity for EMA (fig. 11-15C) (73) and lack of reactivity for S-100 protein (fig. 11-15B), as well as GFAP, Leu-7, and keratin. The ultrastructural features of meningioma were noted in both studies (73,74).

Differential Diagnosis. The differential diagnosis of nerve-associated meningiomas requires knowledge of their operative anatomy. Given the greater frequency with which cranial and spinal meningiomas extend peripherally through dural root sleeves, confirmation of an ectopic origin requires attention to neuroimaging and surgical findings. Rare soft tissue meningiomas unassociated with nerve also enter into the differential (96). Perineurioma may be confused with meningioma, as illustrated by two examples, one mandibular (75) and another of the foot (101). Given the morphologic spectrum of meningiomas, the differential

diagnosis is broad. In the context of a nerve association, it includes mainly schwannoma and an occasional soft tissue perineurioma. Their distinguishing features relative to meningioma are summarized in Table 11-1. A full discussion of the differential diagnosis of meningioma may be found in the Armed Forces Institute of Pathology (AFIP) Fascicle, Tumors of the Central Nervous System (102).

Treatment and Prognosis. Information regarding the treatment and prognosis of peripheral nerve meningiomas is scant. Too few examples have been reported to draw conclusions. The subtotally excised brachial plexus tumor of Coons and Johnson (73) was associated with multiple recurrences despite the absence of atypia. After multiple partial resections and two courses of radiotherapy, the patient is alive at 17 years with persistent disease. The patient that Hallgrimsson et al. (100) treated by nerve-sparing resection was tumor-free at 3 years. Depending upon the nerve affected, total removal or simple debulking of tumor may suffice. In any case, invasion of nerve by meningiomas may underlie recurrences (103). As at other sites, radiation therapy may be required (73).

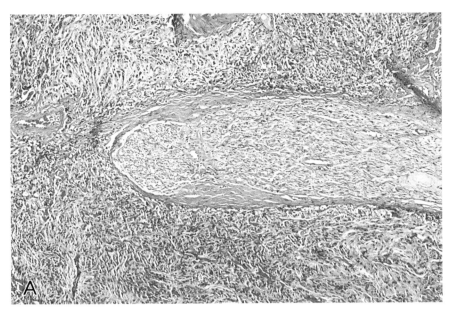

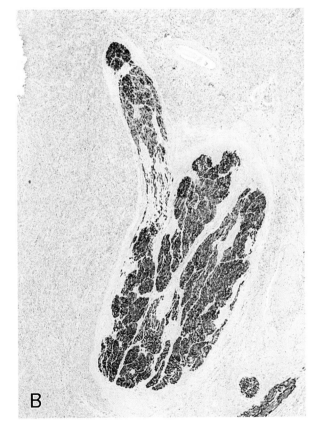

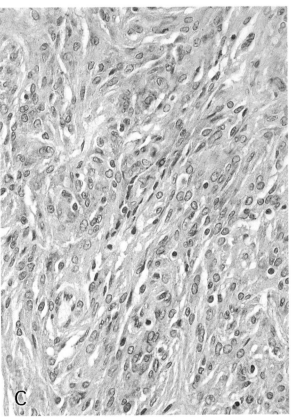

Figure 11-15

MENINGIOMA OF NERVE

This multiple, recurrent, rather cellular meningothelial meningioma arose in the brachial plexus of a 50-year-old female with a long history of pain. It encased nerve fascicles (A), here accentuated on S-100 protein stain (B), and was epithelial membrane antigen (EMA) immunoreactive (C). (Courtesy of Drs. S. Coons, Phoenix, AZ and P. C. Johnson, Tucson, AZ.)

Cutaneous Meningioma

Of meningiomas arising outside the CNS, 45 percent are cutaneous. Some of these are nerve associated. Rare examples, due either to multifocality (104) or to an association with pheochromocytoma (105), are thought to be a manifestation of a phakomatosis.

Cutaneous meningiomas are divided into three clinicopathologic types (80). Likely congenital, those of *type I* occur in children and young adults and involve primarily the scalp, forehead, and paravertebral area. Some are presumed to originate in arachnoidal rests entrapped during development, and have been conceptually linked to rudimentary meningocele of skin (106,107) or to hamartoma of scalp with ectopic meningothelial elements (108). An association with underlying osseous defects or congenital anomalies may be seen. *Type II lesions* often arise along the distribution of cranial or spinal nerves, particularly in the orbital, nasal, aural, and buccal regions. Their genesis may be in arachnoidal cells accompanying nerves as they penetrate the skull. Such tumors occur primarily in adults. *Type III lesions* result from direct extension of intracranial meningiomas into skin, and again affect primarily adults; spinal examples are rare (84).

Cutaneous meningiomas generally show the histologic, immunohistochemical, and ultrastructural features typical of meningioma. Unencapsulated and invasive of connective tissue, some type I lesions are nerve associated (85); the same is true of a significant proportion of type II tumors occurring in cranial nerve distribution. Solid or partly cystic, type I lesions are relatively hypocellular and consist largely of meningothelial cells dissecting between collagen bundles, a pattern that may mimic angiosarcoma (108).

Adrenal Adenoma

Four examples of heterotopic adrenal tissue within the nervous system have been described, including one intracranial rest composed of adrenal cortex and medulla (109), as well as four *adrenal cortical adenomas* of spinal nerve root (32,110,111). The clinicopathologic features of the latter were recently summarized (32). All were discrete tumors (fig. 11-16A) involving either anterior or posterior roots. Unlike the

adrenal rest, an incidental autopsy finding, the four adenomas of nerve root were symptomatic due to pressure effects.

The microscopic features of three of the adenomas were typical of adrenal adenoma (fig. 11-16B); the fourth was oncocytic in appearance (32). In one case, biochemical measurement of adrenal steroid hormones showed high tumoral levels (110). In two other cases, immunohistochemistry demonstrated the presence of adrenal enzymes (fig. 11-16C) (111). Stereogenic factor 1 and alpha-inhibin reactivity were seen (32). Despite these findings, none of the lesions were endocrinologically active. Given their relatively discrete nature, gross total resection with sparing of the involved root was possible in all cases. No recurrences have been reported.

MALIGNANT NON-NEUROGENIC TUMORS

Synovial Sarcoma

General and Clinical Features. *Synovial sarcoma* comprises approximately 10 percent of soft tissue sarcomas. Most involve the extremities of adolescents and young adults, but they may occur at any age and in a variety of soft tissue or even visceral locations. With the discovery that synovial sarcomas carry specific translocations, including t(X;18)(p11.23;q11)(SS18-SSX1) (about 65 percent of cases) or t(X;18)(p11.21;q11) (SS18-SSX2) (about 35 percent of cases), such tumors are now identified in unusual locations (112,113).

Primary synovial sarcomas of nerve are rare. Only 22 cases have been reported to date (114). Most (16 of 22) are small (less than 5 cm). A large example is shown in figure 11-17. Rare intraneural metastases from synovial sarcoma have also been reported (115). The morphologic and immunohistochemical features of intraneural synovial sarcomas are essentially identical to those of their soft tissue counterparts; most are monophasic (figs. 11-18, 11-19). Their early presentation (75 percent) is typically with sensorimotor loss or pain.

Differential Diagnosis. The main entity in the differential diagnosis of primary intraneural synovial sarcoma is conventional malignant peripheral nerve sheath tumor (MPNST). The morphologic features of monophasic synovial sarcoma and conventional, spindle cell MPNST

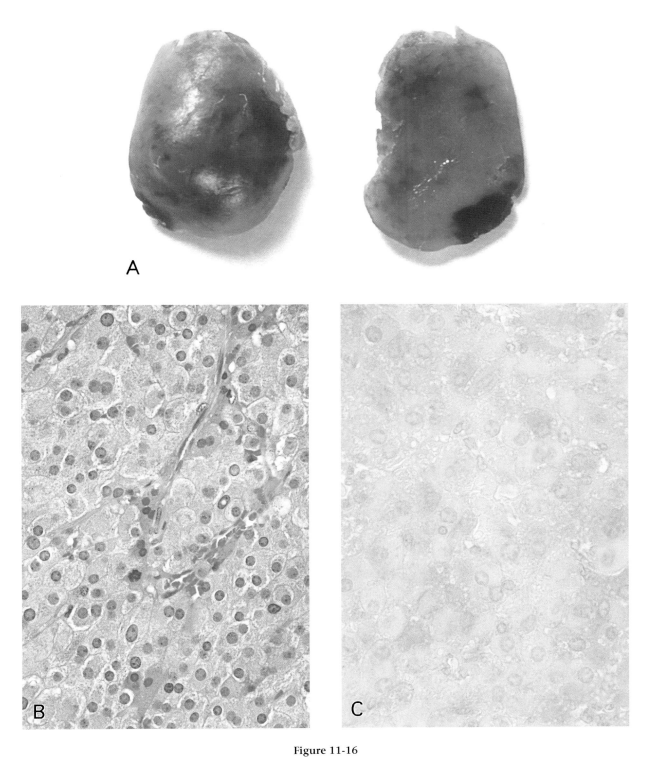

Figure 11-16

ADRENAL CORTICAL ADENOMA OF NERVE ROOT

A: The nodular tumor was delicately encapsulated and readily separated from the parent nerve.

B: Microscopically, it resembled adrenal cortex.

C: Immunohistochemistry shows that it contained cytochrome P450-11b, a steroidogenic adrenal cortical enzyme.

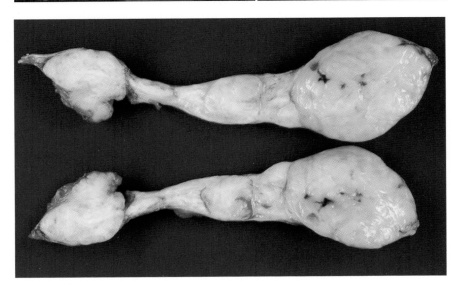

Figure 11-17

SYNOVIAL SARCOMA OF SCIATIC NERVE

Top: This sagittal maximum intensity projection (MIP) fluoro-deoxyglucose (FDG)-positron emission tomography (PET) image shows avid uptake in the multinodular mass within the thigh originating from the peroneal branch of sciatic nerve (arrows).

Bottom: Grossly, this unusual tumor of the peroneal division of the sciatic nerve is multilobed.

are remarkably similar. Features offering significant discriminatory assistance include occurrence in a patient with documented neurofibromatosis type 1 or an origin from a preexisting neurofibroma. Additional morphologic features of help are the presence of wiry collagen and stromal calcifications in synovial sarcoma versus the often greater pleomorphism of MPNST.

Even glandular differentiation may be seen in both tumors, although the glands of biphasic synovial sarcoma tend to be small, lined by cuboidal cells, and filled with eosinophilic debris, in contrast to the cytologically benign-appearing enteric-type glands seen in so-called glandular MPNST (116). Similarly, the immunophenotypes of monophasic synovial sarcoma

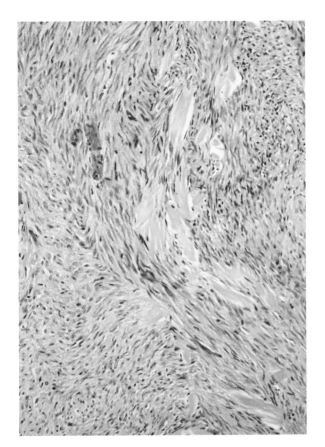 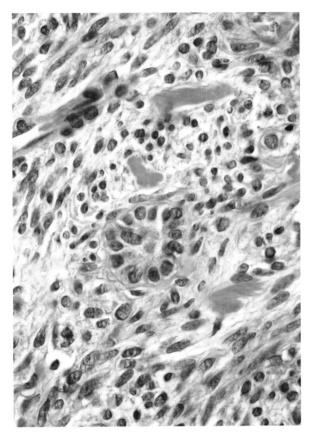

Figure 11-18

SYNOVIAL SARCOMA OF NERVE

Left: Histologically, most lesions are monophasic.
Right: Biphasic tumors are unusual among tumors affecting nerve.

and MPNST also overlap. This is illustrated by: 1) the frequent expression of putative nerve sheath markers such as S-100 protein and CD57 in synovial sarcoma (117); 2) the expression of EMA both in synovial sarcoma and in MPNST with perineurial differentiation; 3) rare reported cytokeratin-positive MPNSTs (118); and 4) very focal or even absent expression of epithelial markers in some monophasic synovial sarcomas. Given these overlapping morphologic and immunophenotypic features, the demonstration of one of the synovial sarcoma-associated fusion genes has come to be regarded as the "gold standard" in the differential diagnosis. Relative to MPNST of the extremities, particularly lower extremity examples, patients with synovial sarcomas of nerve appear to have a more favorable prognosis.

Angiosarcoma

Angiosarcoma primary in nerve is a rare neoplasm. Only two examples have been reported (119,120). A detailed discussion of these and other malignant vascular tumors secondarily affecting nerve is found in chapter 14.

Hemangiopericytoma

Only a single bona fide *hemangiopericytoma* of nerve has been described (121). Involving the sciatic nerve of an adult, it was entirely limited to epineurium. On rare occasion, an MPNST shows a hemangiopericytoma-like histologic pattern (see fig. 12-16C).

Primary Non-Hodgkin Lymphoma

Whereas secondary involvement of nerve by malignant lymphoma is not uncommon

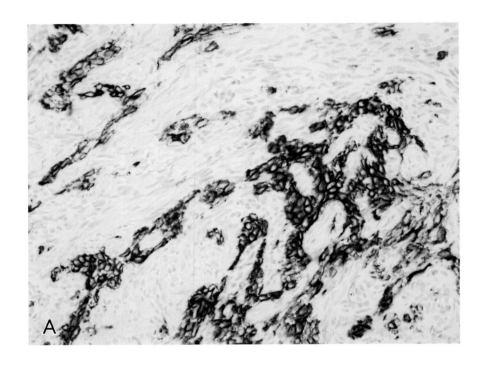

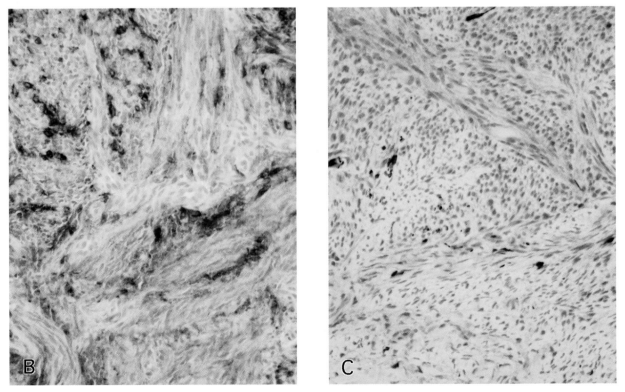

Figure 11-19

SYNOVIAL SARCOMA OF NERVE

The immunophenotype includes reactivity for keratin (A), EMA (B), S-100 protein (C), CD57 (D), and transducer-like enhancer of split 1 (TLE-1) (E). Axons immunoreactive for neurofilament protein indicate endoneurial involvement (F).

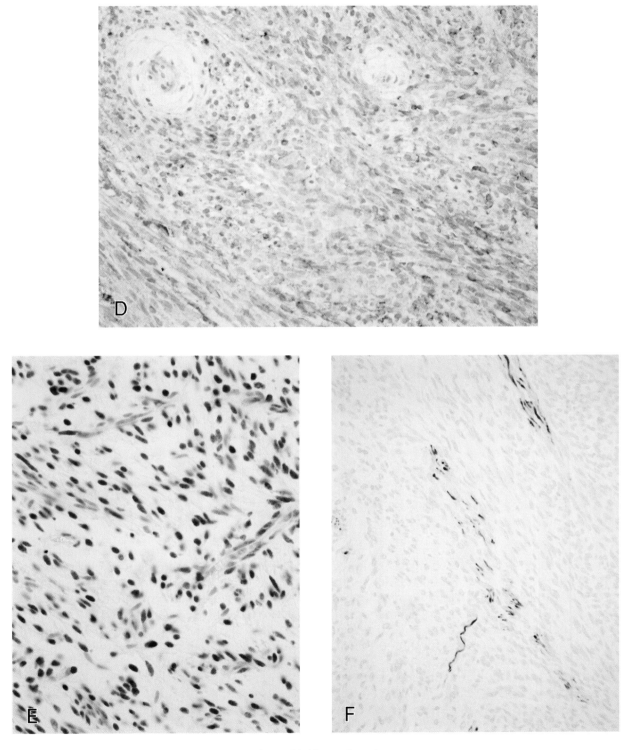

Figure 11-19, continued

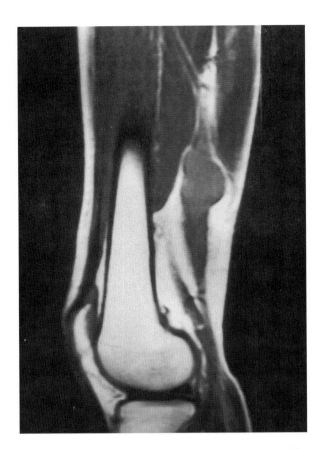 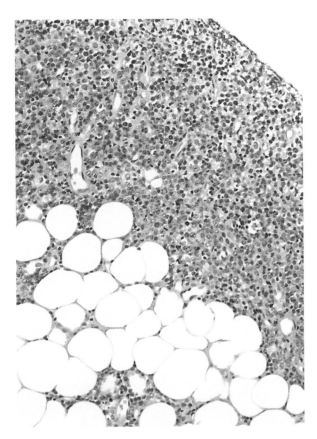

Figure 11-20

PRIMARY LYMPHOMA OF NERVE

Left: An MRI scan clearly shows that the globular tumor arises in the sciatic nerve.

Right: Microsections of the sparing biopsy show infiltration of epineurium; nerve fascicles were not sampled. (Courtesy of Dr. F. Roncaroli, Bologna, Italy.)

(122,123), *primary lymphoma* of peripheral nerve is rare. Of reported, well-characterized examples, all but one (124) arose in the sciatic nerve (fig. 11-20) (125–129). Affected adults ranged in age from 34 to 72 years (mean, 55 years); males were predominantly affected (5 to 1 ratio). No patient had evidence of systemic lymphoma or of immunodeficiency. Symptoms included progressive paresthesia, numbness, weakness, and pain. Involvement was unilateral but varied in terms of the extent and level at which the nerve was involved: three affected the mid-portion of the nerve, one arose at the level of the femoral head, one extended within the sciatic nerve from the level of the ischium to the ankle, and a lumbar nerve root lesion had both intradural and extradural components (124). Most tumors formed fusiform enlargements of the nerve, an appearance resembling nerve sheath tumor. Details regarding the clinicopathologic findings in five of the six reported cases are summarized in a recent article on the subject (129). Three tumors were of B-cell type and two were T-cell lymphomas. Four were diffuse in histologic pattern and one was nodular. Three tumors were intermediate and two were high-grade types. Despite various combinations of resection, radiation, and chemotherapy, three tumors disseminated between 16 and 50 months of presentation.

We have examined a diffuse, large cell lymphoma of B-cell type arising in an intradural lumbar nerve root. Unassociated with systemic disease, it exhibited both an epineurial and intrafascicular pattern of growth (fig. 11-21).

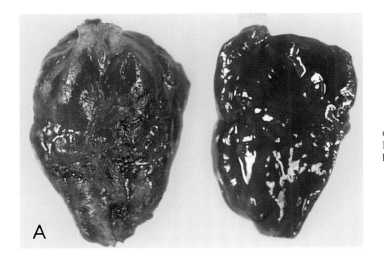

Figure 11-21

PRIMARY LYMPHOMA OF NERVE

A,B: This globular lumbar nerve root tumor of B-cell type was unassociated with disease elsewhere. It replaced the parent nerve (A, top) and infiltrated both epineurium and endoneurium (B).
C: Neurofilament protein stain.

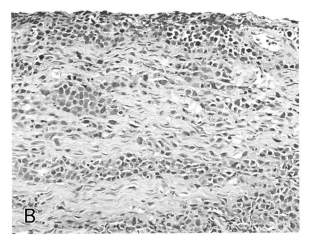

Amyloidoma of Nerve

General Features. Once termed *tumefactive amyloidosis of nerve, amyloidomas* of the peripheral nervous system are extremely rare. Localized lesions, they are composed primarily of amyloid and feature only scant plasma cells. Most lesions involve the trigeminal (Gasserian) ganglion (130–136); in one case, involvement was bilateral (136). Peripheral nerves are less often involved; reported examples have included the infraorbital (137) and sciatic (138) nerves. As in amyloidomas of the CNS, no association with systemic amyloidosis has been reported (134).

Clinical Features. Symptoms related to trigeminal nerve involvement include progressive facial numbness, dysesthesia, and neuralgia (130–134,136–138). In instances in which the lesion also extends into the cerebellopontine angle and jugular foramen, resultant hemifa-

cial spasms, cerebellar signs, and hearing loss may be observed (135). On MRI, a hypodense mass is seen on T1-weighted images, one that enhances upon contrast administration but is unassociated with perilesional edema.

Gross and Microscopic Findings. The gross and histologic features of amyloidomas are typical. They are solitary, appear tan-brown, and are rubbery, waxy, or crumbly in consistency. Small foci of calcification may be observed.

With the hematoxylin and eosin (H&E) stain, the amyloid appears acellular and eosinophilic. Unlike collagen, it is a homogeneous and delicately fibrillar in texture rather than forming coarse bundles. Within ganglia and nerve, interstitial deposits extensively replace parenchyma (fig. 11-22A). Remaining ganglion cells and nerve fibers are widely dispersed. Sparsely scattered lymphocytes and mature plasma cells

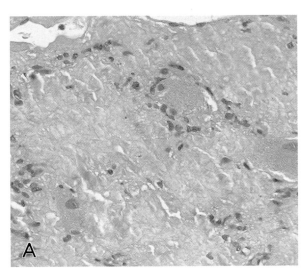

Figure 11-22

AMYLOIDOMA OF NERVE

A: This tumor-like deposit affected the trigeminal (Gasserian) ganglion. A residual ganglion cell is seen.

B,C: Apple green birefringence is seen on polarized light (B), and Igλ immunoreactivity (C).

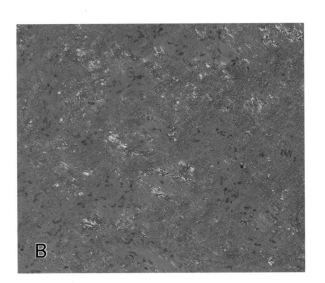

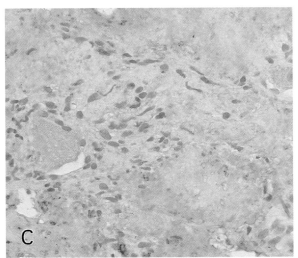

vary in number but are generally scant. In addition to massive interstitial amyloid deposits, the walls of entrapped blood vessels are affected. The substance is Congo red positive and shows apple green birefringence (fig. 11-22B) as well as bright yellow-green fluorescence in thioflavin T preparations.

Although both central and peripheral amyloidomas are sparsely cellular, their localized occurrence and pattern of immunoglobulin light chain expression (134) indicate they are not inflammatory pseudotumors but rather neoplasms, essentially "burned out" plasmacytomas.

Immunohistochemical and Ultrastructural Findings. The amyloid in nerves affected by amyloidoma has been characterized both immunohistochemically and biochemically (131,134,136).

Only AL expression has been observed (fig. 11-22C). With the exception of one case in which AA-protein immunoreactivity was focally observed in the absence of chronic inflammatory disease or circulating antinuclear antibodies, no other amyloid protein subunits, such as AA-protein, amyloid A4 protein, transthyretin, microglobulin, cystatin C, or gelsolin, have been detected (136). Monotypic B lymphocytes and plasma cells are not found in peripheral blood.

At the ultrastructural level, aggregates of amyloid are composed of nonbranching fibrils with a diameter of 8 to 12 nm.

Treatment and Prognosis. Since amyloidomas of peripheral nerves are well demarcated unifocal lesions unassociated with systemic disease, resection is curative.

REFERENCES

Benign Non-Neurogenic Tumors

1. Phalen GS, Kendrick JI, Rodriguez JM. Lipomas of the upper extremity. A series of fifteen tumors in the hand and wrist and six tumors causing nerve compression. Am J Surg 1971;121:298-306.
2. Terzis JK, Daniel RK, Williams HB, Spencer PS. Benign fatty tumors of the peripheral nerves. Ann Plast Surg 1978;1:193-216.
3. Guthikonda M, Rengachary SS, Balko MG, van Loveren H. Lipofibromatous hamartoma of the median nerve: case report with magnetic resonance imaging correlation. Neurosurgery 1994;35:127-132.
4. Chatillon CE, Guiot MC, Jacques L. Lipomatous, vascular, and chondromatous benign tumors of the peripheral nerves: representative cases and review of the literature. Neurosurg Focus 2007;22:E18.
5. Rusko RA, Larsen RD. Intraneural lipoma of the median nerve—case report and literature review. J Hand Surg Am 1981;6:388-391.
6. Spinner RJ, Scheithauer BW, Amrami KK, Wenger DE, Hébert-Blouin MN. Adipose lesions of nerve: the need for a modified classification. J Neurosurg 2012;116:418-431.
7. Sunderland S. The adipose tissue of peripheral nerves. Brain 1945;68:118-122.
8. Burger PC, Scheithauer B, W. Tumors of the central nervous system. AFIP Atlas of Tumor Pathology, 4th Series, Fascicle 7. Washington, DC: American Registry of Pathology; 2007:446-447.
9. Kato T, Sawamura Y, Abe H. Trigeminal neuralgia caused by a cerebellopontine-angle lipoma: case report. Surg Neurol 1995;44:33-35.
10. Singh SP, Cottingham SL, Slone W, Boesel CP, Welling DB, Yates AJ. Lipomas of the internal auditory canal. Arch Pathol Lab Med 1996;120:681-683.
11. Wu SS, Lo WW, Tschirhart DL, Slattery WH 3rd, Carberry JN, Brackmann DE. Lipochoristomas (lipomatous tumors) of the acoustic nerve. Arch Pathol Lab Med 2003;127:1475-1479.
12. Tankere F, Vitte E, Martin-Duverneuil N, Soudant J. Cerebellopontine angle lipomas: report of four cases and review of the literature. Neurosurgery 2002;50:626-631; discussion 631-632.
13. Apostolides PJ, Spetzler RF, Johnson PC. Ectomesenchymal hamartoma (benign "ectomesenchymoma") of the VIIIth nerve: case report. Neurosurgery 1995;37:1204-1207.
14. Rodriguez FJ, Erickson-Johnson MR, Scheithauer BW, Spinner RJ, Oliveira AM. HMGA2 rearrangements are rare in benign lipomatous lesions of the nervous system. Acta neuropathol 2008;116:337-338.
15. Gersdorff MC, Decat M, Duprez T. Neuromuscular hamartoma of the internal auditory canal. Eur Arch Otorhinolaryngol 1996;253:440-442.
16. Vandewalle G, Brucher JM, Michotte A. Intracranial facial nerve rhabdomyoma. Case report. J Neurosurg 1995;83:919-922.
17. Zwick DL, Livingston K, Clapp L, Kosnik E, Yates A. Intracranial trigeminal nerve rhabdomyoma/choristoma in a child: a case report and discussion of possible histogenesis. Hum Pathol 1989;20:390-392.
18. Robertson SC, Traynelis VC, Follett KA, Menezes AH. Idiopathic spinal epidural lipomatosis. Neurosurgery 1997;41:68-74; discussion 74-75.
19. Pasini B, Stratakis CA. SDH mutations in tumorigenesis and inherited endocrine tumours: lesson from the phaeochromocytoma-paraganglioma syndromes. J Intern Med 2009;266:19-42.
20. Kepes JJ, Zacharias DL. Gangliocytic paragangliomas of the duodenum. A report of two cases with light and electron microscopic examination. Cancer 1971;27:61-67.
21. Scheithauer BW, Nora FE, LeChago J, et al. Duodenal gangliocytic paraganglioma. Clinicopathologic and immunocytochemical study of 11 cases. Am J Clin Pathol 1986;86:559-565.
22. Sonneland PR, Scheithauer BW, LeChago J, Crawford BG, Onofrio BM. Paraganglioma of the cauda equina region. Clinicopathologic study of 31 cases with special reference to immunocytology and ultrastructure. Cancer 1986;58:1720-1735.
23. Scheithauer BW, Parameswaran A, Burdick B. Intrasellar paraganglioma: report of a case in a sibship of von Hippel-Lindau disease. Neurosurgery 1996;38:395-399.
24. Wippold FJ, Neely JG, Haughey BH. Primary paraganglioma of the facial nerve canal. Otol Neurotol 2004;25:79-80.
25. Santovito D, Conforti M, Varetto G, Rispoli P. Paraganglioma of the hypoglossal nerve. J Vasc Surg 2009;49:1053-1055.
26. Miller RB, Boon MS, Atkins JP, Lowry LD. Vagal paraganglioma: the Jefferson experience. Otolaryngol Head Neck Surg 2000;122:482-487.
27. Makhdoomi R, Nayil K, Santosh V. Primary spinal paragangliomas: a review. Neurosurg Q 2009;19:196-199.
28. Singh RV, Yeh JS, Broome JC. Paraganglioma of the cauda equina: a case report and review of the literature. Clin Neurol Neurosurg 1993;95:109-113.

29. Wolansky LJ, Stewart VA, Pramanik BK, et al. Giant paraganglioma of the cauda equina in adolescence: magnetic resonance imaging demonstration. J Neuroimaging 1996;6:54-56.

30. Blades DA, Hardy RW, Cohen M. Cervical paraganglioma with subsequent intracranial and intraspinal metastases. Case report. J Neurosurg 1991;75:320-323.

31. Vural M, Arslantas A, Isiksoy S, Adapinar B, Atasoy M, Soylemezoglu F. Gangliocytic paraganglioma of the cauda equina with significant calcification: first description in pediatric age. Zentralbl Neurochir 2008;69:47-50.

32. Schittenhelm J, Ebner FH, Harter P, Bornemann A. Symptomatic intraspinal oncocytic adrenocortical adenoma. Endocr Pathol 2009;20:73-77.

33. Hirose T, Sano T, Mori K, et al. Paraganglioma of the cauda equina: an ultrastructural and immunohistochemical study of two cases. Ultrastruct Pathol 1988;12:235-243.

34. Kliewer KE, Wen DR, Cancilla PA, Cochran AJ. Paragangliomas: assessment of prognosis by histologic, immunohistochemical, and ultrastructural techniques. Hum Pathol 1989;20:29-39.

35. Orrell JM, Hales SA. Paragangliomas of the cauda equina have a distinctive cytokeratin immunophenotype. Histopathology 1992;21:479-481.

36. Erlandson RA. Diagnostic transmission electron microscopy tumors. New York: Raven Press; 1994:616-622.

37. Linnoila RI, Lack EE, Steinberg SM, Keiser HR. Decreased expression of neuropeptides in malignant paragangliomas: an immunohistochemical study. Hum Pathol 1988;19:41-50.

38. Carlsen CS, Godballe C, Krogdahl AS, Edal AL. Malignant vagal paraganglioma: report of a case treated with embolization and surgery. Auris Nasus Larynx 2003;30:443-446.

39. Keith J, Lownie S, Ang LC. Co-existence of paraganglioma and myxopapillary ependymoma of the cauda equina. Acta Neuropathol 2006;111:617-618.

40. Van Gompel JJ, Griessenauer CJ, Scheithauer BW, Amrami KK, Spinner RJ. Vascular malformations, rare causes of sciatic neuropathy: a case series. Neurosurgery 2010;67:1133-1142.

41. Ergin MT, Druckmiller WH, Cohen P. Intrinsic hemangiomas of the peripheral nerves report of a case and review of the literature. Conn Med 1998;62:209-213.

42. Roncaroli F, Scheithauer BW, Krauss WE. Hemangioma of spinal nerve root. J Neurosurg 1999;91:175-180.

43. Vigna PA, Kusior MF, Collins MB, Ross JS. Peripheral nerve hemangioma. Potential for clinical aggressiveness. Arch Pathol Lab Med 1994;118:1038-1041.

44. Matias-Guiu X, Alejo M, Sole T, Ferrer I, Noboa R, Bartumeus F. Cavernous angiomas of the cranial nerves. Report of two cases. J Neurosurg 1990;73:620-622.

45. Stewart SF, Bettin ME. The motor significance of haemangioma with report of a case of plexiform telangiectasis of the sciatic nerve and its branches. Surg Gynecol Obstet 1924;39:307-317.

46. Mastronardi L, Guiducci A, Frondizi D, Carletti S, Spera C, Maira G. Intraneural capillary hemangioma of the cauda equina. Eur Spine J 1997;6:278-280.

47. Giannini C, Wright A, Dyck PJ. Polyneuropathy associated with nerve angiomatosis and multiple soft tissue tumors. A newly recognized syndrome. Am J Surg Pathol 1995;19:1325-1332.

48. Rao VK, Weiss SW. Angiomatosis of soft tissue. An analysis of the histologic features and clinical outcome in 51 cases. Am J Surg Pathol 1992;16:764-771.

49. Smith KA, Mackinnon SE, Macauley RJ, Mailis A. Glomus tumor originating in the radial nerve: a case report. J Hand Surg Am 1992;17:665-667.

50. Calonje E, Fletcher CD. Cutaneous intraneural glomus tumor. Am J Dermatopathol 1995;17:395-398.

51. Kline SC, Moore JR, deMente SH. Glomus tumor originating within a digital nerve. J Hand Surg Am 1990;15:98-101.

52. Mitchell A, Spinner RJ, Ribeiro A, Mafra M, Mouzinho MM, Scheithauer BW. Glomus tumor of digital nerve: case report. J Hand Surg Am 2012;37:1180-1183.

53. Scheithauer BW, Rodriguez FJ, Spinner RJ, et al. Glomus tumor and glomangioma of the nerve. Report of two cases. J Neurosurg 2008;108:348-356.

54. Seizinger BR. Toward the isolation of the primary genetic defect in von Hippel-Lindau disease. Ann N Y Acad Sci 1991;615:332-337.

55. Browne TR, Adams RD, Roberson GH. Hemangioblastoma of the spinal cord. Review and report of five cases. Arch Neurol 1976;33:435-441.

56. Wisoff HS, Suzuki Y, Llena JF, Fine DI. Extramedullary hemangioblastoma of the spinal cord. Case report. J Neurosurg 1978;48:461-464.

57. Brodkey JA, Buchignani JA, O'Brien TF. Hemangioblastoma of the radial nerve: case report. Neurosurgery 1995;36:198-200; discussion 200-201.

58. Giannini C, Scheithauer BW, Hellbusch LC, et al. Peripheral nerve hemangioblastoma. Mod Pathol 1998;11:999-1004.

59. Ismail SM, Cole G. Von Hippel-Lindau syndrome with microscopic hemangioblastomas of the spinal nerve roots. Case report. J Neurosurg 1984;60:1279-1281.

60. Mitchell A, Scheithauer BW, Wharen RE, Franck J, Chan K. Hemangioblastoma of spinal nerve: a report of six cases. Clin Neuropathol 2012 [Epub ahead of print]

61. Krucke W. Pathologie der peripheren nerven. In: Olivecrona H, Tönnis W, Krenkel W, eds. Handbuch der neurochirugie, Vol 7, Part 3. Berlin: Springer-Verlag; 1974.

62. Rohde V, Voigt K, Grote EH. Intra-extradural hemangioblastoma of the cauda equina. Zentralbl Neurochir 1995;56:78-82.

63. Ortega-Martinez M, Cabezudo JM, Fernandez-Portales I, Pineda-Palomo M, Rodriguez-Sanchez JA, Bernal-Garcia LM. Multiple filum terminale hemangioblastomas symptomatic during pregnancy. Case report. J Neurosurg Spine 2007;7:254-258.

64. Roberti F, Jones RV, Wright DC. Cranial nerve hemangioblastomas. Report of a rare case and review of literature. Surg Neurol 2007;67:640-646; discussion 646.

65. Michal M, Vanecek T, Sima R, et al. Primary capillary hemangioblastoma of peripheral soft tissues. Am J Surg Pathol 2004;28:962-966.

66. Patton KT, Satcher RL Jr, Laskin WB. Capillary hemangioblastoma of soft tissue: report of a case and review of the literature. Hum Pathol 2005;36:1135-1139.

67. Smalley SR, Schomberg PJ, Earle JD, Laws ER Jr, Scheithauer BW, O'Fallon JR. Radiotherapeutic considerations in the treatment of hemangioblastomas of the central nervous system. Int J Radiat Oncol Biol Phys 1990;18:1165-1171.

68. Fujimoto Y, Kato A, Taniguchi M, Maruno M, Yoshimine T. Meningioma arising from the trigeminal nerve: a case report and literature review. J Neurooncol 2004;68:185-187.

69. Tatagiba M, Koerbel A, Bornemann A, Freudenstein D. Meningioma of the accessory nerve extending from the jugular foramen into the parapharyngeal space. Acta neurochir (Wien) 2005;147:909-910.

70. Thome C, Grobholz R, Boschert J, Schmiedek P. Bilateral meningiomatous lesions of the spinal accessory nerves. Acta neurochir (Wein) 2003;145:309-313; discussion 313.

71. Smith ER, Ott M, Wain J, Louis DN, Chiocca EA. Massive growth of a meningioma into the brachial plexus and thoracic cavity after intraspinal and supraclavicular resection. Case report and review of the literature. J Neurosurg 2002;96:107-111.

72. Farr HW, Gray GF Jr, Vrana M, Panio M. Extracranial meningioma. J Surg Oncol 1973;5:411-420.

73. Coons SW, Johnson PC. Brachial plexus meningioma, report of a case with immunohistochemical and ultrastructural examination. Acta neuropathol 1989;77:445-448.

74. Harkin JC, Reed RJ. Tumors of the peripheral nervous system. Atlas of Tumor Pathology, 2nd Series, Fascicle 3. Washington, DC: Armed Forces Institute of Pathology; 1969.

75. Landini G, Kitano M. Meningioma of the mandible. Cancer 1992;69:2917-2920.

76. Apatenko AK, Sementsov PN. [Arachnoidendotheliomas (meningiomas, psammomas) of the skin]. Arkh Patol 1974;36:34-42. [Russian]

77. Daugaard S. Ectopic meningioma of a finger. Case report. J Neurosurg 1983;58:778-780.

78. Payano M, Kondo Y, Kashima K, et al. Two cases of nondura-based clear cell meningioma of the cauda equina. APMIS 2004;112:141-147.

79. Wei FY, Wu CT, Lin KL, Wong AM, Wong HF, Ng SH. Childhood atypical meningioma with perineural spread: MR findings. Pediatr Radiol 2005;35:895-898.

80. Lopez DA, Silvers DN, Helwig EB. Cutaneous meningiomas—a clinicopathologic study. Cancer 1974;34:728-744.

81. Smith AT, Selecki BR, Stening WA. Ectopic meningioma. Med J Austr 1973;1:1100-1104.

82. Henderson JW. Meningioma. Orbital Tumors. New York: Raven Press; 1994:377-390.

83. Kulali A, Ilcayto R, Rahmanli O. Primary calvarial ectopic meningiomas. Neurochirurgia 1991;34:174-177.

84. Shuangshoti S, Boonjunwetwat D, Kaoroptham S. Association of primary intraspinal meningiomas and subcutaneous meningioma of the cervical region: case report and review of literature. Surg Neurol 1992;38:129-134.

85. Theaker JM, Fletcher CD, Tudway AJ. Cutaneous heterotopic meningeal nodules. Histopathology 1990;16:475-479.

86. Walters GA, Ragland RL, Knorr JR, Malhotra R, Gelber ND. Posttraumatic cutaneous meningioma of the face. AJNR Am J Neuroradiol 1994;15:393-395.

87. Kershisnik M, Callender DL, Batsakis JG. Extracranial, extraspinal meningiomas of the head and neck. Ann Otol Rhinol Laryngol 1993; 102:967-970.

88. Nichols RD, Knighton RS, Chason JL, Strong DD. Meningioma in the parotid region. Laryngoscope 1987;97:693-696.

89. Simpson MT, Sneddon KJ. Extracranial meningioma of the oral cavity. Br J Oral Maxillofac Surg 1987;25:520-525.

90. Suzuki H, Gilbert EF, Zimmermann B. Primary extracranial meningioma. Arch Pathol 1967;84:202-206.

91. Weinberger JM, Birt BD, Lewis AJ, Nedzelski JM. Primary meningioma of the nasopharynx: case report and review of ectopic meningioma. J Otolaryngol 1985;14:317-322.

92. McCabe JS, Low FN. The subarachnoid angle: an area of transition in peripheral nerve. Anat Rec 1969;164:15-33.

93. Harvey SC, Burr HS, Van Campenhout E. Development of the meninges: further experiments. Arch Neurol Psychiat 1933;29:683-690.
94. Theaker JM, Gatter KC, Esiri MM, Fleming KA. Epithelial membrane antigen and cytokeratin expression by meningiomas: an immunohistological study. J Clin Pathol 1986;39:435-439.
95. Wick MR, Nappi O. Ectopic neural and neuroendocrine neoplasms. Semin Diagn Pathol 2003;20:305-323.
96. Singh RV, Yeh JS, Broome JC, Campbell DA. Primary ectopic intramuscular meningioma of the thigh. Clin Neurol Neurosurg 1993;95:245-247.
97. Drlicek M, Grisold W, Lorber J, Hackl H, Wuketich S, Jellinger K. Pulmonary meningioma. Immunohistochemical and ultrastructural features. Am J Surg Pathol 1991;15:455-459.
98. Falleni M, Roz E, Dessy E, et al. Primary intrathoracic meningioma: histopathological, immunohistochemical and ultrastructural study of two cases. Virchows Arch 2001;439:196-200.
99. Robinson PG. Pulmonary meningioma. Report of a case with electron microscopic and immunohistochemical findings. Am J Clin Path 1992;97:814-817.
100. Hallgrimsson J, Bjornsson A, Gudmundsson G. Meningiona of the neck. Case report. J Neurosurg 1970;32:695-699.
101. Tomaru U, Hasegawa T, Hasegawa F, Kito M, Hirose T, Shimoda T. Primary extracranial meningioma of the foot: a case report. Jpn J Clin Oncol 2000;30:313-317.
102. Burger PC, Scheithauer BW. Tumors of the central nervous system. AFIP Atlas of Tumor Pathology, 4th Series, Fascicle 7. Washington, DC: American Registry of Pathology; 2007:331-362.
103. Larson JJ, van Loveren HR, Balko MG, Tew JM Jr. Evidence of meningioma infiltration into cranial nerves: clinical implications for cavernous sinus meningiomas. J Neurosurg 1995;83:596-599.
104. Winkler M. Uber psammone der haut und des unterhautgewebes. Virchows Arch 1904;178:323-350.
105. Shnitka TK, Bain GO. Cutaneous meningioma (psammoma). Autopsy findings in a previously reported case. Arch Dermatol 1959;80:410-412.
106. Marrogi AJ, Swanson PE, Kyriakos M, Wick MR. Rudimentary meningocele of the skin. Clinicopathologic features and differential diagnosis. J Cutan Pathol 1991;18:178-188.
107. Sibley DA, Cooper PH. Rudimentary meningocele: a variant of "primary cutaneous meningioma." J Cutan Pathol 1989;16:72-80.
108. Suster S, Rosai J. Hamartoma of the scalp with ectopic meningothelial elements. A distinctive benign soft tissue lesion that may simulate angiosarcoma. Am J Surg Pathol 1990;14:1-11.
109. Meyer AW. Spolia anatomica addenda II. Anat Rec 1917;12:43-94.
110. Kepes JJ, O'Boynick P, Jones S, Baum D, McMillan J, Adams ME. Adrenal cortical adenoma in the spinal canal of an 8-year-old girl. Am J Surg Pathol 1990;14:481-484.
111. Mitchell A, Scheithauer BW, Sasano H, Hubbard EW, Ebersold MJ. Symptomatic intradural adrenal adenoma of the spinal nerve root: report of two cases. Neurosurgery 1993;32:658-661; discussion 661-662.

Malignant Non-Neurogenic Tumors
112. Billings SD, Meisner LF, Cummings OW, Tejada E. Synovial sarcoma of the upper digestive tract: a report of two cases with demonstration of the X;18 translocation by fluorescence in situ hybridization. Mod Pathol 2000;13:68-76.
113. Pan CC, Chang YH. Primary synovial sarcoma of the prostate. Histopathology 2006;48:321-323.
114. Scheithauer BW, Amrami KK, Folpe AL, et al. Synovial sarcoma of nerve. Hum Pathol 2011;42:568-588.
115. Matsumine A, Kusuzaki K, Hirata H, Fukutome K, Maeda M, Uchida A. Intraneural metastasis of a synovial sarcoma to a peripheral nerve. J Bone Joint Surg Br 2005;87:1553-1555.
116. Woodruff JM, Christensen WN. Glandular peripheral nerve sheath tumors. Cancer 1993;72:3618-3628.
117. Guillou L, Wadden C, Kraus MD, Dei Tos AP, Fletcher CD. S-100 Protein reactivity in synovial sarcomas—a potentially frequent diagnostic pitfall. Immunohistochemical analysis of 100 cases. Appl Immunohistochem 1996;4:167-175.
118. Smith TA, Machen SK, Fisher C, Goldblum JR. Usefulness of cytokeratin subsets for distinguishing monophasic synovial sarcoma from malignant peripheral nerve sheath tumor. Am J Clin Pathol 1999;112:641-648.
119. Bricklin AS, Rushton HW. Angiosarcoma of venous origin arising in radial nerve. Cancer 1977;39:1556-1558.
120. Conway JD, Smith MB. Hemangioendothelioma originating in a peripheral nerve; report of a case. Ann Surg 1951;134:138-141.
121. Young JN, Friedman AH, Harrelson JM, Rossitch E Jr, Alston S, Rozear M. Hemangiopericytoma of the sciatic nerve. Case report. J Neurosurg 1991;74:512-515.
122. Russell DS, Rubinstein LJ. Nervous system involvement by lymphomas, histiocytoses and leukemias. In: Russell DS, Rubinstein LJ, ed. Pathology of tumours of the nervous system. Baltimore: Williams & Wilkins; 1989:590-638.

123. Scheithauer BW, Woodruff JA, Erlandson RA. Tumors of the peripheral nervous system. AFIP Atlas of Tumor Pathology, 3rd Series, Fascicle 24. Washington, DC: American Registry of Pathology; 1999:293-295.

124. Viswanathan R, Swamy NK, Vago J, Dunsker SB. Lymphoma of the lumbar nerve root: case report. Neurosurgery 1997;41:479-481; discussion 481-482.

125. Eusebi V, Bondi A, Cancellieri A, Canedi L, Frizzera G. Primary malignant lymphoma of sciatic nerve. Report of a case. Am J Surg Pathol 1990;14:881-885.

126. Kanamori M, Matsui H, Yudoh K. Solitary T-cell lymphoma of the sciatic nerve: case report. Neurosurgery 1995;36:1203-1205.

127. Pillay PK, Hardy RW Jr, Wilbourn AJ, Tubbs RR, Lederman RJ. Solitary primary lymphoma of the sciatic nerve: case report. Neurosurgery 1988;23:370-371.

128. Purohit DP, Dick DJ, Perry RH, Lyons PR, Schofield IS, Foster JB. Solitary extranodal lymphoma of sciatic nerve. J Neurol Sci 1986;74:23-34.

129. Roncaroli F, Poppi M, Riccioni L, Frank F. Primary non-Hodgkin's lymphoma of the sciatic nerve followed by localization in the central nervous system: case report and review of the literature. Neurosurgery 1997;40:618-621; discussion 621-622.

130. Borghi G, Tagliabue G. Primary amyloidosis in the Gasserian ganglion. Acta Neurol Scand 1961;37:105-110.

131. Bornemann A, Bohl J, Hey O, et al. Amyloidoma of the gasserian ganglion as a cause of symptomatic neuralgia of the trigeminal nerve: report of three cases. J Neurolog 1993;241:10-14.

132. Daly DD, Love JG, Dockerty MB. Amyloid tumor of the gasserian ganglion; report of case. J Neurosurg 1957;14:347-352.

133. DeCastro S, Sparks JR, Lapey JD, Freidberg SR. Amyloidoma of the gasserian ganglion. Surg Neurol 1976;6:357-359.

134. Laeng RH, Altermatt HJ, Scheithauer BW, Zimmermann DR. Amyloidomas of the nervous system: a monoclonal B-cell disorder with monotypic amyloid light chain lambda amyloid production. Cancer 1998;82:362-374.

135. Matsumoto T, Tani E, Maeda Y, Natsume S. Amyloidomas in the cerebellopontine angle and jugular foramen. Case report. J Neurosurg 1985;62:592-596.

136. O'Brien TJ, McKelvie PA, Vrodos N. Bilateral trigeminal amyloidoma: an unusual case of trigeminal neuropathy with a review of the literature. Case report. J Neurosurg 1994;81:780-783.

137. Kyle RA, Bayrd ED. Amyloidosis: review of 236 cases. Medicine (Baltimore) 1975;54:271-299.

138. Gabet JY, Vital Durand D, Bady B, Kopp N, Sindou M, Levrat R. [Amyloid pseudotumor of the sciatic nerve.] Rev Neurol (Paris) 1989;145:872-876. [French]

12 MALIGNANT TUMORS OF THE PERIPHERAL NERVES

There are two sources of primary malignant tumors of the peripheral nervous system. The first includes nerves and ganglia, which give rise to neural and neuronal tumors, respectively. Common examples of the former are malignant peripheral nerve sheath tumors (MPNSTs) with schwannian and perineurial differentiation. Of the latter, neuroblast-derived tumors (neuroblastoma, ganglioneuroblastoma, and malignant paraganglioma) are best known and are discussed in detail in the 2007 Fascicle, Tumors of the Adrenal Gland (1). The principal source of the tumors discussed in this section is cells of the peripheral nerve sheath. The second source is the interstitial plexus of neuroactive somatic cells of Cajal (see chapter 13).

The outer portion of the peripheral nerve sheath contains an assortment of specialized but not site-specific mesenchymal cells, including fibroblasts, endothelial cells, pericytes, and adipocytes. The functional, inner compartment consists in large part of two cells intrinsic to the nerve, Schwann and perineurial cells. While any of these cells may give rise to a malignant tumor, accumulated histologic, immunohistochemical, ultrastructural, and genetic evidence points to the Schwann cell as the neoplastic cell of the great majority of MPNSTs.

Most MPNSTs arise in patients with neurofibromatosis type 1 (NF1) or from neurofibromas. Both NF1 and neurofibromas exhibit *NF1* gene loss. Neurofibromas and, to a lesser extent (50 to 60 percent), MPNSTs express S-100 protein. MPNSTs exhibit S-100 protein to a varying degree but only rarely in all tumor cells, the reduction in staining attributed to anaplasia. As shown by dual-color fluorescence in situ hybridization, NF1 deletions in plexiform neurofibromas are confined to cells expressing S-100 protein, while in both sporadic and NF1-associated MPNSTs the deletions are found in both S-100 protein-positive and -negative tumor cells (2). In addition to developing in a neurofibroma, MPNST may arise de novo: within a nerve, unassociated with a nerve, and rarely, by malignant transformation of a schwannoma. Only rarely do they originate in ganglioneuroma, ganglioneuroblastoma, or paraganglioma, including pheochromocytoma, presumably from Schwann cells or related sustentacular cells. Since neurofibroma is not the only precursor of MPNST, and an origin in schwannoma is rare, the restrictive terms "malignant schwannoma" and "neurofibrosarcoma" are no longer in use. The all-encompassing designation of malignant peripheral nerve sheath tumor has been adopted.

For MPNSTs developing in nerve, the compartmental anatomy must be considered. The epineurium, in consisting of cellular elements common to all soft tissues but devoid of indigenous nerve sheath cells, is highly unlikely to give rise to a typical MPNST. Since epineurial fibrous tissue is contiguous with surrounding connective tissue, malignant neoplasms involving it may have arisen in extraneural soft tissue. For these reasons, we exclude from the category of MPNST any malignant soft tissue tumor involving epineurium but sparing nerve fascicles. Instead, they are grouped among extrinsic, soft tissue tumors secondarily affecting a peripheral nerve. Although, as a manifestation of metaplastic change, angiosarcoma has been described as a component of MPNST and of neurofibroma, we do not regard as MPNST those pure angiosarcomas arising from the peripheral nerve vasculature (3).

CONVENTIONAL MALIGNANT PERIPHERAL NERVE SHEATH TUMORS

Definition. *Malignant peripheral nerve sheath tumors* (MPNSTs) include any malignant tumor arising from or differentiating toward cells intrinsic to the peripheral nerve sheath. Excluded are tumors of epineurial soft tissue and endoneurial tumors originating from the peripheral nerve vasculature.

General Features. MPNSTs are uncommon: among primary malignant soft tissue tumors they account for 5 percent (4). The majority are high-grade aggressive tumors. This fact alone necessitates careful pathologic assessment, a process often facing impediments. Histologically, most MPNSTs closely resemble one or more other non-neural tumors, including monophasic synovial sarcoma, fibrosarcoma, neurotropic melanoma, and metastatic spindle cell melanoma. There is no histologic hallmark reliably distinguishing MPNST from such mimics. Indeed, some MPNSTs show misleading heterologous differentiation. Conversely, at least two benign peripheral nerve sheath tumors, cellular schwannoma (see chapter 8) and neurofibroma with hypercellularity and/or degenerative nuclear atypia (see chapter 9), may be mistaken for low- or even high-grade MPNST.

The morphologic features alone often are insufficient for distinguishing MPNST from other tumors. Aid comes from the knowledge that MPNSTs differ from most mimics noted above by virtue of three associations: NF1, origin from a nerve, and development from a preexistent benign tumor, usually neurofibroma. Once it is determined that the tumor is histologically malignant and could be a MPNST, the use of the following guidelines diminishes the chance of pathologic misinterpretation: 1) evidence of a nerve origin (exclusive of the epineurium); 2) origin from a neurofibroma, schwannoma, ganglioneuroblastoma, ganglioneuroma, or paraganglioma/pheochromocytoma (or at prior resection site); 3) manifestation in an individual with NF1 and with histologic features compatible with MPNST; and 4) manifestation in an individual without NF1 or nerve association, but with the histologic features of MPNST further confirmed by immunohistochemical and/or ultrastructural study.

The above-mentioned triad of key associations is so helpful in establishing a firm diagnosis of MPNST that in this text studies in which they have been used are preferentially cited. The single most important step in the care of MPNST patients is the pathologist's role in arriving at an accurate diagnosis, which may require consultation with pathologists more aware of the subtleties of peripheral nerve pathology. Just as tumor type guides treatment, reevalu-

ation of histologic specimens enrolled in any long-term study is crucial to the accuracy of its findings. During the past 25 years, strides have been made in the treatment of MPNST, but for an even longer period, advances have come about in its pathologic characterization, most importantly, the distinction from histologic mimics. Some histologic diagnoses in past studies were likely wrong, being based on criteria now known to be insufficient for the diagnosis or simply erroneous. For a retrospective study to be meaningful, the histopathology of included tumors must be reevaluated in light of current knowledge. Thus, studies based strictly on data extracted from long-maintained databases and unaccompanied by a strict pathologic review are not given serious consideration here. Similarly, studies of MPNST comparing differences between syndrome-associated and sporadic tumors, but failing to include relevant data regarding tumor location, size, and nerve or neurofibroma association for each group, have limited citation value. In addition to the responsibility of providing a reliable diagnosis, anatomic pathologists should be able to advise clinicians as to a tumor's potential behavior. When deemed helpful to the reader, some articles we cite may be accompanied by comments as to their accuracy and usefulness.

Clinical Settings. *NF1.* The data we rely upon and that form our conclusions on the association of MPNST and NF1 come from four large studies that followed the above guidelines for a reliable MPNST diagnosis and provided data regarding the triad of associations. Included are MPNSTs arising in: 1) 120 patients treated in a single institution over a 71-year period (5); 2) cranial nerves and intracranial sites (6); 3) central paraspinal area (7); and 4) buttock and lower extremity (8). In all but the cranial nerve/intracranial group, the overall percentages of patients with NF1 ranged from 52 to 60 percent, and in females from 48 to 56 percent. Based on available clinical information, the respective percentages in the cranial nerve/intracranial study were 38.5 percent total and 17 percent in females. The dissimilar findings for cranial/intracranial MPNSTs, explained in part by the relatively high percentage (25 percent) of these tumors arising in conventional schwannomas, require separate evaluation of this tumor group.

Three of the four studies, excluding cranial and intracranial MPNST (6), provide 188 patients for analysis. Of these patients (ranging in age from 7 to 84 years), 53 percent had NF1. Evidence of an associated neurofibroma was noted in 57 percent of the cases overall. In all three studies the neurofibroma association was at least twice as frequent in the NF1 group as in the sporadic, in which the lowest incidence was 20 percent (8). NF1 as the clinical setting for about half of MPNSTs has also been reported by other hospital-based studies (9,10), as well as in one that was population based (11). MPNSTs arising in patients with NF1 are assumed to originate from a neurofibroma; one long-term study indicates the latter are usually of plexiform type (12). Add to this the number of sporadic MPNSTs arising in association with a neurofibroma and it is probable that at least two thirds of MPNSTs share this origin. Most of the remaining sporadic tumors presumably develop de novo or postirradiation.

The lifetime risk of developing MPNST in individuals with NF1 was the focus of two population-based longitudinal studies. In the first, covering a 13-year period, the calculated risk was 8 to 13 percent (13). A follow-up study by McCaughan et al. (11), using the same statistical method but conducted on a different population group and over a 12-year period, estimated a risk of 5.9 to 10.3 percent. The latter calculation is smaller in part because: 1) a shorter lifespan was chosen, one reflecting the observation that individuals with NF1 survive approximately 15 years less than those in the general population (14,15), and 2) because the calculation utilized the birth incidence of NF1 in addition to its prevalence. In cross-sectional studies of NF1, 1 to 2 percent of those affected developed a MPNST (16).

NF2. This far less common form of neurofibromatosis is a tumor-predisposing genetic disorder unassociated with MPNST. Perusal of candidate cases reveals a single histologically confirmed, spontaneous, nonradiation-induced example. Originally misdesignated as "neurofibrosarcoma" (17), the tumor arose in a preexisting conventional schwannoma of the retroperitoneum in a 20-year-old female with unequivocal NF2. An independent review of representative sections revealed a benign schwannoma having undergone extensive malignant change to an

epithelioid MPNST (MPNST ex-schwannoma) (see fig.12-38) (18). A presumed earlier case, reported by Higami et al. (19), was determined by Scheithauer et al. (6) in their review of reported cranial nerve MPNSTs to lack convincing evidence of NF2; the multiple tumors described are best regarded as metastases of a MPNST rather than individual schwannomas. The rarity of MPNST developing spontaneously in NF2, a disorder with an estimated birth incidence of 1/30,000 to 1/40,000 (20), can be attributed to the well-known resistance of nonmelanotic schwannomas to malignant transformation.

Doubtful Association with Xeroderma Pigmentosum. A few reported MPNSTs arising on sun-exposed areas of patients with xeroderma pigmentosum may have been neurotropic melanomas (21,22), thus leading to a false association with this disorder.

Ionizing Radiation. In addition to hereditary factors, radiation plays a role in the induction of MPNST. To qualify, tumors must arise in a field of prior irradiation of malignant or benign tumors. They do not include malignant melanotic schwannomas, no examples of which have been shown to be radiation induced. No minimal dose has been determined to incite tumor development. Most MPNSTs arising after radiotherapy involve nerves of the neck, brachial plexus, and paraspinal area. Treated tumors include lymphomas and carcinomas of breast, uterus, and testes. Less frequent are MPNSTs of the head and neck developing after radiotherapy for benign gliomas (6,24,25) and cranial nerve schwannomas (25,26).

Postirradiation MPNST is a late effect, the latency interval in the two initial series ranging from 4 to 41 years (23,24). In one study, the incidence of postirradiation MPNST among all patients was 11 percent (24). Higher incidences have been reported in the setting of paraspinal (20 percent) (7) and cranial nerve (31 percent) (6) MPNSTs. Neurofibromas with postradiation atypical nuclear changes also have been reported (23), some with contiguous areas of MPNST (24), a finding suggesting radiation-induced malignant transformation of some neurofibromas.

NF1 and non-NF1 patients are about equally affected. Among individuals developing MPNST after radiotherapy of optic tract gliomas are patients with NF1. Concern has been expressed regarding the risk of developing postirradiation MPNSTs in this disorder (25,27), as well as in individuals irradiated for vestibular nerve schwannomas. It has been suggested that of three possible examples of the latter, as indicated by Comey et al. (28), one was a NF2 patient. Our lack of acceptance of additional such examples is attributed to failure to histologically confirm the presence of a schwannoma prior to instituting stereotactic radiosurgery (29–31).

Chemical Induction. Exposure to such chemical carcinogens as ethylnitrosourea, which is known to induce experimental MPNST (32), has not been shown to play a role in human examples.

Age Considerations. The above-noted 1986 study of 120 MPNST patients of all ages (5) found no significant gender predilection and an age range of 7 to 75 years (mean, 35.3 years). Although mainly a disease of adults, the MPNST exhibited characteristic bimodal age distribution: the age range and mean for those with NF1 was 7 to 62 years and 28.7 years, respectively, figures about one decade younger than for patients without the disorder (range, 12 to 75 years; mean, 39.7 years). In other studies, ages at the higher limit extended into the ninth decade, and at the lower end, to below the age of 7 years.

Childhood MPNST. The pathologic criteria underpinning the diagnoses of MPNST in childhood (early first decades), therefore meaningful clinical data, are not as settled upon as in adults. In this young age group, data from two criteria of the triad of associations, namely neurofibroma and NF1, are limited. Neurofibromas infrequently appear before the middle of the first decade: in the study by Boulanger and Larbrisseau (33), cutaneous neurofibromas were not evident before 4 years of age (mean, 7.9 years) and plexiform neurofibromas not before 3.5 years (mean, 5.8 years). The appearance of the latter coincided with the mean age of individuals identified as having NF1, a diagnosis that could be rendered in only 20 percent of NF1-affected infants. If at least half of adults with MPNST have NF1 and most of their tumors arise from neurofibroma, the absence or infrequency of both these clues in early childhood injects uncertainty into the diagnostic process. Thus, it is not readily evident what criteria have been used to make diagnoses of most reported childhood MPNSTs in this early period. Three

series found the number of cases presenting in infancy to be considerable: 16 in ages 0 to 1 years (34), 4 in ages 0 to 2 years (35), and 14 in ages 0 to 1 years (36), figures representing 21 percent, 17 percent, and 8 percent, respectively, of all cases in each study. Two of these reports elaborated on follow-up data. One (34) noted that patients younger than 7 years had a better prognosis than those older. The other (35) found that three of four treated infants were alive and tumor free at 10.3 and 19.1 years. Meis and Enzinger (34) later detailed the histologic findings in four of their earlier reported childhood MPNSTs and included an additional five histologically similar tumors. Another investigation, having examined one of these lesions and five additional tumors with identical histology, concluded they were not MPNSTs but rather plexiform cellular schwannomas (37). The latter often present in childhood, occur at an earlier age than neurofibroma, and are occasionally congenital. Although histologically worrisome and capable of local recurrence, cellular schwannomas are neither malignant nor behave as such (see chapter 8).

As of now, due to the frequent lack of pathologic criteria and paucity of illustrations, much of the existing data regarding childhood MPNSTs is sub judice. Mindful of this, the reliable data on MPNST in childhood are as follows. One large institutional study of MPNST in all age groups found 12.8 percent to occur in children aged 7 to 16 years (38). The mean ages in three major childhood studies ranged from 11.0 to 12.7 years (35,38,39). Combining data from five series and excluding patients older than 20 years (35,38–40), a slight female predilection was observed. The reported incidence of NF1 was either clustered at 30 percent or less (34,35,41), or around 60 percent (38,39).

Tumor Multiplicity. Multiple MPNSTs in the same patient, synchronous or not, are uncommon (7,42,43). Most likely, all examples occur in the setting of NF1. If one tumor is high grade and the other low grade (7), multifocality is a reasonable conclusion, but if both are high grade, the combination could represent metastasis of a primary tumor.

Tumor Location. In all age groups, most MPNSTs are found in the trunk and extremities. In the 120 cases of Ducatman et al. (5), approximate percentages involving the trunk, extremities, and head and neck were 45 percent, 35 percent, and 20 percent, respectively. Of those NF1-associated cases, 55 percent presented in the trunk, 27 percent in the extremities, and 18 percent in the head and neck region. In asyndromic cases, the figures for tumors at comparable locations were 36 percent, 43 percent, and 21 percent, respectively. The high percentage of centrally located tumors in NF1 patients is mirrored in other studies as well (7,44). The distribution of childhood tumors (35,36,38–40) in the trunk (44 percent), extremity (37 percent), and head and neck (19 percent), mostly parallels that for patients of all ages. A noteworthy difference is the decidedly lesser frequency of intracranial MPNSTs in children (6). We are unaware of a convincing primary MPNST of external genitalia in any age group.

Clinical Features. Whether occurring in an adult or a child, syndrome (NF1 or NF2) associated or not, the most common clinical presentations of MPNSTs are pain, mass, and dysesthesia. Frequently, neurologic findings are limited to the affected nerve and its distribution, symptoms being elicited with percussion of that nerve (Tinel sign) (8). The most frequent symptom of sciatic nerve involvement is sciatica, pain radiating distally along the distribution of the affected nerve (8). Patients with central paraspinal MPNSTs below the level of the diaphragm often have pain localized to the back or radiating leg pain; if above the diaphragm, the complaint may be localized chest pain (7). Presentations for head and neck tumors (fig. 12-1) are more varied than for those at other sites and include cough, dysphasia, vocal cord and pharyngeal wall paralysis, headaches, hearing impairment, facial nerve symptoms, and neurologic decline (6).

Nerve Localization. Large and medium-sized nerves are more prone to involvement by MPNST than are small nerves (figs. 12-2–12-4). The sites commonly affected include the buttock and thigh, brachial plexus and upper arm, and paraspinal nerves including sacral plexus. Of the extremities, the lower is more commonly involved (45). The sciatic is the most frequently affected nerve (figs. 12-3, 12-4), particularly at the level of the sciatic notch (fig. 12-4) (46) and distally, near the popliteal fossa (18,46,47).

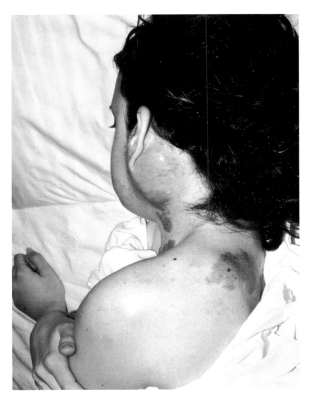

Figure 12-1

NEUROFIBROMATOSIS (NF)1-ASSOCIATED MALIGNANT PERIPHERAL NERVE SHEATH TUMOR (MPNST)

The tumor arose in the neck, elevating the superficial soft tissues and producing erythema of the overlying skin. Evident are multiple café-au-lait macules on the subjacent neck and upper middle back.

Patients with and without NF1 are equally affected, and there is no laterality (8).

Cranial Nerve MPNST. Of the nerves in the head and neck, the vagus, trigeminal (inclusive of gasserian ganglion), and vestibular are most often involved (6). Based on reported cases, their incidence by site is unsettled. Furthermore, many reports antedate immunohistochemistry or lack its support. For this and other reasons, a firm diagnosis is often lacking. The frequency of occurrence of trigeminal MPNST may have been overstated. For those having arisen from distant branches of this nerve, a site of predilection of neurotropic melanoma, the histologic distinction was not always made. Neurotropic melanomas typically arise in skin, lip, and visible mucosa, whereas MPNSTs generally do not. In one report, for example, two cases of presumed MPNST originating as

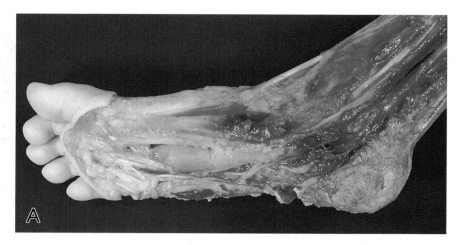

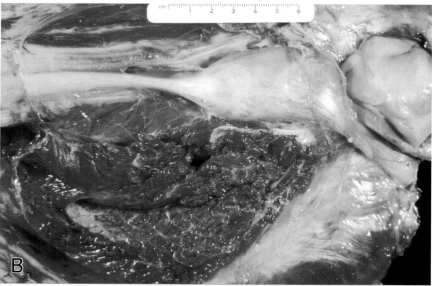

Figure 12-2

FUSIFORM MPNST

A common shape of MPNST, here found in an unusual foot example involving the plantar nerve (A), a neurofibroma with early malignant change (B), and a postirradiation MPNST (C,D). The posterior tibial nerve tumor in B was found in a hemipelvectomy specimen from a 22-year-old woman with NF1 who had a large high-grade MPNST of the thigh that originated in a plexiform neurofibroma of the femoral nerve and spread superior to the inguinal ligament. The MPNST in C and D, not NF1 associated, presented in the proximal median nerve years after radiation therapy given postmastectomy for an ipsilateral mammary carcinoma. In addition to local spread, note intravenous tumor (D, bottom).

superficial orbital lesions (22) and a few more in yet another study of lip or lip/cheek (48) may have been neurotropic melanomas.

Cranial nerve MPNSTs arise sporadically or from a precursor, either neurofibroma or schwannoma. Schwannoma is more often the precursor of intracranial examples and neurofibroma for those synchronously involving both intracranial and extracranial sites. This was shown in the recent series of 17 cranial nerve MPNSTs reported by Scheithauer et al. (6). Exclusive of 1 malignant melanotic schwannoma and 1 intracerebral MPNST, of 10 entirely intracranial examples, 4 arose from a schwannoma, and 1 from a neurofibroma. In contrast, of 3 extracranial MPNSTs and 2 both intracranial and extracranial, 4 arose in association with

a neurofibroma, and none were schwannoma associated. Only 1 patient with MPNST ex-schwannoma had probable NF2, whereas all 5 patients with MPNST developing in neurofibroma had NF1. Only a few intracerebral MPNSTs have been reported (6,49). They are presumed to arise from nerves accompanying cerebral vessels into brain parenchyma (50).

Visceral MPNST. These are rare, usually occur in the setting of NF1, and are often found associated with multiple neurofibromas, from which they appear to arise by malignant transformation (51).

Radiologic Features. Awareness of the gross appearances (see below) goes hand in hand with computerized tomography (CT) and magnetic resonance imaging (MRI) in the evaluation of

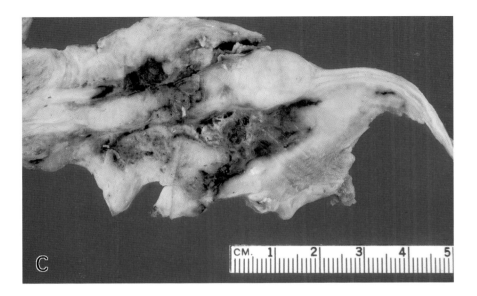

Figure 12-2, continued

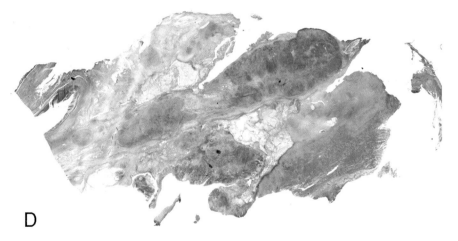

possible MPNST. MRI is the imaging modality of choice (52). Irregular tumor margins and lack of homogeneity, best seen with gadolinium enhancement, are features suggestive of malignancy (fig. 12-5, top), but their occasional absence (fig. 12-5, bottom) makes some MPNSTs indistinguishable from benign nerve sheath tumors. Tissue inhomogeneity may be due to variations in tumoral cellularity, cell-stroma ratio, vascularity, and, of course, necrosis (fig. 12-5). As a rule, MPNSTs lack the target sign so typical of localized intraneural neurofibroma (53). Positron emission tomography (PET) studies, based on ascertaining the presence of increased tumor metabolism, may prove useful in identifying areas of malignant transformation in sizeable plexiform neurofibromas (54). Sometimes radiologic evidence of

bone destruction, as opposed to simple remodeling, is a presenting feature (fig. 12-6).

Gross Findings. Whether associated with a neurofibroma or not, most MPNSTs arise from nerves deep to the superficial fascia (fig. 12-7A–C) and grow predominantly along the course of the nerve to assume a fusiform shape (fig. 12-2), or less often, in an eccentric manner to become globoid (fig. 12-3). Tumor shapes vary depending upon local circumstances. For example, sciatic nerve examples arising in the area of the greater sciatic foramen are often fusiform but may acquire a crook-neck deformity (fig. 12-4). Low-grade MPNSTs are most often fusiform, and even when invasive, generally show limited growth into adjacent soft tissue. The sciatic nerve, also the site of globoid MPNST,

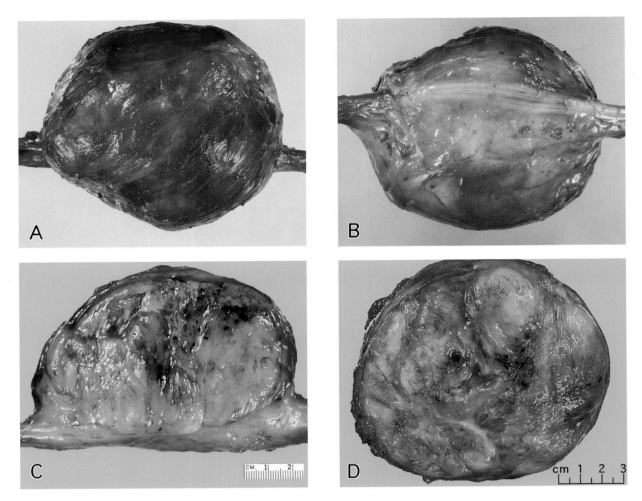

Figure 12-3

GLOBOID DE NOVO MPNST

This 11 x 9 x 6 cm MPNST (A–C), presenting as a painful mass in the hamstring compartment of a 34-year-old man and found arising from the sciatic nerve, is globoid in shape (A). One sciatic nerve segment is stretched over the tumor (B), which on cross section is seen to arise from the other segment and to grow eccentrically from it (C). Paraspinal globoid tumor (D) was shown histologically to be a high-grade MPNST.

Figure 12-4

CROOK-NECK MPNST

The distorted shape is due to origin in the greater sciatic foramen.

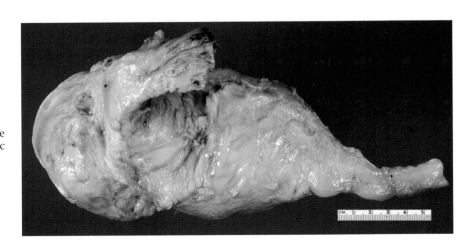

Malignant Tumors of the Peripheral Nerves

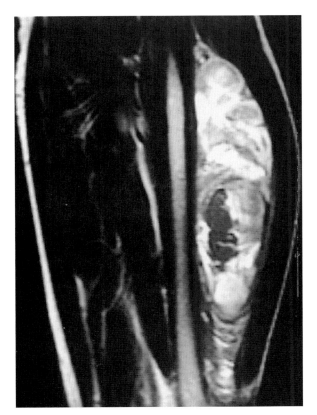

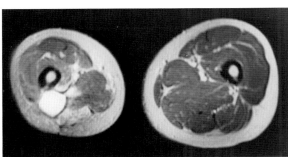

Figure 12-5

IMAGING OF MPNST

Although irregularity and inhomogeneity (top) are strongly suggestive of malignancy, some MPNSTs (bottom) lack these features and resemble benign nerve sheath tumors.

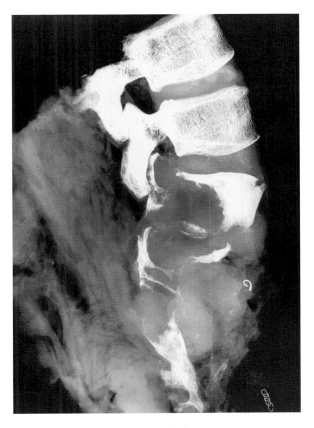

Figure 12-6

BONE INVOLVEMENT IN MPNST

Frank bone involvement, as seen in this specimen X ray showing destruction of sacral bone, may be a presenting feature. The same is also true of soft tissue sarcomas.

has two segments. These give rise to the common peroneal and tibial nerves, each with its own epineurium. MPNSTs arise from one or the other segment. Globoid MPNSTs exhibit eccentric growth directed away from the uninvolved segment (fig. 12-3C). Since small caliber nerves provide limited volume in which to spread longitudinally, MPNSTs arising in them are often globular (fig. 12-3D).

Occasional MPNSTs massively enlarge a body part (8). Of such tumors, most arise in the thigh from either the sciatic or femoral nerve (figs. 12-7, 12-9). Smaller, deep-seated tumors that lift overlying skin or mucosa may also be clinically evident (fig. 12-1). In carefully examined cases, an associated nerve is more often found than not, its involvement constituting an important diagnostic clue. An involved nerve is more readily identified grossly than is an associated neurofibroma, the finding of which often awaits microscopic examination. An exception is a large plexiform neurofibroma (fig. 12-8). On the other hand, some MPNSTs arising within plexiform neurofibromas may be grossly inapparent. Thus, thorough sectioning of all plexiform neurofibromas is recommended. Only an occasional MPNST arises superficial to the fascia. Most MPNSTs are 5 cm or larger (5,8).

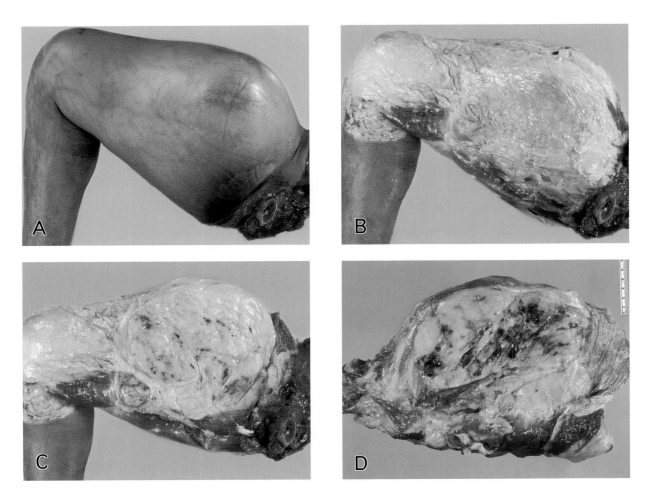

Figure 12-7

MPNST IN AMPUTATION SPECIMEN

Lower extremity of a 47-year-old man (A) after stepwise dissection of a biopsy proven soft tissue malignancy. A 24-cm MPNST of the thigh originated from the femoral nerve (D). The tumor was NF1 unassociated. As with most MPNSTs, it arose deep to the superficial fascia (B,C). On cross section, the cream-tan and extensively necrotic (C,D) MPNST was obviously high grade. Note post-dissection pink discoloration of the tumor (D).

One may be presented with an amputation specimen of a MPNST mistakenly thought on biopsy to be another form of soft tissue tumor. It is customary with such specimens to perform a careful preliminary examination. In the process, cutaneous neurofibromas (fig. 12-9A) and/or café-au-lait spots may be found. The finding of either suggests the tumor may be a MPNST. Attention should then be directed to identifying a nerve of origin (fig. 12-9B,C). If found, it is essential to determine whether it is draped over or enters the tumor (fig. 12-9D).

Sectioning a MPNST is informative. Optimally, observations should be made within

3 minutes. Most often, MPNSTs are opaque, cream-tan, firm, smooth, and fleshy (figs. 12-7C, 12-10). Multinodularity is exceptional and occurs mainly in those originating in plexiform neurofibromas where the tumor spreads unevenly among affected nerve fascicles. The result is an assortment of variably sized benign and malignant tumor nodules (fig. 12-8). In addition, epithelioid MPNSTs often show a nodular or cobblestone growth pattern (see fig. 12-30). Areas of necrosis are grossly apparent in over half of MPNSTs (figs. 12-3C,D; 12-7C,D; 12-8) (8), often in association with hemorrhage.

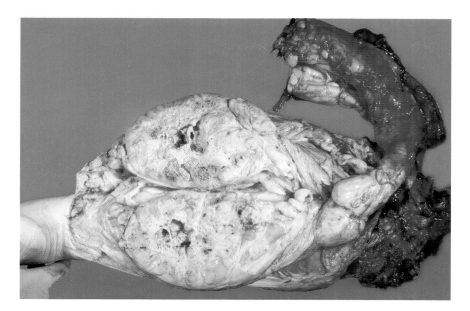

Figure 12-8

MPNST ARISING FROM PLEXIFORM NEUROFIBROMA

A 30 x 14.5 x 12-cm tibial nerve MPNST arose from a 30 x 8-cm plexiform neurofibroma that also involved the sciatic nerve of this 24-year-old male with NF1.

In most cases, the periphery of the tumor consists of a pseudocapsule formed of surrounding, tumor-infiltrated soft tissue (fig. 12-11, left). Infiltration typically elicits a fibrous reaction. For aggressively infiltrative, typically high-grade examples, delineation of a tumor's outline requires sharp dissection from the surrounding soft tissue. In some cases, pseudocapsules measure over 2 cm in thickness (fig. 12-11, right). Thick pseudoencapsulation may be an impediment to preoperative biopsy (18). When MPNSTs involve a nerve not embedded in soft tissue, such as one protruding in the popliteal space, a distinct pseudocapsule often is not formed. Bone in the tumor's path may be invaded and destroyed (fig. 12-9E–G) (8). In low-grade MPNSTs, grossly obvious malignant features often are inconspicuous. These frequently possess a smooth, tan, nonfleshy cut surface that is not opaque, but rather translucent, thus resembling neurofibroma. When low-grade MPNST invades surrounding soft tissue, the pseudocapsule formed usually is thin. While epithelioid MPNSTs are often grossly distinguishable from conventional MPNSTs, those exhibiting divergent heterologous differentiation are not.

The sampling of soft tissue tumors suspected of being MPNSTs should be thorough, not only in order to identify an associated nerve or neurofibroma, but to identify the presence of heterologous elements and to establish an accurate histologic grade. We suggest at least one section per centimeter of greatest tumor dimension. Given the natural growth of MPNSTs within nerve fascicles (see fig. 12-18A–C), it is imperative to intraoperatively assess proximal and distal nerve margins by frozen section. Spread within nerves should particularly be sought in paraspinous tumors, which may show proximal extension with encroachment upon the spinal canal and even intradural extension (7,55).

Microscopic Findings. The most common histology of conventional MPNST is that of hypercellular but orderly, largely back-to-back growth of enlarged elongated tumor cells possessing hyperchromatic spindle nuclei with rounded or tapered ends, moderate amounts of faintly eosinophilic cytoplasm, and indistinct cell membranes (fig. 12-12A,B). Interspersed among the cells are inconspicuous collagen fibers. Tumor nuclei are at least triple the size of most neurofibroma nuclei, and are often sinuous, bent, or buckled. Occasionally, the cells are ovoid (fig. 12-12C). With few exceptions, mitotic figures are found (fig. 12-12A). Significant cellular pleomorphism may be seen, but when present, usually takes the form of scattered tumor giant cells (fig. 12-12D). Of all the findings, uniform hyperchromasia of tumor cells is the most common.

The tumor cells are most commonly seen in arrayed, aligned fascicles or sheaves (figs. 12-12B, 12-13, left), en face (fig. 12-13, right), or

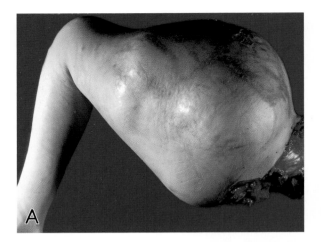

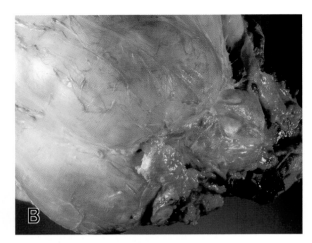

Figure 12-9

MPNST IN AMPUTATION SPECIMEN

The 30-cm MPNST in the lower extremity arose deep to the superficial fascia in a 22-year-old woman with a preoperative diagnosis of liposarcoma of the anterior thigh. Predissection inspection revealed evidence of NF1 in the form of multiple cutaneous neurofibromas on the lower leg (A), raising doubt about the clinical diagnosis. As anterior thigh MPNSTs most often arise from the femoral nerve, attention was directed to where it enters the thigh (B,C). The MPNST grew along and distended the femoral nerve (D), then invaded into adjacent soft tissues and upper femur (E,F). In part conventional spindle cell MPNST (G), the tumor showed extensive divergent chondrosarcomatous differentiation (H). Although of presumed neurofibroma origin, no remnants of neurofibroma were found in the tumor.

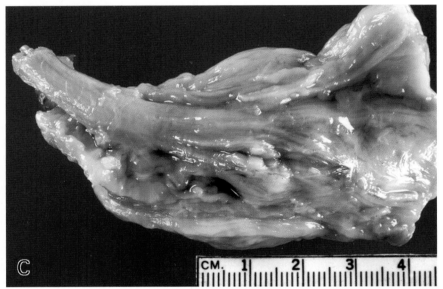

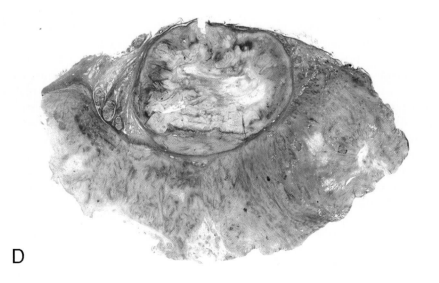

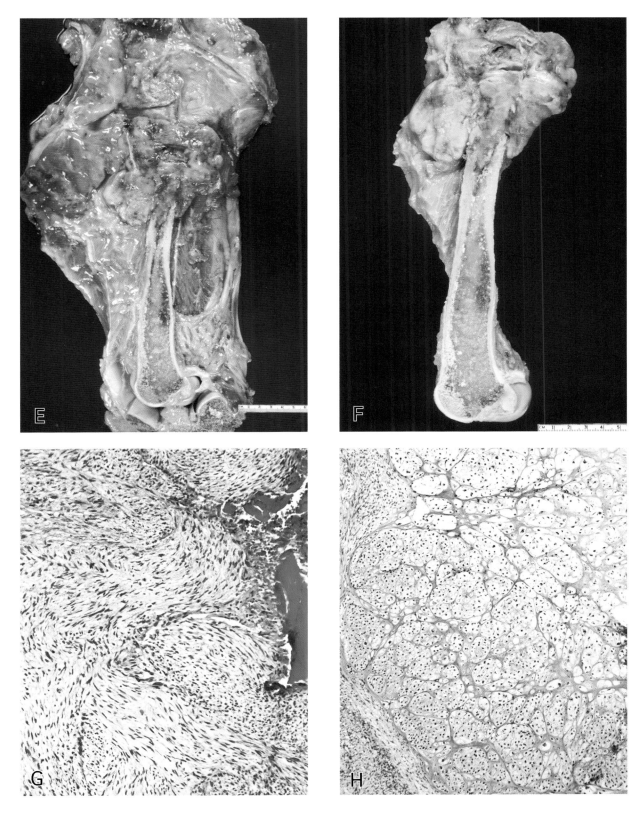

Figure 12-9, continued

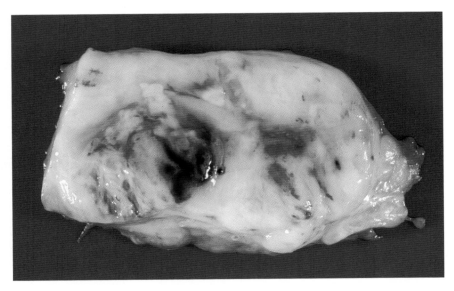

Figure 12-10

MPNST: POSTIRRADIATION

Cross section of a brachial plexus MPNST from a patient treated earlier by radiotherapy for Hodgkin disease but who had no evidence of NF1. The tumor is homogeneously light tan and glistening, but opaque. The hemorrhagic area is the site of biopsy.

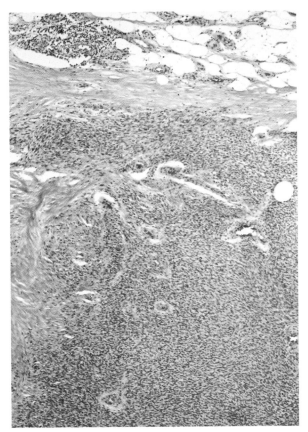

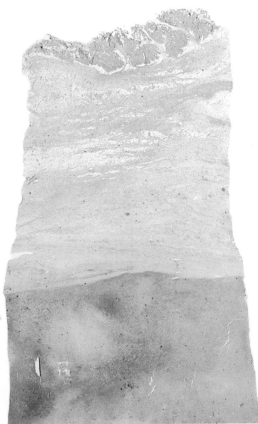

Figure 12-11

MPNST PSEUDOCAPSULE

Left: Fibrous pseudocapsules are formed when MPNST invades surrounding soft tissues.

Right: The pseudocapsule can attain considerable thickness, up to 2 cm in the case illustrated. Multiple frozen section biopsies revealed only fibrotic tissue before the underlying malignant tumor was reached, enabling a diagnosis of malignant soft tissue tumor.

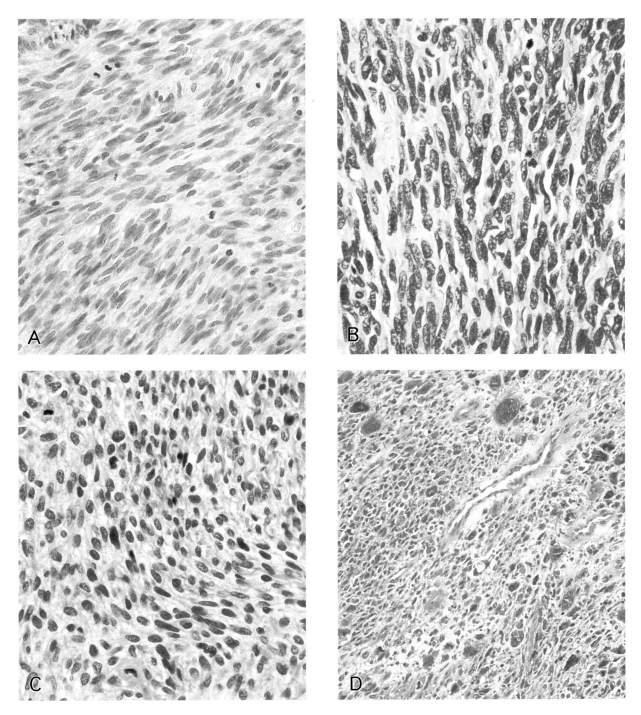

Figure 12-12

CONVENTIONAL MPNST: COMMON HISTOLOGIC FEATURES

A: The cells are spindle-shaped, have nuclei at least triple the size of neurofibroma nuclei, and are uniformly hyperchromatic.

B: Curved or buckled nuclei, a feature not notable with other malignant soft tissue tumors, is a frequent finding.

C: In some cases, the nuclei are ovoid.

D: Some pleomorphic giant cells may be seen in high-grade tumors, as in this postirradiation MPNST (same tumor as in fig.12-2C,D).

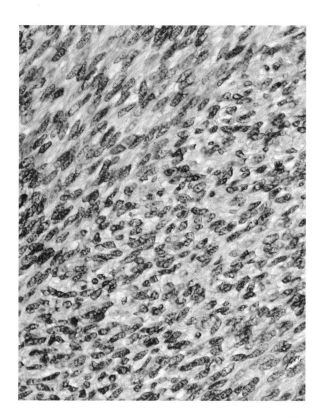
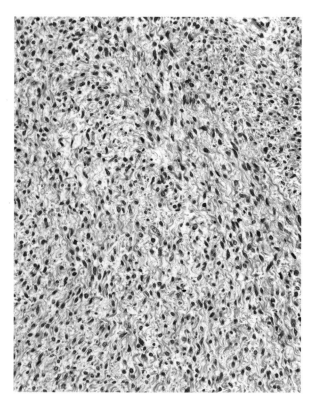

Figure 12-13

CONVENTIONAL MPNST: GROWTH PATTERNS

The tumor cells are usually densely packed and arranged in short fascicles, which when viewed histologically are roughly aligned in the plane of section (left) or en face (right).

at slanting angles (fig. 12-14, right). Resulting dominant histologic patterns are alternating dense fascicles (fig. 12-14, left) or alternating dense and hypodense fascicles (fig. 12-15). Occasionally, dense fascicles cross at 90 degrees to produce a "herringbone" pattern (fig. 12-14, left). Uncommon patterns include storiform arrangements (fig. 12-16A), loose cellular whorls (fig. 12-16B), and a pattern resembling that of hemangiopericytoma (fig. 12-16C). Other features include condensation of tumor cells into cuffs about vessels (fig. 12-17A), geographic tumoral necrosis (fig. 12-17B), and diffuse necrosis with sparing of perivascular tumor cell cuffs (fig. 12-17C).

Particularly helpful to making a diagnosis of MPNST is the finding of nerve fascicles that may (fig. 12-18B) or may not (fig. 12-18A) be overrun by plexiform neurofibroma, with or without perineurium involvement (fig. 12-18A–C), or a nerve symmetrically expanded by infiltrative

tumor (see fig. 12-9D). In addition to soft tissue invasion, vascular (fig. 12-18D) or osseous permeation may be seen.

Most hypercellular MPNSTs exhibit at least 4 mitotic figures per 10 high-power fields, and counts of 10 to 20 are common. We count the greatest number of mitoses in 10 consecutive high-power fields (X400) in the maximally active portion of the tumor. In one study of extensively sampled tumors, pleomorphic giant cells were noted in the hypercellular areas of one third of the MPNSTs (8). Geographic necrosis, a feature of over half the tumors (56), occurs with approximately equal frequency in sporadic and NF1-associated lesions.

A smaller proportion of conventional MPNSTs, only about 15 percent in the authors' experiences, exhibit lower cellularity. These tumors generally fall into one of three groups, all of which are more cellular than ordinary neurofibromas. The first consists of a uniform

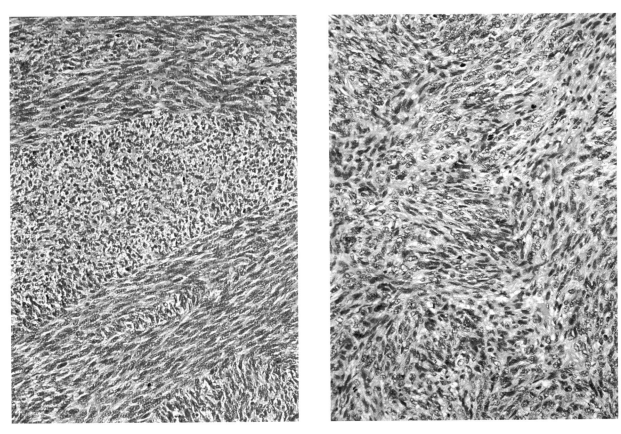

Figure 12-14

CONVENTIONAL MPNST: GROWTH PATTERNS

Left: Perpendicularly aligned fascicles produce a "herringbone" pattern.
Right: In other tumors they slant at varying angles.

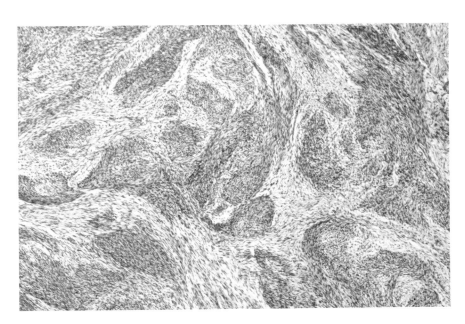

Figure 12-15

CONVENTIONAL MPNST: GROWTH PATTERNS

Alternating dense and hypo-dense fascicles produce a marblized appearance.

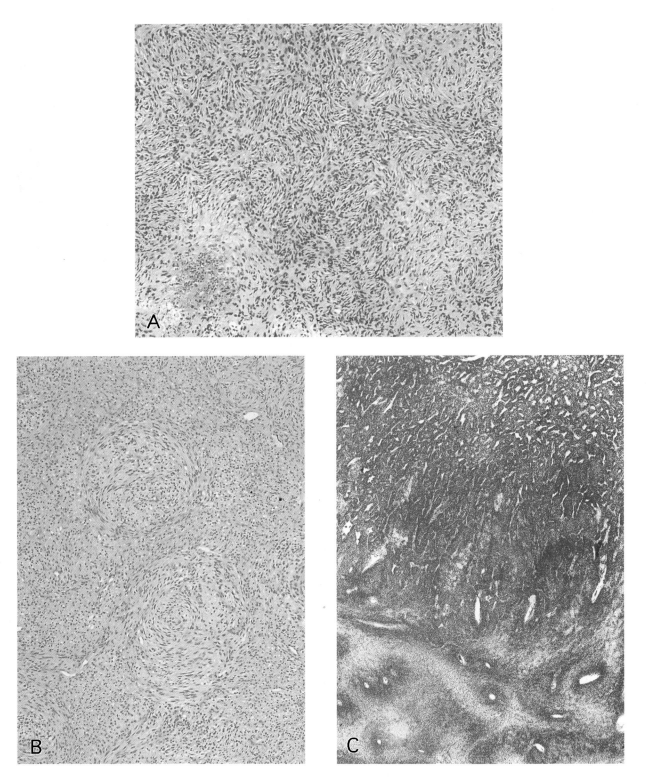

Figure 12-16

CONVENTIONAL MPNST: UNCOMMON HISTOLOGIC PATTERNS

Storiform growth (A), formation of whorls (B), and a "hemangiopericytomatous" pattern (C) are infrequently seen.

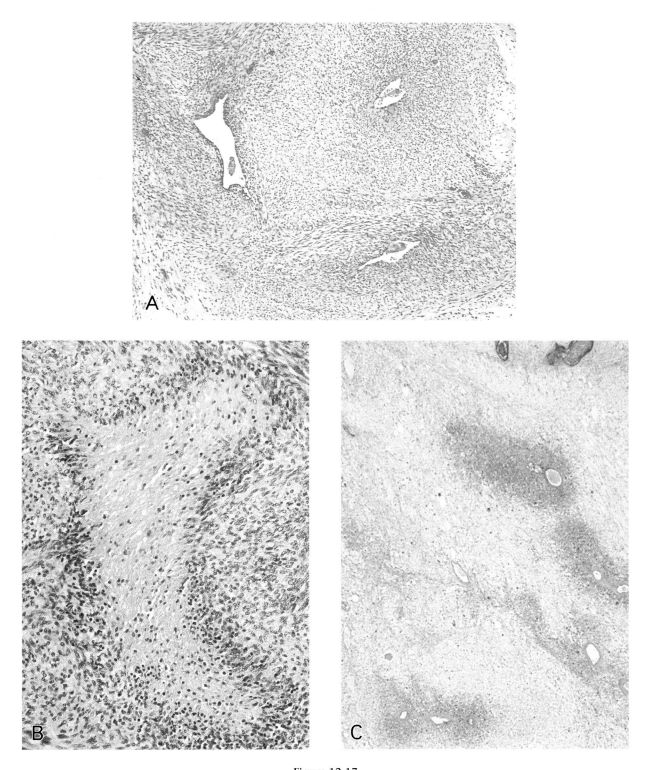

Figure 12-17

CONVENTIONAL MPNST: OTHER COMMON FINDINGS

These include condensation of tumor cells about blood vessels (A), geographic palisaded necrosis (B), and diffuse necrosis with perivascular sparing of tumor cells (C).

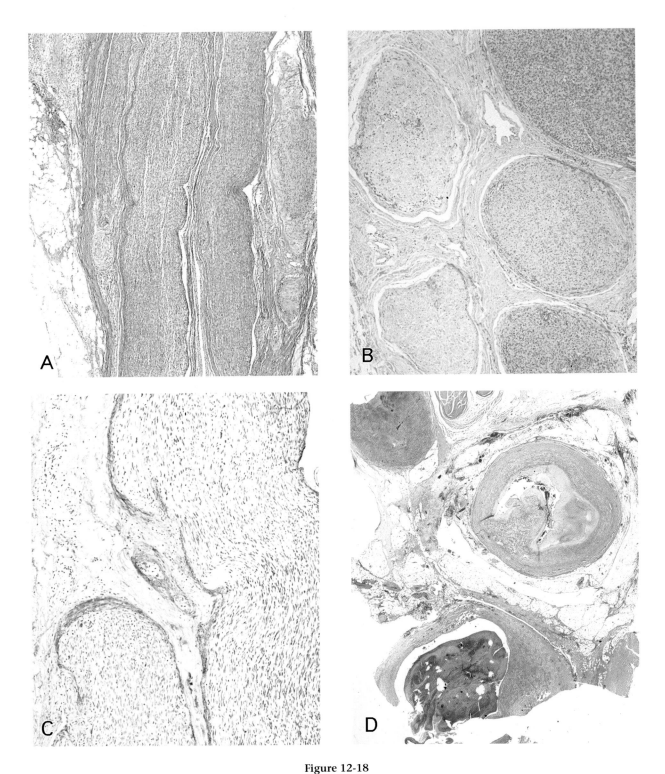

Figure 12-18

MPNST: TUMOR SPREAD

MPNSTs spread by permeation along nerve fascicles, involved or not by neurofibroma, without violation of perineurium (A–C); extension through perineurium and epineurium into surrounding soft tissues (fig. 12-11, left); and by venous invasion (D). (C: epithelial membrane antigen stain.)

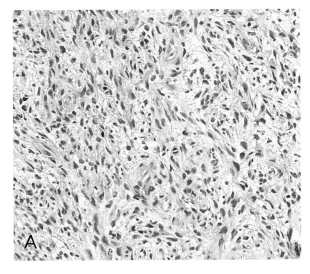

Figure 12-19

LESS CELLULAR MPNST

A,B: The cells in these tumors, although cytologically malignant, vary in size and are loosely arranged.

C: Well-formed fascicles of uniform cytologically malignant cells have a greater cellularity than that in A and B, but not at the level of that in figures 12-12 through 12-14.

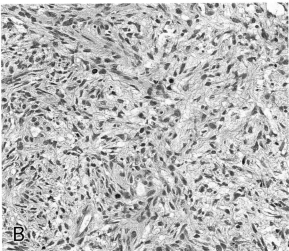

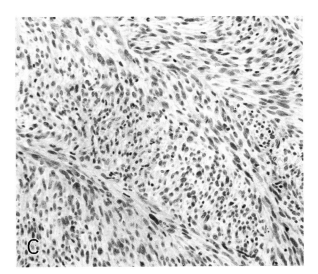

population of enlarged hyperchromatic cells resembling the malignant transformation of neurofibroma, as illustrated in figure 8-37A. The second group features similar cells in a loose arrangement (fig. 12-19A,B). The third consists of moderately cellular tumors in which the cells are arranged in closely woven fascicles (fig. 12-19C). Mitotic figures in the first group are uncommon, and in the latter two sparse, the index often less than 4 per 10 high-power fields. Generally, no necrosis is evident. Elements of all three tumor groups may show remnants of neurofibroma. Focal or extensive fibrosis may be present. Areas of this less cellular tumor may be present in MPNSTs with hypercellular characteristics.

About 10 to 15 percent of MPNSTs (38), usually markedly cellular examples, exhibit an array of heterologous elements, including rhabdomyoblasts, benign or malignant cartilage (see fig. 12-9H) and/or bone, and glandular, squamous, and even neuroendocrine elements. The clinicopathologic aspects of MPNSTs with such divergent differentiation are discussed below.

Cytologic Findings. Given the infrequency of MPNST and the consequent general unfamiliarity with its microscopic features, making a diagnosis on an aspirate, even with supportive clinical information, is rare. This is borne out in the report of Gupta et al. (57), who in a review of eight histologically proven MPNST cases found only three aspiration specimens thought to be malignant or possibly malignant spindle cell tumors. None had been diagnosed as MPNST. In yet another report, most of the specimens

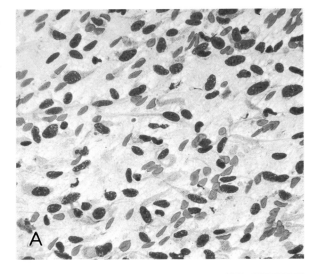

Figure 12-20

CONVENTIONAL MPNST

Aspirate of a subsequent metastasis of the MPNST illustrated in figure 12-8 (A,B, hematoxylin & eosin [H&E]; C, Giemsa stain).

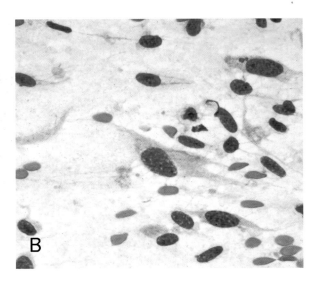

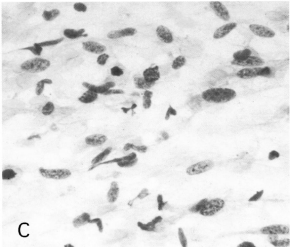

were classified as one of the forms of soft tissue sarcoma often histologically mistaken for MPNST (58). Those MPNSTs most likely to be cytologically interpreted as such are conventional examples devoid of significant pleomorphism. Staining of some smears with hematoxylin and eosin (H&E) is helpful. Commonly seen are spindle cells, both cohesive and clustered, forming short fascicles, or dissociated (fig. 12-20A), set in a sometimes fibrillary background (57,59). Their cytoplasm, best evaluated in areas of dispersion on H&E-stained sections (fig. 12-20A,B), is moderate in quantity, often disposed in bipolar and terminally pointed and sometimes curved processes. Also, scattered throughout may be elongated, thin cytoplasmic processes extending for a distance of more than twice the length of a nucleus and reminiscent of

those seen in neurofibroma cells (fig. 12-20A). Nuclei are ovoid or elongated, smooth contoured, moderately hyperchromatic, with gradually curved rather than pointed ends (fig. 12-20A,B). Bent nuclei are neither routinely found nor conspicuous (57). Pap preparations, in providing greater nuclear detail, commonly reveal a granular chromatin pattern and inconspicuous nucleoli (fig. 12-20C). Unless the tumor happens to be an epithelioid variant of MPNST, the presence of large nucleoli is more suggestive of sarcoma or metastatic melanoma. Mitotic figures are often present. If additional smears are provided, or a cell block made, immunohistochemistry for S-100 protein and other markers can be performed.

Minimal Histologic Criteria of MPNST: the Distinction from Atypical and Premalignant

Changes in Neurofibroma. As the source of most MPNSTs and their almost exclusive precursor, it is important to histologically distinguish between meaningful atypia or premalignant changes in neurofibroma and alterations indicating malignant transformation. A more extensive discussion of these features is found in chapter 8. Aside from finding cytologically malignant epithelioid cells or angiosarcoma arising within an otherwise unremarkable neurofibroma (see below), minimal or focal changes warranting a malignant diagnosis take two forms. Most common and important is diffuse hypercellularity of uniformly hyperchromatic spindle cells with at least three-fold nuclear enlargement compared to ordinary neurofibroma nuclei (see fig. 8-37A). Second in frequency is localized, focal hypercellularity in which a few scattered plump, elongated or ovoid tumor cells with ample cytoplasm and hyperchromatic, pleomorphic nuclei are found (see fig. 8-37B). The presence of mitotic figures does not, of itself, indicate malignant change in a neurofibroma, even if plexiform, cellular, or containing some atypical cells. Determination of malignant change rests on the cytologic characteristics of the atypical cells found. Since malignant changes may be focal or multifocal, adequate sampling of a neurofibroma, especially a plexiform neurofibroma, is recommended.

Immunohistochemical Findings. Although a nonspecific marker of nerve sheath tumors, S-100 protein is the one most sensitive for MPNST. Reactivity is seen 30 to 67 percent of MPNSTs (60–64). Among conventional tumors, staining is most widespread in well-differentiated, low-grade examples (fig. 12-21A), and is considerably diminished in high-grade lesions in which reactivity resides in scattered cells (fig. 12-21B). The latter is attributed to the extensive cellular anaplasia of high-grade tumors, which comprise the large majority of MPNSTs. Far less often, immunopositive cells are patchy in distribution (fig. 12-21C). There is lack of agreement whether both the alpha and beta subunits of S-100 protein are expressed in MPNST (65). Thus, we recommend the use of polyclonal antisera that detect both forms of the protein. MPNSTs may also show variable immunoreactivity for Leu-7 (fig. 12-21D) (64,66). Well-differentiated MPNSTs may stain for basal lamina components,

such as collagen type 4 and laminin (67,68). In most instances, such staining is minor when compared to neurofibroma (68) and particularly schwannoma. The same is true of glial fibrillary acidic protein (GFAP) reactivity. Whereas most MPNSTs are negative, limited staining is seen in occasional cells within better-differentiated, low-grade tumors (fig. 12-21D) (61,64,69). Epithelial membrane antigen (EMA) reactivity in spindle cell MPNST is rare and suggests perineurial differentiation (see fig. 12-28C) (70,71). Like virtually all soft tissue tumors, MPNSTs are vimentin positive (61,69), a finding that serves as little more than evidence of tissue immunoviability. In addition to the above-noted commonly encountered antigens, some MPNSTs reportedly stain for myelin basic protein (66) and nerve growth factor receptor (72), with the significance of the latter still unsettled.

When MPNSTs show no association with neurofibroma, immunohistochemistry plays an important role in the diagnosis. In keeping with the advice of Swanson et al. (73), we recommend a battery approach, employing antisera to both S-100 protein and Leu-7 to maximize the identification of MPNST. Given the distinctly low frequency with which GFAP, EMA, and myelin basic protein staining are observed in MPNST, we see no reason for their routine use.

Ultrastructural Findings. The fine structural features of MPNSTs reflect the type and degree of differentiation of the constituent cells (figs. 12-22–12-24) (62,74–78). Unlike benign PNST in which the cells are consistently well differentiated, those of most MPNSTs are undifferentiated. The next largest group of tumor cells are mainly undifferentiated but there are inconspicuous cytoplasmic processes, rudimentary cell junctions, and wisps of surface basal lamina, features consistent with the Schwann cell origin or differentiation of MPNST. Only a small proportion of MPNSTs, usually low-grade, shows convincing ultrastructural features of Schwann cell differentiation. These include arrays of relatively thick, occasionally intersecting cytoplasmic processes joined by varying numbers of rudimentary cell junctions and coated on their free surfaces by a discontinuous basal lamina. In addition to the usual cytoplasmic organelles, intermediate filaments and microtubules are rarely seen (78). Intercellular long-spacing collagen, or Luse bodies, is lacking.

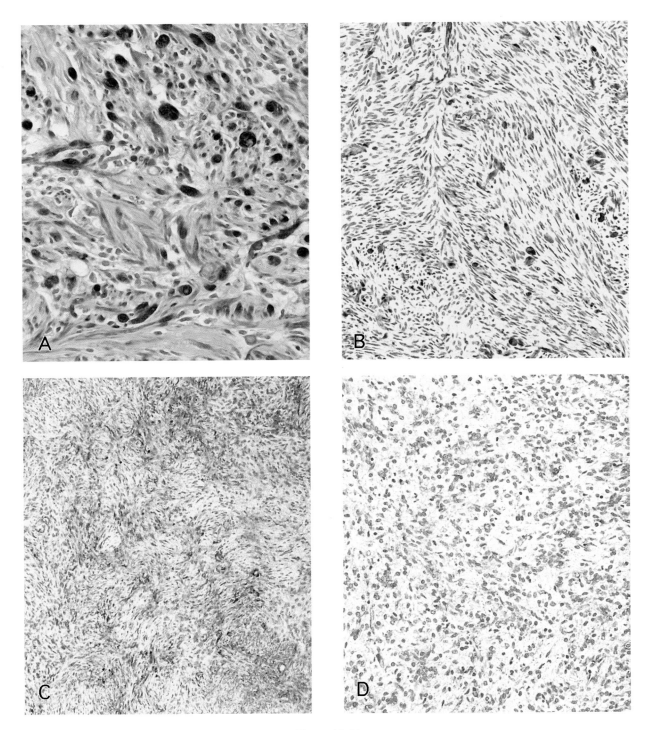

Figure 12-21

CONVENTIONAL MPNST

A: Although staining for S-100 protein is present in just over half of conventional MPNSTs, it represents the most useful marker of nerve sheath differentiation. Well-differentiated tumors show extensive staining.

B,C: Most MPNSTs are high grade and show reactivity in only scattered cells.

D: Staining for Leu-7 (CD57) may be of diagnostic value, but glial fibrillary acid protein (GFAP) reactivity is rarely evident, even in low-grade tumors.

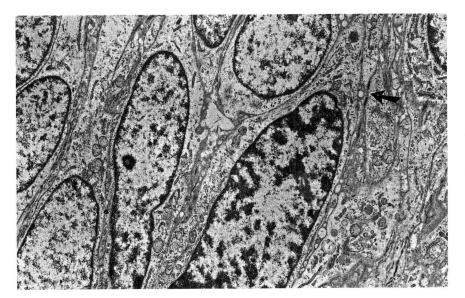

Figure 12-22

CONVENTIONAL MPNST

Spindle-shaped tumor cells with nuclei of varying sizes are joined by rudimentary cell junctions (arrow). Intercellular basal lamina substance is seen. These ultrastructural features are consistent with a diagnosis of MPNST.

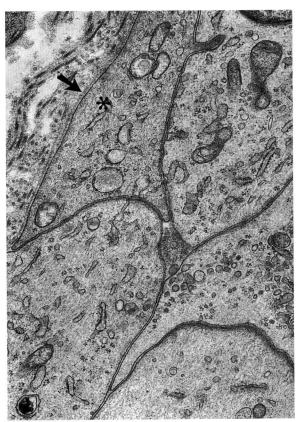

Figure 12-23

CONVENTIONAL MPNST

A cluster of obliquely sectioned cytoplasmic processes are coated by a thin basal lamina (arrow). Diffuse arrays of fine filaments as well as occasional microtubules (asterisk) are evident in the cytoplasm.

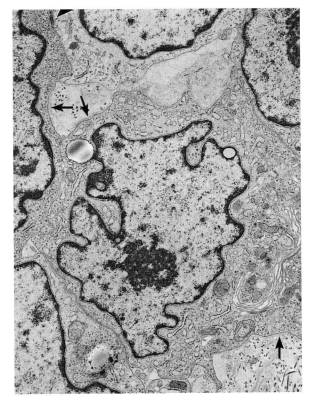

Figure 12-24

CONVENTIONAL MPNST

Cells of this poorly differentiated example with pleomorphic nuclei and large nucleoli show some basal lamina formation (arrows). The cells are joined by scattered rudimentary cell junctions (arrowhead). The presence of basal lamina and cell junctions supports a diagnosis of MPNST in the absence of structures indicating another type of sarcoma.

Other than tumors showing Schwann cell differentiation, subsets of MPNST show the fine structural features of perineurial cells or fibroblasts. Those with perineurial cell features are discussed in the section on MPNST variants, below.

Histologic Grading. It is well known that the clinical behavior of malignant soft tissue tumors is not uniform but varies by tumor type. Unfortunately, the prognostic utility accruing from this observation is diminished by frequent discrepancies in interobserver histologic typing (79). To deal with this problem, histologic grading systems, evaluating the degree of malignancy in terms of probability of distant metastasis for the group as a whole, have been proposed. Among these, the most thoroughly investigated scheme, proposed in 1984 by the French Federation of Cancer Centers (FNCLCC) (80), is based on three microscopic findings. These include cellular differentiation, mitosis count, and absence or degree of tumor necrosis. The scheme was intended for the evaluation of soft tissue sarcomas (STS) as well as MPNSTs. Seventeen years later, on the basis of a study of 1,240 malignant soft tissue tumors, 75 of which were MPNSTs, the group concluded that FNCLCC grade is an independent predictive indicator of metastasis in approximately 90 percent of adult STS, but not MPNST (81). Bearing upon this issue was a subsequent, separate study of 38 NF1-associated and 14 sporadic MPNSTs (82). FNCLCC grading correlated with prognosis only in the sporadic tumors. More recently, however, using the same grading system to study 123 MPNSTs, the large majority being sporadic tumors, no correlation between grade and prognosis was found in either the NF1 or sporadic group. This lack of correlation may be related to fundamental differences between STS and MPNST.

In contrast to sarcomas, MPNSTs are neuroectodermal rather than mesenchymal neoplasms. The majority arise from benign precursors, an association having no precedent in STS. At their time of inception, most STSs are composed of monomorphous cells. This imparts histologic uniformity, which over time is only altered by progressive loss of differentiation. Over time, some STS types also develop marked cellular pleomorphism. In contrast, cells initially comprising most MPNSTs, namely NF1- or neurofibroma-associated ones, are not monomorphous.

At this early stage, many consist of an admixture of typical neurofibroma cells and a population of neurofibroma cells showing hyperchromasia and a variable increase in nuclear size (fig. 12-19A,B). Progressive monomorphism occurs as nuclei of the proliferating cells become triple the size of normal neurofibroma cells (fig. 12-19C). At this point, the cells often still show extensive S-100 protein immunopositivity. In most cases, this sequence of events is followed by a progressive increase in cellularity, the result being a tumor made up of densely packed, uniformly sized malignant cells (see figs. 12-12–12-14). Beyond this point, changes consist mainly of increased mitotic activity and cytologic abnormalities such as the foci of necrosis and least frequently, scattered tumor giant cells. Although not readily evident on conventionally stained material, progressive loss of differentiation ensues, a finding confirmed by significant loss of S-100 protein expression.

In terms of frequency, 80 percent or more of the MPNSTs seen by the authors of this Fascicle have been tumors composed partly or entirely of densely packed tumor cells. One explanation for this is that most MPNSTs, sheltered within an antecedent neurofibroma, pass through the early phases of malignant transformation before being clinically detected, by which time most or all of an affected neurofibroma may have been replaced by a largely monomorphous expansile tumor. We also use strict criteria to: 1) determine whether a neurofibroma with atypia has undergone malignant change and 2) establish a diagnosis of MPNST in tumors not having a demonstrable origin in a nerve. Also of importance is our observation that most MPNSTs that metastasized or were associated with a fatal outcome were partially to entirely composed of densely packed tumor cells. This finding serves as a clear point of separation in histologic grading. We consider that MPNSTs with these findings are high-grade, and those without, low-grade tumors (see fig. 12-19). By considering other histologic parameters, such as mitotic count, modifications of this approach to grading may, of course, be made. Mitoses appear to increase in number in parallel with the extent of anaplasia.

Molecular Findings. *DNA Ploidy.* Ploidy in MPNSTs varies widely from hypodiploid to near tetraploid. Triploid or tetraploid clones are more common in large (over 10 cm) and high-grade tumors (83). In our experience, most MPNSTs are aneuploid. A study of 28 examples, most high grade, and 26 neurofibromas found 64 percent of MPNSTs and 33 percent of neuro-fibromas were aneuploid (84). The difference was statistically significant (p = 0.04), but the frequency of aneuploidy in sporadic and NF1-associated tumors was not.

Cytogenetics. MPNSTs have a complex karyo-type with numerous structural and numerical chromosomal changes (83,85,86). In terms of comparative genomic hybridization studies, losses are more common than gains (83). Especially relevant to MPNST formation are the frequent losses at 17p (83,86,87) and 9p21 (83).

Molecular Genetics. There is no pathogno-monic chromosomal translocation in MPNST. Molecular genetic events associated with the development of both NF1-associated and spo-radic MPNST involve inactivation of the TP53 and RB pathways of cell cycle regulation. For TP53, this is related to deletions and muta-tions in the gene locus on chromosome 17p (86–88). In one study, these led to inactivation of both alleles (89). The resulting presence of a mutant *p53* gene is reflected in nuclear immu-nohistochemical overexpression of the protein (90), a frequent finding in MPNST both NF1-associated and sporadic, but not in ordinary neurofibromas (88,91–93). Inactivation of the RB pathway relates in part to losses on the short arm of chromosome 9 (94,95). This is the site of 9p21 and the tandemly linked tumor sup-pressor genes *p15INK4B (CDKN2B), p14ARF (p19ARF),* and *p16INK4A (CDKN2A).* This gene cluster encodes for the cyclin-dependent kinase inhibitors p16 and p15, and for p14 which acts to prevent MDM2 mediated neutralization of p53. Homozygous deletions of the *p16INK4A* gene have been reported in at least 50 percent of MPNSTs (96,97). In a more recent study of 15 MPNSTs, these homozygous deletions were noted in 3 lesions, heterozygous deletions in 5, and gross gene rearrangements in 5 (98).

A high percentage of deletions has also been found in the *p14ARF* gene (96). Of 11 immunohis-tochemically studied MPNSTs, all but one failed to stain for p16; this contrasted with its presence in all neurofibromas examined (97). A later, mostly PCR-based study of 26 equally sporadic and NF1-associated MPNSTs for deletions at the 9p21 locus found inactivation of the p16, p14, and p15 pathways in 77 percent of the tumors, with co-inactivation of the TP53 and RB pathways in 75 percent (95). Nuclear immunostaining for pRB is found in most neurofibromas and MPNSTs, but in a study of 35 MPNSTs it was overexpressed in 24 (69 percent), compared to typically weak staining in neurofibroma controls (93).

Also frequently lost in MPNST is the tumor suppressor effect of p27, a cyclin-dependent kinase (CDK) inhibitor important in maintain-ing the normal functional status of pRB by inhibiting cyclin E/CDK2 complexes (99). On immunostained sections, this is demonstrated by the frequent nuclear absence of p27 and its appearance instead within the cytoplasm (93,100). Nuclear expression of cyclin E, which after association with CDK2 normally targets pRB phosphorylation, is more pronounced in MPNSTs than in neurofibromas (93).

In support of the diagnosis of MPNST, al-terations most often sought are increased p53 immunoexpression at a nuclear labeling index of 5 percent or more (18); lack of nuclear p16 immunoexpression (93,97) and deletion or inac-tivation of the p16 gene (93,95,97); and loss (93) or decreased (100) nuclear immunoexpression of p27 along with its cytoplasmic increase.

Differential Diagnosis. The list of neoplasms that mimic conventional MPNSTs is sizeable. Benign tumors include schwannomas of cellular and melanotic type, soft tissue perineurioma, and, of course, neurofibromas with increased cellularity, epithelioid cells, mitotic figures, or nuclear atypia. The group of malignant neo-plasms includes synovial sarcoma, leiomyosar-coma, fibrosarcoma, gastrointestinal stromal tumor (GIST), metastatic spindle cell melanoma, and neurotrophic melanoma. Immunohisto-chemistry (Table 12-1) plays an important role in the distinction of these various lesions from MPNST. Alterations induced by irradiation may also cause concern about malignant transforma-tion in nerve tissue (see fig. 12-26).

Cellular schwannoma is frequently mistaken for STS and often low-grade MPNST (espe-cially when presenting in children), given its hypercellularity, moderate hyperchromasia, sometimes brisk mitotic activity, and, rarely, microfoci of necrosis (see Table 7-2). Supportive

Table 12-1

IMMUNOHISTOCHEMISTRY IN THE DIFFERENTIAL DIAGNOSIS OF MALIGNANT PERIPHERAL NERVE SHEATH TUMOR (MPNST)

	Schwannoma	Perineur-ioma	MPNST	Fibrosar-coma/MFH[a]	Leiomyo-sarcoma	Synovial Sarcoma	Epithelioid Sarcoma
Vimentin	+	+	+	+/+	+	+	+
Cytokeratin	–	–	glandular +	–	occ[b]	bi- and mono-phasic +	+
Desmin	–	–	triton +	+/–	+	–	–
GFAP[c]	20%	–	Rare	–	–	–	–
Muscle-specific actin (HHF-35)	–	–	triton +	+/–	+	–	–
HMB45	(melanotic +)	–	–	–	–	–	–
S-100 protein	>95%	–	>50%	–	occ	occ	–
Leu-7	50-60%	–	30-40%	–	10-20%	25-40%	–
EMA	–	+	glandular differentiation +	–	–	bi- and monophasic +	+
CEA	–	–	glandular differentiation +	–	–	glands +/–	–
Chromogranin	–	–	glandular differentiation +	–	–	–	–
Factor VIII, CD31	–	–	angiosarcoma differentiation +	–	–	–	–
CD68 (KP-1)	+	+/–	+/–	–/+	–	–	–
Laminin and collagen 4	+	+	25-30%	–	+	10%	10%

[a]MFH = malignant fibrous histiocytoma.
[b]Occ = occasional.
[c]GFAP = glial fibrillary acidic protein; EMA = epithelial membrane antigen; CEA = carcinoembryonic antigen.

of the diagnosis of cellular schwannoma are cellular whorls, subcapsular lymphocytic infiltrates, and, in many cases, features shared with conventional schwannoma, including a true capsule, hyalinized blood vessels, and clusters of lipid-laden cells. In contrast to most MPNSTs, cellular schwannomas are consistently, diffusely and strongly immunoreactive for S-100 protein; however, a few MPNSTs are diffusely immunopositive. This can lead to the reverse problem, misinterpretation of an MPNST as cellular schwannoma, especially when the pathologist is presented with a limited biopsy or partial excision. In any problematic cases involving this differential, immunohistochemical evaluation for increased nuclear p53 or absence of p16 expression is recommended. The finding of either or both favors a diagnosis of MPNST. Differentiation of epithelioid schwannoma from epithelioid MPNST, admittedly an infrequent problem, is discussed under epithelioid MPNST (see below). We have not encountered a melanotic example of conventional MPNST.

The distinction between MPNST and neurofibroma with cellular areas (see figs. 8-27B,F;

8-28), or with epithelioid cells (see fig. 8-29), is based on the cytologic characteristics of the cells in question. Neurofibromas with benign cytologic atypia (see fig. 8-35) or with cytologic atypia regarded as early changes in malignant transformation (see fig. 8-36) are discussed in chapter 8. As previously stressed, the presence in a neurofibroma of mitotic figures alone is not an indicator of malignant change.

An occasional soft tissue perineurioma may be mistaken for a low-grade conventional MPNST. The principal features serving to differentiate the two are diffuse immunoexpression for EMA rather than S-100 protein in perineuriomas, and lack of an associated nerve. The distinction is complicated by the existence of rare MPNSTs with perineurial cell differentiation (see below).

Monophasic synovial sarcoma, the closest histologic mimic of conventional MPNST, consists of cells that are more densely packed and have plumper nuclei. In addition, the stroma of synovial sarcoma typically features irregularly distributed, dense collagen bands of varying thickness and occasional calcifications. Rare synovial sarcomas, occasionally found around the ankle area, exhibit a myxoid stroma, thus further complicating their distinction (101,102). Nearly 50 percent of monophasic synovial sarcomas express cytokeratin and/or EMA; usually such cells are lacking in conventional MPNST (103). Since S-100 protein staining is seen in about one fourth of monophasic synovial sarcomas (103), it does not reliably distinguish it from MPNST. Ultrastructurally, most monophasic synovial sarcomas differ from MPNSTs by having cells with short bipolar processes and greater numbers of intercellular junctions, as well as featuring occasional small lumens with microvilli and only inconspicuous intercellular spaces. If the distinction remains unsure, molecular genetic evaluation (reverse transcriptase-polymerase chain reaction [RT-PCR] or fluorescence in situ hybridization [FISH]) can be used to seek a distinctive t(x;18) translocation. Found in approximately 90 percent of synovial sarcomas (104), it is lacking in MPNST (105–108). A genetic study may also be needed in rare instances in which synovial sarcomas arise in a peripheral nerve and simulate a primary MPNST (109) (see chapter 11).

In contrast to conventional MPNST, the elongated cells of leiomyosarcoma possess blunt-ended nuclei, more abundant eosinophilic cytoplasm, and longitudinal cytoplasmic fibrils that stain red in trichrome and blue in phosphotungstic acid-hematoxylin (PTAH) preparations. Since occasional leiomyosarcomas express S-100 protein (73), this antibody cannot be relied upon to make the distinction from MPNST. Instead, appropriate muscle markers should be applied. The closest leiomyosarcoma simulator is one arising from a vena comitant of an artery in an extremity. Positioned in a neurovascular bundle, it is also companion to a nerve. The leiomyosarcoma may be fusiform, thus grossly indistinguishable from MPNST. Here, proof of the tumor's type is achieved by histologic demonstration of an origin from a vein.

Fibrosarcoma, when displaying a herringbone and related histologic pattern, closely resembles MPNST, but differs in showing both a greater degree of stromal collagen and lack of S-100 protein immunoreactivity. Although it is uncommon for MPNSTs to contain a myxoid stroma, they occasionally show distinctive myxoid areas such as seen in myxofibrosarcoma and

so-called malignant fibrous histiocytoma, both of which feature cells more plump than those of MPNST. Ultrastructurally, fibrosarcomas often have folded nuclear contours, are devoid of surface basal lamina, and have far better developed rough endoplasmic reticulum. Those exhibiting myofibroblastic differentiation also feature myoid filaments beneath the cell membrane.

Rare examples of MPNST affecting the gastrointestinal tract must be distinguished from GISTs, particularly in the setting of NF1 (110,111). GISTs are discussed in greater detail in chapter 13.

Problems in differential diagnosis arise with two forms of melanoma: spindle and neurotropic. On H&E stain and viewed at low power, spindle cell melanoma can be virtually indistinguishable from conventional MPNSTs (fig. 12-25). There are, however, subtle distinctions. Compared with MPNST (see fig. 12-12A,B), melanoma cells generally have more abundant and denser cytoplasm, irregular nuclear contours, and prominent chromatin clumping. The presence of scattered large cells with extreme pleomorphism or multinucleation is more consistent with MPNST. Additional features of melanoma include sometimes amphophilic cytoplasm, strong diffuse immunoreactivity for S-100 protein, and staining for microphthalmia transcription factor (MiTF). Only a few spindle cell melanomas are positive for HMB45 and Melan-A (112). Although conventional MPNSTs have not been described as arising in lymph nodes and only rarely exhibit metastasis, nodal metastases of melanoma to axillary lymph nodes and perinodal soft tissue have been mistaken for MPNSTs (113). At such sites, findings favoring melanoma include absence of pseudopalisading about foci of necrosis and the knowledge that MPNSTs metastatic to lymph nodes are invariably epithelioid in type (see below for distinction of epithelioid MPNST from melanoma). The last form of melanoma, one to keep in mind when evaluating possible MPNSTs of the head, is neurotropic melanoma. Its distinguishing characteristics are discussed in chapter 14.

Scattered cells exhibiting cytologic atypia, including nuclear enlargement and hyperchromasia, may be seen in a nerve following radiation, even at doses as low as 2 Gy (114). These must not be overinterpreted as evidence of malignant change. This is less a challenge at

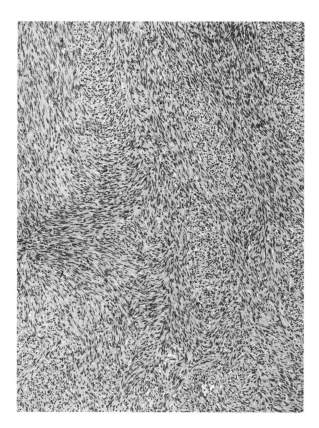
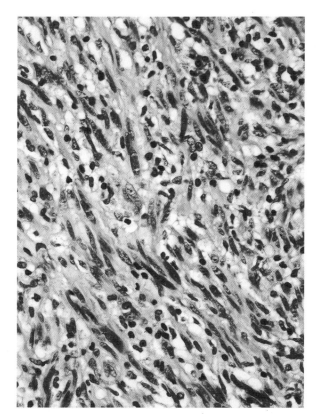

Figure 12-25

METASTATIC MELANOMA HISTOLOGICALLY SIMULATING MPNST

Left: At low magnification, there is a fascicular arrangement of cells not unlike that in MPNST.

Right: In contrast to most MPNSTs, the nuclei of the melanoma cells have a coarse appearance owing to a greater chromatin density and variability in width and length.

sites irradiated for non-neurogenic neoplasms (fig. 12-26A–D) than in the setting of a possibly recurrent MPNST (fig. 12-26E). Although no firm criteria permit the distinction of irradiation-induced atypia in Schwann cells or fibroblasts from isolated residual tumor cells or recurrent sarcoma, we have found no evidence of proliferative activity (mitoses or Ki-67 labeling) in the former. Interestingly, experimental evidence suggests that radiation doses of 10 to 20 Gy may in fact impair the proliferative capacity of Schwann cells (114).

Frozen Section Diagnosis. Prior to definitive therapy, it is essential to determine whether a peripheral nerve tumor is benign or malignant. As a result, a biopsy is often performed. If the surgeon believes he is dealing with a malignant tumor and only benign fibrous tissue is seen, it is advisable to remind him that MPNSTs are often

surrounded by a pseudocapsule that may need to be penetrated by multiple biopsies to obtain diagnostic tissue (see fig. 12-11, right). With regard to a malignant diagnosis, unless the pathologist has extensive experience with peripheral nerve or soft tissue tumors, we do not think frozen sections should be relied upon to report anything other than an obvious malignant soft tissue tumor, with the caveat that an MPNST cannot be ruled out. With this report in hand, the surgeon should be able to determine whether a diagnosis of MPNST fits the clinical presentation.

The resection of an MPNST by a wide en bloc procedure that may necessitate the sacrifice of a sizeable involved nerve is a problematic decision when based upon a frozen section specimen alone. In the mediastinum this approach is acceptable, since sacrifice of one or more thoracic spinal nerves does not produce major

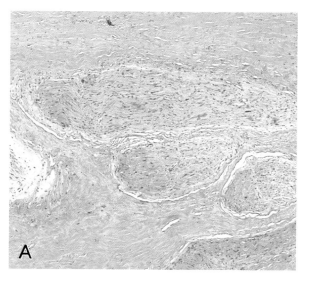

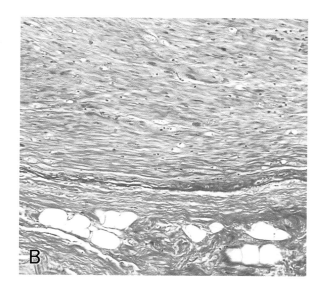

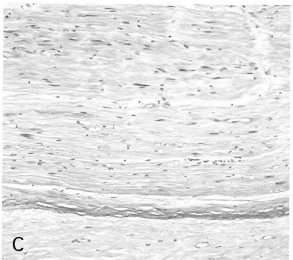

Figure 12-26

RADIATION-INDUCED EFFECT ON NORMAL NERVE

This axillary nerve, a part of the brachial plexus subjected to radiotherapy for breast carcinoma, shows not only extensive perineural and endoneurial fibrosis (A,B) but loss of myelin (C) and axons (D), as well as nuclear atypia of Schwann cells. When seen in the setting of a previously radiation-treated MPNST (E), such atypical cells might be confused with a permeative malignant tumor. Such irradiation-affected non-neoplastic cells lack proliferative activity in terms of mitoses and proliferation marker labeling. (B: trichrome stain; C: luxol fast blue; D: neurofilament protein.)

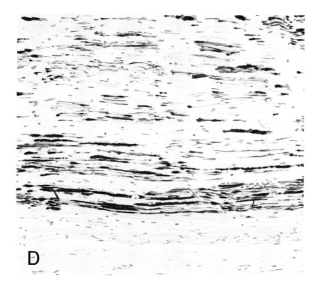

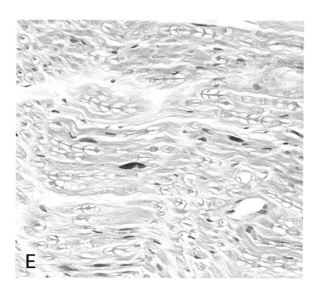

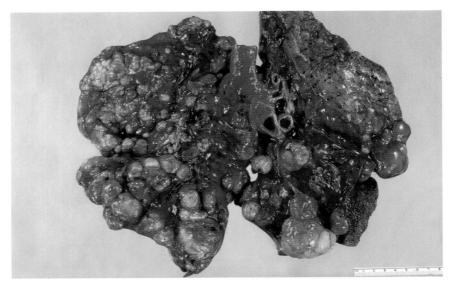

Figure 12-27

MPNST: METASTASIS

Top: MPNST metastatic to lungs, the leading site for distant spread of the tumor.

Bottom: Metastatic MPNST to both lungs and their visceral and parietal pleurae was found on a chest X ray of a 9-year-old girl 5 months after resection of the primary posterior left neck tumor. The patient had familial NF1 with multiple café-au-lait macules since birth and soft tissue masses of the left neck and orbital area since age 2 years, which over the years gradually increased in size. At autopsy, in addition to pleural involvement, there were numerous intra-pulmonary metastases.

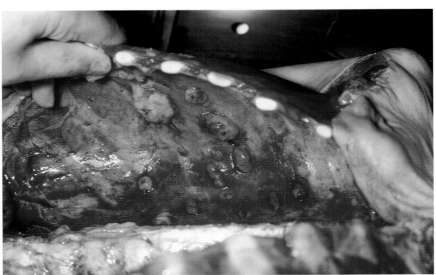

neurologic disability; a similar sacrifice of lumbosacral nerve(s) may result in significant functional deficits. If cellular schwannoma enters into the differential, we recommend resection of the tumor with preservation of functionally important nerves. This is adequate treatment if on permanent sections the well-sampled tumor is a cellular schwannoma. Alternatively, if the tumor is an MPNST, either wide local excision, with or without sacrifice of nerve, or radiation therapy of the tumor bed may be undertaken.

Recurrence and Metastasis. Local and distant metastases of MPNST may be found at initial resection; the local metastasis is sometimes so near as to appear to be part of the primary tumor. Rates of local tumor recurrence after surgical resection are high, ranging from 40 to 65 percent (7,8). For the pediatric age group, the local relapse rate in patients presenting solely with localized tumors is 50 percent (35). The literature has conflicting data regarding the frequency of local recurrence in patients with and without NF1.

MPNSTs metastasize through blood, rarely via lymphatics. The most common sites of metastases are lung (fig. 12-27, top), distantly followed by bone, pleura (fig. 12-27, bottom), soft tissue, liver, and brain. Metastatic rates range from 40 to 68 percent (7,8). A lower rate of distant metastasis (25 percent) has been reported for childhood tumors (35). One study of tumors from diverse sites and in patients varying in age found a higher rate of metastasis in those with NF1 (35 percent) as opposed to those with sporadic tumors (16 percent) (5). This stands in contrast to studies specifically of MPNST of buttock and lower extremities (8) as well as of the paraspinal region (7,8) which reported no significant difference in the metastatic rates for patients with or without the syndrome.

Treatment. Centered upon surgical excision, a multimodality approach is currently used for treating MPNST of both adults and children. Although the type of resection varies with the anatomic location, wide en bloc resection is the procedure of choice for tumors involving soft tissues (8). Primary re-excision has been recommended in cases determined to have inadequate margins at the first operation (36). In one review of childhood cases, this resulted in 32 percent of patients with marginal resections achieving microscopically free margins (36). Postoperative radiation therapy is often administered to the tumor bed. This has led to some reduction in the incidence of locally recurrent MPNSTs in children with completely excised tumors, as well as for those in whom tumors were grossly resected but with microscopic residual disease and/or regional lymph node spread. The local failure is somewhat higher in nonirradiated patients, although not significantly so (36). In a small study of mostly adults, adjuvant irradiation (60 or more Gy) as well as brachytherapy and intraoperative electron irradiation significantly improved local tumor control (115,116).

Whether there is a role for chemotherapy in the treatment of MPNST is currently under investigation. Although MPNST is generally considered poorly responsive to adjuvant chemotherapy (35), Carli et al. (36) reported an overall response rate in children with MPNST of 45 percent, and 28 percent showing a significant response, particularly with the use of primary chemotherapy, which in 65 percent of the cases included ifosfamide.

Prognosis. The overall prognosis for patients with MPNST is poor, comparable to that of rhabdomyosarcoma patients (117), one of the most aggressive soft tissue sarcomas. Two large retrospective studies correlating strict histologic diagnosis with long-term follow-up found that 63 percent (5) and 68 percent (8) of patients died of tumor. In these series, the 5-year survival rate ranged from 34 to 39 percent. It could be argued that having been conducted at referral centers, each with a major interest in cancer care, the studies likely included a high percentage of advanced-stage tumors, thus making the results less representative of the behavior of MPNST as a whole. This same concern could be voiced regarding one study from a children's research hospital that reported a 5-year survival rate of 39 percent (40). Other studies, perhaps with more representative cases, reported 5-year survival rates of 43.7 percent (10) and 51 percent (36). A more recent, but not comparable series (115) reported a 5-year survival rate of 52 percent; the series differed from those above by the 15 percent inclusion of perineurial cell MPNSTs, a MPNST variant known to have a more favorable prognosis. In stark contrast to these various studies is one reporting a survival rate of 85 percent at 11 +/- 5 years (118), leading these authors to conclude that patients with MPNST "have a greater likelihood of long survival than all others with soft tissue tumors except for patients with epithelioid sarcoma." The study included 80 patients, 77.5 percent of whom had sporadic tumors. All data came from an in-house orthopedic oncology database accumulated over a period of 25 years starting in the 1970s, but apparently unaccompanied by a systematic pathologic review prior to publication. If, indeed, original microsections were not reevaluated applying current histologic, there is a high likelihood of tumor misclassifications. The study was further compromised in that specific data regarding tumor location and percentage of small or large (over 5 cm) lesions were not provided.

Tumor Location. The location of a tumor strongly influences patient survival. Early studies showed survival rates to be better for patients with extremity than with head and neck tumors (5). The same was true of lower extremity (8) versus truncal lesions (7). This was thought due to extremity lesions being detected earlier and more amenable to total resection. In a recent study of 123 patients (119), however, although MPNSTs affecting the peripheral portion of the upper limb were associated with the best survival on univariate analysis, the benefit of extremity involvement over other sites disappeared on multivariate analysis. The lower extremity is more often the site of these tumors, and part of the authors' explanation for their finding was that the majority of large volume tumors in their study were located in the distal lower extremity. On the other hand, in a large study of MPNSTs in children (36), multivariate analysis found extremity location to be an independent factor for survival.

Tumor Size. Larger tumor size is an adverse prognostic factor (5,7,8,10,35,36,120,121). In studies specifying the cutoff size, it was most often found to be 5 cm (5,10,36). In one study, the 5 cm cutoff held on multivariate analysis (36). In yet another study focusing upon tumor volume (119), multivariate analysis found less than 200 mL volume was associated with significantly better survival.

Histologic Grade. In our experience, using the two-grade system, high-grade tumors or those with a high-grade component account for most deaths. No acceptable criteria have yet been provided for MPNSTs of intermediate grade.

Resection with a Positive Margin, and Recurrence. In large series, positive margins (7,115) and/or failure to achieve local tumor control (8,36) are associated with a poor outcome. A more recent study (119) noted local recurrence in 30 percent of patients with inadequate margins as compared to 6 percent with adequate surgical margins, and that recurrence tended to be associated with a worse, but not statistically significant, outcome. In another study, this time of 35 patients with MPNST of the extremities, Vauthey et al. (116) found that seven of nine patients with tumor-positive margins died of disease and one was alive with disease. However, only three of the nine had a local recurrence. The authors concluded that the poor outcome associated with positive margins was perhaps related to tumor characteristics other than the inability to achieve adequate margins. Presumably, their reference was to occult distant metastasis.

Distant Metastasis. Most patients with distant metastatic MPNST die of the disease.

NF1 Association. There is a lack of consensus as to whether NF1 is an independent indicator of a poor prognosis in MPNST. Data from multiple series (5,119,122) suggest that patients with NF1 have a worse prognosis than those

with sporadic tumors. In some series, this difference in prognosis may be due to other factors, in particular, tumor location and size. The large series of Ducatman et al. (5) showed significant differences in 5- and 10-year survival rates; NF1-associated tumors were more often central in location (57 versus 36 percent), and large (74 versus 46 percent measuring 5 cm or more). In contrast to the above series are studies showing no significant difference in size or outcome between patients with and without NF1 (7,8,10,123). One of these studies dealt with buttock and lower extremity tumors (8) and the other with central/paraspinal MPNSTs (7).

MPNST Arising Postirradiation. Radiation-associated MPNSTs are known to be associated with a poor prognosis. In the first reported series (23) of seven patients, all died of tumor, survival periods ranging from 2 months to 2 years. A subsequent series describing 12 cases (24) confirmed the association with poor outcome: of 11 patients whose disease courses were followed, 9 died of tumor, having survived from 2 months to 23 years after diagnosis, all but 1 within 5 years. Of the remainder, 1 patient was alive at 15 months and another at 12 years. Combining data from both series, 16 of 19 (84 percent) patients with follow-up died of disease. As with the presence of NF1, this outcome may have been influenced by tumor site; all but one of the MPNSTs arose in the trunk or in an axial location. Tumor size was provided in too few cases to permit evaluation of its effect upon survival.

PERINEURIAL CELL MPNST

A small group of MPNSTs, designated *perineurial MPNST*, exhibit the characteristics of this second intrinsic element of nerve sheath (124,125). Their cells, often spindled with long cell processes, are arranged in whorls (fig. 12-28A) or in a storiform pattern (fig. 12-28B), embedded in a variable amount of myxoid matrix, and show immunoexpression for EMA (fig. 12-28C) rather than S-100 protein. Reactivity for Leu-7 may also be seen. Ultrastructural study reveals interdigitating cytoplasmic processes with surface pinocytotic vesicles, discontinuous basal lamina, and primitive cell junctions (fig. 12-29). Since no examples have been shown to arise directly from a conventional MPNST or neurofibroma, a case cannot be made for their representing divergent differentiation.

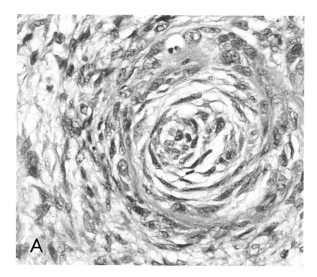

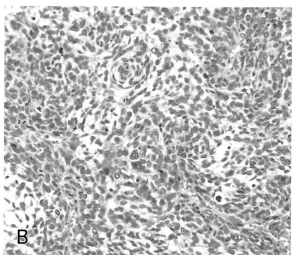

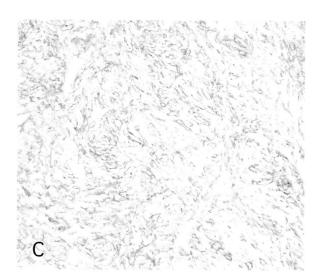

Figure 12-28

PERINEURIAL MPNST

A: Occasional MPNSTs show perineurial cell rather than Schwann cell differentiation, such as this example with focal whorl formation.

B: The cytoplasm of the tumor cells is less apparent than with conventional MPNST.

C: Typically, the tumors express epithelial membrane antigen (EMA), and not S-100 protein. (Courtesy of Dr. T. Hirose, Saitama, Japan.)

Figure 12-29

PERINEURIAL MPNST

The ultrastructural findings of the case illustrated in figure 12-28 include thin cytoplasmic processes with variable numbers of pinocytotic vesicles, discontinuous basal lamina, and occasional primitive junctions, features consistent with perineurial cell differentiation. (Courtesy of Dr. T. Hirose, Saitama, Japan.)

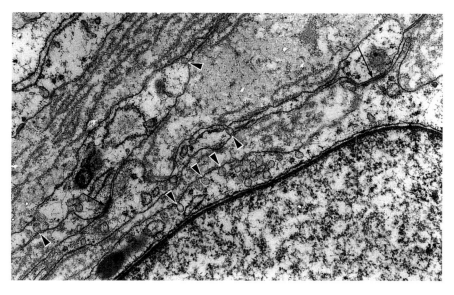

There are too few reported cases for a meaningful demographic study, but nine patients, representing both sexes and ranging in age from 11 to 83 (mean, 51.8) years, had acceptable tumors that included appropriate immunostaining (124,124a,125,125a). Soft tissue was the main site of origin, only one tumor was nerve associated, and none had arisen from a benign soft tissue perineurioma. No tumor was found to be encapsulated. The tumor cells were generally uniform in size and shape, with some pleomorphic cells in a few cases (124a,125a). There was limited to extensive high cellularity, varying degrees of anaplasia, mitotic activity ranging from 1 to 85/10 high-power fields and, in three cases, tumor necrosis. Based on high cellularity in most areas, frank anaplasia, frequent mitoses, and necrosis, four tumors were classified as high-grade malignant. Of eight followed cases, four tumors recurred locally and two (both high grade) metastasized distantly, but there were no tumor-related deaths. Thus far, the prognosis of patients with perineurial cell MPNST appears to be more favorable than with conventional spindle cell MPNST. Not included in this assessment because of an expressed diagnostic uncertainty, which possibly might have been resolved by an ultrastructural evaluation, was a fatal presumed high-grade perineurial cell MPNST with spindle and epithelioid cell features (125b).

Due to its EMA expression the tumor needs to be distinguished from monophasic synovial sarcoma. As with conventional spindle cell MPNST, differences include the usual presence of plumper nuclei, shorter cell processes, and intercellular dense collagen bands in synovial sarcoma, the cells of which also often immunostain for keratin. If needed, a molecular study for the t(x;18) translocation, specific to synovial sarcoma, can be performed.

VARIANTS OF SCHWANN CELL–DERIVED MPNST

Neoplastic Schwann cells exhibit a remarkable repertoire of cellular differentiation. This is reflected in MPNST variants with an epithelioid cell component and divergent differentiation.

EPITHELIOID MPNST

Epithelioid MPNSTs (Table 12-2) are composed of cytologically malignant cells extensively or exclusively epithelioid. They account for only a small percentage of MPNSTs and are unassociated with NF1. Most originate de novo within nerve, while a few arise from conventional schwannoma or neurofibroma. The tumors represent more than simple histologic variants of MPNST since their prognosis differs somewhat depending upon the histology of the underlying peripheral nerve tumor.

Deep Epithelioid MPNST

Definition and General Features. The most thoroughly studied epithelioid MPNSTs are the deeply situated ones. Although often nerve associated (fig. 12-30), they are unassociated with schwannoma, neurofibroma or, for that matter, NF1. Based on data from 27 cases (47,126–129), patient age at diagnosis ranged from 6 to 74 years (mean, 36 years), with no gender predilection. Generally peripheral in location, 70 percent were situated in an extremity, most in a lower extremity. The brachial plexus and sciatic, peroneal, and tibial nerves were most often affected.

Gross Findings. Grossly, the tumor ranges from 1.5 to 15.0 cm (mean, 5.9 cm). Most are fusiform in configuration, although in the above studies, two were plexiform, one involving multiple nerves of a brachial plexus (128) and the other multiple fascicles of a single nerve; neither was NF1 associated. The cut surface, generally described as gray-white, is usually tan-brown on quick examination (within 3 minutes of sectioning). The partial or extensive, nodular or cobblestone texture differs from conventional MPNST (fig. 12-30). Necrosis and hemorrhage are often present.

Microscopic Findings. Microscopically, most epithelioid MPNSTs have a spindle cell element, and only a few are purely epithelioid (47,126,128). In epithelioid tumor areas, there is noticeable compartmentalization, and the tumor is divided into lobules by thick fibrovascular and thin fibrous septa (fig. 12-31). The cells are cytologically malignant; round, oval to polygonal or oblong; and disposed in compact nests (fig. 12-32A), sheets (fig. 12-32B), anastomosing strings or cords (fig. 12-33), and micropapillae. The cytoplasm is abundant and most often eosinophilic to plum-colored. Nuclei are typically vesicular and of varying size with sometimes prominent nucleoli (fig. 12-32). The

Table 12-2

COMPARATIVE FINDINGS FOR EPITHELIOID MPNST SUBSETS

Subtype	Deep Epithelioid MPNST	Superficial Epithelioid MPNST	Schwannoma with Epithelioid MPNST	Neurofibroma with Epithelioid MPNST
Association	Nerve	Small nerve or neurofibroma	One tumor in a patient with NF2	No patient with NF1 but one tumor post-irradiation
Ages (years), gender ratio	6-74 (mean, 36), M=2F	19-81 (mean, 36), M=F	20-75 (mean, 51), 6M:4F	21-74 (mean, 48), 6M:2F
Location	Brachial plexus, sciatic, peroneal, tibial nerves	Mostly in extremities	Widely distributed	Mostly in extremities
Gross	51.8% ≥5 cm (mean, 5.95 cm); most often fusiform; tan, brown, and nodular	80% ≥ 5 cm (mean, 4.8 cm)	63.6% ≥ 5 cm (mean, 6 cm); malignant component crumbly, dirty white or cheesy gray	All but one < 5 cm; sizes of epithelioid component, when measured, < 2.1 cm
Microscopic	Most arise in spindle cell MPNSTs; compartmentalized, with oval, polygonal, string-like cells; often with myxoid matrix; usually S-100 protein +	Uni- or multinodular; nested molded cells; little stroma; no mucinous component; 75% S-100 protein +	Relatively circumscribed but infiltrative growth of epithelioid cells with eosinophilic cytoplasm and prominent nucleoli; cells sometimes S-100 protein and keratin +	Malignant epithelioid cells form oval circumscribed lesions; cells rounded and closely packed, have faintly eosinophilic to amphophilic cytoplasm and indistinct cell borders; nuclei with prominent nucleoli; cells usually strongly S-100 protein +
Outcome	Similar to that of conventional MPNST	Follow-up data insufficient for a reliable statement	Of 7 patients followed for at least 1 year, 5 (71.4%) died of disease	Of 5 of 8 patients with some follow-up, 2 had recurrent tumors, and 1 died of an unrelated disorder

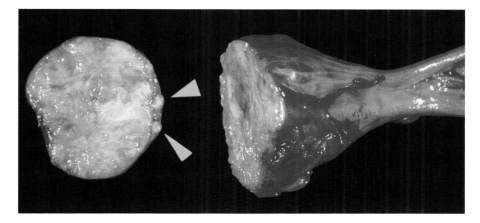

Figure 12-30

DEEP EPITHELIOID MPNST

Epithelioid MPNSTs are frequently nerve related, as is this example arising from the sciatic nerve of a 43-year-old man. In contrast to the relatively smooth cut surfaces of conventional MPNST, the surfaces of epithelioid MPNST generally have a cobblestone appearance. (Courtesy of Dr. W.F. Ballinger, Gainesville, FL.)

cytologic variations include both rhabdoid cells with eccentric nuclei and dense eosinophilic cytoplasm as well as clear cells (fig. 12-32B) (129). Although mainly mononuclear, occasional cells in a syncytial arrangement mimic multinucleation. Hyaluronic acid-rich mucin accumulation (fig. 12-31A,C) can be striking, even forming pools of matrix (fig. 12-31D). A reliable diagnosis of a purely epithelioid MPNST depends upon demonstrating a nerve of origin as well as distinctive immunoreactivities.

Immunohistochemical Findings. In addition to diffuse vimentin immunoreactivity (fig. 12-34A), most deep epithelioid MPNSTs express S-100 protein in the form of cytoplasmic and nuclear reactivity, which may be diffuse (fig. 12-34B,C) or localized. We have also observed Leu-7 (CD57) staining. Occasional tumors show cytokeratin or EMA reactivity (130). In our experience, collagen 4 or laminin staining highlights the basal lamina around individual or clustered cells. Unlike melanomas, epithelioid

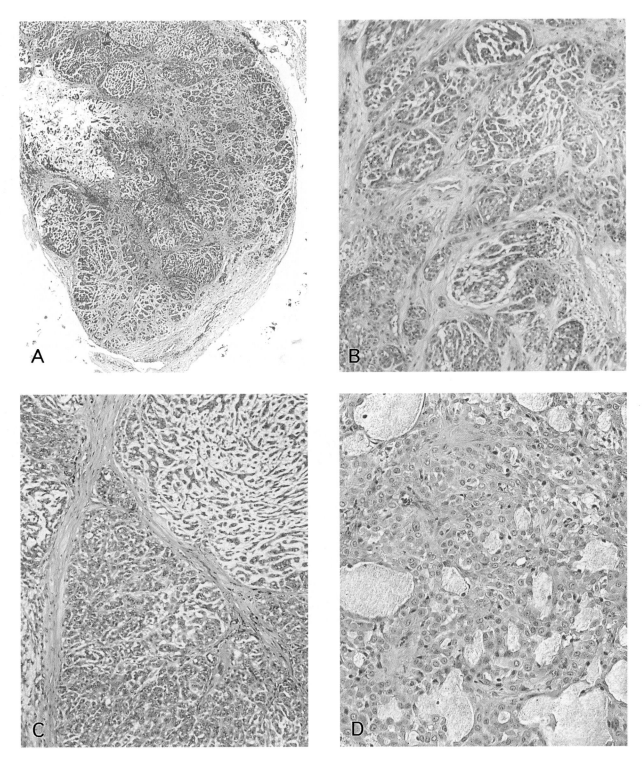

Figure 12-31

DEEP EPITHELIOID MPNST

Low-power microscopy of an epithelioid cell area reveals lobulation (A–C), with the lobules separated by fibrous septa (B,C). The tumor cells often are embedded in mucin (A–C), which sometimes pools in microcysts (D).

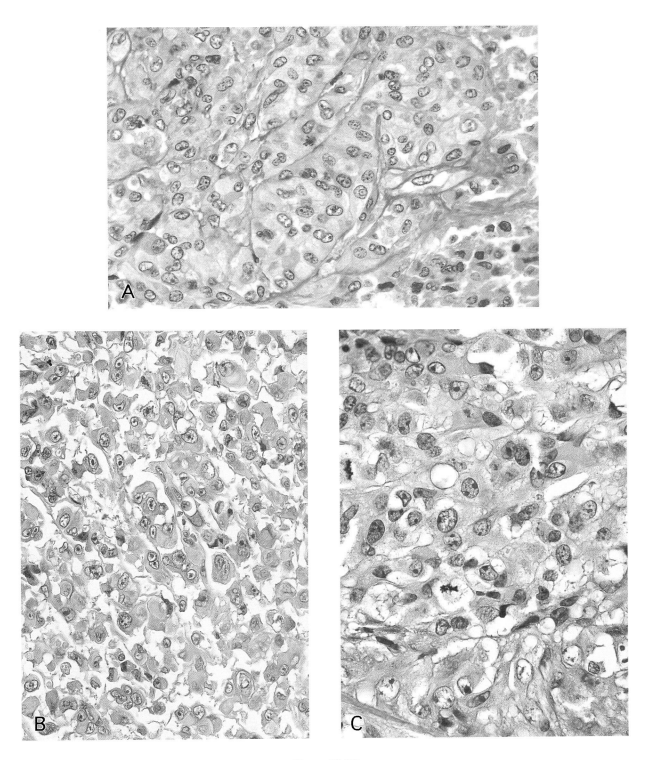

Figure 12-32

DEEP EPITHELIOID MPNST

Epithelioid cells, often growing in nests (A) or sheets (B), are round, oval, or polygonal, and sometimes oblong. Each contains abundant eosinophilic or plum-colored cytoplasm, and some show mucin production (C). The nuclei are variably sized, and the epithelioid tumor cells in which they are eccentrically placed may have a rhabdoid appearance (B).

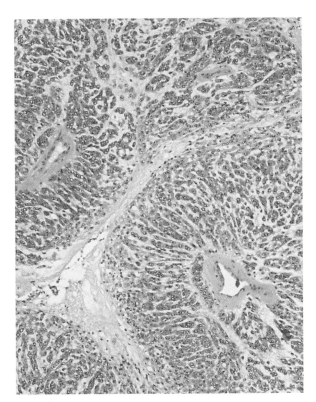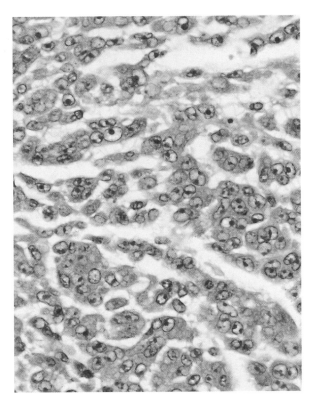

Figure 12-33

DEEP EPITHELIOID MPNST

The tumor cells are arranged in strings and cords.

MPNSTs are immunonegative for the melanoma-associated antigen HMB45 (129).

Ultrastructural Findings. Ultrastructural studies may be useful when results of immunostains are inconclusive, or when differentiation from carcinoma or extraskeletal myxoid chondrosarcoma is unresolved. Key findings include epithelioid cells (fig. 12-35) with delicate interdigitating cytoplasmic projections, varying numbers of cytoplasmic intermediate filaments and microtubules, moderate numbers of rudimentary and tight junctions, discontinuous basal lamina which, when present, varies from scant to reduplicated (fig. 12-36), and diffuse intercellular accumulations of external lamina substance (47,78,128,131,132). Rhabdoid cell forms contain large numbers of cytoplasmic intermediate filaments that are usually vimentin (fig. 12-37). Features of true epithelial differentiation, such as tonofilaments, secretory granules, microvilli, and lumen formation, are absent. An exception was one reported epithelioid MPNST with squamous differentiation, as evidenced by tonofilament formation (130).

Differential Diagnosis. The differential diagnosis of deep epithelioid MPNST includes clear cell sarcoma, extraskeletal myxoid chondrosarcoma, and carcinoma. Its distinction from melanoma and clear cell sarcoma rests on the absence in epithelioid MPNST of melanin on histochemical stains, immunoexpression of melanoma-associated antigens (HMB45, Melan-A, tyrosinase), and ultrastructurally identifiable melanosomes. Clear cell sarcomas have characteristic multinucleated tumor giant cells, and in about 90 percent of the cases, a characteristic t(12;22) on molecular analysis. Extraskeletal myxoid chondrosarcoma differs in containing hyaluronidase-resistant stromal mucin, exhibiting different ultrastructural features, and showing a distinctive t(9;22) translocation. The near total removal of mucin from epithelioid MPNST by hyaluronidase treatment also distinguishes it from extraskeletal myxoid chondrosarcoma. While extraskeletal myxoid

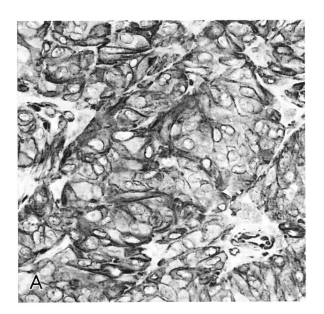

Figure 12-34

DEEP EPITHELIOID MPNST

In addition to vimentin reactivity (A), such tumors reveal strong, diffuse S-100 protein immunostaining (B,C). Occasionally, an otherwise typical example stains for cytokeratin as well.

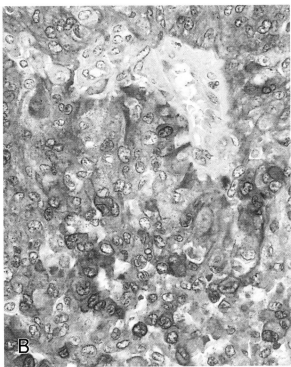

chondrosarcoma may stain for S-100 protein, it lacks keratin reactivity and an association with nerve. The exclusion of carcinoma may prove difficult but is based on a general lack of widespread keratin and EMA immunoreactivity as well as of ultrastructural features of epithelial cells.

Treatment and Prognosis. The clinical outcome for patients with deep epithelioid

MPNST is little different than that for those with conventional MPNST. Of the above-mentioned group of 27 patients (both of the patients reported by DiCarlo et al. [47] subsequently died of disease), 37 percent had distant metastases and 48 percent died of tumor, that figure rising to 66.7 percent if only patients followed for at least 5 years were included. Sites of metastasis

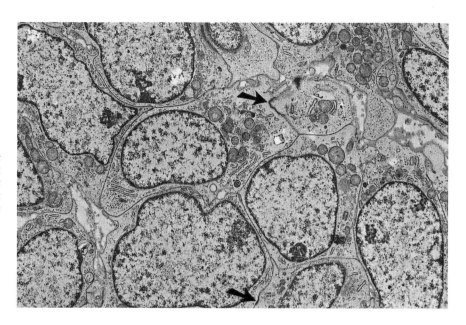

Figure 12-35

DEEP EPITHELIOID MPNST

Clustered epithelioid tumor cells are joined by scattered tight junction-like intercellular junctions (arrows). Flocculent basal lamina substance is in the intercellular space.

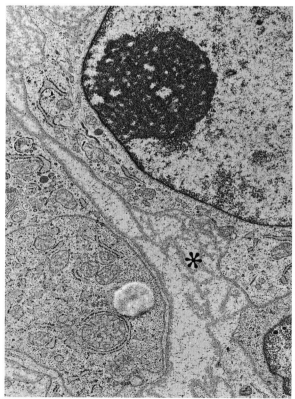

Figure 12-36

DEEP EPITHELIOID MPNST

A round tumor cell nucleus contains a large nucleolus and prominent reduplicated basal lamina (asterisk).

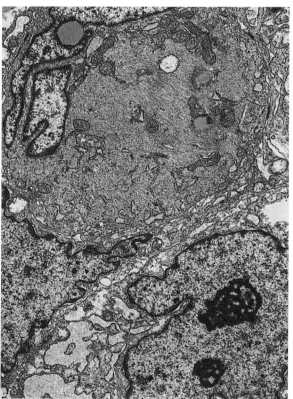

Figure 12-37

DEEP EPITHELIOID MPNST

A tumor cell has a "rhabdoid" appearance due to a peripherally displaced nucleus and cytoplasm distended with intermediate filaments, shown immunohistochemically to be vimentin.

were similar to those for conventional MPNST, with one exception: 18.5 percent of the patients developed lymph node metastases.

Superficial Epithelioid MPNST

Definition and General Features. *Superficial epithelioid MPNSTs*, defined as arising above the superficial fascia, specifically in the skin and subcutaneous tissue, are in need of more investigation and a more precise histologic definition. The reasons for this include the obvious difficulty of demonstrating an origin from a small nerve, frequent lack of close histologic resemblance to deep epithelioid MPNST, and greater difficulty in distinguishing the tumor from melanocytic lesions. With respect to the latter, some presumed examples of superficial epithelioid MPNST from the head have exhibited clinical and histologic features more in keeping with neurotropic melanoma (133).

Clinical and Microscopic Findings. In the largest reported series of nine tumors (129), patients ranged in age from 19 to 81 years (mean, 39 years) with no gender predilection. The tumors presented below the head and neck and involved mostly an extremity, preferentially an arm. There was an association with nerve in six cases, nerve and neurofibroma in two, and a neurofibroma alone in one. Three tumors were 5 cm or larger (mean, 4.8 cm). Histologically, the tumors were typically uninodular rather than multinodular. Except in two cases, the cells were not discrete but molded one to another in nests or tight clusters with little or no intervening stroma or mucinous matrix. To the authors, this appearance was reminiscent of cell nests in nevi. Of the two remaining tumors, the cells were aligned in cords in one instance and pleomorphic in the other. There was some nucleolar prominence and mitotic activity. Three fourths of the tumors stained for S-100 protein. Follow-up of more than 1 year, available in 37 percent of cases, revealed one instance of pulmonary metastasis and no tumor-related deaths. In view of such limited follow-up, no reliable assessment of outcome could be made.

Differential Diagnosis. Primary considerations in the differential diagnosis of superficial epithelioid MPNST are epithelioid schwannoma, a tumor not uncommonly exhibiting worrisome

cellular atypia; large intradermal nevi; and melanoma. Melanoma in particular must be ruled out for any presumed epithelioid MPNST arising in or nearby mucous membranes in the head. The tumor is less likely to be mistaken for epithelioid sarcoma, the cells of which have dense eosinophilic cytoplasm and are often embedded in dense collagen. In addition, epithelioid sarcomas tend to be multifocal rather than unifocal, superficially resemble necrobiotic granulomas, usually lack S-100 protein immunoreactivity in the face of a positive keratin reaction, show loss of INI-1 expression, and ultrastructurally feature tonofilaments.

Conventional Schwannoma with Epithelioid Malignancy

These are unusual tumors given the long-held notion that schwannomas are always benign, a view fostered by Stout's inability to find any convincing reports of malignant change (134). The almost universally benign histology and behavior of conventional schwannomas, coupled with the extreme rarity of frank anaplastic transformation (see below), have slowed its recognition. Instead of a spindle cell proliferation, malignant transformation most often takes the form of epithelioid cells (135). The lesion is rare and may occur in an incipient as well as the fully developed form.

We know of only 11 convincing cases of frank *malignant epithelioid MPNST evolving from schwannoma,* also referred to as *epithelioid MPNST ex-schwannoma* (17,135,136). In addition to the above cases, there is data regarding nine schwannomas showing similar cytologic changes, albeit focal and microscopic. Originally reported by Nayler (137), it was termed *epithelioid malignant change* (EMC) (136).

Epithelioid MPNST Ex-Schwannoma. The general profile of epithelioid MPNST arising in schwannomas includes occurrence in adulthood (range, 20 to 75 years; mean, 51 years) and male predominance (1.5 to 1.0). Of the 11 reported cases, the youngest patient was NF2-affected (fig. 12-38), and the remainder had sporadic lesions. One tumor arose following radiotherapy of the schwannoma (26). Three tumors were clinically present from 3 to 20 years. Three tumors were painful, one painful and associated with paresthesias, and two rapidly enlarging.

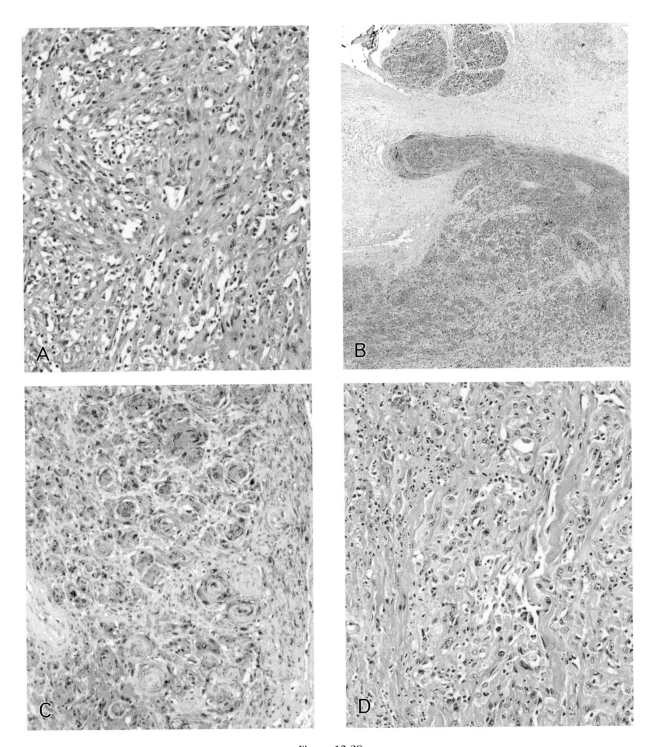

Figure 12-38

EPITHELIOID MPNST EX-SCHWANNOMA: IN PATIENT WITH NF2

Among reported examples of epithelioid MPNST arising from schwannomas, one developed in a patient with NF2. This schwannoma, identified by the presence of Antoni A tissue (A) and cell whorls (C), was strongly S-100 protein immunoreactive (B,C). It arose in the retroperitoneum, measured 10 cm in greatest dimension, had a malignant epithelioid cell component (D), and was extensively necrotic (17).

They were widely distributed, involving the cerebellopontine angle, neck, lower spinal and pelvis region, retroperitoneum, and upper and lower extremities. Stated maximal sizes of 10 of the lesions were 4 to less than 5 cm (4 cases), and from 5 to 10 cm (6 cases); the overall mean size was 6 cm. Gross descriptions indicated that the tumors were totally or partly encapsulated, some of the latter showing focal capsular invasion. With respect to their sectioned appearance, one report mentioned an area of rough and crumbly dirty white tissue (138), and another, an eccentric 2-cm diameter, irregularly defined, cheesy, gray focus distinct from the adjacent brown tissue (139).

Microscopically, features of the parent schwannoma, including Antoni A (figs. 12-38A,B; 12-39A,B) and Antoni B (fig. 12-39A) tissue, Verocay bodies, and in one case cellular whorls (fig. 12-38C), were found. All were diffusely immunoreactive for S-100 protein (fig. 12-38B,C). Each schwannoma was altered by invasive, cytologically malignant epithelioid cells (figs. 12-38D, 12-39A–C) characterized by polygonal, round, and less frequently, oblong shapes; abundant, sometimes dense eosinophilic cytoplasm; somewhat pleomorphic nuclei with vesicular nuclei; and often prominent nucleoli. Occasional binucleation or multinucleation was seen (136). Mitotic figures were usually seen, and focal to extensive necrosis (fig. 12-39B) was present in 6 of 11 tumors. Intercellular mucin was noted in only a single case (129). The immunotype included focal S-100 protein expression in 5 of 7 cases (fig. 12-39D) and more diffuse staining for keratin in at least 3 of 4 (fig. 12-39E).

Follow-up data indicate a poor outcome for patients with this form of MPNST: of 7 patients followed for at least 1 year or who had not died before that time of unrelated cause, 5 (71.4 percent) died of tumor. The tumors recurred locally and/or metastasized to lung, lymph nodes, adrenal gland, and liver. Survival was no longer than 1 year.

Epithelioid Malignant Change (EMC). Ten conventional schwannomas with what was interpreted as microfocal epithelioid malignant change (EMC) have been reported (136). As stated by the authors, EMC denotes the presence of scattered, large epithelioid cells resembling,

to varying degree, those seen in epithelioid MPNST ex-schwannoma. They are distinguished from ordinary tumoral Schwann cells by their larger size and plump shape, open chromatin, and prominent nucleoli (fig. 12-40). They differ from schwannoma cells showing degenerative atypia with its characteristic smudgy chromatin (see figs 7-11D, 7-39C). They are disposed singly, scattered, or clustered. Only in one case did they form a minute (5 mm) nodule. One of the 10 schwannomas featured coexistent invasive epithelioid MPNST. In contrast with the cells of invasive malignant epithelioid MPNST, those of EMC are strongly immunoreactive for S-100 protein. Further, there is no uniform MIB-1 staining.

The clinical findings in this group of patients are of great interest. Among the 9 having solely EMC, ages ranged from 16 to 53 years (mean, 31 years), fully 20 years younger than the mean age of patients with epithelioid MPNST ex-schwannoma. The gender distribution was near equal. The tumors with EMC had most often been present for months as compared to years for the fully malignant tumors.

According to McMenamin and Fletcher (136), the above findings suggest that EMC may represent an "in-situ" phase for the formation of epithelioid MPNST ex-schwannoma. Unfortunately, four of their patients with EMC lacked follow-up and one presented with additional nodules 9 and 48 months after diagnosis. This led to a cautionary recommendation to consider a modest but wider re-excision of the tumor area as long as it had no significant adverse functional or cosmetic effect, until such time as the biologic implications of EMC are better understood. The authors further suggested designating such tumors as "atypical schwannoma with epithelioid cells." A distinction should be made here with epithelioid schwannoma in which the epithelioid cells show atypia (see chapter 7).

Differential Diagnosis. The two main tumors in the differential diagnosis of epithelioid MPNST ex-schwannoma are schwannoma with angiosarcomatous transformation and epithelioid schwannoma. Clearly the more important, angiosarcoma arising in schwannoma consists of epithelioid malignant endothelial cells lining haphazardly arranged channels and sheet-like growth. Cytologically, the angiosarcoma cells so closely resemble those of epithelioid MPNST that

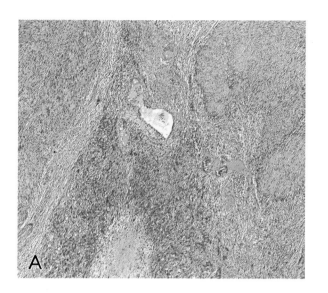

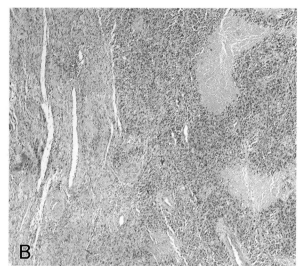

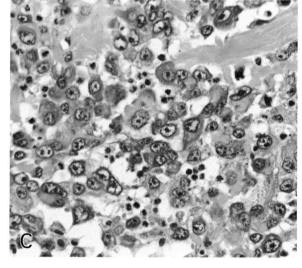

Figure 12-39

EPITHELIOID MPNST EX-SCHWANNOMA

The presence of Antoni A tissue (A) and Verocay bodies (B) allows classification of both tumors as conventional schwannomas. Each is involved by an infiltrative and destructive neoplasm consisting of epithelioid cells with dense eosinophilic cytoplasm and round nuclei having prominent nuclear membranes and variably sized conspicuous nucleoli (C). The malignant neoplasm arising in one of the schwannomas (B) is partly necrotic. In some cases malignant epithelioid cells express S-100 protein (D) and keratin CAM 5.2 (E).

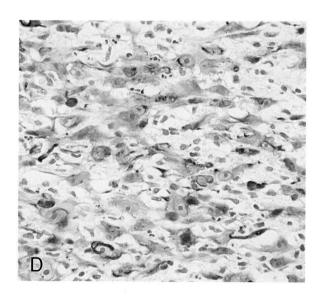

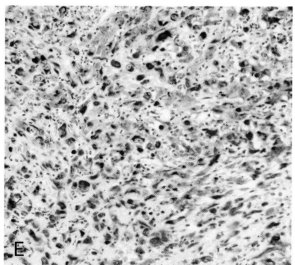

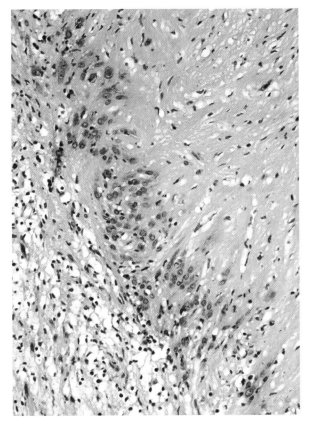

Figure 12-40

**EPITHELIOID MALIGNANT CHANGE (EMC)
IN CONVENTIONAL SCHWANNOMA**

Schwann cells showing change line the rim of Antoni A tissue, and differ cytologically from those with post-irradiation atypia (see fig. 12-26E).

their distinction often rests upon the demonstration of the endothelial cell markers CD31 (see fig. 12-46G) and Fli1. Compared with the cells of epithelioid MPNST, the cells of epithelioid schwannoma are smaller, lack pleomorphism, and possess nuclei more uniformly round, non-vesicular and without nucleolar enlargement (see fig. 7-19). This is not to say that epithelioid schwannomas do not, on occasion, exhibit minor cellular atypia. The distinction may be difficult, but it is one of importance.

Neurofibroma with Malignant Epithelioid Cell Differentiation

Neurofibroma with malignant epithelioid cell differentiation is equally as rare as epithelioid MPNST ex-schwannoma. In a group of nine,

almost entirely nonplexiform neurofibromas, seven previously reported (128,129,140) and two that we have seen in consultation, seven occurred in males and two in females. The patient age ranged from 21 to 74 (mean, 48 years). No patient had NF1, but the tumor in one arose in a plexiform neurofibroma and in another was radiation related. Equally distributed between superficial and deep sites, nearly half involved an upper extremity; the remainder involved the neck, brachial plexus, sciatic nerve, thigh, and calf. Maximal tumor sizes, known in eight instances and presumably reflecting the dimensions of the parent neurofibroma, ranged from 2 to 8 cm, all but one being smaller than 5 cm.

Unlike spindle cell MPNST arising in neurofibroma in which the malignant cells infiltrate linearly, in our own experience and that of others (128,129,140), the malignant epithelioid cells form circumscribed, cellular lesions (fig. 12-41A). This would facilitate sizing the malignant component of the lesion, if routinely performed and reported. In our two cases, the malignant component in one measured 0.7 x 0.3 cm within a 2.0 x 0.7-cm tumor (fig. 12-41A) and 2.1 x 1.7 cm within a neurofibroma measuring 2.5 x 1.7 x 1.7 cm (fig. 12-41D). Currently accepted cytologic criteria useful in the identification of malignant epithelioid cells are illustrated by Allison et al. (140) and in our two examples (fig. 12-41B,D). In each of these three tumors, the malignant component formed a roughly oval, generally circumscribed aggregate of crowded, sometimes nested, rounded or polygonal epithelioid cells with indistinct cell borders, eosinophilic to amphophilic cytoplasm, and oval nuclei containing prominent nucleoli. None of the tumors exhibited myxoid change, a feature of many deep epithelioid MPNST, nor was it mentioned in other reports. Mitoses were readily evident and in one of our tumors, the epithelioid cells had high MIB-1 labeling index. Uniform, strong S-100 protein immunoreactivity (fig. 12-41C) was noted in eight of nine cases, and only one tumor was negative for this marker. Follow-up of at least 3 years and as many as 18 years was obtained in five cases. Two tumors, the high-power histology of which was not illustrated, recurred locally (128,129), one affecting a patient dying of unrelated disease at 18 years (128). No patient died of tumor. The excellent outcome

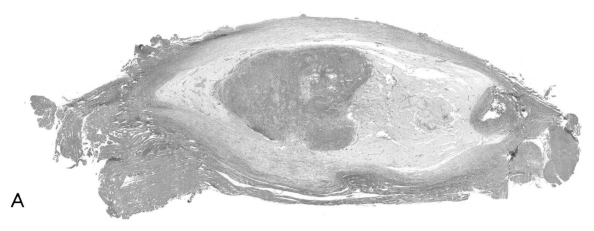

A

Figure 12-41

NEUROFIBROMA WITH EPITHELIOID MPNST

A 2.5 x 1.7 x 1.7-cm neurofibroma from the neck of a 43-year-old man had harbored a 0.7 x 0.3-cm well-circumscribed epithelioid MPNST (A,B). The epithelioid cells were strongly and diffusely reactive for S-100 protein (C). Another epithelioid MPNST, found within a 2.5 x 1.7-cm neurofibroma removed from a 31-year-old man exhibited a higher degree of cytologic atypia (D). Neither neurofibroma was plexiform.

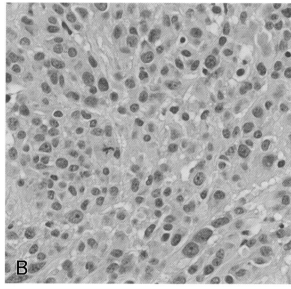

B

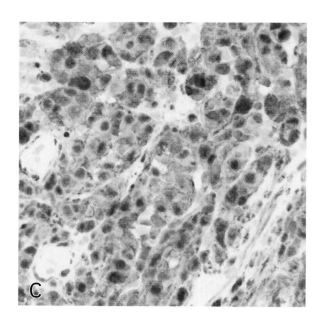

C

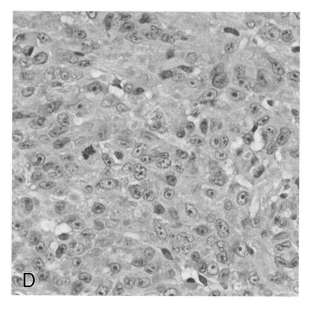

D

Table 12-3

FORMS OF DIVERGENT DIFFERENTIATION IN PNST TYPES

PNST Type	Rhabdomyosarcoma, Chondrosarcoma, or Osteosarcoma	Angiosarcoma	Glandular Differentiation	Squamous Differentiation	Primitive Neuroepithelium
Schwannoma	One case with rhabdomyosarcoma	+	−	+	+
Neurofibroma	−	+	+	−	−
Conventional spindle cell MPNST	+	+	+	+	+
Ganglioneuroblastoma with MPNST	−				
Ganglioneuroma with MPNST	One case with rhabdomyosarcoma		−	−	−
Pheochromocytoma with MPNST	One case with rhabdomyosarcoma		−	−	−

may be attributable to the often small size of the malignant element which permits initial complete or wide tumor resection.

With respect to the differential diagnosis, we know of no reported instances of malignant epithelioid neoplasms metastatic to neurofibroma. It is important that a neurofibroma with a benign epithelioid cell component (see chapter 8) not be misinterpreted as neurofibroma with epithelioid MPNST. Discerning the differences rests on identifying malignant cytologic features. More remote is the likelihood that a giant nevus with both neurofibroma-like areas and a nodule of melanoma is mistaken for a neurofibroma-derived epithelioid MPNST.

MPNST WITH DIVERGENT DIFFERENTIATION

Schwann cell-derived MPNSTs possess a capacity for divergent differentiation unsurpassed by all but germ cell tumors. The spectrum includes various types of mesenchymal cells and epithelial cells, each representing subclonal divergent differentiation. The currently accepted explanation for this is the capacity of migrating neural crest cells to form not only melanocytes, ganglion cells, and Schwann cells, but to contribute to the formation of head and truncal mesenchymal tissue (141–143). Migrating neural crest tissue capable of such variation is referred to as "ectomesenchyme" (142). Schwann cells apparently retain this developmental program which can be activated in neoplastic states. Possible factors underlying the transition are discussed by Pytel et al. (144). That the capac-

ity for divergent differentiation is a feature of neuroectoderm in general is supported by the finding of skeletal muscle in leptomeninges (145), and by reports of myogenesis in gliomas (146), medulloblastoma (147), and intraocular malignant medulloepithelioma (148). Given no developmental counterpart to epithelial differentiation in PNST, its presence in primarily malignant examples has yet to be explained.

Although elements of divergent differentiation in MPNST are all Schwann cell derived, they vary in type and somewhat predictably occur in certain tumors. In schwannomas, the progenitor is well-differentiated neoplastic Schwann cells; in neurofibroma and most conventional MPNSTs, it may be either the same or neoplastic Schwann cells with perineurial-like ultrastructural features. It is, therefore, not surprising that the repertoire of divergent phenotypic changes and their frequency vary to some degree with the parent tumor type (Table 12-3). Glandular epithelium is rare in neurofibroma, having been reported only twice (see figs. 8-34, 12-45A), and one neurofibroma was clearly plexiform (18,78,149). Glandular epithelium is not formed by schwannomas. Rhabdomyosarcomas and a variety of epithelia are almost exclusively seen in otherwise conventional MPNSTs. Such variants represent around 15 percent of MPNSTs. Awareness of the morphologic spectrum of divergent differentiation in MPNST is essential in distinguishing such tumors from histologically similar soft tissue tumors. Understandably, phenotypically compound tumors represent fertile

Malignant Tumors of the Peripheral Nerves

429

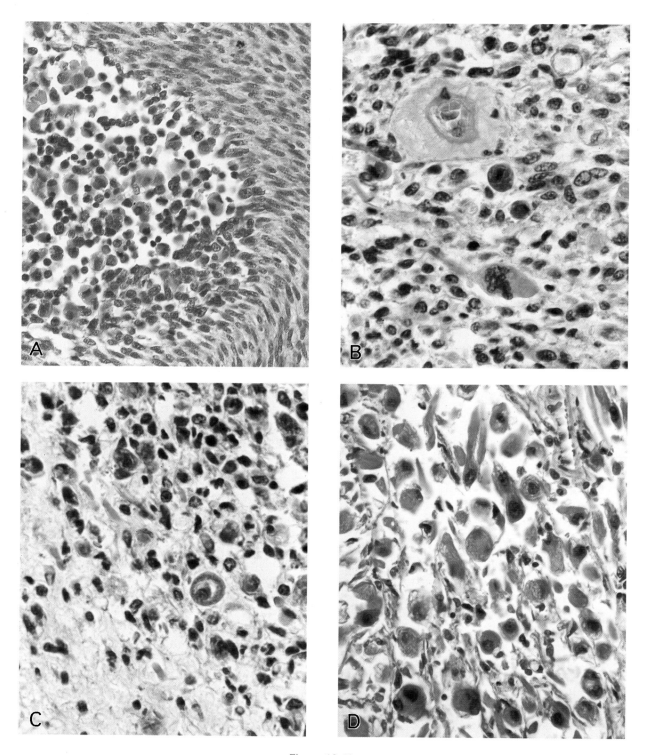

Figure 12-42

MPNST WITH RHABDOMYOBLASTIC DIFFERENTIATION

In malignant triton tumors, the appearance of skeletal muscle elements varies. The sarcoma is most often focal (A) and the rhabdomyosarcoma cells are small with little or no myoplasm (A–C); round (C) or strap-shaped (B,D) with abundant myoplasm; or round with a myoplasmic ring (C,D).

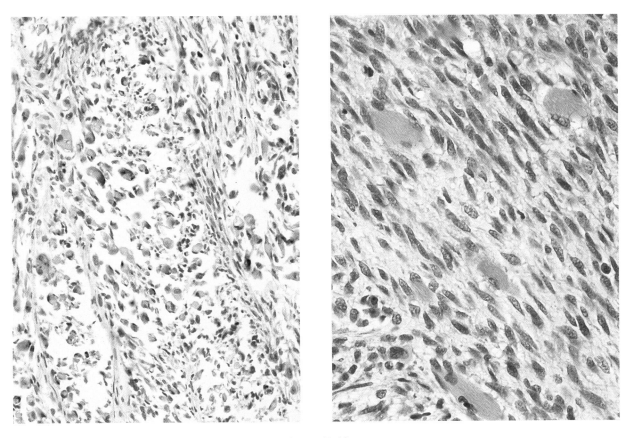

Figure 12-43

MPNST WITH RHABDOMYOSARCOMATOUS DIFFERENTIATION

Left: If required for a diagnosis, proof of skeletal muscle differentiation can be established by immunostaining for alpha sarcomeric actin, myogenin, and as illustrated, muscle-specific actin (HHF-35).

Right: When MPNST is infiltrative of skeletal muscle, distinction must be made between divergent myosarcomatous differentiation and trapped skeletal muscle cells, the latter characterized by a uniform distribution in the tumor and within the cells a uniform distribution of fibers.

ground for diagnostic misinterpretation, a problem we encountered in several published reports and in selected instances call to the reader's attention. On balance, the treatment of MPNST exhibiting divergent differentiation is no different from that of conventional MPNST.

MPNST with Divergent Mesenchymal Differentiation

Among tumors in this category are examples featuring rhabdomyosarcoma (figs. 12-42–12-44), chondrosarcoma (fig. 12-9H), osteosarcoma (see fig. 12-51C), and angiosarcoma (figs. 12-45, 12-46), either singly or in combination. In most instances, the underlying MPNST is conventional spindle cell MPNST.

PNSTs with Rhabdomyosarcoma. This most common form of MPNST with divergent differentiation has been referred to as *malignant triton tumor* (150), a term recalling its original description by Masson in 1932 (151). Using the experimental formation of supernumerary limbs at the site of implantation of sciatic nerve into the back of salamanders of the genus Triturus, Masson suggested that one possible explanation for skeletal muscle differentiation in "neuromas" was the inductive influence of motor nerves. The other, and current, explanation is that mesenchymal differentiation is due to autonomous transformation (151) of neoplastic Schwann cells into striated muscle cells (152). This interpretation is in keeping with the pattern

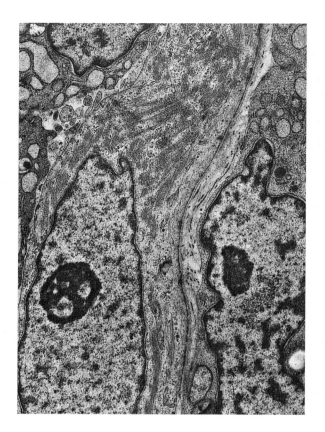 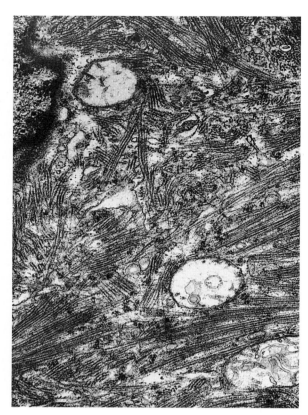

Figure 12-44

MPNST WITH RHABDOMYOBLASTIC DIFFERENTIATION

Ultrastructural findings in rhabdomyoblasts include arrays of rudimentary sarcomeres (left) and disarrayed myosin filaments (right).

of mesenchymal differentiation of neural crest cells observed in embryogenesis.

To qualify as a malignant triton tumor, the underlying nerve sheath tumor should display convincing features of a benign or malignant PNST. To date, with the exception of one schwannoma (153), all have arisen in MPNSTs. In both the above schwannoma and in conventional MPNSTs, the cells giving rise to the rhabdomyoblasts are assumed to be subclones of malignant cells.

In a 1994 review (154), the clinical features of reported cases included a wide age range from newborn to 75 years (mean, 34 years) with no sex predilection and little pediatric representation. Males and females were equally represented. The head, neck, and thigh were most frequently involved. A small majority of patients (57 percent) had NF1 and at least five examples were radiation induced (154,155).

Grossly indistinguishable from a high-grade conventional MPNST, the tumors may or may not be nerve associated. Histologically, there must be convincing histologic evidence of tumor origin in a benign or malignant PNST. Accepting only marginal evidence leads to potential misclassification. In the majority of cases, rhabdomyoblasts are only a minor or localized tumor component (fig. 12-42A) and resemble embryonal rhabdomyosarcoma. The cells vary from small with little cytoplasm and hyperchromatic spindle-shaped nuclei to rounded, ring, strap, or a mixture of these cells (fig. 12-42B–D) (150), often with ample dense to brightly eosinophilic cytoplasm and centrally situated hyperchromatic nuclei. Multinucleated cells are uncommonly encountered (fig. 12-42B). Although concentric perinuclear fibrils and cross striations are often evident with the H&E stain (150), they are accentuated on phosphotungstic acid-hematoxylin (PTAH) preparations. When the myogenic nature of the cells is inapparent, it can be confirmed by immunoreactivity for muscle markers (see below). The rhabdomyoblasts often congregate about dilated blood vessels. Entrapped normal muscle (fig. 12-43, right) is readily distinguished from tumor by its geometric fiber arrangement and uniform orientation of sarcomeres. Some malignant triton tumors contain additional tumor elements, such as osteosarcoma, chondrosarcoma, or epithelial cells (see fig. 12-51). MPNSTs with proliferation of more than one subclone of neoplastic cells are referred to as *MPNST with pluridirectional differentiation*. Whereas mesenchymal components of a MPNST typically appear malignant, epithelial cells most often exhibit benign cytologic features.

The immunoprofile of most malignant triton tumors corresponds to that of conventional MPNST with the addition of some neoplastic cells immunoreactive for muscle markers such as desmin, muscle-specific antigen (HHF-35) (fig. 12-43, left), alpha sarcomeric antigen, and myogenin. Like other MPNSTs, at least 50 percent express S-100 protein. A definitive ultrastructural feature of striated muscle cells is the formation of rudimentary sarcomeres with stacks of myosin filaments (fig. 12-44).

There have been few cytogenetic studies of malignant triton tumor. Examining two tumors, one study found both to show trisomy 22 and structural rearrangements of chromosomes 2, 7, and 21 at identical or closely related breakpoints (156). Specifically, the chromosomal breakpoint 7p22 was altered in both tumors, a finding reported earlier by Riccardi et al. (157) in one unusual tumor said to have a liposarcomatous component. Other abnormalities involved chromosomes 1, 5, 6, 8, 9, 14, and 16. More recently, the analysis of one example revealed breakpoints common to those previously reported in malignant triton tumor, conventional MPNSTs, and rhabdomyosarcoma: 7p22, 7q36, 11p15, 12p13, 13p11.2, and 19q13.1 (158).

Malignant triton tumors must be distinguished from rhabdomyosarcoma and leiomyosarcoma. When it is not obvious that the tumor is of peripheral nerve origin, a histologic clue useful in distinguishing it from rhabdomyosarcoma is the presence of scattered S-100 protein–positive cells in areas remote from those showing myogenic differentiation. Since S-100 protein staining may be seen in embryonal rhabdomyosarcoma (159), caution is required when dealing with a possible malignant triton tumor in children, since a large proportion of the reported examples are said to be predominantly myosarcomatous. How then is the conventional MPNST component of a tumor identified when on H&E-stained sections the less differentiated cells of childhood rhabdomyosarcoma may be identical in appearance, and S-100 protein staining is an unreliable discriminator? Given the association of rhabdomyosarcoma and NF1 (160), knowledge that a child has this disorder is also of little utility. Thus, the final diagnosis in possible pediatric examples of malignant triton tumor often rests upon the tumor's clinical presentation and routine histology. If, for example, the tumor location is typical for and gross and histologic features are characteristic of botryoid sarcoma, the simple finding of some S-100 protein–reactive cells is insufficient for concluding otherwise.

Leiomyosarcomas are more readily distinguished from malignant triton tumors. Like embryonal rhabdomyosarcoma, they occasionally express S-100 protein but, as discussed under the differential diagnosis of conventional MPNST, the cytology of the two tumors differs on routine stains. In addition, leiomyosarcomas lack round or strap-shaped cells with brightly eosinophilic cytoplasm, cytoplasmic cross striations, and immunoreactivity for myogenin or alpha sarcomeric actin. Lastly, we have seen malignant triton tumors presenting as an undifferentiated spindle cell soft tissue tumor in which the principal clue to the diagnosis of a MPNST was focal rhabdomyosarcomatous differentiation.

Patients with malignant triton tumor have a poor prognosis, which may be worse than that of conventional MPNST. Of the 84 cases summarized by Woodruff and Perino (154), 63 percent of the patients with available follow-up either died of or were dying of tumor. Death usually occurred within 2 years of diagnosis.

PNST with Angiosarcoma. Less common than malignant triton tumors are PNSTs with angiosarcoma. The neural component may be schwannoma, neurofibroma, or conventional MPNST, each showing distinct, sometimes multifocal areas of angiosarcoma. These must be distinguished from the rare occurrence of angiosarcoma within non-neoplastic peripheral nerve. Bricklin and Rushton (3) described an angiosarcoma originating in a vein within the radial nerve of a 51-year-old man. The origin of an angiosarcoma reported by Conway and Smith (161) involving a sciatic nerve of a 47-year-old man is unclear; although focal proliferation of "schwannian cells" was noted, the authors concluded that it represented a reaction to the sarcoma.

With regard to proving that both PNST and angiosarcoma elements are present in the same tumor, not all reported cases hold up to scrutiny. Histologically, angiosarcoma features a disorderly array of slit-like spaces or channels lined by cytologically malignant, often epithelioid cells immunoreactive for endothelial markers. There may also appear to be intracytoplasmic lumens containing red blood cells. Whether the growth pattern is diffuse or nodular, the cytologic appearance is the same. No benign vascular component is present. Based on the described and illustrated findings of organized growths more consistent with an angiomatous than an angiosarcomatous process, there is reason to doubt the diagnosis of angiosarcoma in the first three cases of the series of Morphopoulos et al. (162).

Findings in 21 convincing cases in the literature (78,136,163–165), including the fourth case of Morphopoulos et al. (162) and those personally reviewed by the authors (18), indicate the existence of two clinicopathologic forms. In the first, 14 tumors representing about two thirds of the cases, the angiosarcoma arises from neurofibroma in 5 (fig.12-45), conventional MPNST originating in neurofibroma in 6, or pure conventional MPNST in 3 cases. The second is represented by seven examples of angiosarcoma developing in conventional schwannoma (fig. 12-46). The first group were all NF1 associated. Patient ages ranged from 6 to 55 years, the low mean (23 years) reflecting the NF1 association. Patients were predominantly male (11 of 14), a gender bias typical of angiosarcomas as a whole. The tumor of the youngest patient, aged 6 years, arose in a neurofibroma. In contrast, patient age in the second tumor group ranged from 17 to 73 years (mean, 50 years), with no gender predilection. No patient had NF2. Sites of origin for neurofibroma/conventional MPNST with angiosarcoma were widely distributed, whereas

schwannomas with angiosarcoma were situated either in the neck or nearby, the vagus nerve (fig. 12-46A), or buttock and lower extremity.

Grossly, the external appearance of angiosarcoma originating in a PNST is generally unremarkable (fig. 12-46A). It is on cut surface that their often focally hemorrhagic nature is evident (164).

Microscopically, whether the underlying lesion is a neurofibroma, MPNST, or schwannoma, it is altered by the presence of a tumor exhibiting the histology of angiosarcoma, including round or polygonal epithelioid cells lining slit-like spaces or channels (figs. 12-45C, 12-46C,D) and, in some cases, spreading beyond them to grow in sheets and nests. Such epithelioid cells are mildly pleomorphic, possess well-defined margins and copious eosinophilic cytoplasm, and sometimes feature lumens containing red blood cells. Their large nuclei are vesicular and sometimes contain prominent eosinophilic nucleoli (fig. 12-46E). Mitotic figures are usually evident (165). Immunohistochemically, the cells fail to stain for S-100 protein but typically react for endothelial markers such as CD31 (fig. 12-46G) (165) and Fli-1. Confirmatory ultrastructural findings include the presence of cytoplasmic Weibel-Palade bodies and red blood cells (165).

The clinical outcome of the two clinicopathologic forms discussed above differ. Follow-up information, available for 11 group one patients with the tumor combination of neurofibroma and/or MPNST with angiosarcoma, consistently revealed aggressive behavior with local recurrence and/or metastasis as well as a uniformly fatal outcome by 2 years; 7 of the 11 patients died within 1 year. The prognosis of group two patients in whom the underlying tumor is schwannoma appears to be better. Of five affected patients followed for at least 1 year, two died of tumor at 5 and 14 months, and three were alive without evidence of disease at 27, 43, and 90 months. The patient alive and well at 27 months (fig. 12-46) had undergone amputation of a thumb at 15 months for metastatic angiosarcoma (164).

The primary tumor in the differential diagnosis is schwannoma with infiltrating epithelioid MPNST (epithelioid MPNST ex-schwannoma), a distinction most reliably made by the demonstration of CD31 or Fli-1 immunoexpression in angiosarcoma.

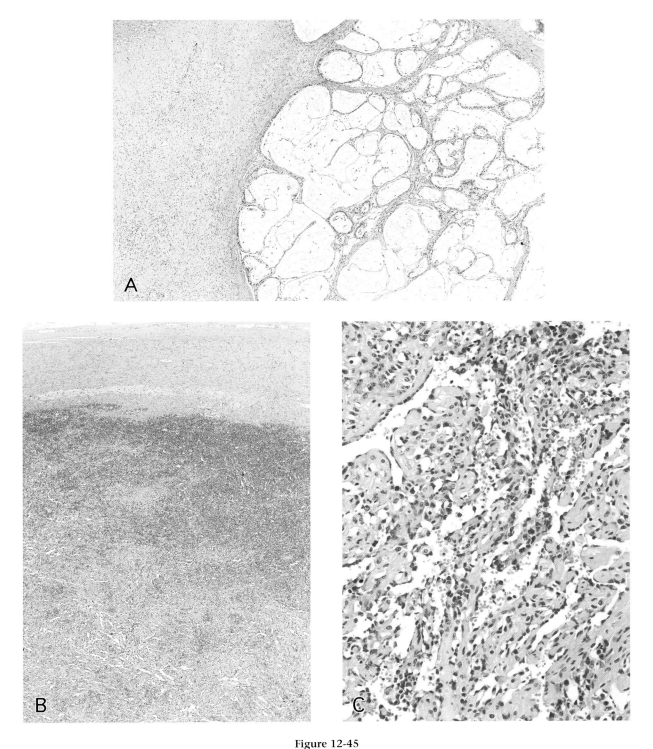

Figure 12-45

NEUROFIBROMA WITH ANGIOSARCOMA

A 10-cm popliteal fossa neurofibroma in a 21-year-old male with NF1 contained both epithelial glands (A) and angiosarcoma (B,C). After treatment by surgical resection and postoperative radiotherapy (64 GY), metastases appeared 5 months later in lung, brain, and liver. The patient died with tumor within 8 months of the initial diagnosis. (Case courtesy of Drs. J. Prat and S. Bague, Barcelona, Spain.)

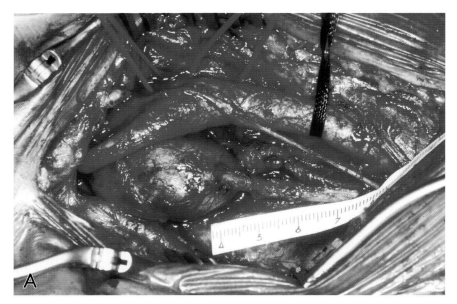

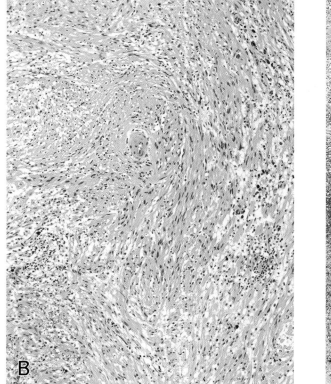

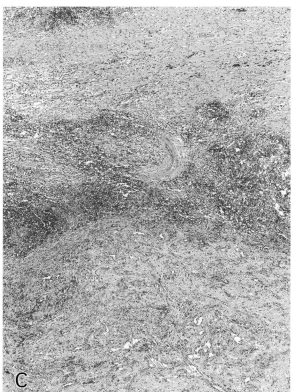

Figure 12-46

SCHWANNOMA WITH ANGIOSARCOMA

A 4.5 x 3.5 x 3.5-cm vagus nerve schwannoma (A) from a 50-year-old man. S-100 protein positive Antoni A tissue (B, F), and angiosarcoma (C–E) are present. Mainly lining disorganized vascular-like channels (D), the angiosarcoma cells were epithelioid in type (E) and expressed CD31 (G). A thumb metastasis was discovered 15 months later but the patient was alive and well at 27 months. (A,B: figs. 3 and 6a from Ruckert RI, Fleige B, Rogalla P, Woodruff JM. Schwannoma with angiosarcoma. Report of a case and comparison with other types of nerve tumors with angiosarcoma. Cancer 2000;89:1580-1582.)

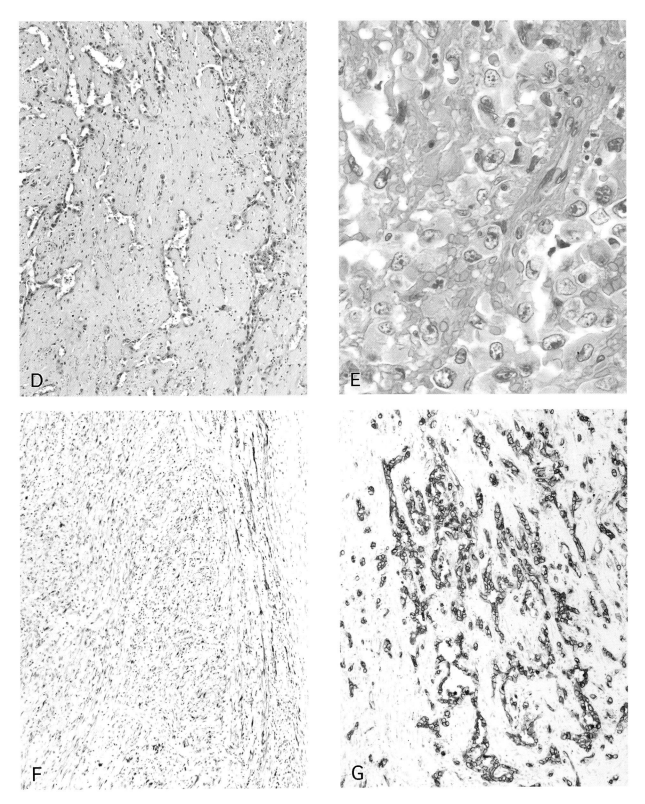

Figure 12-46, continued

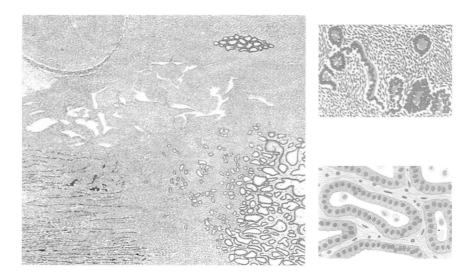

Figure 12-47

MPNST WITH GLANDULAR DIFFERENTIATION

Glandular differentiation in PNST as first depicted in 1892 by Garre (166).

PNST with Divergent Epithelial Differentiation

These rare PNSTs feature glandular epithelium, sometimes accompanied by squamous or neuroendocrine cells.

PNSTs with Glandular Differentiation. The first report of this type of divergent differentiation in PNST (fig. 12-47) (166) preceded Masson's description of malignant triton tumor (151) by 40 years. Unlike most other divergent cell types, there is no known counterpart in the repertoire of normal neural crest cell differentiation. In 1993, a summary of 25 reported cases (167) found the parent tumor to be conventional MPNST in 96 percent of cases and neurofibroma in the remainder. The authors also provided histologic evidence indicating that reported examples of "glandular schwannomas" actually represented cutaneous schwannomas entrapping normal sweat glands (see chapter 7). Patients ranged in age from 19 months to 68 years (mean, 29 years), and the sexes were equally affected. An NF1 association was noted in 74 percent. The thigh and retroperitoneum were preferentially affected.

Grossly, the tumors range in size from 4 to 30 cm (mean, 10 cm). With the exception of one case (see fig. 8-34A) in which the glands arose in a retroperitoneal plexiform neurofibroma elsewhere showing transition to MPNST, the glands are not grossly evident. In that exceptional example, cysts were apparent both on sonography and on cut section.

Microscopically, PNSTs featuring glandular differentiation are either neurofibromas or a conventional spindle cell MPNST. Islands of epithelial glands are distributed singly (fig. 12-48, left), or in nests (fig. 12-48, right) (149). The earliest recognizable indicator of glandular differentiation in MPNST is the presence of slit-like spaces mimicking vascular channels among the spindle cells (fig. 12-49A). Instead of being lined by cells with eosinophilic cytoplasm, however, the hyperchromatic, elongated nuclei often appear bare or misshapen and are accompanied by clear or gray cytoplasm (fig. 12-49B) (149). Adjacent slits often show a single layer of cuboidal cells (fig. 12-49C). Dominant are fully developed glands composed in large part of mucin-producing columnar cells (figs. 8-34C, 12-49D). Mucin not only fills but frequently distends their lumens (figs. 8-34B,C; 12-45A; 12-48, right; 12-49D). Sometimes it is also found in pools in the spindle cell component. Toward the base of the glands, scattered smaller neuroendocrine cells may also be seen. Frank squamous differentiation is uncommon (fig. 12-49E). In most instances, including all neurofibromas with divergent glandular differentiation, the glands exhibit benign histologic features (fig. 12-50, left). Infrequently, the glandular cells are cytologically malignant (fig. 12-50, right). One fourth of glandular MPNSTs show pluridirectional differentiation, most often rhabdomyosarcoma, but in one instance, osteosarcoma as well (fig. 12-51).

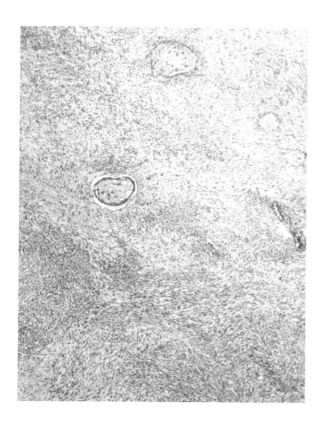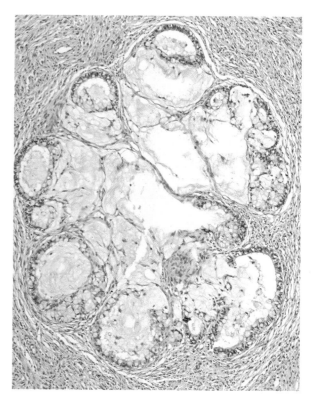

Figure 12-48

MPNST WITH GLANDULAR DIFFERENTIATION

Left: A few isolated epithelial glands with intraluminal mucin were found in this high-grade conventional MPNST that arose in a 27-year-old man years after radiotherapy to the area as treatment for a malignant lymphoma. For further details see case 4 in Tables 2 and 3 in Woodruff and Christensen (167).

Right: A cluster of epithelial glands in a conventional MPNST.

Immunohistochemically, the glandular epithelium stains for cytokeratin (fig. 12-52A,B), EMA, and carcinoembryonic antigen (fig. 12-52C) (167,168). Whether cytologically benign or malignant, the glands in most examples feature basally positioned, often flask-shaped, chromogranin-positive neuroendocrine cells (fig. 12-52D) which are also reactive for somatostatin (fig. 12-52E) and serotonin.

Ultrastructural studies (168–170) show the glands to be of intestinal type, with microvilli with a glycocalyx and core, as well as microfilaments featuring rootlets rather than cilia, which would be the case if the glands were ependymal in nature. The goblet cells contain mucin droplets varying in morphology. Neuroendocrine cells contain dense core neurosecretory granules.

The only primary tumor or soft tissue tumor of nerve that may be histologically confused with PNST with glandular differentiation is biphasic synovial sarcoma (109,168). There are multiple distinguishing features (Table 12-4). Finding goblet and neuroendocrine cells in the former but not the latter provides irrefutable evidence on which to base the distinction. In approximately 20 percent of synovial sarcomas, the spindle cell component shows some degree of immunoreactivity for S-100 protein (103). As a result, this marker is not a reliable determinant in differentiating the two tumors. Spindle cell staining for keratin and EMA as well as strong staining for TLE1 are more useful in the identification of synovial sarcoma. This distinction is important because of the more favorable prognosis of synovial sarcoma.

The treatment of patients with PNST with divergent glandular differentiation differs according to the nature of the underlying tumor.

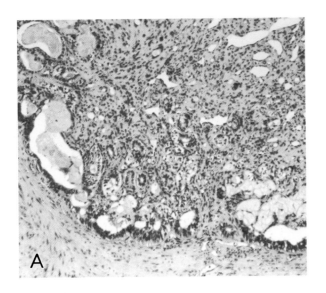

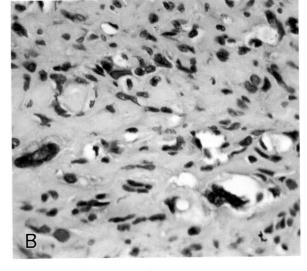

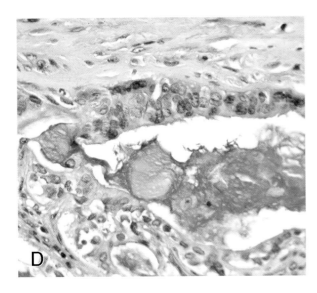

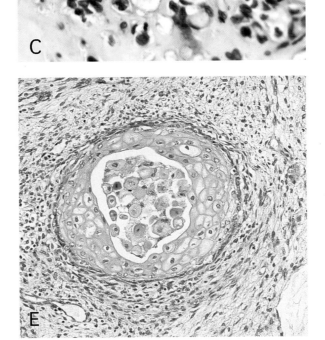

Figure 12-49

GLAND DEVELOPMENT IN CONVENTIONAL MPNST

Epithelial glands in a low-grade MPNST arising from a paraspinal neurofibroma in a 15-year-old girl with NF1.

A: Demarcated from the surrounding spindle cell MPNST and bordered by well-formed epithelial glands is a dense collection of irregularly shaped cells with hyperchromatic, sometimes pleomorphic nuclei.

B,C: These nuclei surround and in some instances partially line intervening slit-like spaces. Some lining cells are cuboidal, suggesting early gland formation.

D: Rarely, luminal mucin is obvious flanking large glands where it is associated with luminal dilatation (mucicarmine stain). For further details, see case 2 in Woodruff (149).

E: Squamous differentiation rarely occurs in conventional MPNST, and when it does, usually presents as cell nests likely formed within glands.

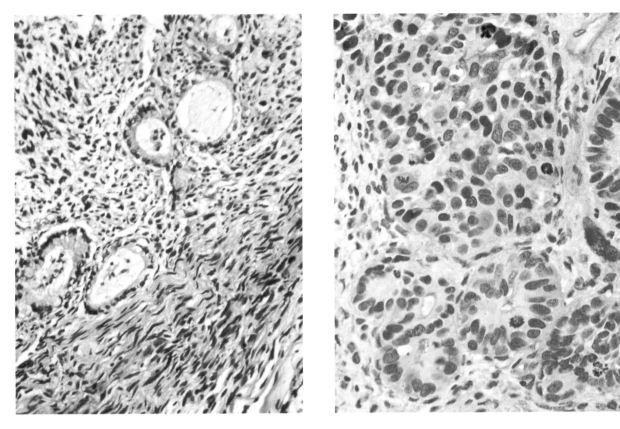

Figure 12-50

EPITHELIAL GLANDS IN PNST

Left: Most epithelial glands formed in PNSTs, including MPNSTs, are histologically benign.

Right: Less frequent are histologically malignant glands. Thus far, malignant epithelial glands have not been described in benign PNSTs. There is no report of a PNST with both histologically benign and malignant glands.

If there is a benign neurofibroma or a neurofibroma with malignant changes in a microscopic area, all that is necessary is total resection. For tumors arising within conventional MPNST, the treatment is no different than for other conventional MPNSTs. For patients in the latter group, 79 percent die of tumor, with a mean survival period of only 2 years (167).

PNST with Primitive Neuroepithelial Tumor. Primitive neuroepithelial differentiation along a neuronal rather than a nerve sheath cell line has been observed in some conventional spindle cell MPNSTs and in a few schwannomas. We are not aware of its occurrence in neurofibromas. The primitive cells are histologically and immunohistochemically identical to those of primitive neuroectodermal tumor (PNET), a neoplasm most often encountered in soft tissue and bone. Historically, morphologically similar tumors were first reported

as nerve-associated lesions (see below). In the setting of PNST, such PNET cells likely represent subclonal divergent differentiation of neoplastic Schwann cells. The finding of primitive neuronal differentiation in tumors of supportive elements of the nervous system is not peculiar to Schwann cell lesions or, for that matter, to normal peripheral nerves. It has also been documented among central nervous system tumors, for example, in glioblastoma (GBM) with PNET components (171). Evidence supporting the transition from glioma cells is the demonstration of the genetic signature of GBM in the PNET element, seen in about half of GBMs with a PNET component.

A histologic diagnosis of neuroepithelial neural differentiation is more readily established in schwannomas than in conventional MPNSTs, where it represents the least well-characterized PNST with divergent differentiation. Part of the

441

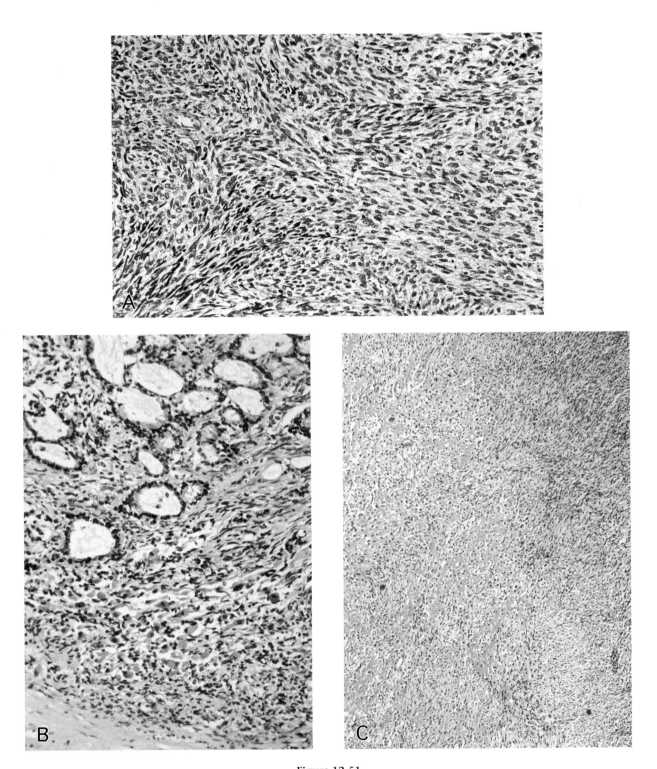

Figure 12-51

PLURIPOTENTIAL DIVERGENT DIFFERENTIATION IN PNST

This example, a head and neck high-grade conventional MPNST (A) resected from a NF1 patient, contained histologically benign epithelial glands (B), rhabdomyosarcoma (B), and osteosarcoma (C). For further details see case 5, Table 2 in Woodruff and Christensen (167).

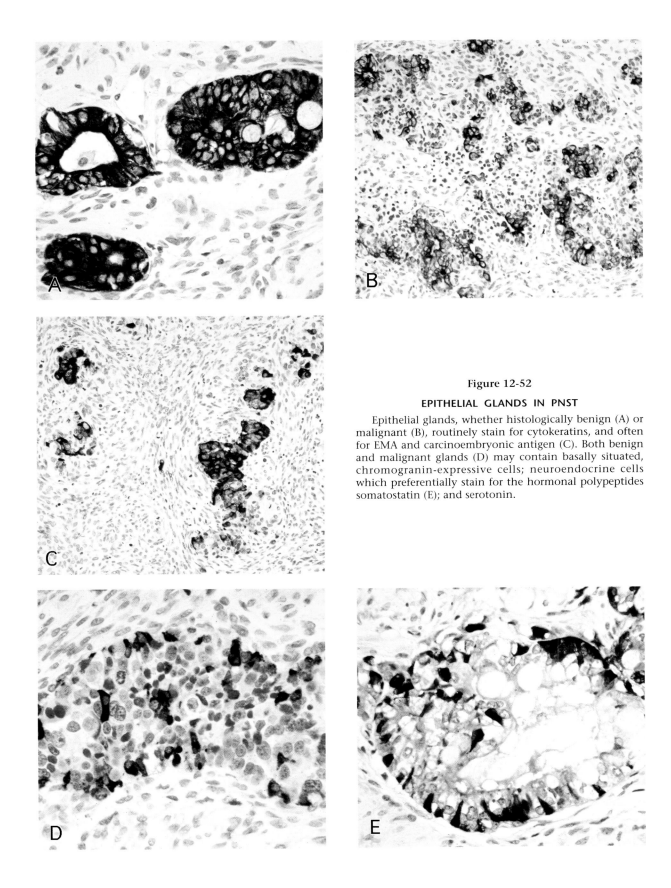

Figure 12-52

EPITHELIAL GLANDS IN PNST

Epithelial glands, whether histologically benign (A) or malignant (B), routinely stain for cytokeratins, and often for EMA and carcinoembryonic antigen (C). Both benign and malignant glands (D) may contain basally situated, chromogranin-expressive cells; neuroendocrine cells which preferentially stain for the hormonal polypeptides somatostatin (E); and serotonin.

Table 12-4

GLANDULAR MPNST VERSUS BIPHASIC SYNOVIAL SARCOMA: DIFFERENTIAL DIAGNOSIS

Features	Glandular MPNST	Biphasic Synovial Sarcoma
Evidence of neurofibroma or origin from a nerve	Often	No[a]
Cytologic resemblance between glandular and nonglandular cells	No	Yes
Goblet cells in glands	At least 50%	No
Neuroendocrine cell differentiation (chromogranin staining)	91%	No
Cytokeratin	Usually present and only in glands; CK20 positive, CK7 negative	Present in glandular and often nonglandular cells; CK7 positive, CK20 negative
EMA[b]	In glandular cells in the majority; not present in nonglandular cells	Often present in both glandular and nonglandular cells
CEA[b]	Present in glands	Infrequently present in glands

[a]One known example arose in epineurium of nerve (see chapter 11).
[b]EMA = epithelial membrane antigen; CEA = carcinoembryonic antigen.

problem is distinguishing anaplastic MPNST cells from those of PNET in routinely stained tissue. In the past, the finding in MPNST of cells with small, rounded to angulated nuclei possessing evenly distributed, finely clumped chromatin, inconspicuous nucleoli, and scant cytoplasm may have been too readily interpreted as PNET cells. The cells of PNET may be arranged in sheets, cords, or nests. More specific histologic evidence for PNET differentiation, such as Homer-Wright rosettes (see fig. 12-55), is rarely present. One early study, conducted before the routine use of such immunomarkers as synaptophysin and CD99, concluded that the predominant histologic component of 15 percent of 78 childhood MPNSTs with a limited spindle cell component resembled PNET (34). A more recent attempt, in our view not convincing, was made to introduce a deep soft tissue, nerve, and NF1-unassociated, predominantly small cell variant of MPNST. It exhibits cellular heterogeneity, lacks both S-100 protein or CD99 expression, and features variation in histology, immunohistochemistry, and ultrastructure (172).

Schwannoma with PNET, first convincingly described by Carstens and Schrodt (fig. 12-53) (173), has been documented in three cases (153,173,174). All were adult females, their ages ranging from 48 to 93 years. In two, the mass had been present for many years. Locations and maximum sizes of the schwannomas were thumb (2.5 cm), posterior-apical mediastinum (14 cm), and spinal intradural-extramedullary just distal to the conus medullaris in the cauda equina region (2.8 x 2.3 x 1.4 cm). In the third case, a 3.5 x 1.7 cm

recurrence resected 14 months later had become clinically apparent due to severe, intractable low back pain worsened by movement. The initial specimen was a schwannoma featuring clustered atypical cells, whereas the recurrence consisted entirely of PNET cells. Histologically, the PNET component in the three cases varied from a microscopic finding (fig. 12-53A,B) (173) to extensive replacement of the schwannoma (174) or, in the last case, comprising the entire recurrence (153). In two, the PNET cells were S-100 protein negative, but in one (174), were focally positive. The metastases from the latter tumor were histologically more characteristic of PNET than was the primary tumor. The recurrent spinal tumor showed pluridirectional differentiation: the majority of the malignant cells were uniformly small and synaptophysin immunoreactive (fig. 12-54C,D), but were admixed with foci of small, mildly pleomorphic rhabdomyoblasts with scant eosinophilic cytoplasm immunoreactive for muscle markers, including myogenin (fig. 12-54E,F). A subsequent ultrastructural study of the tumor revealed both neurosecretory-type granules and striated muscle differentiation (153). Follow-up was available in all cases. Postoperatively, the sites of the mediastinal and spinal tumors were irradiated, and chemotherapy was administered. Both these patients died due to tumor, the first at 16 months having developed a local recurrence and lung, bone, adrenal gland, and lymph node metastases, and the second at 19 months. The patient with the thumb lesion died of other causes months later.

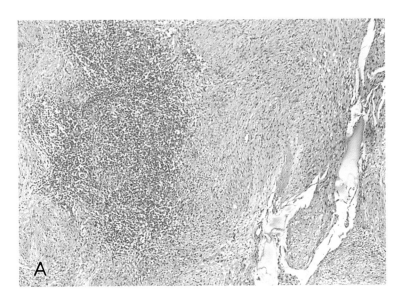

Figure 12-53

SCHWANNOMA WITH PRIMITIVE NEUROECTODERMAL TUMOR (PNET)

This 2.5-cm conventional schwannoma arose at a thumb base in a 93-year-old female and had been present for years. An unexpected tumor component was hyperchromatic, mitotically active small round cells, similar to those in PNETs (A,B). The malignant cells formed a nodule 0.7 cm in greatest dimension, but were also dispersed throughout the Antoni A tissue in the form of irregularly shaped microscopic nests. No rosettes were identified. Ultrastructural findings confirmed that the underlying tumor was a schwannoma (C) but failed to reveal specific differentiation by the small cell component. The patient died of unrelated causes 11 months after the tumor's removal (173). (Courtesy of Dr. P. Carstens, Louisville, Kentucky.)

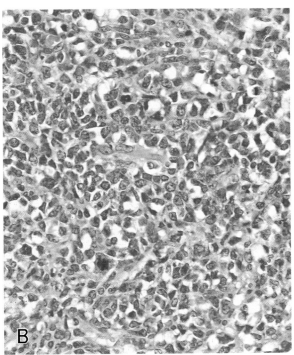

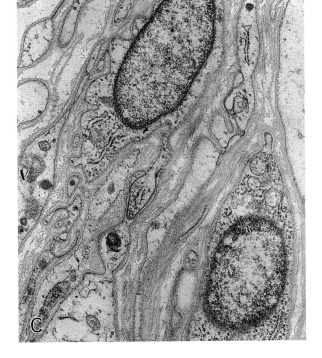

Differentiation toward PNET, or at least PNET-like cells, is most often encountered in conventional MPNST. Features include Homer-Wright rosettes in areas in which cells have rounded up and decreased in size. This is easily overlooked if unaware of the rare occurrence of such differentiation or if only microscopic foci of PNET are present (fig. 12-55) (47). To our knowledge, no sizeable immunohistochemical studies of MPNST for cells expressing synaptophysin,

CD99, and other neuronal markers of ongoing PNET differentiation have been conducted. That conventional MPNST with a PNET component, like soft tissue PNET, is a high-grade malignancy is illustrated by an example we encountered in a 33-year-old male (18). The fusiform 7 x 4 x 3 cm, focally hemorrhagic MPNST arose in a sciatic nerve and contained an unequivocal PNET element in a background of conventional spindle cell MPNST (fig. 12-56, left). That the

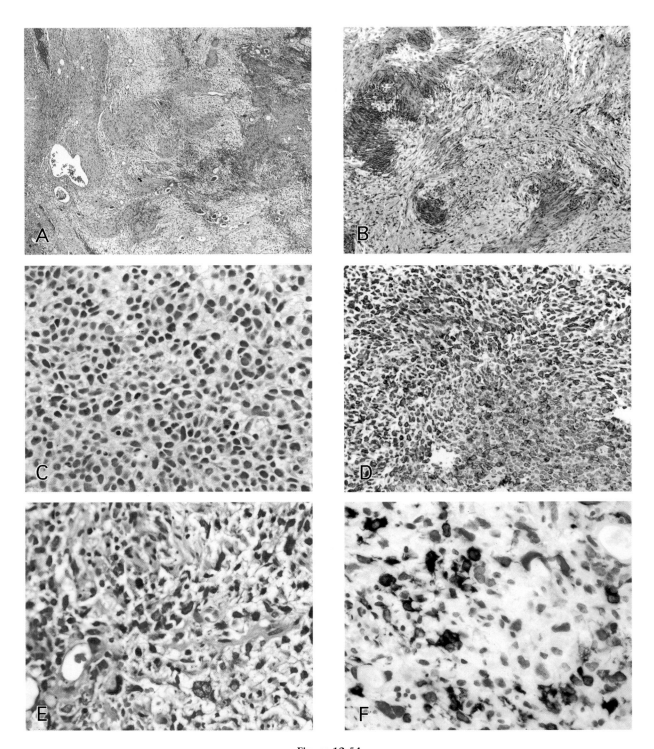

Figure 12-54

SCHWANNOMA WITH PNET

An intramedullary spinal canal tumor, proven by the demonstration of Antoni A and B tissue (A) and expression of S-100 protein (B), to be a conventional schwannoma, in a local recurrence showed pluridirectional malignant divergent differentiation in the forms of synaptophysin-positive PNET (C,D) and myogenin-positive rhabdomyoblasts (E,F). Ultrastructural study confirmed the nature of both divergent cell types (153).

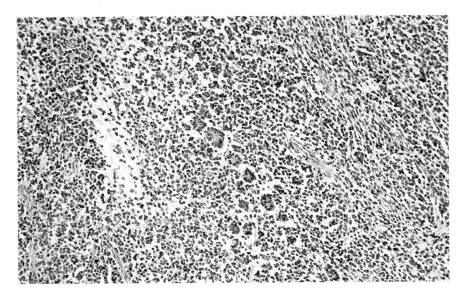

Figure 12-55

**CONVENTIONAL
MPNST WITH PNET**

The presence of Homer-Wright rosettes in a MPNST is definitive evidence of PNET differentiation.

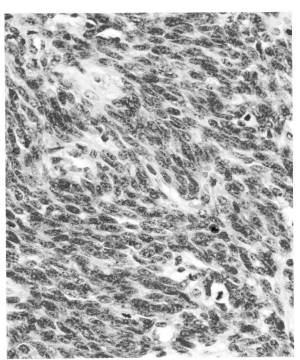

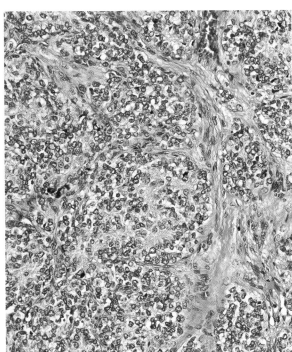

Figure 12-56

CONVENTIONAL MPNST WITH PNET

This fusiform malignant neoplasm of the distal sciatic nerve, composed of cytologically malignant spindle cells consistent with MPNST and a population of small cells that formed confluent Homer-Wright rosettes, fulfills the definition of a MPNST with PNET.

nested primitive neuroepithelial cells (fig. 12-56, right) represented PNET was evidenced by numerous rosettes and the reverse transcriptase-polymerase chain reaction (RT-PCR) identifica-tion of a t(12;22) translocation in these cells. The patient eventually developed pulmonary metastases of PNET and died of disease 7 years and 11 months after the original diagnosis.

Figure 12-57

PROBLEM TUMOR WITH RESPECT TO DIAGNOSIS OF MPNST WITH PNET

A large, extensively necrotic mediastinal tumor adherent to the vagus nerve was found to have two different histologic components: a diffusely S-100 protein- (E) and Leu-7 (CD57)- (F) expressive spindle cell component (A,B), and a synaptophysin-expressive (D) small cell malignancy consistent with PNET (A-C). Subsequent study revealed some cells with abundant eosinophilic cytoplasm (G), a few strips of medullary-type epithelium (H), and diffuse expression of the spindle cell component for GFAP (I).

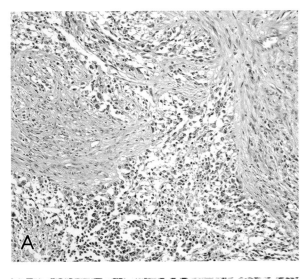

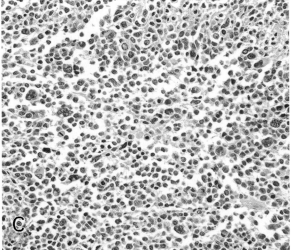

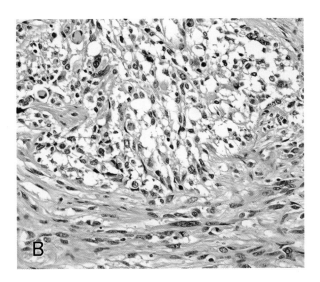

The main entity in the differential diagnosis of schwannoma with PNET is lymphoma, a distinction readily made on the basis of immunohistochemical markers. Some poorly differentiated peripheral neurepithelial or similar tumors arising in or intimately associated with otherwise normal nerve may be misinterpreted as MPNST with PNET due to the presence of a malignant spindle cell component. A relevant illustration involves an egg-shaped, "encapsulated," largely necrotic and hemorrhagic posterior mediastinal mass that appeared connected to a vagus nerve in an adult man (fig. 12-57). Histologically, it was adherent to the nerve but did not enter its substance. Two histologically different components were apparent, one variously bland (fig. 12-57A) with atypical spindle cells (fig. 12-57B) and the

other a histologically malignant proliferation of PNET-like cells with abortive rosettes and focal significant pleomorphism (fig. 12-57B). The PNET-like cells grew in sheets (fig. 12-57C), spread between spindle cells (fig. 12-57A), and immunoexpressed synaptophysin (fig. 12-57D), but not MIC2 (CD99). An interpretation of MPNST was made when the spindle cells were shown to be diffusely, strongly immunoreactive for S-100 protein (fig. 12-57E) and Leu-7 (CD57) (fig. 12-57F). A final diagnosis of "MPNST of small cell type with pleomorphic spindle cell sarcomatous areas" was made. In actuality, the finding of diffuse strong S-100 protein expression in MPNST is rare, particularly in high-grade examples. We are also unaware of reported MPNSTs showing a similar degree of CD57 reactivity. Significantly, in the

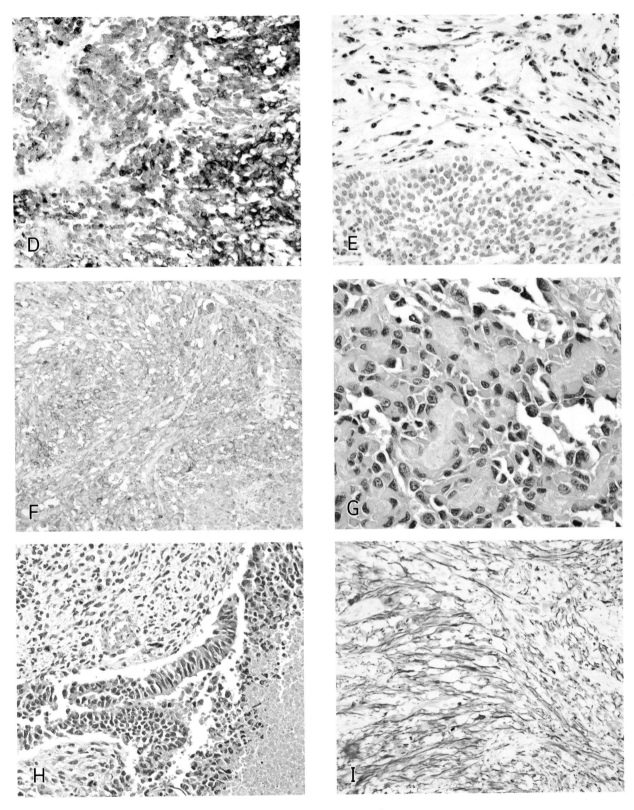

Figure 12-57, continued

Table 12-5

MPNST PRESENTING POSTIRRADIATION IN GANGLIONEUROBLASTOMA (GNB) OR GANGLIONEUROMA (GN)

Author, Year (ref #)	Patient Age/Sex	Site	Histology, Size	Treatment	Prior History	Outcome
Foley et al. 1980, Ricci et al. 1984 (23,175)	18 years 9 months/F	Adrenal, left	GN with MPNST, 13 cm	Surgical resection and chemotherapy	Retroperitoneal NB[a] at age 1 year, treated with radiation (2,500 cGy)	Pulmonary mets at 14 months; received chemotherapy; DOD[b] at 2 years with widespread mets
Ricci et al. 1984 (175)	10 years/M	Supra-nasal intraos-seous mass	GN with MPNST, 2.5 cm	Surgical resection and chemotherapy	Adrenal GNB at age 21 months; tumor thought to spread to regional lymph nodes; treated with chemotherapy and radiation; supranasal GN found at age 34 months, treated with radiation (2,000 cGy and a 970 cGy boost) and chemotherapy	DOD at age 9 months
Keller et al. 1984 (176)	20 years/F	Retro-gastric mass	GN with MPNST, 10 x 8 cm	Surgical resection and radiation therapy (4,500 cGy)	Retrogastric NB at age 14 months; treated with radiation (1,500 cGy)	Local recurrence at 6 months; no further FU
Navarro et al. 2000 (177)	14 years/F	Retroperi-toneum	MPNST in tissue taken from site of original tumor	Chemotherapy	Retroperitoneal NB on biopsy when patient was 6 months old, treated with chemotherapy and radiation (1,600 cGy); another biopsy 6 months later showed GNB	DOD
Navarro et al. 2000 (177)	13.5 years/F	Cervico-thoracic	GN with MPNST	Chemotherapy	Cervico-thoracic GNB at age 19 months; treated with radiation (2,700 cGy) and chemotherapy	DOD at 22 months with metastatic tumor

[a]NB = neuroblastoma; GN = ganglioneuroma.
[b]DOD = dead of disease; FU = follow-up.

above case, gemistocytic cells suggesting glial differentiation were also identified (fig. 12-57B,G), as was rare medullary epithelium (fig. 12-57H). Collectively, these features indicate differentiation to central nervous system elements, which is confirmed by strong GFAP reactivity in the spindle cell component (fig. 12-57I). This finding, consistent with glia but incompatible with the spindle cells of MPNST, equates with a diagnosis of monodermal epithelial malignant teratoma featuring central nervous system elements. We have never observed such differentiation in MPNSTs.

MPNST ARISING IN PERIPHERAL NEUROBLASTIC TUMORS

MPNST Presenting in Ganglioneuroma or Ganglioneuroblastoma

Normal ganglia, ganglioneuroma (GN), and ganglioneuroblastoma (GNB) contain Schwann cells. In normal ganglia, they encircle ganglionic cells (see chapter 2) and ensheath their numer-ous axonal processes. Their relation to ganglion cells in GN and particularly GNB is less apparent, but Schwann cells contribute significantly to the bulk of both tumors. On rare occasion, they serve as the source of a MPNST. There are two situations in which MPNST occurs in GN or GNB. One is when, in pure form, such tumors undergo transformation to MPNST. The other is when, on rare occasion, a ganglioneuromatous portion of an ectomesenchymoma does the same (see below).

The occurrence of MPNST in GN or GNB was first reported in detail by Foley et al. in 1980 (23); additional aspects of the case were provided 4 years later (fig. 12-58) (175). There are now at least 13 known cases. These fall into two clinical groups. The first consisted of five patients (one male, four females), ranging in age from 10 to 20 years and presenting with a presumed radiation-induced MPNST (Table 12-5). At initial presentation, they were 21 months of age or younger, having an intra-abdominal and one a cervicothoracic neuroblastoma (NB)

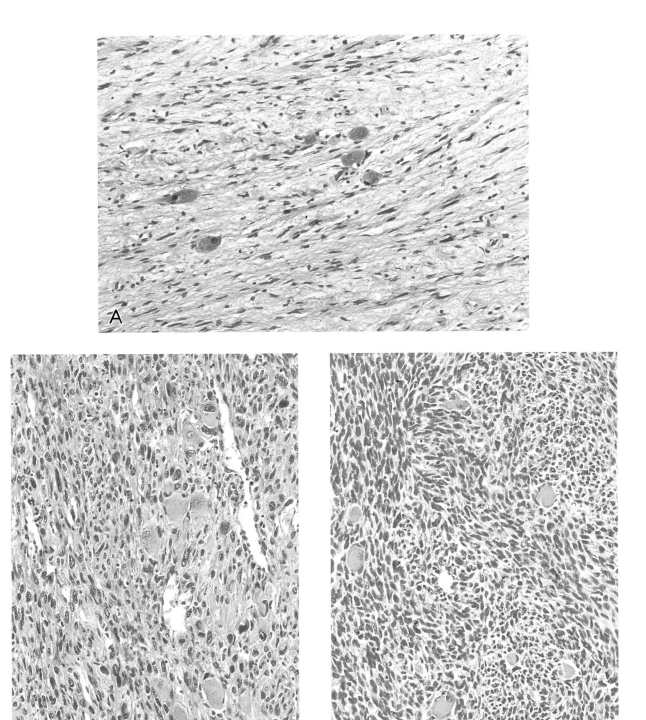

Figure 12-58

MPNST ARISING POSTIRRADIATION OF A NEUROBLASTOMA

A high-grade spindle cell MPNST was found 17 years and 9 months after radiotherapy of an adrenal neuroblastoma in an 18-year-old female (C). The MPNST involved a ganglioneuroma (A,B). For more details see Table 12-5, case 1.

Table 12-6

MPNST PRESENTING DE NOVO IN GANGLIONEUROMA (GN)

Author, Year (ref. #)	Patient Age/Sex	Site	Histology, Size	Treatment	Outcome
Chandrasoma et al. 1986 (176)	30 years/ M	Adrenal	GN[a] with S-100 protein+ MPNST, 11 x 10 cm	Resection	Local recurrence at 4 months, treated with chemotherapy, resection, and radiation; at 10 months metastatic MPNST found in three thoracic vertebrae
Fletcher et al. 1988 (178)	23 years/ F	Thorax, paraspinal	GN with S-100 protein+ MPNST, 11 x 7 x 6 cm	Resection and radiation therapy (4000 cGy)	NED[a] at 14 months
Banks et al. 1989 (179)	15 years/ M	Paratesticular	GN with S-100 protein+ MPNST that was metastatic to 2 retroperitoneal lymph nodes, 8 x 4 x 3.5 cm	Resection, retro-peritoneal lymph node dissection and chemotherapy	NED at 3 years
Damiani et al. 1991 (184)	18 years/ F	Retroperi-toneum	16-cm GN with a 4-cm well-circumscribed S-100 protein+ MPNST	Resection	NED at 4 years
Ghali et al. 1992 (180)	25 years/ M	Retroperi-toneum	GN S-100 protein+ MPNST, 21 x 16 x 12 cm	Resection	Local recurrence at 16 months; DOD at 2 years
Grippari et al. 1996 (185)	21 years/ M	Posterior mediastinum	GN with malignant triton tumor	Resection and radiation	NED 12 months
Drago et al. 1997 (181)	11.5 years/ F	Posterior mediastinum, paravertebral	GN with S-100 protein + MPNST, 9 x 7.5 x 5 cm	Resection, chemo-therapy and radi-ation (40 cGy)	NED 27 months
DeChadare-vian et al. 2004 (182)	6 years/ M	Adrenal	GN with S-100 pro-tein+ MPNST, 8 cm	Chemotherapy for 5 months, then total resection	No follow-up beyond 5 months

[a]NED = no evidence of disease; DOD = dead of disease.

or GNB which was then treated by irradiation. After a postirradiation interval ranging from 7 to 19 years, a high-grade malignant spindle cell tumor consistent with MPNST was found, either in a GN within the treatment field (four cases) (fig. 12-59) or in a small sample of the previously treated tumor (one case). The second group (Table 12-6) consisted of eight patients, including four males and three females, aged 6 to 25 years, without a history of prior irradiation. All had MPNST presenting in a GN (fig. 12-60). It is not possible to determine whether in any of these cases the MPNST arose in a tumor at a time when the precursor was perhaps at a GNB stage.

The locations of the tumors in both groups (13 patients) varied, including the retroperitoneum (4 patients), adrenal gland (3), thorax-mediastinum (3), skull (1), cervico-thoracic area (1), and para-testicular region (1). Tumor size, provided in 9 of the 13 cases, ranged from 2.5 to 13.0 cm; only 2 lesions were smaller than 5.0 cm. Most were grossly encapsulated. The degree of replacement

of the parent lesion by MPNST generally was difficult to determine grossly, but in at least 1 example the two components were clearly distinguishable (183). In this case (fig. 12-60), the ganglioneuromatous element was uniformly firm, tan-white, and glistening. It surrounded circumscribed, round, focally necrotic and cream-white tissue representing the MPNST. In another case, the malignant component was also circumscribed and said to be friable (184). Several other tumors were focally necrotic and hemorrhagic. Microscopically, in all cases, this was a spindle cell tumor consistent with MPNST. In 5 cases, S-100 protein was positive. Divergent differentiation to rhabdomyosarcoma, confirmed by immunohistochemistry and electron microscopy, was evident in 1 tumor (185).

The clinical outcome in the first patient group was poor. Three of the five died of tumor within 2 years of the diagnosis, another died without mention of a cause of death, and the fifth was alive with locally recurrent MPNST 6 months

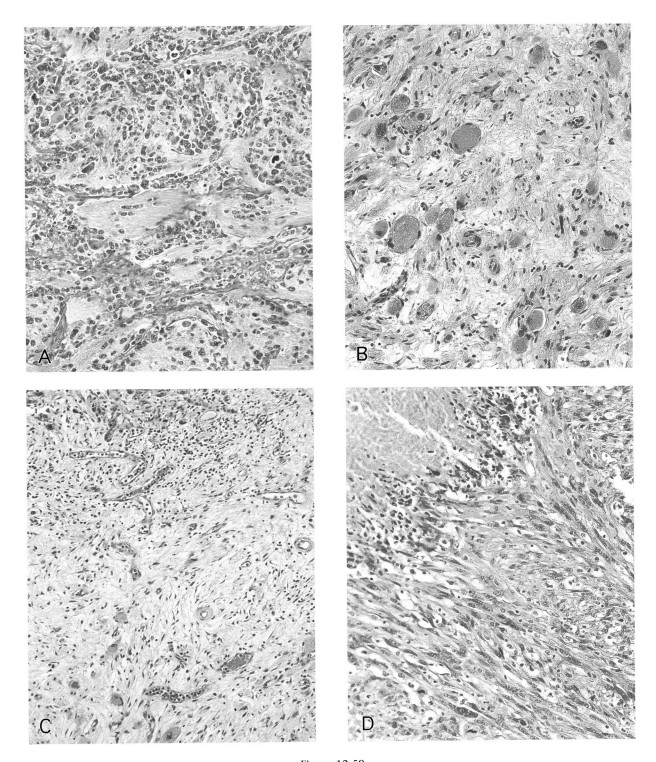

Figure 12-59

MPNST PRESENTING POSTIRRADIATION IN A GANGLIONEUROMA

The primary tumor, an adrenal ganglioneuroblastoma (A), treated with chemotherapy and radiotherapy, metastasized to the skull. Upon skull biopsy, it had matured to a ganglioneuroma (B,C). Treated by local radiotherapy, after 76 months the skull lesion was discovered to have transformed to a MPNST (D). For more details see Table 12-5, case 2.

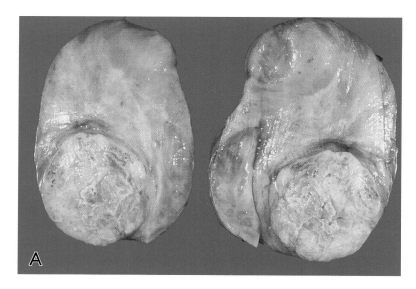

Figure 12-60

**MPNST PRESENTING
IN GANGLIONEUROMA**

This large, glistening adrenal ganglioneuroma (A) had circumscribed round, fleshy growth at one pole. The latter proved to be a high-grade MPNST (B,C). The interface of ganglioneuroma with MPNST is abrupt (B). For more details see Table 12-6, case 1. (Courtesy of Dr. P. Chandrasoma, Los Angeles, CA.)

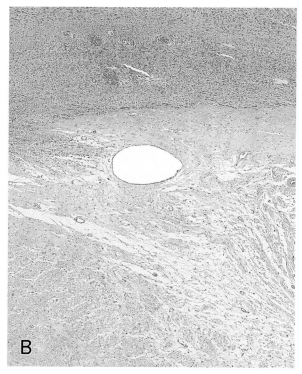

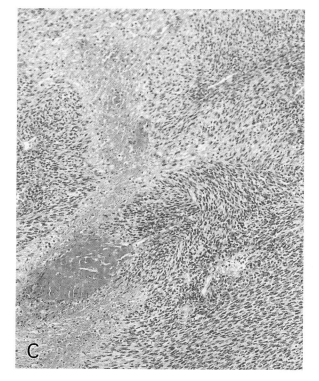

after the onset of treatment. For patients in the second, nonirradiated group, seven of the eight were followed from 1 year and 4 months to 4 years. Six were alive without tumor, and one was alive with metastatic tumor. Although follow-up periods for the second patient group were limited, it appears that MPNST arising postradiation in peripheral neuroblastic tumors carries a worse prognosis than those arising de novo.

The main tumor in the differential diagnosis of a GN with MPNST is a MPNST overrunning normal ganglionic tissue, typically dorsal root ganglion. Among other findings (see chapter 10), the distinction is aided by the lack of orderly arrangement and uniform cytology of tumoral ganglion cells, which are often multinucleated and vacuolated, and may contain spherical, eosinophilic cytoplasmic inclusions.

Table 12-7

MPNST ARISING IN PHEOCHROMOCYTOMA

Author, Year (Ref#)	Patient Age/ Sex	NF1	Gross Features	Microscopic Features	Immunohistochemistry/Ultrastructure of Sarcoma	Treatment Follow-up
Min et al. 1988 (183)	39 years/ F	No	Left adrenal; 35-cm encapsulated, partly hemorrhagic and necrotic tumor	Components intermingled; anaplastic spindle cell tumor with minor low-grade component	Occasional S-100 protein positivity in low-grade element; immuno-negative in predominant anaplastic element; EM[a]: some schwannian features but mainly undifferentiated	Combination chemotherapy; DOD[b] at 8 months; autopsy; regional "sarcomatosis" but no distant metastases
Miettinen and Saari 1988 (182)	38 years/ F	No	Left adrenal; 18-cm encapsulated tumor	Spindle to round cells with some hemangiopericytoma-like pattern	Primary: many S-100 protein-positive cells; EM: schwannoma-like features; metastases; only vimentin reactive; EM: undifferentiated	Widespread metastases (liver, retroperitoneum); alive with metastases at 18 months
Sakaguchi et al. 1996 (111)	48 years/ M	Yes	Left adrenal, 2-cm tumor; right adrenal region, 8-cm tumor adherent to adrenal gland; mediastinal metastasis	Left: MPNST in center of pheo; right: both tumor components; intermingled MPNST mainly anaplastic with chondro-osseous divergent differentiation	Primary: some S-100 protein-positive cells in associated "neurofibromatous nodules," tumor negative; EM: osteosarcomatous differentiation	Mediastinal and lung metastases; radio- and chemotherapy; DOD at 3 months; autopsy: widespread metastases (lungs, lymph nodes, pleura, diaphragm, spleen), cardiac tamponade; associated gastrointestinal stromal tumors
Lack 1997 (1)	27 years/ F	No	Right adrenal; 10-cm partly hemorrhagic and necrotic tumor	N/A[c]	N/A	N/A
Gupta et al. 2009 (184)	26 years/ M	No	Right adrenal; 27 x 22 x 9 cm hemorrhagic, red-brown; focal gray-white myxoid areas	Spindle cell tumor with myxoid background; in a few areas spindle cells had densely eosinophilic cytoplasm and cross striations	Spindle cells with focal S-100 protein staining; cells with cross striations, and positive staining for desmin and myogenin	Adrenalectomy; no FU[b]

[a]EM = electron microscopy.
[b]DOD = dead of disease; FU = follow-up.
[c]N/A = not available.

Far from convincing are reports of MPNST arising in ectomesenchymomas with a GN component. Ectomesenchymomas are complex tumors containing neuroblasts or ganglion cells as well as mesenchymal elements, often rhabdomyosarcoma, and are assumed to originate from pluripotential tissue derived from neural crest (186). Presenting mainly in infants, they are widely distributed throughout the body. Their identification is important because typical examples are histologically malignant and associated with a poor outcome (187). Of 13 ectomesenchymomas listed in one literature review (188), 7 had a ganglioneuromatous component. In 2 of these there was said to be an MPNST component.

Unfortunately, neither report clearly illustrates features of MPNST and one fails to prove the presence of even a ganglioneuromatous element.

MPNST Arising in Pheochromocytoma

The least common of the MPNSTs arising in transition from neuronal tumors of the sympathetic nervous system develop from pheochromocytoma. Their likely source is the modified Schwann cells or sustentacular cells so much a part of paraganglionic tumors. Less likely candidates are normal Schwann cells in nearby nerves. The five reported examples (Table 12-7) all occurred in young to middle-aged adults (age range, 26 to 48 years), with no gender bias

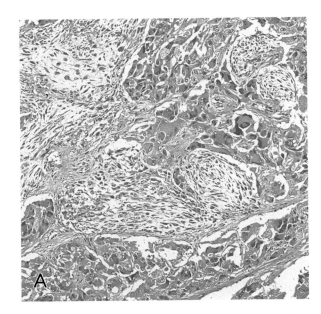

Figure 12-61

MPNST ARISING IN PHEOCHROMOCYTOMA

A mass in the right adrenal gland region microscopically had two components which were in part admixed (A), a feature best appreciated on chromogranin immunostained tissue (B). The MPNST demonstrated chondro-osseous differentiation (C). For clinical details see Table 12-7, case 3. (Courtesy of Dr. K. Sano, Matsumoto, Japan.)

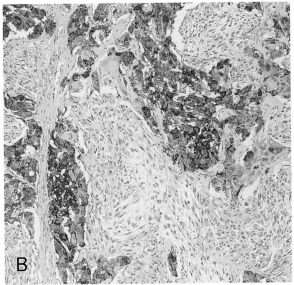

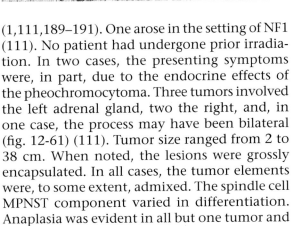

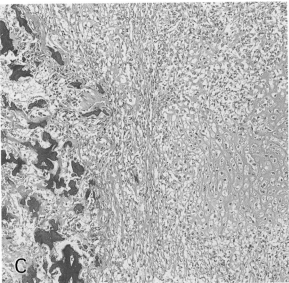

(1,111,189–191). One arose in the setting of NF1 (111). No patient had undergone prior irradiation. In two cases, the presenting symptoms were, in part, due to the endocrine effects of the pheochromocytoma. Three tumors involved the left adrenal gland, two the right, and, in one case, the process may have been bilateral (fig. 12-61) (111). Tumor size ranged from 2 to 38 cm. When noted, the lesions were grossly encapsulated. In all cases, the tumor elements were, to some extent, admixed. The spindle cell MPNST component varied in differentiation. Anaplasia was evident in all but one tumor and

featured a minor low-grade element (190). Varying numbers of S-100 protein–immunoreactive spindle cells were said to be present in three cases. One tumor featured divergent chondro-osseous differentiation (fig. 12-61), and another rhabdomyosarcoma (190,191). Ultrastructural studies, when performed, showed some degree of schwannian differentiation.

Clinical follow-up, provided in three cases, revealed widespread metastases of MPNST in two (111,189). Two patients died of disease 3 and 8 months after presentation; the third was alive at 18 months.

Table 12-8

NEUROBLASTOMA AND PRIMITIVE NEUROECTODERMAL TUMOR (PNET): DIFFERENTIAL DIAGNOSIS

Feature	Neuroblastoma	PNET
Patient Age	<5 years	>10 years
Location	Adrenal, sympathetic ganglia	Soft tissue, thoracopulmonary region, bone
Neurotransmitters	Adrenergic	Cholinergic
Metabolite Excretion	Present	Absent
Immunohistochemistry		
Vimentin	<5%	+
O13	–	+
Chromogranin A	~10%	–
Synaptophysin	+	Occasional
Nerve growth receptor	+	+
Neuron specific enolase	+	+
Neurofilament protein	+	Rare
Keratin	–	20%
S-100 protein	–	Occasional
Leu-7	+40%	+40%
MHC[a] (beta2 microglobulin)	–	Frequent
Ultrastructure	Frequent long neurites, few to numerous neurosecretory granules	Abortive neurites, few pleomorphic granules
Chromosomal Abnormalities	Del 1(q-), HSRs[b], DMs	Reciprocal translocation t(11;22)
Oncogenes	N-*myc* amplification	–
Survival		
Local disease	80%	50%
Disseminated disease	20%	10%

[a]MHC = major histocompatibility complex.
[a]HSRs = homogeneously stained regions. DMs = double minutes.

PRIMITIVE NEUROECTODERMAL TUMOR OF PERIPHERAL NERVE

Definition. *Primitive neuroectodermal tumor* (PNET) of peripheral nerve is a tumor of peripheral nerve featuring the characteristics of PNET of soft tissues, but no features of MPNST.

General Features. The peripheral nerve tumor, once referred to as peripheral neuroepithelioma, has come to be equated with PNET of nerve. The term "neural" has been loosely used to denote both nerve sheath and neuroblastic/neuronal differentiation. With respect to PNET, it implies the latter. Like neuroblastoma cells, those of PNET appear to be derived from migrating neural crest cells. Both exhibit early neuronal differentiation as evidenced ultrastructurally by primitive neurite formation and the presence of neurosecretory granules. The degree of neuronal differentiation differs significantly, thus permitting their distinction (Table 12-8). That PNETs composed of rosette-forming, seemingly undifferentiated small round cells may arise in nerves unassociated with conventional MPNST is attributed to Stout, who in 1918, de-

scribed an ulnar nerve tumor with some of these features (192). Stout refrained from specifically labeling his tumor. Over time, the term "peripheral neuroepithelioma" came to be applied to PNET of nerve. Beginning with Stout's 1942 description of a radial nerve example, there have been at least five additional reports (192–196). Mention was made of yet another 13 examples (197–199). Affected nerves include the sciatic, ulnar, median, radial, intercostal, and popliteal, as well as an S-1 nerve root.

In the 1970s, it became evident that a tumor histologically identical to peripheral neuroepithelioma arises far more often in extraneural soft tissues. Lattes (200) reported an example occurring in the chest wall. Thereafter, Seemayer et al. (201) described two such tumors, one featuring rosette formation; neither patient had a primary NB elsewhere. Two large series of similar cases were reported in 1979. One of 15 cases was by Lieberman (202) who chose the now-preferred designation of PNET. The other was a series of 20 cases by Askin et al. (203) of a "malignant small cell tumor of the thoracopulmonary region of children." Subsequent supportive evidence showed the neural nature of this soft tissue form of the tumor (204,205). Rare morphologically similar tumors also arise from conventional MPNST (see figs. 12-55, 12-56).

Gross Findings. The tumor size varies depending upon location, with those of nerve often smaller than 5 cm and those of soft tissue larger. At both sites, the sectioned tumor is gray and often hemorrhagic or focally necrotic.

Microscopic Findings. PNET is a small cell tumor with neuronal features closely resembling, but less well differentiated than NB (fig. 12-62). Low-power examination may reveal extensive involvement of a nerve (fig. 12-62A). At higher power, the cells are somewhat round with poorly defined cell borders and scanty cytoplasm (fig. 12-62B,C). The latter, best seen in optimally fixed tissue, contains glycogen. Nuclei are round, with granular nucleoplasm and inconspicuous nucleoli (206,207). The nuclear to cytoplasmic ratio is high. The cells are often disposed in a lobular pattern and in a somewhat fibrillar background resembling neuropil (fig.12-62C). Some degree of Homer-Wright rosette formation may be seen (fig. 12-62B,C), but rosettes of the Flexner type are not. Ganglion cell differentiation is rarely observed (204,208–212).

Immunohistochemical Findings. Most PNETs express neuron-specific enolase, a less than reliable neuronal marker, and the glycoprotein CD99 (p30/32MIC2) as identified by the monoclonal antibody O13 (212–214). In the appropriate setting, CD99 reactivity (fig. 12-62D) is a more specific marker of PNET than neuron-specific enolase. Its expression is also seen in Ewing sarcoma, the osseous counterpart of PNET (215,216), and in a variety of other tumors (217,218). Occasional synaptophysin and rare neurofilament protein reactivity may be seen.

Ultrastructural Findings. The fine structural features include rounded cells with variable numbers of short, microtubule-containing neuritic processes (fig. 12-63, left). The cytoplasm is typically scant and contains few, occasionally pleomorphic, dense-core granules (fig. 12-63, right). Glycogen is present in some cases (219).

Molecular Findings. Most soft tissue PNETs demonstrate the characteristic reciprocal translocation t(11;22)(q21;q12) (220), an alteration also seen in Ewing sarcoma (221). To date, no cytogenetic evaluation of a nerve-based PNET

has been reported, but the same translocation has been identified in one case of MPNST with divergent PNET formation (18).

Differential Diagnosis. The principal tumor in the differential diagnosis of nerve-based PNET is PNET of soft tissue secondarily invading nerve. The distinction is usually based upon finding a dominant extraneural soft tissue tumor and streak-like invasion of the adjacent or encompassed nerve (see fig. 14-9). We have not yet seen a NB primarily involving nerve; but if ever suspected, the differences listed in Table 12-8 should aid in clarifying which of the two tumors is present.

Treatment and Prognosis. PNET is locally aggressive (196) and capable of widespread metastasis. Common sites of metastatic spread include lungs, bone, and lymph nodes (222). The reported 3-year, disease-free survival rate of patients with initially localized tumors is 50 percent (223).

MALIGNANT GRANULAR CELL TUMOR

Definition. The malignant counterpart of benign granular cell tumor, *malignant granular cell tumor* (GCT) is a lesion of assumed Schwann cell origin. In addition to consistent immunoreactivity for S-100 protein, the tumor cells feature large numbers of secondary lysosomes.

General Features. Since Ravisch and Stout's (224) original description of a GCT, numerous bona fide examples have been reported (78) but their number represents only a tiny percentage of all GCTs. Critical reviews of the literature (225,226) have rejected many of the early reported cases which, given their morphologic features, were more consistent with alveolar soft part sarcoma or myosarcoma. GCTs are classified as malignant when their constituent cells are cytologically malignant or when a morphologically benign GCT metastasizes or otherwise directly results in the patient's death.

Clinical Features. The age and sex distribution of patients with benign and malignant GCTs coincide. The peak incidence of malignant GCT is in the fourth to sixth decades, with a mean patient age of 50 years and a slight female predilection (1.4 to 1.0). It has not been reported to occur in children; the youngest reported patient was 23 years of age (227). Malignant GCTs occur at almost all sites. The

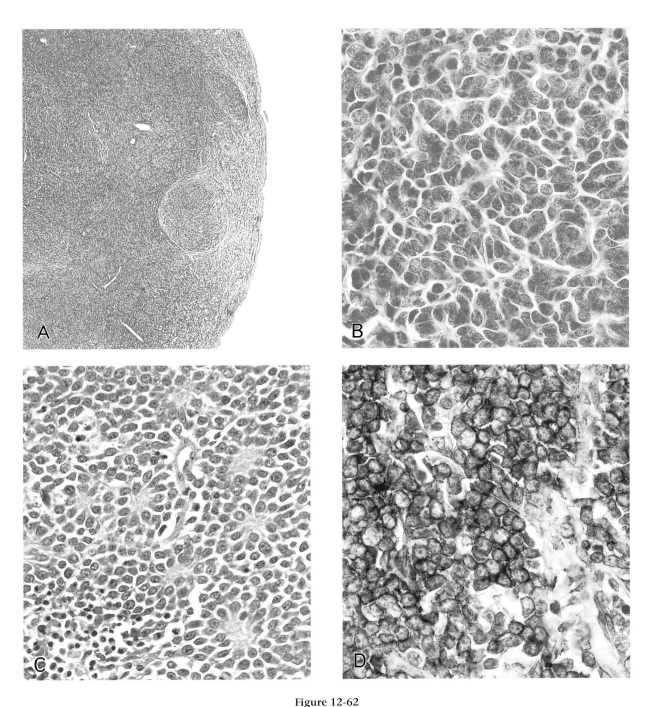

Figure 12-62

PNET OF NERVE

A: This cervical root PNET developed in a 20-year-old female. Dumbbell-shaped with both an intradural and extradural foraminal component, it involves both nerve fascicles and epineurium.

B: Its histologic features are typical and include poorly defined cell borders, scant cytoplasm, and vague rosette formation.

C,D: Another, more readily diagnosed example arose in the left S-1 nerve root of a 40-year-old male. Features include coarser chromatin and more prominent nucleoli than in neuroblastomas of comparable cellularity. There are well-formed Homer-Wright rosettes (C) and a strong membrane immunoreactivity for CD99 (D). Such immunoreactivity is lacking in neuroblastoma. (Courtesy of Dr. P.C. Burger, Baltimore, MD.)

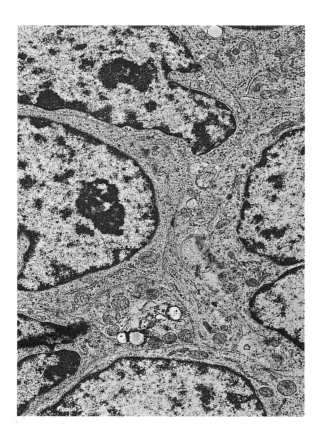
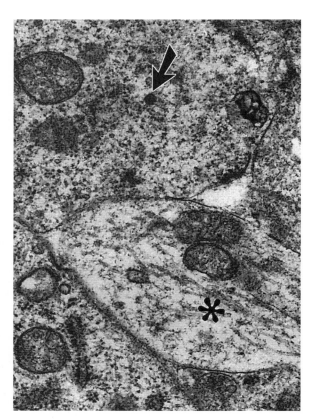

Figure 12-63

PNET ULTRASTRUCTURE

The ultrastructural features of this poorly differential tumor (left) include formation of occasional microtubule-containing processes (*) and the presence of rare dense core granules (arrow) (right).

trunk and extremities are most often affected, the thigh being the single most common site. Several tumors involved deep soft tissues; at least one was intrapelvic (228). Two tumors were vulvar (229,230). Oral mucosal examples are uncommon. Two malignant GCTs involved identifiable large nerves, specifically the sciatic and radial (230,231). Little information is available regarding the imaging characteristics of malignant GCTs (232).

Gross Findings. Grossly, malignant GCTs present either as fairly circumscribed or clearly infiltrative masses (fig. 12-64A,B). Most measure 4 to 15 cm in greatest dimension (233), but examples as small as 1 cm have been reported (234). Gross association with a nerve is rare. Firm to hard on palpation, their cut surface is gray, white, or yellow. On occasion, necrosis is apparent.

Microscopic Findings. Malignant GCTs microscopically consist of sheets or irregular accumulations of polygonal to somewhat spindle-shaped cells with abundant eosinophilic, granular cytoplasm and scattered prominent eosinophilic spherical globules (fig. 12-64C). Both the granules and globules are periodic acid–Schiff (PAS) positive (fig. 12-64D). Angulate bodies, PAS-positive crystalloids, may be seen within stromal histiocytes. Although some malignant CGTs are indistinguishable from their benign counterpart, histologically malignant examples often show at least three of the following: marked cellularity, pleomorphism (fig. 12-65A), a high nuclear to cytoplasmic ratio, nucleolar prominence, readily identifiable mitoses (fig. 12-65B), prominent spindling of tumor cells (fig. 12-65C), and frequent foci of necrosis (fig. 12-65D) (234). Vesicular nuclei (fig. 12-65B) are also a common finding. Mitotic figures and areas of necrosis are generally absent in benign GCTs.

Clinically malignant but histologically benign GCTs cannot be diagnosed on the basis of their microscopic features alone. Although

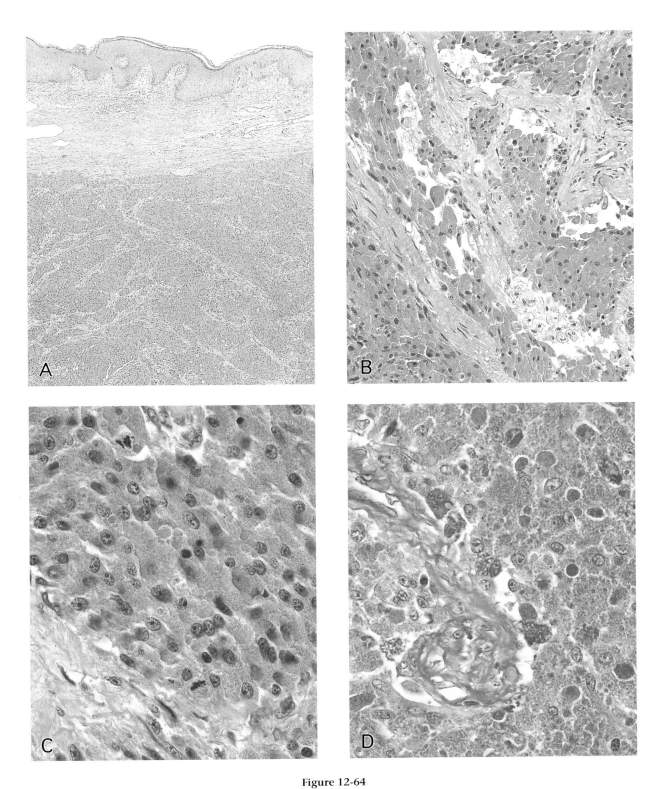

Figure 12-64

MALIGNANT GRANULAR CELL TUMOR

This cellular infiltrative example (A,B) arose in the thigh of a 31-year-old female. On careful examination, most examples of this tumor type have eosinophilic spherical cytoplasmic globules (C), which are periodic acid–Schiff (PAS) positive (D).

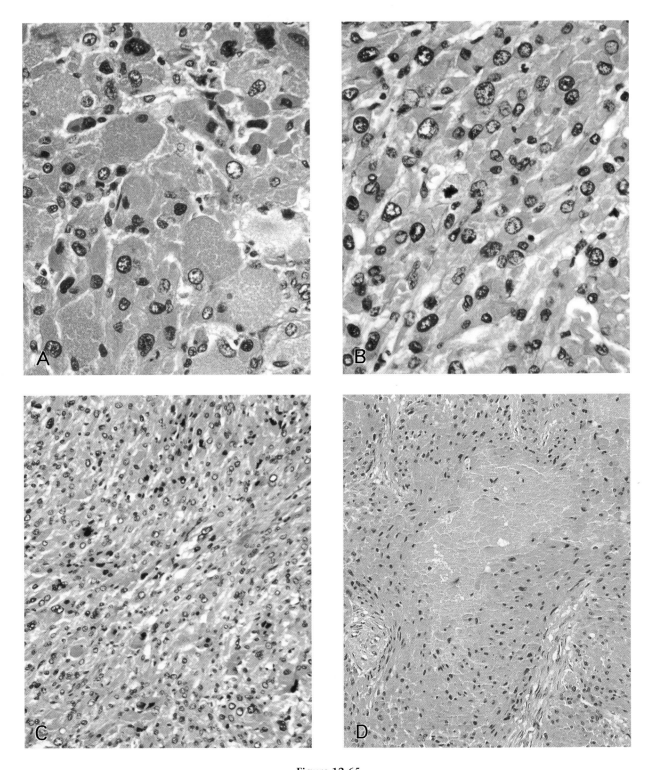

Figure 12-65

MALIGNANT GRANULAR CELL TUMOR

Histologic features commonly found are marked cellularity with nuclear pleomorphism (A) and readily identified mitotic figures (B). There may also be spindle cell growth of the tumor (C), and it may be focally necrotic (D).

benign GCTs generally consist of a uniform population of cytologically bland granular cells, it has been suggested that mild to moderate pleomorphism in such tumors should prompt consideration of malignancy (230). This may be true. Given the implications of treatment, we are reluctant to make a diagnosis of malignant GCT in such instances unless there are two or more low-power fields in which most cells possess large, pleomorphic, vesicular or hyperchromatic nuclei with prominent nucleoli. Mitotic figures may or may not be present but, in our view, mitoses alone do not indicate malignant change. Fortunately, the histologic changes upon which a diagnosis of malignant GCT can be made in this setting are often obvious and widespread. Attention to tumor growth characteristics is also of diagnostic utility. Although limited invasion of surrounding soft tissue cannot be interpreted as malignant behavior, destructive growth and lymphatic or vascular invasion can.

Cytologic Findings. In a comparative study of cytologic material from 3 malignant GCTs and 17 benign GCTs, Wieczorek et al. (235) were able to identify distinguishing features. They determined that when found throughout the cytologic sample as a group of findings, hyperchromasia, coarse chromatin, increased nuclear to cytoplasmic ratio, nuclear pleomorphism, vesicular nuclei with enlarged nucleoli, and spindle cell morphology were associated with malignancy. All these criteria were present diffusely in malignant GCTs, but vesicular nuclei with enlarged nucleoli as well as spindle cell morphology were diffusely present in only 2 tumors and focally in 1. One to five of these features were present focally in 8 benign GCTs. In addition to focal nuclear pleomorphism and hyperchromasia, 1 benign tumor had diffuse vesicular nuclei, large nucleoli, and coarse chromatin. Mitotic figures, present in 2 of 3 malignant GCTs, were absent in benign tumors.

Immunohistochemical Findings. Like their benign counterparts, the cells of malignant GCT consistently express vimentin, S-100 protein (fig. 12-66, left) (236), and neuron-specific enolase (234). Reactivity for carcinoembryonic antigen has also been reported (237). The frequency and significance of this unexpected finding are unclear, but the finding may be nonspecific and related to the abundance of cytoplasmic lysosomes. Stains for muscle markers are negative. Despite uniform immunoreactivity of benign GCTs for CD68 (238), only some malignant GCTs are reactive (fig. 12-66, right) (234). Collagen 4 reactivity occasionally outlines cell lobules (78).

Immunoreactivity for proliferation markers may help identify malignant GCTs. In one large series, half of histologically malignant tumors exhibited labeling indices of 10 to 50 percent (234); nearly 70 percent showed extensive p53 protein staining.

Ultrastructural Findings. Aside from the presence of large pleomorphic nuclei (fig. 12-67), marginated chromatin, and often multiple nucleoli (236), the ultrastructural features of morphologically malignant GCT are identical to those of benign examples. Lysosomes fill the cells. Specialized junctions are lacking and individual or grouped cells are often surrounded by basement membrane.

Differential Diagnosis. Major considerations in the differential diagnosis of morphologically malignant GCT are leiomyosarcoma and alveolar soft part sarcoma. Early concerns regarding the distinction of malignant GCT from pleomorphic rhabdomyosarcoma were largely negated by the definition of GCT as immunonegative for muscle markers. Conversely, rhabdomyosarcomas are, with few exceptions (167,239,240), S-100 protein negative. Granular cell leiomyosarcoma (241), on the other hand, may be indistinguishable from malignant GCT with routine immunohistochemical stains. Whenever muscle differentiation is suspected we recommend the use of selected antibodies from a panel designed to identify smooth or striated muscle cells. These include desmin, muscle common actin (HHF 35), smooth muscle actin, myogenin, and sarcomeric actin. Alveolar soft part sarcoma poses little differential difficulty since its distinctive organoid or alveolar growth pattern is lacking in GCT (242). Alveolar soft part sarcoma also lacks S-100 protein expression, and may contain diastase-resistant crystalline structures (243). Ultrastructurally, such crystalloids have a distinctive rhomboid appearance (244).

Treatment and Prognosis. Wide en-bloc excision is the treatment of choice for malignant GCT. There is no evidence indicating that radiotherapy and chemotherapy are effective modalities.

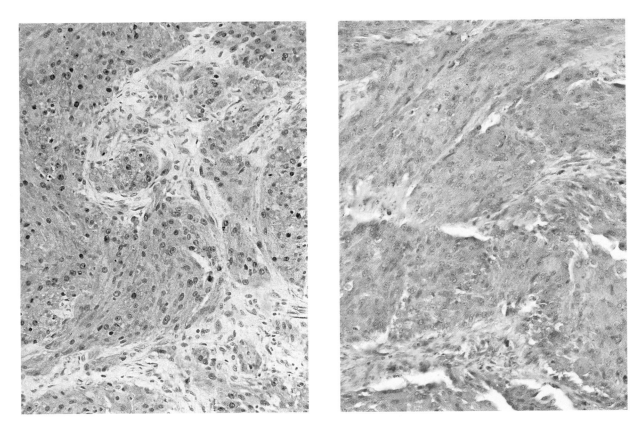

Figure 12-66

MALIGNANT GRANULAR CELL TUMOR

These tumors consistently and uniformly immunostain for S-100 protein (left), but infrequently express CD68 (right).

Figure 12-67

MALIGNANT GRANULAR CELL TUMOR

A portion of a neoplastic cell with a pleomorphic nucleus and numerous cytoplasmic secondary lysosomes, features consistent with a granular cell tumor.

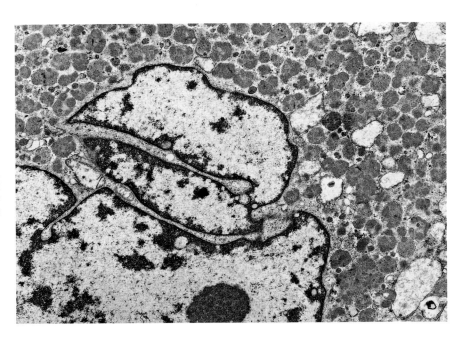

Malignant GCTs are aggressive tumors that often recur locally before metastasizing to regional lymph nodes or other sites. The lung is the most common site of distant spread, and is involved in nearly half of all cases. In most instances, metastases developed within 2 years of initial resection; in one case, however, it occurred at 5 years. Generalized metastases may occur, in which case the prognosis is poor. In a literature review of 31 clinically malignant GCTs with available follow-up, 58 percent of the patients died of tumor (78). Most died within 3 years, although one survived for 6 years, and two died after 8 years. Of five patients with his-

tologically malignant but nonmetastatic tumors (245–249), none died of tumor.

In a large Armed Forces Institute of Pathology (AFIP) series (234), features adversely affecting the survival of patients with malignant GCT included old age, larger tumor size, vesicular nuclei with large nucleoli, increased mitotic activity, and necrosis. When subject to multivariate analysis, only advancing age and Ki-67 labeling indices greater than or equal to 10 percent were adverse survival factors; older age was the only factor significantly related to metastases. None were significantly related to tumor recurrence.

REFERENCES

Malignant Peripheral Nerve Sheath Tumor

1. Lack EE. Tumors of the adrenal gland and extra-adrenal paraganglia. AFIP Atlas of Tumor Pathology. 3rd Series, Fascicle 19. Washington, DC: American Registry of Pathology; 1997.
2. Perry A, Roth KA, Banerjee R, Fuller CE, Gutmann DH. NF1 deletions in S-100 protein-positive and negative cells of sporadic and neurofibromatosis 1 (NF1)-associated plexiform neurofibromas and malignant peripheral nerve sheath tumors. Am J Pathol 2001;159:57-61.
3. Bricklin AS, Rushton HW. Angiosarcoma of venous origin arising in radial nerve. Cancer 1977;39:1556-1558.
4. Lewis JJ, Brennan MF. Soft tissue sarcomas. Curr Probl Surg 1996;33:817-872.
5. Ducatman BS, Scheithauer BW, Piepgras DG, Reiman HM, Ilstrup DM. Malignant peripheral nerve sheath tumors. A clinicopathologic study of 120 cases. Cancer 1986;57:2006-2021.
6. Scheithauer BW, Erdogan S, Rodriguez FJ, et al. Malignant peripheral nerve sheath tumors of cranial nerves and intracranial contents: A clinicopathologic study of 17 cases. Am J Surg Pathol 2009;33:325-338.
7. Kourea HP, Bilsky MH, Leung DH, Lewis JJ, Woodruff JM. Subdiaphragmatic and intrathoracic paraspinal malignant peripheral nerve sheath tumors: a clinicopathologic study of 25 patients and 26 tumors. Cancer 1998;82:2191-2203.
8. Hruban RH, Shiu MH, Senie RT, Woodruff JM. Malignant peripheral nerve sheath tumors of the buttock and lower extremity. A study of 43 cases. Cancer 1990;66:1253-1265.
9. Doorn PF, Molenaar WM, Buter J, Hoekstra HJ. Malignant peripheral nerve sheath tumors in patients with and without neurofibromatosis. Eur J Surg Oncol 1995;21:78-82.
10. Wanebo JE, Malik JM, VandenBerg SR, Wanebo HJ, Driesen N, Persing JA. Malignant peripheral nerve sheath tumors. A clinicopathologic study of 28 cases. Cancer 1993;71:1247-1253.
11. McCaughan JA, Holloway SM, Davidson R, Lam WW. Further evidence of the increased risk for malignant peripheral nerve sheath tumour from a scottish cohort of patients with neurofibromatosis type 1. J Med Genet 2007;44:463-466.
12. King AA, Debaun MR, Riccardi VM, Gutmann DH. Malignant peripheral nerve sheath tumors in neurofibromatosis 1. Am J Med Genet 2000;93:388-392.
13. Evans DG, Baser ME, McGaughran J, Sharif S, Howard E, Moran A. Malignant peripheral nerve sheath tumours in neurofibromatosis 1. J Med Genet 2002;39:311-314.
14. Rasmussen SA, Yang Q, Friedman JM. Mortality in neurofibromatosis 1: an analysis using U.S. death certificates. Am J Hum Genet 2001;68:1110-1118.
15. Zoller M, Rembeck B, Akesson HO, Angervall L. Life expectancy, mortality and prognostic factors in neurofibromatosis type 1. A twelve-year follow-up of an epidemiological study in Goteborg, Sweden. Acta Derm Venereol 1995;75:136-140.

16. Huson SM, Compston DA, Harper PS. A genetic study of von Recklinghausen neurofibromatosis in south east Wales. II. Guidelines for genetic counselling. J Med Genet 1989;26:712-721.

17. Chen Y, Diamond AS, Vaheesan KR, Schneider S, Valderrama E. Retroperitoneal neurofibrosarcoma in a patient with neurofibromatosis type 2: A case report and review of the literature. Pediatr Pathol Mol Med 2003;22:375-381.

18. Antonescu CR, Woodruff JM. Primary tumors of cranial, spinal and peripheral nerves. In: Russell and Rubinstein's pathology of tumors of the nervous systems. London: Hodder Arnold; 2006:787-835.

19. Higami Y, Shimokawa I, Kishikawa M, et al. Malignant peripheral nerve sheath tumors developing multifocally in the central nervous system in a patient with neurofibromatosis type 2. Clin NeuroPathol 1998;17:115-120.

20. Evans DG, Huson SM, Donnai D, et al. A genetic study of type 2 neurofibromatosis in the United Kingdom. I. Prevalence, mutation rate, fitness, and confirmation of maternal transmission effect on severity. J Med Genet 1992;29:841-846.

21. Yamashiro S, Nagahiro S, Mimata C, Kuratsu J, Ushio Y. Malignant trigeminal schwannoma associated with xeroderma pigmentosum—case report. Neurol Med Chir (Tokyo) 1994;34:817-820.

22. Jakobiec FA, Font RL, Zimmerman LE. Malignant peripheral nerve sheath tumors of the orbit: a clinicopathologic study of eight cases. Trans Am Ophthalmol Soc 1985;83:332-366.

23. Foley KM, Woodruff JM, Ellis FT, Posner JB. Radiation-induced malignant and atypical peripheral nerve sheath tumors. Ann Neurol 1980;7:311-318.

24. Ducatman BS, Scheithauer BW. Postirradiation neurofibrosarcoma. Cancer 1983;51:1028-1033.

25. Evans DG, Birch JM, Ramsden RT, Sharif S, Baser ME. Malignant transformation and new primary tumours after therapeutic radiation for benign disease: Substantial risks in certain tumour prone syndromes. J Med Genet 2006;43:289-294.

26. Rasbridge SA, Browse NL, Tighe JR, Fletcher CD. Malignant nerve sheath tumour arising in a benign ancient schwannoma. Histopathology 1989;14:525-528.

27. Sharif S, Ferner R, Birch JM, et al. Second primary tumors in neurofibromatosis 1 patients treated for optic glioma: Substantial risks after radiotherapy. J Clin Oncol 2006;24:2570-2575.

28. Comey CH, McLaughlin MR, Jho HD, Martinez AJ, Lunsford LD. Death from a malignant cerebellopontine angle triton tumor despite stereotactic radiosurgery. Case report. J NeuroSurg 1998;89:653-658.

29. McLean CA, Laidlaw JD, Brownbill DS, Gonzales MF. Recurrence of acoustic neurilemoma as a malignant spindle-cell neoplasm. Case report. J NeuroSurg 1990;73:946-950.

30. Hanabusa K, Morikawa A, Murata T, Taki W. Acoustic neuroma with malignant transformation. Case report. J NeuroSurg 2001;95:518-521.

31. Shin M, Ueki K, Kurita H, Kirino T. Malignant transformation of a vestibular schwannoma after gamma knife radiosurgery. Lancet 2002;360:309-310.

32. Koestner A, Swenberg JA, Wechsler W. Transplacental production with ethylnitrosourea of neoplasms of the nervous system in Sprague-Dawley rats. Am J Pathol 1971;63:37-56.

33. Boulanger JM, Larbrisseau A. Neurofibromatosis type 1 in a pediatric population: Ste-Justine's experience. Can J Neurol Sci 2005;32:225-231.

34. Meis JM, Enzinger FM, Martz KL, Neal JA. Malignant peripheral nerve sheath tumors (malignant schwannomas) in children. Am J Surg Pathol 1992;16:694-707.

35. Casanova M, Ferrari A, Spreafico F, et al. Malignant peripheral nerve sheath tumors in children: A single-institution twenty-year experience. J Pediatr Hematol Oncol 1999;21:509-513.

36. Carli M, Ferrari A, Mattke A, et al. Pediatric malignant peripheral nerve sheath tumor: The italian and german soft tissue sarcoma cooperative group. J Clin Oncol 2005;23:8422-8430.

37. Woodruff JM, Scheithauer BW, Kurtkaya-Yapicier O, et al. Congenital and childhood plexiform (multinodular) cellular schwannoma: a troublesome mimic of malignant peripheral nerve sheath tumor. Am J Surg Pathol 2003;27:1321-1329.

38. Ducatman BS, Scheithauer BW, Piepgras DG, Reiman HM. Malignant peripheral nerve sheath tumors in childhood. J NeuroOncol 1984;2:241-248.

39. Raney RB Jr, Littman P, Jarrett P, Waldman MT, Chatten J. Results of multimodal therapy for children with neurogenic sarcoma. Med Pediatr Oncol 1979;7:229-236.

40. deCou JM, Rao BN, Parham DM, et al. Malignant peripheral nerve sheath tumors: The St. Jude children's research hospital experience. Ann Surg Oncol 1995;2:524-529.

41. Ferrari A, Casanova M, Collini P, et al. Adult-type soft tissue sarcomas in pediatric-age patients: experience at the Istituto Nazionale Tumori in Milan. J Clin Oncol 2005;23:4021-4030.

42. Krumerman MS, Stingle W. Synchronous malignant glandular schwannomas in congenital neurofibromatosis. Cancer 1978;41:2444-2451.

43. Leslie MD, Cheung KY. Malignant transformation of neurofibromas at multiple sites in a case of neurofibromatosis. Postgrad Med J 1987;63:131-133.

44. Guccion JG, Enzinger FM. Malignant schwannoma associated with von Recklinghausen's neurofibromatosis. Virchows Arch A Pathol Anat Histol 1979;383:43-57.

45. Vauthey JN, Woodruff JM, Brennan MF. Extremity malignant peripheral nerve sheath tumors (neurogenic sarcomas): a 10-year experience. Ann Surg Oncol 1995;2:126-131.

46. Thomas JE, Piepgras DG, Scheithauer B, Onofrio BM, Shives TC. Neurogenic tumors of the sciatic nerve. A clinicopathologic study of 35 cases. Mayo Clin Proc 1983;58:640-647.

47. DiCarlo EF, Woodruff JM, Bansal M, Erlandson RA. The purely epithelioid malignant peripheral nerve sheath tumor. Am J Surg Pathol 1986;10:478-490.

48. Robertson I, Cook MG, Wilson DF, Henderson DW. Malignant schwannoma of cranial nerves. Pathology 1983;15:421-429.

49. Tanaka M, Shibui S, Nomura K, Nakanishi Y, Hasegawa T, Hirose T. Malignant intracerebral nerve sheath tumor with intratumoral calcification. Case report. J Neurosurg 2000;92:338-341.

50. Casadei GP, Komori T, Scheithauer BW, Miller GM, Parisi JE, Kelly PJ. Intracranial parenchymal schwannoma. A clinicopathological and neuroimaging study of nine cases. J Neurosurg 1993;79:217-222.

51. Levy D, Khatib R. Intestinal neurofibromatosis with malignant degeneration: report of a case. Dis Colon Rectum 1960;3:140-144.

52. Fuchs B, Spinner RJ, Rock MG. Malignant peripheral nerve sheath tumors: an update. J Surg Orthop Adv 2005;14:168-174.

53. Bhargava R, Parham DM, Lasater OE, Chari RS, Chen G, Fletcher BD. MR imaging differentiation of benign and malignant peripheral nerve sheath tumors: use of the target sign. Pediatr Radiol 1997;27:124-129.

54. Ferner RE, Golding JF, Smith M, et al. [18F]2-fluoro-2-deoxy-D-glucose positron emission tomography (FDG PET) as a diagnostic tool for neurofibromatosis 1 (NF1) associated malignant peripheral nerve sheath tumours (MPNSTs): a long-term clinical study. Ann Oncol 2008;19:390-394.

55. Vieta J, Pack GT. Malignant neurilemomas of peripheral nerves. Am J Surg 1951;82:416-431.

56. Chen KT, Latorraca R, Fabich D, Padgug A, Hafez GR, Gilbert EF. Malignant schwannoma: a light microscopic and ultrastructural study. Cancer 1980;45:1585-1593.

57. Gupta K, Dey P, Vashisht R. Fine-needle aspiration cytology of malignant peripheral nerve sheath tumors. Diagn Cytopathol 2004;31:1-4.

58. Klijanienko J, Caillaud JM, Lagace R, Vielh P. Cytohistologic correlations of 24 malignant peripheral nerve sheath tumor (MPNST) in 17 patients: The Institut Curie experience. Diagn Cytopathol 2002;27:103-108.

59. Jimenez-Heffernan JA, Lopez-Ferrer P, Vicandi B, Hardisson D, Gamallo C, Viguer JM. Cytologic features of malignant peripheral nerve sheath tumor. Acta Cytologica 1999;43:175-183.

60. Daimaru Y, Hashimoto H, Enjoji M. Malignant peripheral nerve-sheath tumors (malignant schwannomas). An immunohistochemical study of 29 cases. Am J Surg Pathol 1985;9:434-444.

61. Gray MH, Rosenberg AE, Dickersin GR, Bhan AK. Glial fibrillary acidic protein and keratin expression by benign and malignant nerve sheath tumors. Hum Pathol 1989;20:1089-1096.

62. Herrera GA, de Moraes HP. Neurogenic sarcomas in patients with neurofibromatosis (von Recklinghausen's disease). Light, electron microscopy and immunohistochemistry study. Virchows Arch A Pathol Anat Histopathol 1984;403:361-376.

63. Weiss SW, Langloss JM, Enzinger FM. Value of S-100 protein in the diagnosis of soft tissue tumors with particular reference to benign and malignant Schwann cell tumors. Lab Invest 1983;49:299-308.

64. Johnson TL, Lee MW, Meis JM, Zarbo RJ, Crissman JD. Immunohistochemical characterization of malignant peripheral nerve sheath tumors. Surg Pathol 1991;4:121-135.

65. Kikuchi A, Akiyama M, Han-Yaku H. Solitary cutaneous malignant schwannoma. Immunohistochemical and ultrastructural studies. Am J Dermatopathol 1993;15:15-19.

66. Wick MR, Swanson PE, Scheithauer BW, Manivel JC. Malignant peripheral nerve sheath tumor. An immunohistochemical study of 62 cases. Am J Clin Pathol 1987;87:425-433.

67. Ogawa K, Oguchi M, Yamabe H, Nakashima Y, Hamashima Y. Distribution of collagen type IV in soft tissue tumors. An immunohistochemical study. Cancer 1986;58:269-277.

68. Chanoki M, Ishii M, Fukai K, et al. Immunohistochemical localization of type I, III, IV, V, and VI collagens and laminin in neurofibroma and neurofibrosarcoma. Am J Dermatopathol 1991;13:365-373.

69. Gould VE, Moll R, Moll I, Lee I, Schwechheimer K, Franke WW. The intermediate filament complement of the spectrum of nerve sheath neoplasms. Lab Invest 1986;55:463-474.

70. Hirose T, Hasegawa T, Kudo E, Seki K, Sano T, Hizawa K. Malignant peripheral nerve sheath tumors: an immunohistochemical study in relation to ultrastructural features. Hum Pathol 1992;23:865-870.

71. Hirose T, Scheithauer BW, Sano T. Giant plexiform Schwannoma: a report of two cases with soft tissue and visceral involvement. Mod Pathol 1997;10:1075-1081.

72. Yasuda T, Sobue G, Ito T, et al. Human peripheral nerve sheath neoplasm: expression of Schwann cell-related markers and their relation to malignant transformation. Muscle Nerve 1991;14:812-819.

73. Swanson PE, Stanley MW, Scheithauer BW, Wick MR. Primary cutaneous leiomyosarcoma. A histological and immunohistochemical study of 9 cases, with ultrastructural correlation. J Cutan Pathol 1988;15:129-141.

74. Dickersin GR. The electron microscopic spectrum of nerve sheath tumors. Ultrastruct Pathol 1987;11:103-146.

75. Erlandson RA, Woodruff JM. Peripheral nerve sheath tumors: An electron microscopic study of 43 cases. Cancer 1982;49:273-287.

76. Taxy JB Battifora H. Epithelioid schwannoma: diagnosis by electron microscopy. Ultrastruct Pathol 1981;2:19-24.

77. Tsuneyoshi M, Daimaru Y, Enjoji M. Malignant hemangiopericytoma and other sarcomas with hemangiopericytoma-like pattern. Pathol Res Pract 1984;178:446-453.

78. Scheithauer BW, Woodruff JM, Erlandson RA. Tumors of the peripheral nervous system. AFIP Atlas of Tumor Pathology, 3rd Series, Fascicle 24. Washington, DC: American Registry of Pathology; 1999.

79. Coindre JM, Trojani M, Contesso G, et al. Reproducibility of a histopathologic grading system for adult soft tissue sarcoma. Cancer 1986;58:306-309.

80. Trojani M, Contesso G, Coindre JM, et al. Soft-tissue sarcomas of adults; study of pathological prognostic variables and definition of a histopathological grading system. Int J Cancer 1984;33:37-42.

81. Coindre JM, Terrier P, Guillou L, et al. Predictive value of grade for metastasis development in the main histologic types of adult soft tissue sarcomas: a study of 1240 patients from the French Federation of Cancer Centers Sarcoma Group. Cancer 2001;91:1914-1926.

82. Hagel C, Zils U, Peiper M, et al. Histopathology and clinical outcome of NF1-associated vs. sporadic malignant peripheral nerve sheath tumors. J Neurooncol 2007;82:187-192.

83. Mertens F, Dal Cin P, De Wever I, et al. Cytogenetic characterization of peripheral nerve sheath tumours: a report of the CHAMP Study Group. J Pathol 2000;190:31-38.

84. Scheithauer BW, Halling KC, Nascimento AG, Hill EM, Sim F, Katzmann JA. Neurofibroma and malignant peripheral nerve sheath tumor: A proliferation index and DNA ploidy study [abstract]. Path Res Pract 1995;19:771.

85. Fletcher JA, Kozakewich HP, Hoffer FA, et al. Diagnostic relevance of clonal cytogenetic aberrations in malignant soft-tissue tumors. N Engl J Med 1991;324:436-442.

86. Jhanwar SC, Chen Q, Li FP, Brennan MF, Woodruff JM. Cytogenetic analysis of soft tissue sarcomas. Recurrent chromosome abnormalities in malignant peripheral nerve sheath tumors (MPNST). Cancer Genet Cytogenet 1994;78:138-144.

87. Menon AG, Anderson KM, Riccardi VM, et al. Chromosome 17p deletions and p53 gene mutations associated with the formation of malignant neurofibrosarcomas in von Recklinghausen neurofibromatosis. Proc Natl Acad Sci U S A 1990;87:5435-5439.

88. Birindelli S, Perrone F, Oggionni M, et al. Rb and TP53 pathway alterations in sporadic and NF1-related malignant peripheral nerve sheath tumors. Lab Invest 2001;81:833-844.

89. Legius E, Dierick H, Wu R, et al. TP53 mutations are frequent in malignant NF1 tumors. Genes Chromosomes Cancer 1994;10:250-255.

90. Baas IO, Mulder JW, Offerhaus GJ, Vogelstein B, Hamilton SR. An evaluation of six antibodies for immunohistochemistry of mutant p53 gene product in archival colorectal neoplasms. J Pathol 1994;172:5-12.

91. Kindblom LG, Ahlden M, Meis-Kindblom JM, Stenman G. Immunohistochemical and molecular analysis of p53, MDM2, proliferating cell nuclear antigen and Ki67 in benign and malignant peripheral nerve sheath tumours. Virchows Arch 1995;427:19-26.

92. Halling KC, Scheithauer BW, Halling AC, et al. P53 expression in neurofibroma and malignant peripheral nerve sheath tumor. An immunohistochemical study of sporadic and NF1-associated tumors. Am J Clin Pathol 1996;106:282-288.

93. Kourea HP, Cordon-Cardo C, Dudas M, Leung D, Woodruff JM. Expression of p27(kip) and other cell cycle regulators in malignant peripheral nerve sheath tumors and neurofibromas: the emerging role of p27(kip) in malignant transformation of neurofibromas. Am J Pathol 1999;155:1885-1891.

94. Berner JM, Sorlie T, Mertens F, et al. Chromosome band 9p21 is frequently altered in malignant peripheral nerve sheath tumors: studies of CDKN2A and other genes of the pRB pathway. Genes Chromosomes Cancer 1999;26:151-160.

95. Perrone F, Tabano S, Colombo F, et al. P15INK4b, p14ARF, and p16INK4a inactivation in sporadic and neurofibromatosis type 1-related malignant peripheral nerve sheath tumors. Clin Cancer Res 2003;9:4132-4138.

96. Kourea HP, Orlow I, Scheithauer BW, Cordon-Cardo C, Woodruff JM. Deletions of the INK4a gene occur in malignant peripheral nerve sheath tumors but not in neurofibromas. Am J Pathol 1999;155:1855-1860.

97. Nielsen GP, Stemmer-Rachamimov AO, Ino Y, Moller MB, Rosenberg AE, Louis DN. Malignant transformation of neurofibromas in neurofibromatosis 1 is associated with CDKN2A/p16 inactivation. Am J Pathol 1999;155:1879-1884.

98. Agesen TH, Florenes VA, Molenaar WM, et al. Expression patterns of cell cycle components in sporadic and neurofibromatosis type 1-related malignant peripheral nerve sheath tumors. J Neuropathol Exp Neurol 2005;64:74-81.

99. Weinstein IB. Disorders in cell circuitry during multistage carcinogenesis: the role of homeostasis. Carcinogenesis 2000;21:857-864.

100. Zhou Y, Coffin CM, Perkins S, et al. Malignant peripheral nerve sheath tumor: a comparison of grade, immunophenotype, and cell cycle/growth activation marker expression in sporadic and neurofibromatosis-1-related lesions. Am J Surg Pathol 2003;27:1337-1345.

101. Vang R, Biddle DA, Harrison WR, Heck K, Cooley LD. Malignant peripheral nerve sheath tumor with a t(X;18). Arch Pathol Lab Med 2000;124:864-867.

102. Krane JF, Bertoni F, Fletcher CD. Myxoid synovial sarcoma: An underappreciated morphologic subset. Mod Pathol 1999;12:456-462.

103. Ordonez NG, Mahfouz SM, Mackay B. Synovial sarcoma: An immunohistochemical and ultrastructural study. Hum Pathol 1990;21:733-749.

104. Fligman I, Lonardo F, Jhanwar SC, Gerald WL, Woodruff J, Ladanyi M. Molecular diagnosis of synovial sarcoma and characterization of a variant SYT-SSX2 fusion transcript. Am J Pathol 1995;147:1592-1599.

105. Ladanyi M, Woodruff JM, Scheithauer BW, et al. Re: O'Sullivan MJ, Kyriakos M, Zhu X, et al. Malignant peripheral nerve sheath tumors with t(X;18). A pathologic and molecular genetic study. Mod Pathol 2000;13:1336-46. Mod Pathol 2001;14:733-737.

106. Coindre JM, Hostein I, Benhattar J, Lussan C, Rivel J, Guillou L. Malignant peripheral nerve sheath tumors are t(X;18)-negative sarcomas. Molecular analysis of 25 cases occurring in neurofibromatosis type 1 patients, using two different RT-PCR-based methods of detection. Mod Pathol 2002;15:589-592.

107. Fletcher CD, Fletcher JA, Dal Cin P, Ladanyi M, Woodruff JM. Diagnostic gold standard for soft tissue tumours: Morphology or molecular genetics? Histopathology 2001;39:100-103.

108. Tamborini E, Agus V, Perrone F, et al. Lack of SYT-SSX fusion transcripts in malignant peripheral nerve sheath tumors on RT-PCR analysis of 34 archival cases. Lab Invest 2002;82:609-618.

109. Scheithauer BW, Amrami KK, Folpe AL, et al. Synovial sarcoma of nerve. Hum Pathol 2011;42:568-577.

110. Min KW, Balaton AJ. Small intestinal stromal tumors with skeinoid fibers in neurofibromatosis: report of four cases with ultrastructural study of skeinoid fibers from paraffin blocks. Ultrastruct Pathol 1993;17:307-314.

111. Sakaguchi N, Sano K, Ito M, Baba T, Fukuzawa M, Hotchi M. A case of von Recklinghausen's disease with bilateral pheochromocytoma-malignant peripheral nerve sheath tumors of the adrenal and gastrointestinal autonomic nerve tumors. Am J Surg Pathol 1996;20:889-897.

112. Koch MB, Shih IM, Weiss SW, Folpe AL. Microphthalmia transcription factor and melanoma cell adhesion molecule expression distinguish desmoplastic/spindle cell melanoma from morphologic mimics. Am J Surg Pathol 2001;25:58-64.

113. King R, Busam K, Rosai J. Metastatic malignant melanoma resembling malignant peripheral nerve sheath tumor: report of 16 cases. Am J Surg Pathol 1999;23:1499-1505.

114. Cavanagh JB. Effects of X-irradiation on the proliferation of cells in peripheral nerve during wallerian degeneration in the rat. Br J Radiol 1968;41:275-281.

115. Wong WW, Hirose T, Scheithauer BW, Schild SE, Gunderson LL. Malignant peripheral nerve sheath tumor: analysis of treatment outcome. Int J Radiat Oncol Biol Phys 1998;42:351-360.

116. Vauthey JN, Woodruff JM, Brennan MF. Extremity malignant peripheral nerve sheath tumors (neurogenic sarcomas): a 10-year experience. Ann Surg Oncol 1995;2:126-131.

117. Coindre JM, Terrier P, Bui NB, et al. Prognostic factors in adult patients with locally controlled soft tissue sarcoma. A study of 546 patients from the French Federation of Cancer Centers Sarcoma Group. J Clin Oncol 1996;14:869-877.

118. Cashen DV, Parisien RC, Raskin K, Hornicek FJ, Gebhardt MC, Mankin HJ. Survival data for patients with malignant schwannoma. Clin Orthop Relat Res 2004(426):69-73.

119. Porter DE, Prasad V, Foster L, Dall GF, Birch R, Grimer RJ. Survival in malignant peripheral nerve sheath tumours: a comparison between sporadic and neurofibromatosis type 1-associated tumours. Sarcoma 2009;2009:756395.

120. Anghileri M, Miceli R, Fiore M, et al. Malignant peripheral nerve sheath tumors: prognostic factors and survival in a series of patients treated at a single institution. Cancer 2006;107:1065-1074.

121. Okada K, Hasegawa T, Tajino T, et al. Clinical relevance of pathological grades of malignant peripheral nerve sheath tumor: a multi-institution TMTS study of 56 cases in Northern Japan. Ann Surg Oncol 2007;14:597-604.

122. Nambisan RN, Rao U, Moore R, Karakousis CP. Malignant soft tissue tumors of nerve sheath origin. J Surg Oncol 1984;25:268-272.

123. Storm FK, Eilber FR, Mirra J, Morton DL. Neurofibrosarcoma. Cancer 1980;45:126-129.

Perineurial Cell MPNST

124. Hirose T, Sumitomo M, Kudo E, et al. Malignant peripheral nerve sheath tumor (MPNST) showing perineurial cell differentiation. Am J Surg Pathol 1989;13:613-620.

124a. Hirose T, Scheithauer BW, Sano T. Perineurial malignant peripheral nerve sheath tumor (MPNST): a clinicopathologic, immunohistochemical, and ultrastructural study of seven cases. Am J Surg Pathol 1998;22:1368-1378.

125. Hirose T, Maeda T, Furuya K, Kiyasu Y, Kawasaki H. Malignant peripheral nerve sheath tumor of the pancreas with perineurial cell differentiation. Ultrastruct Pathol 1998;22:227-231.

125a. Rosenberg AS, Langee CL, Stevens GL, Morgan MB. Malignant peripheral nerve sheath tumor with perineurial differentiation: "malignant perineurioma." J Cutan Pathol 2002;29:362-367.

125b. Karaki S, Mochida J, Lee YH, Nishimura K, Tsutsumi Y. Low-grade malignant perineurioma of the paravertebral column, transforming into a high-grade malignancy. Pathol Int 1999;49:820-825.

Epithelioid MPNST

126. Honma K, Watanabe H, Ohnishi Y, Tachikawa S, Tachikawa K. Epithelioid malignant schwannoma. A case report. Acta Pathol Jpn 1989;39:195-202.

127. McCormack LJ, Hazard JB, Dickson JA. Malignant epithelioid neurilemoma (schwannoma). Cancer 1954;7:725-728.

128. Lodding P, Kindblom LG, Angervall L. Epithelioid malignant schwannoma. A study of 14 cases. Virchows Arch A Pathol Anat Histopathol 1986;409:433-451.

129. Laskin WB, Weiss SW, Bratthauer GL. Epithelioid variant of malignant peripheral nerve sheath tumor (malignant epithelioid schwannoma). Am J Surg Pathol 1991;15:1136-1145.

130. Axiotis C. Nerve sheaths and keratin. Am J Surg Pathol 1998;22:1544.

131. Alvira MM, Mandybur TK, Menefee MG. Light microscopic and ultrastructural observations of a metastasizing malignant epithelioid schwannoma. Cancer 1976;38:1977-1982.

132. Taxy JB, Battifora H, Trujillo Y, Dorfman HD. Electron microscopy in the diagnosis of malignant schwannoma. Cancer 1981;48:1381-1391.

133. Tsuchiya D, Takamura H, Saito K, Kashiwa H, Maeda K, Yamashita H. Immunohistochemical diagnosis of a rare case of epithelioid malignant peripheral nerve sheath tumor with multiple metastases. Jpn J Ophthalmol 2004;48:565-569.

134. Stout A. The peripheral manifestations of the specific nerve sheath tumor (neurilemoma). Am J Cancer 1935;24:751-796.

135. Woodruff JM, Selig AM, Crowley K, Allen PW. Schwannoma (neurilemoma) with malignant transformation. A rare, distinctive peripheral nerve tumor. Am J Surg Pathol 1994;18:882-895.

136. McMenamin ME, Fletcher CD. Expanding the spectrum of malignant change in schwannomas: Epithelioid malignant change, epithelioid malignant peripheral nerve sheath tumor, and epithelioid angiosarcoma. A study of 17 cases. Am J Surg Pathol 2001;25:13-25.

137. Nayler SJ, Leiman G, Omar T, Cooper K. Malignant transformation in a schwannoma. Histopathology 1996;29:189-192.

138. Fowler M. A malignant neurilemmoma. Med J Aust 1955;42, 1:236-237.

139. Yousem SA, Colby TV, Urich H. Malignant epithelioid schwannoma arising in a benign schwannoma. A case report. Cancer 1985;55:2799-2803.

140. Allison KH, Patel RM, Goldblum JR, Rubin BP. Superficial malignant peripheral nerve sheath tumor: a rare and challenging diagnosis. Am J Clin Pathol 2005;124:685-692.

MPNST with Divergent Differentiation

141. Graham A, Begbie J, McGonnell I. Significance of the cranial neural crest. Dev Dyn 2004;229:5-13.

142. Horstadius S. The neural crest: its properties and derivations in the light of experimental research. New York: Hafner Publishing Co.; 1969.

143. Le Douarin NM, Smith J. Development of the peripheral nervous system from the neural crest. Annu Rev Cell Biol 1988;4:375-404.

144. Pytel P, Taxy JB, Krausz T. Divergent differentiation in malignant soft tissue neoplasms: The paradigm of liposarcoma and malignant peripheral nerve sheath tumor. Int J Surg Pathol 2005;13:19-28.

145. Ambler MW. Striated muscle cells in the leptomeninges in cerebral dysplasia. Acta Neuro-Pathol 1977;40:269-271.

146. Tomlinson FH, Scheithauer BW, Kelly PJ, Forbes GS. Subependymoma with rhabdomyosarcomatous differentiation: Report of a case and literature review. Neurosurgery 1991;28:761-768.

147. Russell DS, Rubinstein LJ. Tumours of the cranial, spinal, and peripheral nerve sheaths. Pathology of tumours of the nervous system. Baltimore: William & Wilkins; 1989:533-589.

148. Zimmerman LE, Font RL, Andersen SR. Rhabdomyosarcomatous differentiation in malignant intraocular medulloepitheliomas. Cancer 1972;30:817-835.

149. Woodruff JM. Peripheral nerve tumors showing glandular differentiation (glandular schwannomas). Cancer 1976;37:2399-2413.

150. Woodruff JM, Chernik NL, Smith MC, Millett WB, Foote FW Jr. Peripheral nerve tumors with rhabdomyosarcomatous differentiation (malignant "triton" tumors). Cancer 1973;32:426-439.

151. Masson P. Recklinghausen's neurofibromatosis, sensory neuromas and motor neuromas. In: Contributions to the medical sciences in honor of Dr. Emanuel Libman, Vol. 2. New York: The International Press; 1932:793-802.

152. Masson P. Human tumors: histology, diagnosis, and technique. Detroit: Wayne State University Press.; 1970.

153. Kurtkaya-Yapicier O, Scheithauer BW, Woodruff JM, Wenger DD, Cooley AM, Dominique D. Schwannoma with rhabdomyoblastic differentiation: a unique variant of malignant triton tumor. Am J Surg Pathol 2003;27:848-853.

154. Woodruff JM, Perino G. Non-germ-cell or teratomatous malignant tumors showing additional rhabdomyoblastic differentiation, with emphasis on the malignant triton tumor. Semin Diagn Pathol 1994;11:69-81.

155. Yakulis R, Manack L, Murphy AI Jr. Postradiation malignant Triton tumor. A case report and review of the literature. Arch Pathol Lab Med 1996;120:541-548.

156. Travis JA, Sandberg AA, Neff JR, Bridge JA. Cytogenetic findings in malignant triton tumor. Genes Chromosomes Cancer 1994;9:1-7.

157. Riccardi VM, Elder DW. Multiple cytogenetic aberrations in neurofibrosarcomas complicating neurofibromatosis. Cancer Genet Cytogenet 1986;23:199-209.

158. Haddadin MH, Hawkins AL, Long P, et al. Cytogenetic study of malignant Triton tumor: a case report. Cancer Genet Cytogenet 2003;144:100-105.

159. Schmidt D, Steen A, Voss C. Immunohistochemical study of rhabdomyosarcoma: Unexpected staining with S-100 protein and cytokeratin [letter]. J Pathol 1989;157:83.

160. Matsui I, Tanimura M, Kobayashi N, Sawada T, Nagahara N, Akatsuka J. Neurofibromatosis type 1 and childhood cancer. Cancer 1993;72:2746-2754.

161. Conway JD, Smith MB. Hemangioendothelioma originating in a peripheral nerve; report of a case. Ann Surg 1951;134:138-141.

162. Morphopoulos GD, Banerjee SS, Ali HH, et al. Malignant peripheral nerve sheath tumour with vascular differentiation: A report of four cases. Histopathology 1996;28:401-410.

163. Meis-Kindblom JM, Enzinger FM. Plexiform malignant peripheral nerve sheath tumor of infancy and childhood. Am J Surg Pathol 1994;18:479-485.

164. Ruckert RI, Fleige B, Rogalla P, Woodruff JM. Schwannoma with angiosarcoma. Report of a case and comparison with other types of nerve tumors with angiosarcoma. Cancer 2000;89:1577-1585.

165. Trassard M, Le Doussal V, Bui BN, Coindre JM. Angiosarcoma arising in a solitary schwannoma (neurilemoma) of the sciatic nerve. Am J Surg Pathol 1996;20:1412-1417.

166. Garre C. Uber sekundar maligne neurome. Beitr Z Klin Chir 1892;9:465-495.

167. Woodruff JM, Christensen WN. Glandular peripheral nerve sheath tumors. Cancer 1993;72:3618-3628.

168. Christensen WN, Strong EW, Bains MS, Woodruff JM. Neuroendocrine differentiation in the glandular peripheral nerve sheath tumor. Pathologic distinction from the biphasic synovial sarcoma with glands. Am J Surg Pathol 1988;12:417-426.

169. Uri AK, Witzleben CL, Raney RB. Electron microscopy of glandular Schwannoma. Cancer 1984;53:493-497.

170. Warner TF, Louie R, Hafez GR, Chandler E. Malignant nerve sheath tumor containing endocrine cells. Am J Surg Pathol 1983;7:583-590.

171. Perry A, Miller CR, Gujrati M, et al. Malignant gliomas with primitive neuroectodermal tumor-like components: a clinicopathologic and genetic study of 53 cases. Brain Pathol 2009;19:81-90.

172. Abe S, Imamura T, Park P, et al. Small round-cell type of malignant peripheral nerve sheath tumor. Mod Pathol 1998;11:747-753.

173. Carstens PH, Schrodt GR. Malignant transformation of a benign encapsulated neurilemoma. Am J Clin Pathol 1969;51:144-149.

174. Hanada M, Tanaka T, Kanayama S, Takami M, Kimura M. Malignant transformation of intrathoracic ancient neurilemoma in a patient without von Recklinghausen's disease. Acta Pathol Jpn 1982;32:527-536.

MPNST Arising in Peripheral Neuroblastic Tumors

175. Ricci A Jr, Parham DM, Woodruff JM, Callihan T, Green A, Erlandson RA. Malignant peripheral nerve sheath tumors arising from ganglioneuromas. Am J Surg Pathol 1984;8:19-29.

176. Keller SM, Papazoglou S, McKeever P, Baker A, Roth JA. Late occurrence of malignancy in a ganglioneuroma 19 years following radiation therapy to a neuroblastoma. J Surg Oncol 1984;25:227-231.

177. Navarro O, Nunez-Santos E, Daneman A, Faria P, Daltro P. Malignant peripheral nerve-sheath tumor arising in a previously irradiated neuroblastoma: report of 2 cases and a review of the literature. Pediatr Radiol 2000;30:176-180.

178. Fletcher CD, Fernando IN, Braimbridge MV, McKee PH, Lyall JR. Malignant nerve sheath tumour arising in a ganglioneuroma. Histopathology 1988;12:445-448.

179. Banks E, Yum M, Brodhecker C, Goheen M. A malignant peripheral nerve sheath tumor in association with a paratesticular ganglioneuroma. Cancer 1989;64:1738-1742.

180. Ghali VS, Gold JE, Vincent RA, Cosgrove JM. Malignant peripheral nerve sheath tumor arising spontaneously from retroperitoneal ganglioneuroma: A case report, review of the literature, and immunohistochemical study. Hum Pathol 1992;23:72-75.

181. Drago G, Pasquier B, Pasquier D, et al. Malignant peripheral nerve sheath tumor arising in a "de novo" ganglioneuroma: a case report and review of the literature. Med Pediatr Oncol 1997;28:216-222.

182. de Chadarevian JP, MaePascasio J, Halligan GE, et al. Malignant peripheral nerve sheath tumor arising from an adrenal ganglioneuroma in a 6-year-old boy. Pediatr Dev Pathol 2004;7:277-284.

183. Chandrasoma P, Shibata D, Radin R, Brown LP, Koss M. Malignant peripheral nerve sheath tumor arising in an adrenal ganglioneuroma in an adult male homosexual. Cancer 1986;57:2022-2025.

184. Damiani S, Manetto V, Carrillo G, Di Blasi A, Nappi O, Eusebi V. Malignant peripheral nerve sheath tumor arising in a "de novo" ganglioneuroma. A case report. Tumori 1991;77:90-93.

Primitive Neuroectodermal Tumor of Peripheral Nerve

185. Grippari JL, Neveux Y, Arborio M, et al. [Tumor of the peripheral nerve sheath with rhabdomyoblastic differentiation arising in a ganglioneuroma: neurilemmoma? A fortuitously detected case.] Ann Pathol 1996;16:128-132. [French]

186. Karcioglu Z, Someren A, Mathes SJ. Ectomesenchymoma. A malignant tumor of migratory neural crest (ectomesenchyme) remnants showing ganglionic, schwannian, melanocytic and rhabdomyoblastic differentiation. Cancer 1977;39:2486-2496.

187. Hajlvassiliou C, Carachi E, Simpson W, Young DG. Ectomesenchymoma: One or two tumors? Case report and review of literature. J Pediatr Surg 1997;32:1351-1355.

188. Kawamoto EH, Weidner N, Agostini RM Jr, Jaffe R. Malignant ectomesenchymoma of soft tissue. Report of two cases and review of the literature. Cancer 1987;59:1791-1802.

189. Miettinen M, Saari A. Pheochromocytoma combined with malignant schwannoma: unusual neoplasm of the adrenal medulla. Ultrastruct Pathol 1988;12:513-527.

190. Min KW, Clemens A, Bell J, Dick H. Malignant peripheral nerve sheath tumor and pheochromocytoma. A composite tumor of the adrenal. Arch Pathol Lab Med 1988;112:266-270.

191. Gupta R, Sharma A, Arora R, Vijayaraghavan M. Composite phaeochromocytoma with malignant peripheral nerve sheath tumour and rhabdomyosarcomatous differentiation in a patient without von Recklinghausen disease. J Clin Pathol 2009;62:659-661.

192. Stout AP. A tumor of the ulnar nerve. Proceedings of the New York Pathology Society. 1918;18:2-12.

193. Bolen JW, Thorning D. Peripheral neuroepithelioma: a light and electron microscopic study. Cancer 1980;46:2456-2462.

194. Harper PG, Pringle J, Souhami RL. Neuroepithelioma—a rare malignant peripheral nerve tumor of primitive origin: Report of two new cases and a review of the literature. Cancer 1981;48:2282-2287.

195. Nesbitt KA, Vidone RA. Primitive neuroectodermal tumor (neuroblastoma) arising in sciatic nerve of a child. Cancer 1976;37:1562-1570.

196. Stout AP, Murray MR. Neuroepithelioma of the radial nerve with a study of its behavior in vitro. Rev Canad de Biol 1942;1:651-659.

197. Abell MR, Hart WR, Olson JR. Tumors of the peripheral nervous system. Hum Pathol 1970;1:503-551.

198. Stout AP. Case 6. In: Seminar on tumors of the soft tissue. American Society of Clinical Pathologists, October 19, 1951. Chicago: American Society of Clinical Pathologists; 1953:18-19.

199. Stout A. Tumors of the peripheral nervous system. In: Ackerman LV, ed. Atlas of tumor pathology. Washington, DC: Armed Forces Institute of Pathology; 1949.

200. Lattes R, Enzinger FM, Hartmann WH. Soft tissue tumors. Case 9. Proceedings of the thirty-ninth Annual Anatomic Pathology Slide Seminar of the American Society of Clinical Pathologists, October 26, 1973. Chicago: American Society of Clinical Pathologists; 1973:49-42.

201. Seemayer TA, Thelmo WL, Bolande RP, Wiglesworth FW. Peripheral neuroectodermal tumors. Perspect Pediatr Pathol 1975;2:151-172.

202. Lieberman P. Case 21. Proceedings of the forty-fifth Annual Anatomic Pathology Slide Seminar of the American Society of Clinical Pathologists. Chicago: American Society of Clinical Pathologists; 1979:100-105.

203. Askin FB, Rosai J, Sibley RK, Dehner LP, McAlister WH. Malignant small cell tumor of the thoracopulmonary region in childhood: A distinctive clinicopathologic entity of uncertain histogenesis. Cancer 1979;43:2438-2451.

204. Hashimoto H, Enjoji M, Nakajima T, Kiryu H, Daimaru Y. Malignant neuroepithelioma (peripheral neuroblastoma). A clinicopathologic study of 15 cases. Am J Surg Pathol 1983;7:309-318.

205. Linnoila RI, Tsokos M, Triche TJ, Marangos PJ, Chandra RS. Evidence for neural origin and PAS-positive variants of the malignant small cell tumor of thoracopulmonary region ("Askin tumor"). Am J Surg Pathol 1986;10:124-133.

206. Erlandson RA. Diagnostic transmission electron microscopy of tumors: with clinicopathologigica, immunohistochemical, and cytogenetic correlations. New York: Raven Press; 1994.

207. Nesland JM, Sobrinho-Simoes MA, Holm R, Johannessen JV. Primitive neuroectodermal tumor (peripheral neuroblastoma). Ultrastruct Pathol 1985;9:59-64.

208. Enzinger FM. Case 12. In: Proceedings of Forty-ninth Annual Anatomic Pathology Slide Seminar of the American Society of Clinical Pathologists. Chicago: American Society of Clinical Pathologists; 1983:90-96.

209. Gonzalez-Crussi F, Wolfson SL, Misugi K, Nakajima T. Peripheral neuroectodermal tumors of the chest wall in childhood. Cancer 1984;54:2519-2527.

210. Schmidt D, Harms D, Burdach S. Malignant peripheral neuroectodermal tumours of childhood and adolescence. Virchows Arch A Pathol Anat Histopathol 1985;406:351-365.

211. Voss BL, Pysher TJ, Humphrey GB. Peripheral neuroepithelioma in childhood. Cancer 1984;54:3059-3064.

212. Fellinger EJ, Garin-Chesa P, Su SL, DeAngelis P, Lane JM, Rettig WJ. Biochemical and genetic characterization of the HBA71 Ewing's sarcoma cell surface antigen. Cancer Res 1991;51:336-340.

213. Garin-Chesa P, Fellinger EJ, Huvos AG, et al. Immunohistochemical analysis of neural cell adhesion molecules. Differential expression in small round cell tumors of childhood and adolescence. Am J Pathol 1991;139:275-286.

214. Pappo AS, Douglass EC, Meyer WH, Marina N, Parham DM. Use of HBA 71 and anti-beta 2-microglobulin to distinguish peripheral neuroepithelioma from neuroblastoma. Hum Pathol 1993;24:880-885.

215. Fellinger EJ, Garin-Chesa P, Glasser DB, Huvos AG, Rettig WJ. Comparison of cell surface antigen HBA71 (p30/32MIC2), neuron-specific enolase, and vimentin in the immunohistochemical analysis of Ewing's sarcoma of bone. Am J Surg Pathol 1992;16:746-755.

216. Fellinger EJ, Garin-Chesa P, Triche TJ, Huvos AG, Rettig WJ. Immunohistochemical analysis of Ewing's sarcoma cell surface antigen p30/32MIC2. Am J Pathol 1991;139:317-325.

217. Hess E, Cohen C, DeRose P, Yost B, Costa M. Non-specificity of p30/32MIC2 immunolocalization with the 013 monoclonal antibody in the diagnosis of Ewing sarcoma: application of an algorithmic immunohistochemical analysis. Appl Immunohistochem 1997;5:94-103.

218. Stevenson A, Chattan J, Bertoni F, Miettinen M. Cd99 (p30/32MIC2) neuroectodermal/Ewing's sarcoma antigen as an immunohistochemical marker. Review of more than 600 tumors and the literature experience. Appl Immunohistochem 1994;2:231-240.

219. Papierz W, Alwasiak J, Kolasa P, et al. Primitive neuroectodermal tumors: ultrastructural and immunohistochemical studies. Ultrastruct Pathol 1995;19:147-166.

220. Whang-Peng J, Triche TJ, Knutsen T, et al. Cytogenetic characterization of selected small round cell tumors of childhood. Cancer Genet Cytogenet 1986;21:185-208.

221. Turc-Carel C, Aurias A, Mugneret F, et al. Chromosomes in ewing's sarcoma. I. An evaluation of 85 cases of remarkable consistency of t(11;22)(q24;q12). Cancer Genet Cytogenet 1988;32:229-238.

222. Marina NM, Etcubanas E, Parham DM, Bowman LC, Green A. Peripheral primitive neuroectodermal tumor (peripheral neuroepithelioma) in children. A review of the St. Jude experience and controversies in diagnosis and management. Cancer 1989;64:1952-1960.

223. Jurgens H, Bier V, Harms D, et al. Malignant peripheral neuroectodermal tumors. A retrospective analysis of 42 patients. Cancer 1988;61:349-357.

Malignant Granular Cell Tumor

224. Ravich A, Stout AP, Ravich RA. Malignant granular cell myoblastoma involving the urinary bladder. Ann Surg 1945;121:361-372.

225. Gamboa LG. Malignant granular-cell myoblastoma. AMA Arch Pathol 1955;60:663-668.

226. Mackenzie DH. Malignant granular cell myoblastoma. J Clin Pathol 1967;20:739-742.

227. Obiditsch-Mayer I, Salzer-Kuntschik M. [Malignant "granular cell neuroma," so-called "myoblastmyoma" of the esophagus.] Beitr Pathol Anat 1961;125:357-373. [German]

228. O'Donovan DG, Kell P. Malignant granular cell tumour with intraperitoneal dissemination. Histopathology 1989;14:417-419.

229. Magori A, Szegvari M. [Abrikossoffs tumour of the vulva with recurrence and metastasis (author's transl).] Zentralbl Allg Pathol 1973;117:265-273. [German]

230. Robertson AJ, McIntosh W, Lamont P, Guthrie W. Malignant granular cell tumour (myoblastoma) of the vulva: Report of a case and review of the literature. Histopathology 1981;5:69-79.

231. Shimamura K, Osamura RY, Ueyama Y, et al. Malignant granular cell tumor of the right sciatic nerve. Report of an autopsy case with electron microscopic, immunohistochemical, and enzyme histochemical studies. Cancer 1984;53:524-529.

232. Hurrell MA, McLean C, Desmond P, Tress BM, Kaye A. Malignant granular cell tumour of the sciatic nerve. Australas Radiol 1995;39:86-89.

233. al-Sarraf M, Loud AV, Vaitkevicius VK. Malignant granular cell tumor. Histochemical and electron microscopic study. Arch Pathol 1971;91:550-558.

234. Fanburg-Smith JC, Meis-Kindblom JM, Fante R, Kindblom LG. Malignant granular cell tumor of soft tissue: diagnostic criteria and clinicopathologic correlation. Am J Surg Pathol 1998;22:779-794.

235. Wieczorek TJ, Krane JF, Domanski HA, et al. Cytologic findings in granular cell tumors, with emphasis on the diagnosis of malignant granular cell tumor by fine-needle aspiration biopsy. Cancer 2001;93:398-408.

236. Troncoso P, Ordonez NG, Raymond AK, Mackay B. Malignant granular cell tumor: immunocytochemical and ultrastructural observations. Ultrastruct Pathol 1988;12:137-144.

237. Geisinger KR, Kawamoto EH, Marshall RB, Ahl ET, Cooper MR. Aspiration and exfoliative cytology, including ultrastructure, of a malignant granular-cell tumor. Acta Cytologica 1985;29:593-597.

238. Kurtin PJ, Bonin DM. Immunohistochemical demonstration of the lysosome-associated glycoprotein CD68 (KP-1) in granular cell tumors and schwannomas. Hum Pathol 1994;25:1172-1178.

239. Chang Y, Dehner LP, Egbert B. Primary cutaneous rhabdomyosarcoma. Am J Surg Pathol 1990;14:977-982.

240. Mierau GW, Berry PJ, Orsini EN. Small round cell neoplasms: Can electron microscopy and immunohistochemical studies accurately classify them? Ultrastruct Pathol 1985;9:99-111.

241. Suster S, Rosen LB, Sanchez JL. Granular cell leiomyosarcoma of the skin. Am J Dermatopathol 1988;10:234-239.

242. Christopherson WM, Foote FW Jr., Stewart FW. Alveolar soft-part sarcomas; structurally characteristic tumors of uncertain histogenesis. Cancer 1952;5:100-111.

243. Shipkey FH, Lieberman PH, Foote FW Jr, Stewart FW. Ultrastructure of alveolar soft part sarcoma. Cancer 1964;17:821-830.

244. Lieberman PH, Brennan MF, Kimmel M, Erlandson RA, Garin-Chesa P, Flehinger BY. Alveolar soft-part sarcoma. A clinico-pathologic study of half a century. Cancer 1989;63:1-13.

245. Hunter DT Jr, Dewar J. Malignant granular cell myoblastoma: Report of a case and review of literature. Am Surg 1960;26:554-559.

246. Kirschner H. [On a case of malignant degeneration of myoblasticmyoma of the breast.]. Bruns Beitr Klin Chir 1962;204:87-94. [German]

247. Madhaven M, Aurora AL, Sen SB. Malignant granular cell myoblastoma—report of a case. Indian J Cancer 1974;11:360-363.

248. Ross RC, Miller TR, Foote FW Jr. Malignant granular-cell myoblastoma. Cancer 1952;5:112-121.

249. Salvadori B, Talamazzi F. [Malignant granular cell myoblastomyoma.] Tumori 1967;53:645-649. [Italian]

13
TUMORS OF THE NEURAL TRANSMITTING MESENCHYMAL CELL COMPONENT OF THE PERIPHERAL NERVOUS SYSTEM

Investigations spanning the past few decades have characterized a network of mesenchymal cells (1) exhibiting neuronal characteristics. First identified in 1893 by the Spanish neuroanatomist, Santiago Ramón y Cajal, and thereafter referred to as "interstitial cells of Cajal" (ICC), they lie intercalated between enteric autonomic nerves and intestinal smooth muscle (2). These cells relay normal neural activity to smooth muscle cells (3–5) and complement the action of enteric nerves in augmenting gastrointestinal function by self-generating pacemaker signals (6,7). The ICCs are the pathologic substrate of potentially malignant neoplasms referred as gastrointestinal stromal tumors (GISTs).

GASTROINTESTINAL STROMAL TUMOR

Definition. *Gastrointestinal stromal tumor* (GIST) is a tumor composed of spindle to epithelioid cells exhibiting the immunohistochemical and ultrastructural features of ICCs. In most cases, the tumors possess an activated mutation in either the *KIT* or *PDGFRA* gene. As expected, they are geographically related to the intestinal myenteric plexus.

General Features. Although a poorly understood pathologic entity, GIST is the most common mesenchymal tumor of the intestinal tract. Some 4,500 to 6,000 new cases present each year in the United States (8). Until recently, GISTs were classified as a form of smooth muscle tumor. The subsequent application of electron microscopy and immunohistochemistry provided evidence of only partial or no smooth muscle differentiation. This led to the adoption of the noncommittal designation, gastrointestinal stromal tumor (9,10). Subsequent ultrastructural studies (11,12) and immunohistochemical findings (12) showed that some GISTs possess neuronal features. The terms *plexosarcoma* (11) and

gastrointestinal autonomic nerve tumor (GANT) (12,13) were applied to these tumors.

The confirmation that a GIST exhibits a Cajal cell phenotype includes molecular genetic studies revealing mutations in KIT receptor tyrosine kinase (14). Other findings regarding the nature of GISTs are listed in Table 13-1. KIT expression by GISTs not only furnishes a molecular signature facilitating pathologic diagnosis, but also provides a therapeutic target for a tumor largely unresponsive to any therapy.

Clinical Features. In the gastrointestinal tract, GISTs arise anywhere ICCs are found. Fifty to 60 percent occur in the stomach, 20 to 30 percent in the small bowel, 10 percent in the colon and rectum, and 5 percent in the esophagus (15). GISTs also occur at sites outside the gastrointestinal tract, including in mesentery, omentum, retroperitoneum, and pelvis. Similar tumors have been identified in the gallbladder and pancreas, sites also containing ICCs (16). Unexpectedly, ICCs are even encountered in fallopian tube, myometrium, portal vein, and mammary stroma (16).

GISTs present over a wide patient age range, from childhood to senescence, but most occur in older adults (mean and median ages of 63 and 58 years, respectively) (8,17). Males are slightly more often affected (18).

The clinical setting of GISTs is variable, and includes sporadic, familial, syndrome-associated, and solitary and multiple examples with or without ICC hyperplasia. Tumors appearing in older adults are primarily sporadic and solitary. About 3 percent of sporadic examples occur in children and in young adults aged 30 years or less, show a female predilection, typically affect the stomach, are multifocal and small, and are unassociated with ICC hyperplasia (19–21). Both the molecular genetic findings and the

Table 13-1

EVIDENCE ESTABLISHING A HISTOGENETIC CONNECTION BETWEEN
GASTROINTESTINAL STROMAL TUMOR (GIST) AND INTESTINAL CELLS OF CAJAL (ICC)

Discovery of the proto-oncogene, *c-kit*, which encodes the receptor tyrosine kinase KIT (43). The latter is activated by the KIT ligand, stem cell factor (SCF) (43,66).

An effort to identify cell lineages, beyond those for which KIT is shown to play a developmental role, leads to demonstration of KIT immunoexpression by ICC (45).

KIT gain of function mutations are detected in 5 of 6 studied GISTs. Corresponding mutant KIT proteins are constitutively activated, independent of KIT ligand (14).

Germline *KIT* mutations, similar to ones found in sporadic GIST, are identified in inherited examples (56). Familial GIST is characterized by multiple tumors and ICC hyperplasia within the myenteric plexus.

GIST and ICC are immunopositive for KIT and CD34, while intestinal leiomyomas and leiomyosarcomas are not (34,67).

Ultrastructurally, GIST cells resemble ICCs (33).

KIT mutation in a knock-in mouse model is associated with GIST and ICC hyperplasia, a finding faithfully recapitulating the human familial GIST syndrome (56).

disease course in these two age groups differ. Mutations in the *KIT* or *PDGFRA* genes characterize tumors of older patients, but are lacking in those of the young (21).

Most patients with GIST have symptoms associated with satiety, bloating, and fatigue due to anemia related to gastrointestinal bleeding. In one population-based study, a number of tumors were incidental findings: 21 percent at surgery and another 10 percent at autopsy (22). Upon presentation, the tumors may already exhibit intra-abdominal spread or liver metastasis. Pediatric GISTs are more prone to metastasize to lymph nodes than are those of adults; conversely, they follow a more indolent course.

Aside from these major patient groups with sporadic GISTs, others have tumors that are 1) associated with neurofibromatosis 1 (NF1) (23); 2) sporadic, but associated with other neoplasms of Carney triad (24); 3) simply familial (25,26); or 4) familial and associated with paraganglioma (Carney-Stratakis dyad) (27). Details regarding these clinical variations are presented in Table 13-2.

Gross Findings. GISTs vary considerably in size, ranging from less than 1 cm in incidental lesions to masses as large as 35 cm (24) and weighing over 5,000 g (12). Most are solitary and well-circumscribed. These involve the wall of the gastrointestinal tract, often protrude toward the serosa as sessile or pedunculated lesions (figs. 13-1, 13-2), or extend transmurally. Occasionally, lesions are associated with

mucosal ulcerations, intraluminal extension, or obstruction of the viscus. On cut section, the surface of the tumor is usually tan, soft, or friable. It usually lacks a whorled appearance, but is often lobulated and hemorrhagic (fig. 13-2) (12). Large tumors are often centrally cystic and necrotic (fig. 13-3).

Microscopic Findings. Histologic variation typifies GIST (28,29). Some 70 percent are nonpleomorphic spindle cell tumors (fig. 13-4A,E,F) (29), with pale eosinophilic and finely fibrillar cytoplasm and ill-defined cell borders (fig. 13-4B,C). Nuclei are elongated or ovoid, typically shorter than those of smooth muscle tumors; they possess delicate chromatin as well as inconspicuous nucleoli (fig. 13-4B,C). Juxtanuclear vacuoles (fig. 13-4F) are present in some cases, particularly in gastric tumors (29). The cells generally do not "stand alone," but rather assume a syncytial appearance (fig. 13-4B,C). Cellular arrangement also varies. Although most often forming short fascicles (fig. 13-4C,I), they may lie clustered (fig. 13-4A), whorled (fig. 13-4E), lobulated, storiform, or palisaded (fig. 13-4D) (12). The palisaded pattern differs from that of schwannomas by the confluence of the cell palisades. Of the patterns encountered in GISTs, the spindle cell form is histologically most uniform (30).

About 20 percent of GISTs exhibit an epithelioid cytology (fig. 13-5, left) (31): rounded or polygonal cells possessing variably eosinophilic or even clear cytoplasm, the latter being considered a retraction artifact. Unlike in spindle

Table 13-2

GISTS IN FAMILIAL AND SYNDROMIC SETTINGS

Familial GISTs	
Clinical Setting/ Findings	A familial autosomal dominant condition is identified in at least 11 families (25). No gender bias; mean age in 5th decade. Gastric and small intestinal sites affected. Tumors usually multiple. Metastases rare.
Pathology	Tumors usually small. Background of ICC[a] hyperplasia in myenteric plexus.
Genetics	Germline mutations in either *KIT* or *PDGFRA*. Patients with *KIT* exon 11 mutations often have cutaneous hyperpigmentation in perineum, groin, face, neck, digits, axillae, and knees. Occasional urticaria pigmentosa or diffuse mastocytosis in infancy (25). Inherited *PDGFRA* mutations may be cause of familial GISTs previously erroneously referred to as intestinal neurofibromatosis (69). All members of one family with *PDGFRA* mutations had large hands (67).
NF1-Associated GISTs	
Clinical Setting/ Findings	Three-quarters of patients 50 years of age or older. Preferential involvement of small intestine; occasionally stomach and colon. Most patients have multiple GISTs. Tumors uncommonly metastasize or result in mortality (69–71).
Pathology	Wide range of tumor size; many 2 cm or smaller. Microscopically, most spindle cell type; 86 percent feature skeinoid fibers. Over 90% express KIT and many weakly reactive for S-100 protein. One third associated with ICC hyperplasia. Mitotic index usually low (70,71).
Genetics	The molecular event underlying tumor development is a somatic inactivation of wild-type NF1 allele (72). Although most GISTs are wild type, a small subset (11.5 percent) may show mutations in either *KIT* or *PDGFRA* (69–71,73).
Carney Triad	
Clinical Setting/ Findings	Nonfamilial sporadic disorder with multifocal antral-based, gastric GISTs. In addition, one or more of the following: pulmonary chondroma, multicentric functioning extra-adrenal paragangliomas, adrenal adenoma, and esophageal leiomyoma. Female predilection (88%). Mean age at diagnosis of first tumor component 22 years. Often new GISTs after subtotal gastric resection (21 percent). Metastasis (47 percent); often to gastric lymph nodes and liver. Tumor-associated mortality low (13 percent). Estimated 10- and 40-year survival rates of 100% and 73%, respectively. Median survival 26.5 years (74,75).
Pathology	Intramural circumscribed, multicentric tumors expanding gastric wall. Often protruding as polypoid lesions into gastric lumen or as bulging masses from the serosal surface. Tumors 0.2 to 18.0 cm (mean, 6.3 cm). Histologically, 68 percent epithelioid. Immunohistochemistry: 100 percent positive for KIT, 75 percent for CD34, and 90 percent for PDGFRA (75).
Genetics	No coding sequence abnormalities found in *KIT*, *PDGFRA*, or *SDHB-D* genes of familial paraganglioma and GIST-paraganglioma dyad (see below) (75).
Carney-Stratakis Syndrome (Dyad)	
Clinical Setting/ Findings	Familial autosomal disorder with incomplete penetrance, characterized by multifocal gastric GISTs and multicentric paraganglioma. Original report of 12 patients from 5 families showed no gender predilection; mean age, 32 years. Lymph node metastases in 3 (of 12) and, in 2 of the 3, peritoneal spread. Prognosis excellent (27).
Pathology	Tumor size 2 to 8 cm. Microscopically, polygonal and/or spindle cells expressing KIT and CD34.
Genetics	Germline mutations of succinate dehydrogenase genes *SDHB*, *SDHC*, or *SDHD*, encoding subunits B, C or D, in 8 patients from 7 unrelated families. Three patients showed no identifiable mutations. Specifically, no *KIT* or *PDGFRA* mutations found (76,77)

[a]ICC = interstitial cells of Cajal.

cell tumors, the nuclei in epithelioid GISTs are more often pleomorphic with frequent binucleated and multinucleation (8). Most epithelioid GISTs are gastric tumors (31). In the small bowel, epithelioid tumors feature a distinctly nested,

paraganglioma- or carcinoid-like growth pattern (fig. 13-5, right).

Least frequent are mixed spindle and epithelioid GISTs featuring either abrupt transition between zones of spindle and epithelioid cells,

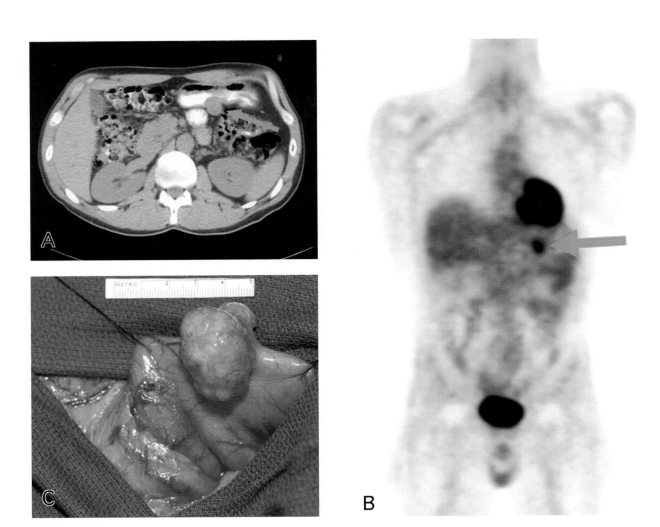

Figure 13-1

GASTROINTESTINAL STROMAL TUMOR (GIST)

Computerized tomography (A), positron emission tomography (B), and intraoperative view (C) of a primary gastric GIST.

or blending of the two cell types. The result is an overall "intermediate" ovoid cytologic appearance (29). Most of these GISTs occur in the stomach (30).

Stromal changes are encountered in GISTs. These include hyalinization of blood vessels and interstitial myxoid change (12), microcystic degeneration, and minor stromal lymphocytic infiltrates (fig. 13-4C). The occasional accumulation of lymphocytes differs from that seen in intestinal schwannomas, where they form characteristic peripheral cuffs (see chapter 7). Also notable is the presence of intercellular skeinoid fibers (fig. 13-4B), especially in spindle cell GISTs

of the small bowel and less often of the stomach and large bowel. This unusual sausage-shaped form of collagen deposit is periodic acid–Schiff (PAS) positive (fig. 13-4G), but best characterized by its ultrastructure (see fig. 13-8D). The fibers are particularly frequent in small bowel GISTs in patients with NF1 (32).

Cytologic Findings. Fine needle aspirates often reveal clusters of abundant, cohesive, nonpleomorphic spindle cells with elongated nuclei and eosinophilic cytoplasm (fig. 13-6, left). The cells are frequently syncytial in arrangement (fig. 13-6, right). To confidently distinguish the cells from those of a schwannoma or smooth

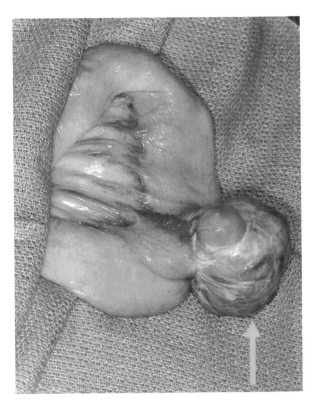
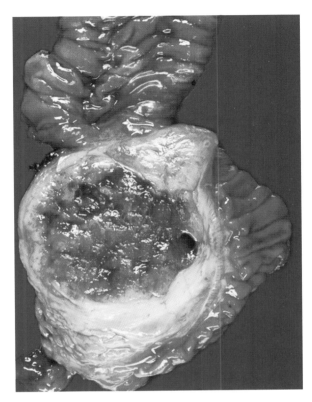

Figure 13-2

GASTROINTESTINAL STROMAL TUMOR (GIST)

Intraoperative view (left) and gross specimen (right) of a pedunculated, small bowel GIST with a hemorrhagic, friable cut surface.

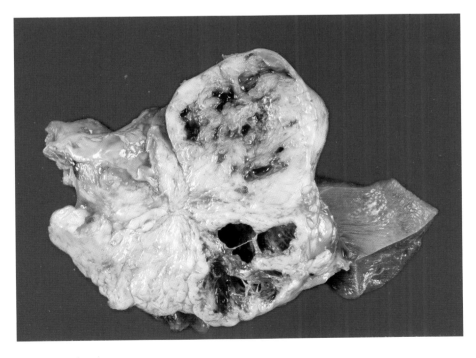

Figure 13-3

GASTROINTESTINAL STROMAL TUMOR (GIST)

Cross section of a large gastric GIST with a tan fleshy cut surface and central cystic-hemorrhagic changes. A complete resection required distal pancreatectomy, splenectomy, and partial gastrectomy.

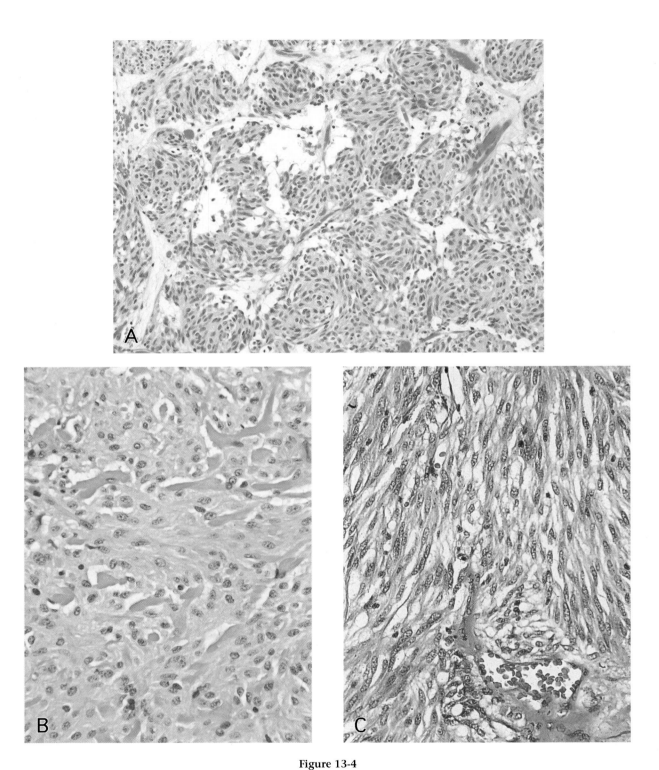

Figure 13-4

SPINDLE CELL GIST

This spindle cell GIST shows morphologically uniform cells, most often arranged in short fascicles (A,C) and having a syncytial appearance (B). Infrequently, tumor cells may be clustered (A), palisaded (D), or whorled (E). Juxtanuclear vacuoles (F) are sometimes found, notably in gastric examples. Eosinophilic interstitial skeinoid fibers (B), most commonly seen in small bowel tumors, are best demonstrated using a periodic acid–Schiff (PAS) stain (G).

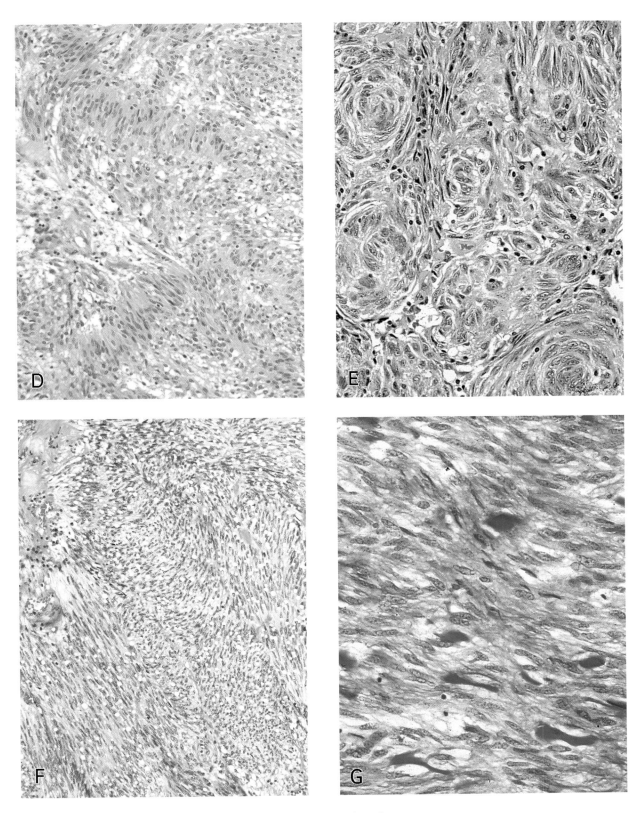

Figure 13-4, continued

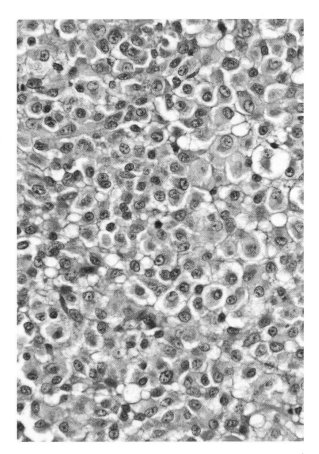 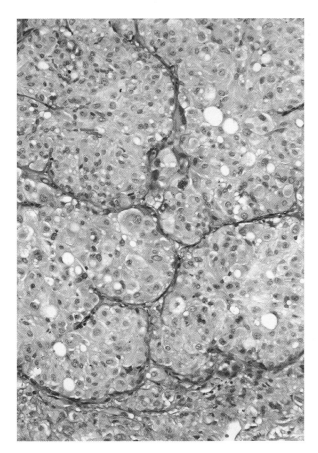

Figure 13-5

EPITHELIOID GIST

Left: Gastric examples may exhibit a diffuse growth pattern and consist of somewhat round, plasmacytoid cells with well-defined cell borders and eosinophilic cytoplasm.

Right: Alternatively, small bowel lesions often feature nested growth reminiscent of paraganglioma.

muscle tumor, immunohistochemistry on cell block sections is often necessary (8).

Immunohistochemical Findings. When sizeable tissue sections are studied, as opposed to those comprising tissue arrays, two sensitive and reliable markers for GISTs have been found useful. The first, CD117 (KIT protein), is the marker most commonly used to confirm the diagnosis (33,34). The reaction is cytoplasmic and commonly both diffuse and strong (fig. 13-7A). Concurrent dot-like or occasionally weak staining is also seen (fig. 13-7B). Weak KIT immunoreactivity may sometimes be seen in other mesenchymal neoplasms, including leiomyosarcoma and desmoid tumor, both of which are, however, routinely reactive for calponin. Leiomyosarcoma is also desmin immunoreactive. Aside from a few with

epithelioid features (30), GISTs are typically non-reactive for both calponin and desmin markers (35). In contrast to schwannoma, GISTs usually do not express S-100 protein; when some staining is evident, it is focal and weak. Most GISTs also express CD34, a marker not usually found in other intestinal tumors.

KIT expression in GISTs is not a constant: approximately 4 percent of GISTs diagnosed by other means are KIT negative (36). These often exhibit a complete or partial epithelioid morphology and arise either in the stomach or outside the gastrointestinal tract (30). Since some GISTs in this group still feature *KIT* or *PDGFRA* mutations, these patients should not be denied tyrosine kinase inhibitor therapy based simply upon a negative immunoreaction.

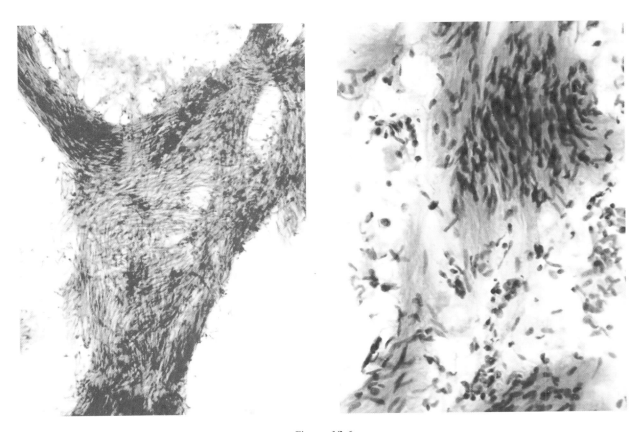

Figure 13-6

SPINDLE CELL GIST

This aspiration cytology specimen of a gastric, spindle cell GIST shows uniform bland spindle cells (left) arranged in short fascicles (right).

The second reliable marker of ICCs and GISTs is DOG1, also known as Ano1 (37–40), which stains GISTs in both a membranous and cytoplasmic pattern (38). Although not immunoexpressed in all GISTs, it labels about one third of KIT-negative tumors (fig. 13-7C) (38). Therefore, it may be used to resolve the typing of a KIT-negative presumed GIST, or distinguish a GIST from other KIT-positive tumors, such as a melanoma and germ cell tumors. Both KIT and DOG1 are equally sensitive in identifying GIST subgroups lacking *KIT* or *PDGFRA* mutations. These include childhood and NF1-associated examples (38).

If after immunohistochemical evaluation the diagnosis remains unproven, *KIT/PDGFRA* mutations may be sought by molecular genetic analysis.

Ultrastructural Findings. The ultrastructural features of GISTs (fig. 13-8) are abundantly illustrated in the literature and summarized by Kindblom et al. (33). They resemble the fine structure of ICCs (2,41), but lack sufficient specificity to play a key role in routine diagnosis.

Molecular Findings. Most GISTs are KIT-expressing and KIT-signaling driven mesenchymal tumors. Many have *KIT*-activating mutations (14). A small subset shows activating mutations in the *PDGFRA* gene, which encodes for a related member of the type III receptor tyrosine kinase family (42). KIT was originally identified as the cellular homolog of the retroviral oncogene *v-kit* in the Hardy-Zuckerman 4-feline sarcoma virus (43). Its receptor plays a critical role in the normal development and function of ICCs (7,44,45), as well as in hematopoiesis, gametogenesis, and melanogenesis during embryonic development and the postnatal period. *KIT* receptor gain of function mutations have been implicated in the pathogenesis of several human tumors, including seminomas (46),

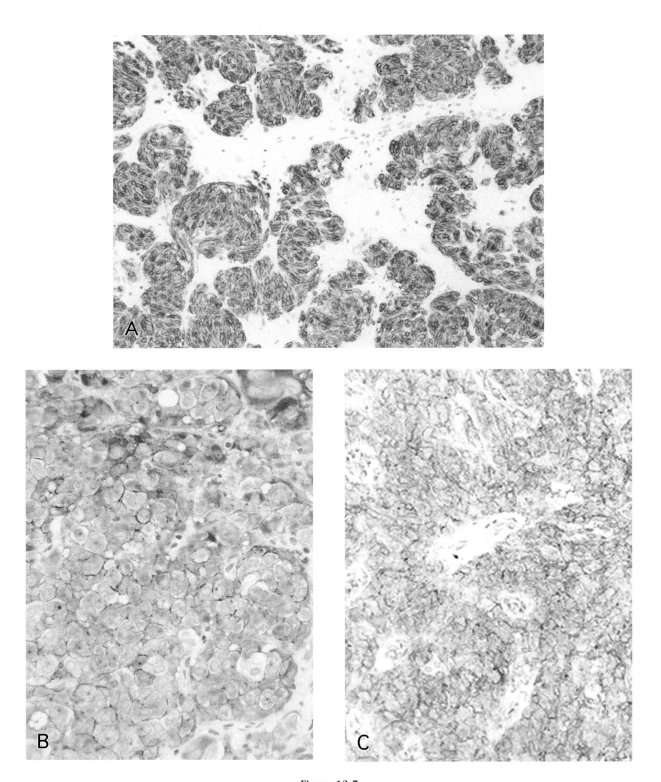

Figure 13-7

GIST: IMMUNOPROFILE

Immunostaining for CD117 (KIT) is strong and diffuse in this spindle cell GIST (A) and is weak and focal in an epithelioid example (B). Diffuse reactivity for DOG1 in an epithelioid gastric GIST. (C, Courtesy Dr. C. Fletcher, Boston, MA.)

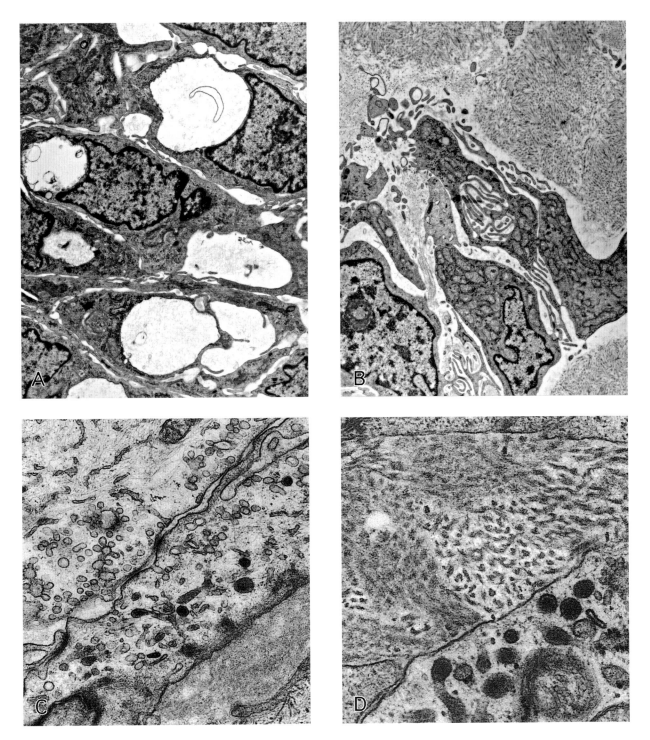

Figure 13-8

GIST: ULTRASTRUCTURE

Among ultrastructural findings in GIST are subnuclear vacuoles (A); elongated cell processes (B); neuritic processes, possibly of innervating enteric neurons, containing variable numbers of fine filaments, vesicles, and neurosecretory granules (C); and intercellular masses of skeinoid fibers seen here to consist of tangles or skeins of collagen fibers of varying thickness with an average periodicity of 45 nm (D).

mastocytosis (47), acute myelogenous leukemias (48), and melanomas (49). Collectively, this suggests a role for *KIT* in oncogenesis.

Ligand-independent activation of the *KIT* receptor by gain of function mutations plays a central role in the pathogenesis of GIST, since up to 90 percent of tumors harbor either *KIT*- or *PDGFRA*-activating mutations (50,51). The majority of mutations occur in the juxtamembrane domain (exon 11) of *KIT*. However, this hotspot does not translate into a specific clinicopathologic presentation. In contrast, mutations in the extracellular domain (exon 9) correlate with both a small bowel location and more aggressive clinical behavior (52). Rarely, mutations have been described in the kinase domain (exons 13 and 17) (50,53). Approximately one third of GISTs lacking *KIT* mutations exhibit a mutation in *PDGFRA* (exons 12, 14 or 18) (42,54). Most *PDGFRA*-mutated GISTs are associated with a distinct clinicopathologic phenotype, including a gastric location, epithelioid morphology, variable or absent KIT immunoexpression, and more indolent behavior (51,55). In about 10 percent of GIST patients, no detectable mutations in either *KIT* or *PDGFRA* are identified.

In the adult population, the wild-type GIST subset represents a heterogeneous group of patients with no particular tumor location or clinical outcome. In contrast, GISTs occurring in children or in those with NF1 are nearly always wild type (19,20,23). Pediatric GISTs represent a distinct clinicopathologic and molecular subset affecting mainly females and presenting as multifocal gastric tumors (21).

The finding that *KIT* activating mutations may be inherited suggested the possibility of developing a murine model featuring a germline gain of function mutation, permitting the study of *KIT* oncogenic signaling mechanisms. Using a knock-in strategy that introduced a *KIT* exon 11 mutation into the murine genome, a mutation identified by Nishida et al. (26) in the familial GIST syndrome, Sommer et al. (56) developed a faithful mouse model of human familial GIST. Heterozygous mutant KIT^V558Δ/+ mice develop, with complete penetrance, a variably distended distal ileum caused by obstructive masses in the cecum. Histologically, the cecal neoplasms are indistinguishable from human GIST, including diffuse immunoreactivity for KIT. In addition,

patchy hyperplasia of KIT-positive cells resembling ICCs is seen in the myenteric plexus throughout the gastrointestinal tract.

Differential Diagnosis. Histologically, the tumors most closely resembling GIST are schwannoma, leiomyosarcoma, leiomyoma, and desmoid tumor. Unlike GIST, all are negative for CD117. Spindle cell GISTs need to be distinguished from inflammatory myofibroblastic tumor, inflammatory fibroid polyp, and solitary fibrous tumor, and epithelioid GIST from carcinoid tumor, glomus tumor, and intestinal clear cell sarcoma. Aside from CD117 immunoreactivity, additional distinguishing features are mentioned in the current literature (30). Establishing a firm diagnosis of GIST is so important to treatment that the demonstration of KIT or DOG1 expression is necessary in virtually all cases. In some instances, genetic analysis is needed to seek relevant mutations.

Treatment. Before the development of imatinib mesylate, the treatment of GIST consisted of resection of the primary tumor, a procedure fairly ineffective in preventing recurrence (57). GISTs were also notoriously refractory to conventional chemotherapy, with a response rate to various agents of 5 percent (58,59).

The discovery of constitutive KIT activation as the central mechanism of GIST pathogenesis suggested that blocking KIT signaling might be therapeutically effective. Indeed, imatinib mesylate (Gleevec™, Novartis Pharmaceutical, Basel, Switzerland) was found to inhibit KIT kinase activity, and currently is the frontline drug for the targeted treatment of unresectable and metastatic GISTs. Imatinib treatment achieves either a partial response or disease stability in about 80 percent of patients with metastases. Its use has resulted in a 75 to 80 percent 2-year survival rate in patients with advanced disease. While the association of *KIT* mutation to clinical outcome remains unresolved, a relationship between *KIT* genotype and response to imatinib has been established in multi-institutional clinical trials (60,61). Tumors with the most common (exon 11) mutation show the highest shrinkage rates and are associated with the most prolonged survival, whereas those with an exon 9 mutation or with wild-type KIT are less likely to respond to imatinib.

About half of the patients initially benefitting from treatment eventually develop resistance.

Table 13-3

RISK STRATIFICATION OF PRIMARY GIST BY MITOTIC INDEX, SIZE, AND SITE[a]

Tumor Parameters		Risk for Progressive Disease (%) by Location[b]			
Mitotic Index	Size	Gastric	Jejunum/Ileum	Duodenum	Rectum
≤ 5 per 50 HPF[c]	≤ 2 cm	None (0%)	None (0%)	None (0%)	None (0%)
	> 2 ≤ 5 cm	Very low (1.9%)	Low (4.3%)	Low (8.3%)	Low (8.5%)
	> 5 ≤ 10 cm	Low (3.6%)	Moderate (24%)	Insufficient data	Insufficient data
	> 10 cm	Moderate (10%)	High (52%)	High (34%)	High (57%)
> 5 per 50 HPF	< 2 cm	None[d]	High[d]	Insufficient data	High (52%)
	> 2 ≤ 5 cm	Moderate (16%)	High (73%)	High (50%)	High (54%)
	> 5 ≤ 10 cm	High (55%)	High (85%)	Insufficient data	Insufficient data
	> 10 cm	High (86%)	High (90%)	High (86%)	High (71%)

[a] Adapted from reference 18. Data based on long-term follow-up of 1,055 gastric, 629 small intestinal, 144 duodenal, and 111 rectal GISTs.
[b] Defined as metastasis or tumor-related death.
[c] HPF = high-power field.
[d] Denotes small numbers of cases.

The most common mechanism of resistance is the acquisition of second site mutations in the kinase domain, an event that poses the main challenge to salvaging affected patients who fail kinase inhibitor monotherapies (62). More recently, sunitinib (Sutent, Pfizer, New York, NY), which shows antiangiogenic effects in addition to KIT and PDGFRA inhibition, has proven efficacious in patients who are intolerant of, or refractory to, imatinib (63).

Prognosis. GIST is a frequently malignant neoplasm. Studies based upon GISTs histologically diagnosed in a single laboratory during the pre-imatinib era found the tumor-related mortality in gastric tumors to be 17 percent (31) and in small intestinal examples, 39 percent (18). The percentage of fatal outcome among patients both with and without metastatic disease and seen at a tertiary referral center is understandably higher. In one group of 200 patients followed for a median of 14 months (range, 1 to 75 months), half died of tumor, their disease-specific survival rate at 5 years being 35 percent (57).

Disease-related mortality is linked to recurrence and metastasis. For GISTs not treated with tyrosine kinase inhibitors (TKI), independent factors in determining the risk of progression

(30) or recurrence-free survival following complete resection (64) include mitotic rate in 50 high-power fields, tumor size, and anatomic location (Table 13-3). The most significant finding predictive of poor outcome is a high mitotic rate (5 or more mitoses per 50 high-power fields) (28,29,64). In different studies, tumor size either greater than 5 cm (28,29) or 10 cm or more (64), as well as small bowel location (28,29), are predictive of an unfavorable outcome. Although the presence of a mutation does not predict recurrence, the type of mutation does correlate with recurrence-free survival. Patients with *KIT* exon 11 deletion 557 or 558 do less well than patients with other *KIT* exon 11 deletions, *KIT* point mutations, or insertions (64).

Using the three parameters of mitotic rate, tumor size, and tumor location, relative risk groups have been created (18,30) that could serve to determine the need for adjuvant TKI therapy. A suggested alternative is referring to a continuous variable prognostic nomogram for recurrence-free survival (65), an approach that might offer flexibility and greater precision in identifying a risk level at which therapy would be most beneficial.

REFERENCES

1. Lecoin L, Gabella G, Le Douarin N. Origin of the c-kit-positive interstitial cells in the avian bowel. Development 1996;122:725-733.
2. Daniel EE, Posey-Daniel V. Neuromuscular structures in opossum esophagus: role of interstitial cells of Cajal. Am J Physiol 1984;246(Pt 1):G305-315.
3. Sanders KM, Ordog T, Koh SD, Torihashi S, Ward SM. Development and plasticity of interstitial cells of Cajal. Neurogastroenterol Motil 1999;11:311-338.
4. Burns AJ, Lomax AE, Torihashi S, Sanders KM, SM. W. Interstitial cells of Cajal mediate inhibitory neurotransmission in the stomach. Proc Nat Acad Sci U S A 1996;93:12008-12013.
5. Ward SM, Beckett EA, Wang X, Baker F, Khoyi M, Sanders KM. Interstitial cells of Cajal mediate cholinergic neurotransmission from enteric motor neurons. J Neurosci 2000;20:1393-1403.
6. Ward SM, Burns AJ, Torihashi S, Harney SC, Sanders KM. Impaired development of interstitial cells and intestinal electrical rhythmicity in steel mutants. Am J Physiol 1995;269(Pt 1):C1577-1585.
7. Huizinga JD, Thuneberg L, Kluppel M, Malysz J, Mikkelsen HB, Bernstein A. W/kit gene required for interstitial cells of Cajal and for intestinal pacemaker activity. Nature 1995;373:347-349.
8. Rubin BP. Gastrointestinal stromal tumours: an update. Histopathology 2006;48:83-96.
9. Mazur MT, Clark HB. Gastric stromal tumors. Reappraisal of histogenesis. Am J Surg Pathol 1983;7:507-519.
10. Miettinen M. Gastrointestinal stromal tumors. An immunohistochemical study of cellular differentiation. Am J Clin Pathol 1988;89:601-610.
11. Herrera GA, Pinto de Moraes H, Grizzle WE, Han SG. Malignant small bowel neoplasm of enteric plexus derivation (plexosarcoma). Light and electron microscopic study confirming the origin of the neoplasm. Dig Dis Sci 1984;29:275-284.
12. Lauwers GY, Erlandson RA, Casper ES, Brennan MF, Woodruff JM. Gastrointestinal autonomic nerve tumors. A clinicopathological, immunohistochemical, and ultrastructural study of 12 cases. Am J Surg Pathol 1993;17:887-897.
13. Walker P, Dvorak AM. Gastrointestinal autonomic nerve (GAN) tumor. Ultrastructural evidence for a newly recognized entity. Arch Pathol Lab Med 1986;110:309-316.
14. Hirota S, Isozaki K, Moriyama Y, et al. Gain-of-function mutations of c-kit in human gastrointestinal stromal tumors. Science 1998;279:577-580.
15. Dei Tos AP. The reappraisal of gastrointestinal stromal tumors: from Stout to the KIT revolution. Virchows Arch 2003;442:421-428.
16. Bussolati G. Of GISTS and EGISTS, ICCS and ICS. Virchows Arch 2005;447:907-908.
17. Parfitt JR, Streutker CJ, Riddell RH, Driman DK. Gastrointestinal stromal tumors: a contemporary review. Pathol Res Pract 2006;202:837-847.
18. Miettinen M, Lasota J. Gastrointestinal stromal tumors: pathology and prognosis at different sites. Semin Diagn Pathol 2006;23:70-83.
19. Prakash S, Sarran L, Socci N, et al. Gastrointestinal stromal tumors in children and young adults: a clinicopathologic, molecular, and genomic study of 15 cases and review of the literature. J Pediatr Hematol Oncol 2005;27:179-187.
20. Miettinen M, Lasota J, Sobin LH. Gastrointestinal stromal tumors of the stomach in children and young adults: A clinicopathologic, immunohistochemical, and molecular genetic study of 44 cases with long-term follow-up and review of the literature. Am J Surg Pathol 2005;29:1373-1381.
21. Agaram NP, Laquaglia MP, Ustun B, et al. Molecular characterization of pediatric gastrointestinal stromal tumors. Clin Cancer Res 2008;14:3204-3215.
22. Nilsson B, Bumming P, Meis-Kindblom JM, et al. Gastrointestinal stromal tumors: the incidence, prevalence, clinical course, and prognostication in the preimatinib mesylate era—a population-based study in western sweden. Cancer 2005;103:821-829.
23. Miettinen M, Fetsch JF, Sobin LH, Lasota J. Gastrointestinal stromal tumors in patients with neurofibromatosis 1: a clinicopathologic and molecular genetic study of 45 cases. Am J Surg Pathol 2006;30:90-96.
24. Carney JA, Sheps SG, Go VL, Gordon H. The triad of gastric leiomyosarcoma, functioning extraadrenal paraganglioma and pulmonary chondroma. N Engl J Med 1977;296:1517-1518.
25. Antonescu CR. Gastrointestinal stromal tumor (GIST) pathogenesis, familial GIST, and animal models. Semin Diagn Pathol 2006;23:63-69.
26. Nishida T, Hirota S, Taniguchi M, et al. Familial gastrointestinal stromal tumours with germline mutation of the KIT gene. Nat Genet 1998;19:323-324.
27. Carney JA, Stratakis CA. Familial paraganglioma and gastric stromal sarcoma: a new syndrome distinct from the Carney triad. Am J Med Genet 2002;108:132-139.
28. Miettinen M, Makhlouf H, Sobin LH, Lasota J. Gastrointestinal stromal tumors of the jejunum and ileum: A clinicopathologic, immunohistochemical, and molecular genetic study of 906 cases before imatinib with long-term follow-up. Am J Surg Pathol 2006;30:477-489.
29. Fletcher CD, Berman JJ, Corless C, et al. Diagnosis of gastrointestinal stromal tumors: A consensus approach. Hum Pathol 2002;33:459-465.

30. Liegl B, Hornick JL, Lazar AJ. Contemporary pathology of gastrointestinal stromal tumors. Hematol Oncol Clin North Am 2009;23:49-68, vii-viii.

31. Miettinen M, Sobin LH, Lasota J. Gastrointestinal stromal tumors of the stomach: A clinicopathologic, immunohistochemical, and molecular genetic study of 1765 cases with long-term follow-up. Am J Surg Pathol 2005;29:52-68.

32. Min KW. Small intestinal stromal tumors with skeinoid fibers. Clinicopathological, immunohistochemical, and ultrastructural investigations. Am J Surg Pathol 1992;16:145-155.

33. Kindblom LG, Remotti HE, Aldenborg F, Meis-Kindblom JM. Gastrointestinal pacemaker cell tumor (GIPACT): gastrointestinal stromal tumors show phenotypic characteristics of the interstitial cells of Cajal. Am J Pathol 1998;152:1259-1269.

34. Sarlomo-Rikala M, Kovatich AJ, Barusevicius A, Miettinen M. CD117: a sensitive marker for gastrointestinal stromal tumors that is more specific than CD34. Mod Pathol 1998;11:728-734.

35. Miettinen MM, Sarlomo-Rikala M, Kovatich AJ, Lasota J. Calponin and h-caldesmon in soft tissue tumors: consistent h-caldesmon immunoreactivity in gastrointestinal stromal tumors indicates traits of smooth muscle differentiation. Mod Pathol 1999;12:756-762.

36. Medeiros F, Corless CL, Duensing A, et al. Kit-negative gastrointestinal stromal tumors: proof of concept and therapeutic implications. Am J Surg Pathol 2004;28:889-894.

37. Gomez-Pinilla PJ, Gibbons SJ, Bardsley MR, et al. Ano1 is a selective marker of interstitial cells of Cajal in the human and mouse gastrointestinal tract. Am J Physiol Gastrointest Liver Physiol 2009;296:G1370-1381.

38. Liegl B, Hornick JL, Corless CL, Fletcher CD. Monoclonal antibody DOG1.1 shows higher sensitivity than kit in the diagnosis of gastrointestinal stromal tumors, including unusual subtypes. Am J Surg Pathol 2009;33:437-446.

39. Espinosa I, Lee CH, Kim MK, et al. A novel monoclonal antibody against DOG1 is a sensitive and specific marker for gastrointestinal stromal tumors. Am J Surg Pathol 2008;32:210-218.

40. West RB, Corless CL, Chen X, et al. The novel marker, DOG1, is expressed ubiquitously in gastrointestinal stromal tumors irrespective of KIT or PDGFRA mutation status. Am J Pathol 2004;165:107-113.

41. Rumessen JJ, Mikkelsen HB, Qvortrup K, Thuneberg L. Ultrastructure of interstitial cells of Cajal in circular muscle of human small intestine. Gastroenterology 1993;104:343-350.

42. Heinrich MC, Corless CL, Duensing A, et al. PDGFRA activating mutations in gastrointestinal stromal tumors. Science 2003;299:708-710.

43. Besmer P, Murphy JE, George PC, et al. A new acute transforming feline retrovirus and relationship of its oncogene v-kit with the protein kinase gene family. Nature 1986;320:415-421.

44. Maeda H, Yamagata A, Nishikawa S, et al. Requirement of c-kit for development of intestinal pacemaker system. Development 1992;116:369-375.

45. Torihashi S, Ward SM, Nishikawa S, Nishi K, Kobayashi S, Sanders KM. C-kit-dependent development of interstitial cells and electrical activity in the murine gastrointestinal tract. Cell Tissue Res 1995;280:97-111.

46. Tian Q, Frierson HF Jr, Krystal GW, Moskaluk CA. Activating c-kit gene mutations in human germ cell tumors. Am J Pathol 1999;154:1643-1647.

47. Nagata H, Worobec AS, Oh CK, et al. Identification of a point mutation in the catalytic domain of the protooncogene c-kit in peripheral blood mononuclear cells of patients who have mastocytosis with an associated hematologic disorder. Proc Natl Acad Sci U S A 1995;92:10560-10564

48. Gari M, Goodeve A, Wilson G, et al. C-kit proto-oncogene exon 8 in-frame deletion plus insertion mutations in acute myeloid leukaemia. Br J Haematol 1999;105:894-900.

49. Willmore-Payne C, Holden JA, Tripp S, Layfield LJ. Human malignant melanoma: detection of BRAF- and c-kit-activating mutations by high-resolution amplicon melting analysis. Hum Pathol 2005;36:486-493.

50. Rubin BP, Singer S, Tsao C, et al. KIT activation is a ubiquitous feature of gastrointestinal stromal tumors. Cancer Res 2001;61:8118-8121.

51. Wardelmann E, Hrychyk A, Merkelbach-Bruse S, et al. Association of platelet-derived growth factor receptor alpha mutations with gastric primary site and epithelioid or mixed cell morphology in gastrointestinal stromal tumors. J Mol Diagn 2004;6:197-204.

52. Antonescu CR, Sommer G, Sarran L, et al. Association of KIT exon 9 mutations with non-gastric primary site and aggressive behavior: Kit mutation analysis and clinical correlates of 120 gastrointestinal stromal tumors. Clin Cancer Res 2003;9:3329-3337.

53. Lasota J, Corless CL, Heinrich MC, et al. Clinicopathologic profile of gastrointestinal stromal tumors (GISTs) with primary KIT exon 13 or exon 17 mutations: a multicenter study on 54 cases. Mod Pathol 2008;21:476-484.

54. Hirota S, Ohashi A, Nishida T, et al. Gain-of-function mutations of platelet-derived growth factor receptor alpha gene in gastrointestinal stromal tumors. Gastroenterology 2003;125:660-667.

55. Lasota J, Dansonka-Mieszkowska A, Sobin LH, et al. A great majority of GISTS with PDGFRA mutations represent gastric tumors of low or no malignant potential. Lab Invest 2004;84:874-883.

56. Sommer G, Agosti V, Ehlers I, et al. Gastrointestinal stromal tumors in a mouse model by targeted mutation of the KIT receptor tyrosine kinase. Proc Nat Acad Sci U S A 2003;100:6706-6711.

57. DeMatteo RP, Lewis JJ, Leung D, et al. Two hundred gastrointestinal stromal tumors: recurrence patterns and prognostic factors for survival. Ann Surg 2000;231:51-58.

58. Demetri GD. Targeting c-kit mutations in solid tumors: scientific rationale and novel therapeutic options. Semin Oncol 2001;28(Suppl 17):19-26.

59. Edmonson JH, Ryan LM, Blum RH, et al. Randomized comparison of doxorubicin alone versus ifosfamide plus doxorubicin or mitomycin, doxorubicin, and cisplatin against advanced soft tissue sarcomas. J Clin Oncol 1993;11:1269-1275.

60. Heinrich MC, Corless CL, Demetri GD, et al. Kinase mutations and imatinib response in patients with metastatic gastrointestinal stromal tumor. J Clin Oncol 2003;21:4342-4349.

61. Debiec-Rychter M, Dumez H, Judson I, et al. Use of C-KIT/PDGFRA mutational analysis to predict the clinical response to imatinib in patients with advanced gastrointestinal stromal tumours entered on phase I and II studies of the EORTC Soft Tissue and Bone Sarcoma Group. Eur J Cancer 2004;40:689-695.

62. Antonescu CR, Besmer P, Guo T, et al. Acquired resistance to imatinib in gastrointestinal stromal tumor occurs through secondary gene mutation. Clin Cancer Res 2005;11:4182-4190.

63. Demetri G, Desai J, Flecther JA, et al. SU11248, a multi-targeted tyrosine kinase inhibitor, can overcome imatinib (IM) resistance caused by diverse genomic mechanisms in patients (pts) with metastatic gastrointestinal stromal tumor (GIST). J Clin Oncol 2004;22:3301.

64. Dematteo RP, Gold JS, Saran L, et al. Tumor mitotic rate, size, and location independently predict recurrence after resection of primary gastrointestinal stromal tumor (GIST). Cancer 2008;112:608-615.

65. Gold JS, Gonen M, Gutierrez A, et al. Development and validation of a prognostic nomogram for recurrence-free survival after complete surgical resection of localised primary gastrointestinal stromal tumour: a retrospective analysis. Lancet Oncol 2009;10:1045-1052.

66. Williams DE, Eisenman J, Baird A, et al. Identification of a ligand for the c-kit proto-oncogene. Cell 1990;63:167-174.

67. Chompret A, Kannengiesser C, Barrois M, et al. PDGFRA germline mutation in a family with multiple cases of gastrointestinal stromal tumor. Gastroenterology 2004;126:318-321.

68. de Raedt T, Cools J, Debiec-Rychter M, et al. Intestinal neurofibromatosis is a subtype of familial GIST and results from a dominant activating mutation in PDGFRA. Gastroenterology 2006;131:1907-1912.

69. Andersson J, Sihto H, Meis-Kindblom JM, Joensuu H, Nupponen N, Kindblom LG. NF1-associated gastrointestinal stromal tumors have unique clinical, phenotypic, and genotypic characteristics. Am J Surg Pathol 2005;29:1170-1176.

70. Takazawa Y, Sakurai S, Sakuma Y, et al. Gastrointestinal stromal tumors of neurofibromatosis type I (von Recklinghausen's disease). Am J Surg Pathol 2005;29:755-763.

71. Yantiss RK, Rosenberg AE, Sarran L, Besmer P, Antonescu CR. Multiple gastrointestinal stromal tumors in type I neurofibromatosis: a pathologic and molecular study. Mod Pathol 2005;18:475-484.

72. Maertens O, Prenen H, Debiec-Rychter M, et al. Molecular pathogenesis of multiple gastrointestinal stromal tumors in NF1 patients. Hum Mol Genet 2006;15:1015-1023.

73. Mussi C, Schildhaus HU, Gronchi A, Wardelmann E, Hohenberger P. Therapeutic consequences from molecular biology for gastrointestinal stromal tumor patients affected by neurofibromatosis type 1. Clin Cancer Res 2008;14:4550-4555.

74. Carney JA. Gastric stromal sarcoma, pulmonary chondroma, and extra-adrenal paraganglioma (Carney Triad): natural history, adrenocortical component, and possible familial occurrence. Mayo Clin Proc 1999;74:543-552.

75. Zhang L, Smyrk TC, Young WF Jr, Stratakis CA, Carney JA. Gastric stromal tumors in Carney triad are different clinically, pathologically, and behaviorally from sporadic gastric gastrointestinal stromal tumors: findings in 104 cases. Am J Surg Pathol 2010;34:53-64.

76. McWhinney SR, Pasini B, Stratakis CA. Familial gastrointestinal stromal tumors and germ-line mutations. N Engl J Med 2007;357:1054-1056.

77. Pasini B, McWhinney SR, Bei T, et al. Clinical and molecular genetics of patients with the Carney-Stratakis syndrome and germline mutations of the genes coding for the succinate dehydrogenase subunits SDHB, SDHC, and SDHD. Eur J Hum Genet 2008;16:79-88.

14 SECONDARY NEOPLASIA

This chapter deals primarily with the involvement of peripheral nerves by neoplasms other than primary ones. The spectrum of lesions is broad, ranging from carcinoma, sarcoma, and melanoma to hematopoietic tumors. The mechanism underlying nerve involvement varies from direct extension of nearby neoplasms to metastasis from a remote primary. Also included is a discussion of metastasis to nerve sheath tumors.

METASTASES AND DIRECT EXTENSION OF NEOPLASMS TO NERVE

Involvement of a nerve occurs by direct extension from a nearby tumor or by metastasis from a distant primary. A tumor may involve one or more compartments of a nerve.

Since the early descriptions of nerve involvement by infiltrating or metastatic neoplasms (1,2), involvement by carcinoma, sarcoma, neurotropic melanoma, and leukemia-lymphoma has become increasingly recognized. Depending in large part upon the nature of the tumor, the patterns of nerve involvement vary, from simple compression or encompassment of an otherwise intact nerve, infiltration of epineurial tissue, and spread within the potential epineurial-perineurial space, to involvement of perineurium or endoneurium (3). Small nerves are commonly involved, while large nerves, such as the sciatic, are not.

The potential epineurial-perineurial space is the main conduit for secondary spread of malignant tumors within peripheral nerve. It is the microanatomic region most often involved when invasion of small nerves is noted in surgical specimens. Although only a potential space, it is readily accessed by infiltrating tumor cells because of the loose attachment of perineurium to surrounding epineurium. Although the space was once thought to be lymphatic (4), no lining cells are demonstrable. This potential space has been shown to communicate with the subarachnoid space in experiments involving the injection of dyes (5,6) and local anesthetics (7). Malignant cells, notably carcinoma cells, may also pass into endoneurium by infiltrating the perivascular sleeve of the transperineurial arterial system whereby arterioles link with the endoneurial capillary plexus (8). It is by this route that neoplastic cells, particularly lymphoma-leukemia cells, gain direct access to endoneurium; carcinoma and sarcoma far less often involve endoneurium.

Carcinoma

General Features. *Carcinomas* are the most common neoplasms secondarily involving nerve. In most instances, neural involvement is by direct extension into perineurium or the potential space surrounding it. Although most commonly observed in association with adenocarcinoma of the prostate, adenoid cystic carcinoma of salivary glands (fig. 14-1), and ductal carcinoma of the breast, perineurial invasion may be seen with almost any type of carcinoma (9). One study of head and neck carcinomas (10) found the incidence of perineurial invasion by squamous carcinoma of the skin, lip, and oral mucosa was as high as that of adenoid cystic carcinoma. Particularly detailed descriptions of tumor spread are found in the literature (9–15).

Having gained access to the potential epineurial-perineurial space, tumors may track proximal or distal, i.e., toward or away from the central nervous system (CNS). A study of 83 squamous cell carcinomas of the head and neck associated with neural invasion (11) found the size of the primary tumor to be at least 2.5 cm, and its extent of perineurial spread to be a distance of 1 cm or less. Growth and spread of tumor within the space, whether proximal, distal, or both, are continuous and unassociated with "skip areas." Extensive proximal spread is of particular clinical importance in that it brings the tumor within reach of the CNS, thus setting the stage for leptomeningeal spread (*meningeal carcinomatosis*) (10,16).

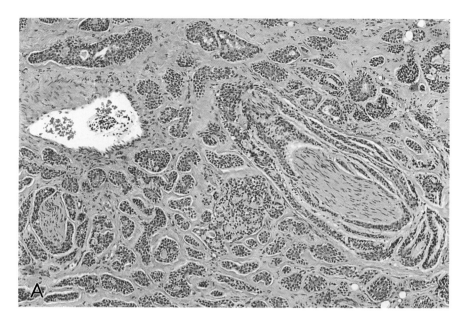

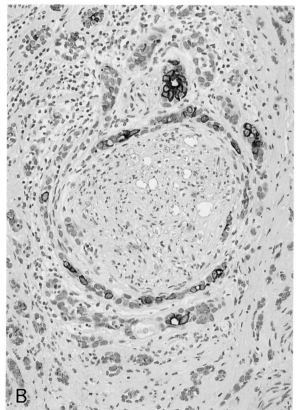

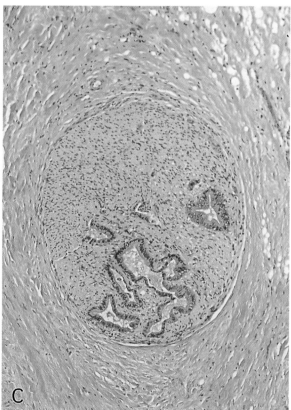

Figure 14-1

ADENOID CYSTIC CARCINOMA INVOLVING PERIPHERAL NERVE

Invasion of the nerve was through the potential epineurial-perineurial space, here taking the form of perifascicular rings of tumor (A,B), a feature of secondary tumor involvement and a conspicuous feature of this neoplasm. Focal endoneurial spread is most apparent with a cytokeratin stain (B). Cholangiocarcinoma extends within the endoneurium (C).

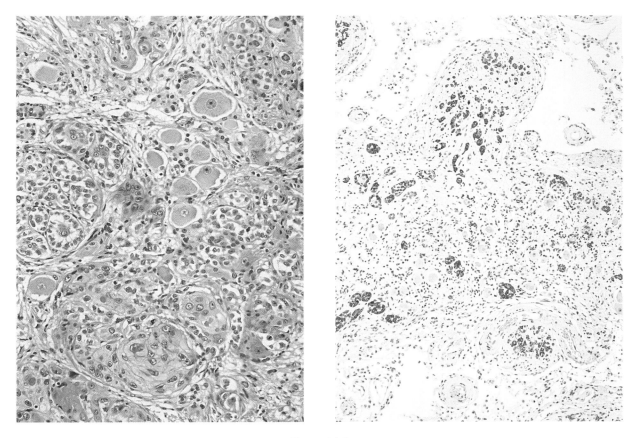

Figure 14-2

CARCINOMA INVOLVING SENSORY GANGLION

The carcinoma (left) extends into an exiting nerve fascicle and immunostains for keratin (right).

Carcinomas uncommonly involve the endoneurium (9,10,15,17). Possible routes of endoneurial invasion include direct extension through perineurium and growth of tumor within perivascular sleeves of the transperineurial arteriolar system (8). Tumoral compression of such vessels may underlie the occasional finding of associated nerve necrosis (13). Although the endoneurium of peripheral nerves is infrequently involved by carcinoma (fig. 14-1), sensory ganglia are less resistant (fig. 14-2) (18). Their susceptibility to metastasis is attributed to their fenestrated vasculature, a feature that also underlies the lack of a blood-ganglion barrier in ganglia.

Clinical Features. Carcinomatous involvement of nerves may or may not be clinically apparent. Subjective complaints of burning, stinging, and shooting pain in a region known to be affected by a primary tumor are highly suggestive of neoplastic involvement of nerve

(10). Numbness in the distribution of a nerve is even more significant (10). Sensory symptoms may precede the recognition of a primary tumor by months. Conversely, the relatively asymptomatic persistence of carcinoma within nerves has been reported to occur years after removal of the primary tumor (10).

Differential Diagnosis. Perineurial or endoneurial nerve involvement by benign proliferative epithelial processes has also been reported. Examples include florid fibrocystic disease of breast (19), benign prostatic hypertrophy (20), vasitis nodosa (21), and benign gallbladder lesions (22). Glandular inclusions of nerve within normal tissues are also seen on occasion, such as in prostate gland (20) or pancreas (23). The process may occur spontaneously or, as in the case of vasitis nodosa (fig. 14-3), postoperatively when reactive epithelial cells presumably gain access to the nerve through the traumatically

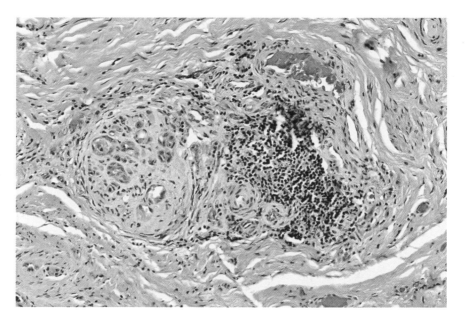

Figure 14-3

BENIGN INTRANEURAL GLANDULAR INCLUSIONS

Glandular inclusions of vasitis nodosa. (Courtesy of Dr. P. Johnson, Tucson, AZ.)

disrupted perineurial sheath. Nerves affected by these processes are usually small.

Sarcoma

Not surprisingly, *sarcomas* secondarily affecting peripheral nerve most often originate in surrounding soft tissues. The frequency and mechanism of nerve involvement were addressed by Barber et al. (3) in a study of 98 extremities amputated for soft tissue sarcoma. Thirty-nine percent were found to grossly affect peripheral nerve. The manner in which they did so ranged from simple displacement, to firm adherence, encasement without invasion, and in 10 percent of cases, presumed nerve invasion based on the presence of localized or diffuse nerve enlargement. Histologic confirmation of neural invasion was apparent in 11 percent of histologically studied cases, and invasion was limited to the epineurium in over half. No correlation could be made with specific symptoms such as pain, numbness, weakness, palsy, and paresthesias. Of the 50 patients with such complaints, symptoms could be explained on the basis of gross and microscopic findings in only 46 percent; in 27 percent of cases with histologically documented neural invasion, there were no corresponding neurologic symptoms.

Invasion of the fascicles of large peripheral nerves by soft tissue sarcoma is generally associated with high-grade tumors. In most in-

stances, they destroy the epineurium and enter the epineurial-perineurial space. Endoneurial involvement is far less common (fig. 14-4). Sarcomas may extend a great distance within the epineurial-perineurial space. Barber et al. (3) described a high-grade fibrosarcoma affecting the median nerve, which extended from the level of the wrist to within 2.5 cm of the brachial plexus. We observed a similar remarkable case (fig. 14-5), an angiosarcoma presenting in the rectum, which extended within the epineurial-perineurial space of small nerves into the right sciatic nerve above the level of the sciatic foramen, descended along the sciatic nerve in the buttock and thigh for a distance of 25 cm, and continued within the tibial nerve to a point 2 cm above the ankle. As a result, both nerves were markedly circumferentially enlarged. There was also limited invasion of epineurium and perineurium (fig. 14-5). In the few examples of extensive transneural spread we have studied, all nerve compartments, including endoneurium, were to some degree involved by sarcoma. Secondary involvement of nerve by high-grade sarcoma may also result in hemorrhage and necrosis of nerve. On rare occasion, the result is focal, near-total destruction of a major nerve and profound functional deficit.

Sarcomas primary of the epineurium are rare. We have observed an example of clear cell sarcoma of the sciatic nerve grossly resembling

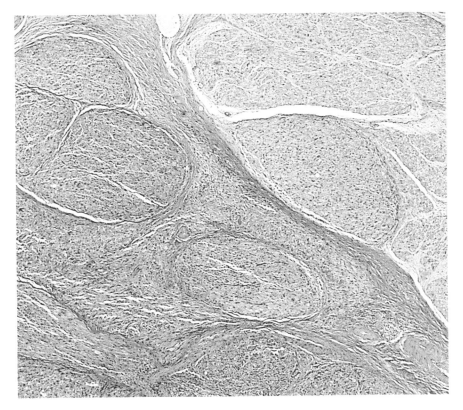

Figure 14-4

SARCOMA WITH PRIMARILY EPINEURIAL INVOLVEMENT

Involvement of the epineurium is more common from a surrounding soft tissue tumor than a primary process. This mode of secondary involvement is illustrated by a leiomyosarcoma of the pelvis in a 54-year-old female, which additionally extended into the endoneurium.

a malignant peripheral nerve sheath tumor (MPNST), but growing exclusively in an extrafascicular manner (fig. 14-6).

Synovial sarcomas arising in surrounding soft tissues may invade nerve, but this is of little diagnostic challenge compared to synovial sarcomas arising within epineurium. The latter is discussed at the length in chapter 11.

Neurotropic Melanoma

Definition and General Features. Of neoplasms secondarily involving nerves, the histologically most diagnostically challenging is *neurotropic melanoma*, a form of desmoplastic melanoma described in 1979 by Reed and Leonard (24) that has "neuroid" features and a propensity to involve nerves. Their observations have been corroborated by several investigators in a review of 46 cases (25). Like desmoplastic melanomas, the lesions show a predilection for the head and neck, are mostly cutaneous in origin, and arise either from precursor melanocytic lesions or de novo. A few present in exposed mucosal surfaces (26). The main challenges confronting pathologists are the deceptively innocent appearance of the tumor in its initial growth phase, the similarities to other spindle cell tumors of skin, and distinguishing tumors that involve nerve from MPNST.

Clinical Features. Neurotropic melanomas almost always occur in sun-exposed skin of older, light-complexioned adults (24). In Mack and Gomez's review of 46 neurotropic melanomas (25), the mean patient age was 60 years (range, 28 to 86 years); 68 percent were men. The head and neck region was involved by 78 percent of the tumors, including face, lip, neck, and ear. Facial sites included the cheeks, temples, chin, forehead, and nose. Yet other head and neck sites have been reported by others. The remainder of tumors involved the trunk and extremities; one arose in the vulva. Over 50 percent of the patients had a pigmented lesion, most often lentigo maligna.

Other reported clinical presentations include a gradually enlarging black lesion; an indurated plaque, lump, or nodule found either alone or developing in a long-standing nevus; and cranial neuropathy. It is possible that some persons diagnosed with xeroderma pigmentosum have instead neurotropic melanoma (see chapter 12) (27,28).

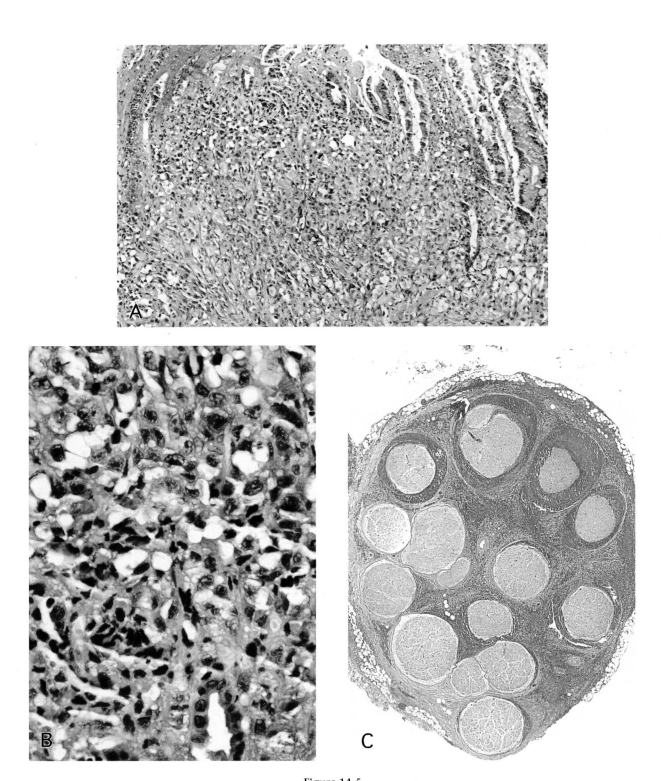

Figure 14-5

ANGIOSARCOMA INVOLVING NERVE

This example arising in the rectal wall (A,B) of an 34-year-old male showed dramatic distal extension within the potential epineurial-perineurial space of the sciatic and upper portion of the tibial nerves (C), where it ringed nerve fascicles (D) and invaded the perineurium (E). The patient died shortly after resection of the tumor.

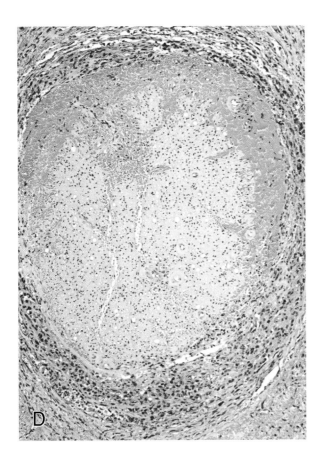
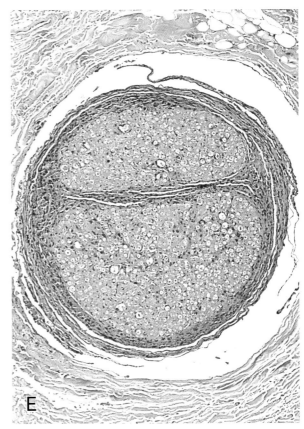

Figure 14-5, continued

Typically, neurotropic melanoma is difficult to diagnose, clinically and histologically, because of inconsistent pigmentation, ill-defined margins, frequent lack of an intraepithelial melanocytic lesion, and a subepithelial spindle cell growth pattern common to various spindle cell lesions of skin. Given their frequent location in the head and neck, where for cosmetic considerations, therapy is likely conservative, neurotropic melanomas are often inadequately treated. For these various reasons, the tumors show a propensity to recur. Reported rates of local recurrence range from 22 to 77 percent (29). Most lesions reappear before 3 years (29) and are amelanotic and often multifocal (24). Recurrent tumors invade local tissues, including nerves, along which they may track to produce neuropathy. Head and neck examples may extend directly to the CNS (24). Nerves most commonly affected include the trigeminal and radial (30). There is evidence suggesting that neurotropic melanomas have a higher rate of recurrence than ordinary desmoplastic melanomas. In a detailed study comparing 12 nerve-centered and 33 ordinary desmoplastic melanomas, respective recurrence rates were 91 and 42 percent (26). In addition to recurring locally, neurotropic tumors may metastasize to regional lymph nodes and to distant sites, such as lung, brain, liver, and bone. Mortality varies. Reported survival rates range from 34 to 89 percent (mean, 60 percent) (29). In one review (25), 30 percent of patients were dead of, and 40 percent alive with, disease. Tumor-related deaths occurred between 15 months and 10 years after diagnosis.

Microscopic Findings. The morphologic features of neurotropic melanoma include strands, fascicles, or nodules of variably atypical, amelanotic spindle cells that form a dermal and sometimes subcutaneous infiltrate. Lesions early in development show an increased number of spindle cells in the upper dermis,

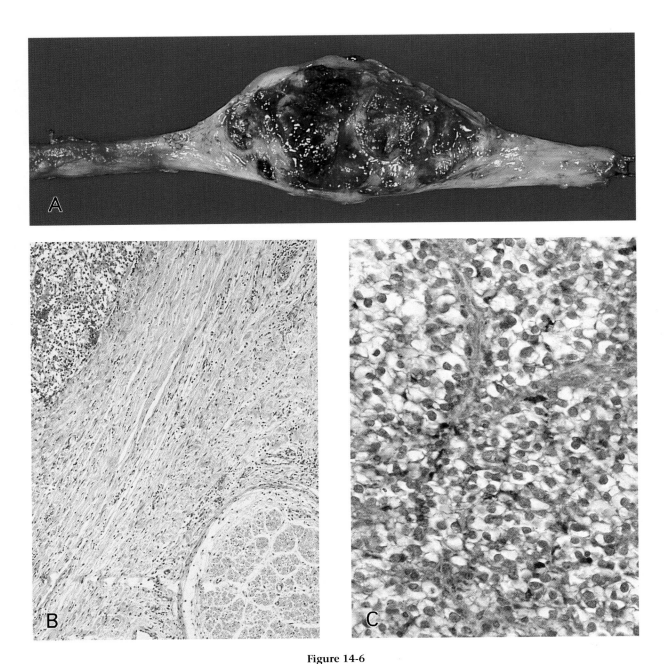

Figure 14-6

SARCOMA WITHIN EPINEURIUM

A clear cell sarcoma arose in the sciatic nerve of a 13-year-old female. Although the tumor grossly resembled MPNST (A), its pattern of growth was almost entirely extrafascicular (B). The histology and HMB45 immunoreactivity were typical of clear cell sarcoma (C). The lesion subsequently metastasized to an adrenal gland.

with the cells arrayed in aligned, gently curved and distinct fascicles (24). Overlying epidermis or mucosal epithelium may contain atypical melanocytes. These are single or aggregated in small nests at the dermo-epidermal junction or above it (31). Upper dermal fascicles of spindle cells often blend with basal portions of the epidermis (24). When extensive, spindle cells involve the entire thickness of the dermis, and extend to or deeply into the subcutaneous fat (31). In the mid-dermis, infiltrates of spindle cells are often dense and variably collagenized (fig. 14-7A,B). Interlaced, the cells often assume a vaguely storiform arrangement (fig. 14-7B). Deeper still, the spindle cells take the form of dispersed, loose fascicles. They appear to be randomly distributed, but on closer inspection, often contact, enwrap (fig. 14-7C,D), and invade the endoneurium of nerves (fig. 14-7D–H) (31). The enwrapment, sometimes of near uniform thickness and circumferential, resembles a perifascicular ring. Invaded nerves are variably hypercellular and enlarged, but retain their overall shape. The tumor cells may also form nodules, notably in recurrences.

The spindle cells comprising neurotropic melanoma have moderate to abundant, faintly eosinophilic, afibrillar cytoplasm (fig. 14-7A). The cell margins are often ill-defined. The nuclei are elongated, of irregular width, and exhibit either uniformly dense or marginated chromatin (fig. 14-7A). Given their hyperchromasia and large nuclear size, the tumor cells are readily distinguishable from normal Schwann cells (fig. 14-7D). Reed and Leonard (24) described a case in which the tumor cells had nevoid cell features. Epithelioid tumor cells are occasionally seen, and may be conspicuous in many metastases.

Since most neurotropic melanomas are amelanotic, the Fontana-Masson stain used to confirm the presence of melanin is negative (32,33).

Immunohistochemical Findings. Usually, but not invariably, the tumor cells of neurotropic melanoma are immunoreactive for S-100 protein (fig. 14-7E,G) (29,34). Unlike in cutaneous melanomas, HMB45 reactivity is infrequent and focal; it is present in the junctional component or in epithelioid tumor cells, usually in the superficial papillary dermis (29). In questionable cases, proof of endoneurial involvement by tumor can be provided by staining for S-100 and neurofilament proteins (fig. 14-7G,H).

Ultrastructural Findings. In their summary of reported ultrastructural findings in desmoplastic neurotropic melanomas, Carlson et al. (29) described long entwining processes, intermediate-type junctions, and some basal lamina. Such features can be found in both Schwann cells and melanocytes, although the presence of basal lamina is uncommon in the latter. In some reports melanosomes or putative melanosomes were said to be present, but none were of stage 2

or 3. Also infrequently mentioned were features suggestive of myofibroblastic differentiation, such as subplasmalemmal dense bodies (35). In one case, long-spacing collagen was identified in both the primary tumor and in lymph node metastases (29). Overall, the ultrastructural findings suggest a tumor with overlapping melanocytic and Schwann cell features (29).

Differential Diagnosis. In early or evolving neurotropic melanoma, the dermal pattern may be deceptively bland and mistaken for neurofibroma, blue nevus, or reactive fibroplasia (24). Dermal neurofibromas feature diffuse rather than fascicular growth, and their nuclei are smaller than those of neurotropic melanoma. Reactive fibroplasia is not immunoreactive for S-100 protein. Although blue nevi also exhibit features of neurotropism, desmoplasia, and fasciculation, they are usually pigmented and show prominent regional variation in patterns (24). It has been suggested that some neurotropic melanomas of the lower lip are mistaken for spindle cell carcinoma (24), a distinction readily settled by immunostaining for keratins and S-100 protein.

The closest histologic simulator of neurotropic melanoma, especially those with unequivocal cranial nerve involvement, is conventional MPNST. In the past, some neurotropic melanomas of cranial nerves were mistaken for MPNST (30,36). The distinction is important since, although both tumors are malignant, neurotropic melanoma is generally associated with a more prolonged disease course and better survival. The pathologist is guided by the many differences between these entities, both in clinical presentation and histologic findings. Neurotropic melanomas are often associated with an overlying, longstanding pigmented skin lesion. In contrast to neurotropic melanoma, MPNST almost always arises at sites distant from the termination of the affected nerve. Furthermore, MPNSTs show no predilection for light-complexioned individuals and may develop postirradiation, an association not reported for neurotropic melanoma. The appearance of the cells of the two tumors differs. Those of MPNST have faintly eosinophilic cytoplasm, elongated nuclei with uniform shapes that gracefully taper to nonpointed ends, and most often contain stippled chromatin. Spindle neurotropic

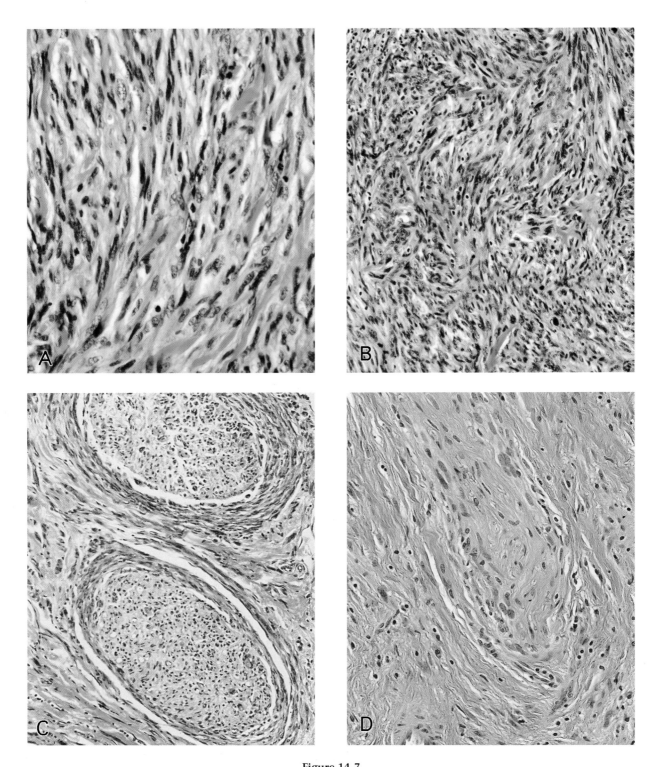

Figure 14-7

NEUROTROPIC MELANOMA

A dense collection of spindle neurotropic melanoma cells are embedded in a variably collagenized stroma (A) and at lower magnification have a storiform arrangement (B). Tumor involvement of nerves is evidenced by perifascicular ringing (C) and endoneurial spread (D).

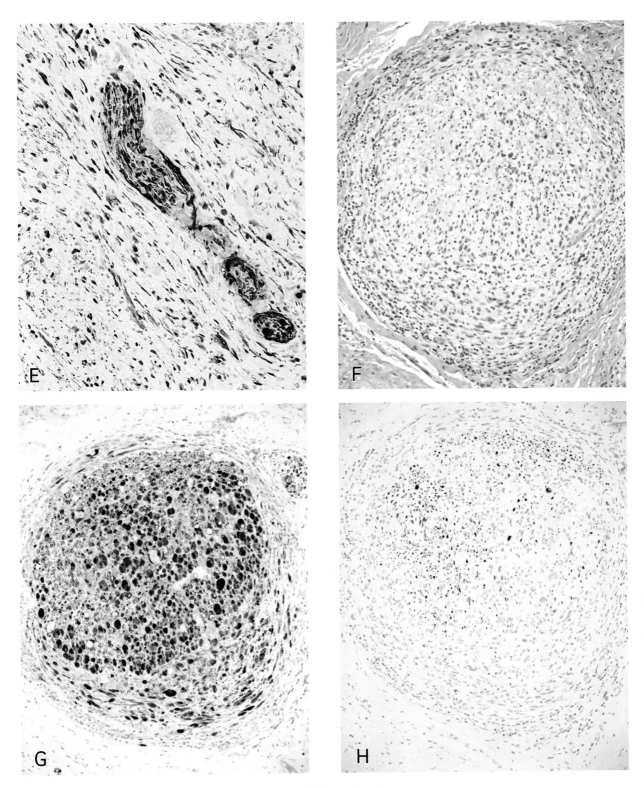

Figure 14-7, continued

The extent of tumor infiltration is clearly evident in material stained for S-100 protein (E). Endoneurial spread leads to enlargement of nerve fascicles (F), confirmed by sections stained for S-100 protein (G) and neurofilament (H).

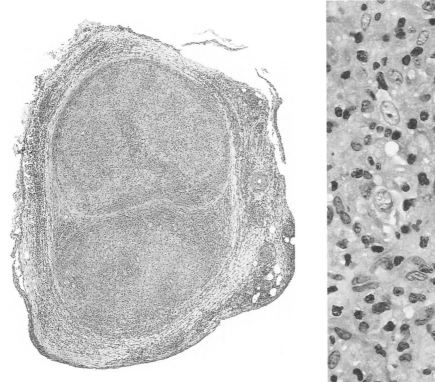 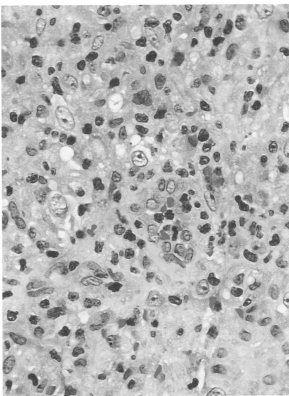

Figure 14-8

LYMPHOMA INVOLVING NERVE

Nerve roots (left) and ganglia are most often involved. Lymphoma infiltrates all compartments of these structures (right).

melanoma cells possess denser cytoplasm, longer, often thinner and more pointed nuclei, and often dense chromatin. It is uncommon to encounter an MPNST confined to a nerve and lacking extrafascicular extension. Early-phase MPNSTs spread within endoneurium and then breach perineurium to involve epineurium and surrounding soft tissues. In numerous studies of MPNST, including our series of cranial nerve tumors (37), we have not seen an example tracking as a sleeve along perineurium to form what, in cross section, appear as perifascicular rings, such as are found in neurotropic melanoma. Since both conventional MPNST and most neurotropic melanomas are amelanotic, the Fontana-Masson stain for melanoma is useless in their distinction. However, most MPNSTs show only patchy or no immunoreactivity for S-100 protein, while neurotropic melanomas typically show diffuse positivity.

Invasion of a peripheral nerve by a soft tissue sarcoma usually represents direct extension from a nearby, sizable, high-grade tumor. Thus, it is not readily mistaken for a tumor of cutaneous origin, and neurotropic melanomas are rarely larger than 2 to 3 cm. Furthermore, most sarcomas invading nerve destroy neural tissue rather than cause nerve enlargement with preservation of its contour, as with neurotropic melanoma. Lastly, when subject to immunohistochemical and ultrastructural study, the differentiation of most sarcomas becomes apparent.

Lymphoma-Leukemia

Mononeuropathies or polyneuropathies are often associated with hematopoietic tumors. Localized or widespread, they may involve nerve roots, ganglia, and cranial or peripheral nerves (fig. 14-8) (38,39). Microscopically, the process

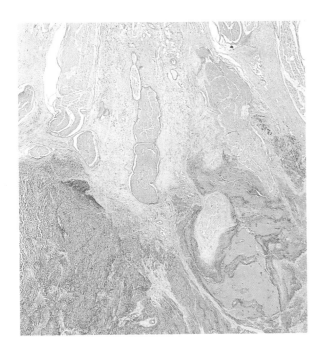 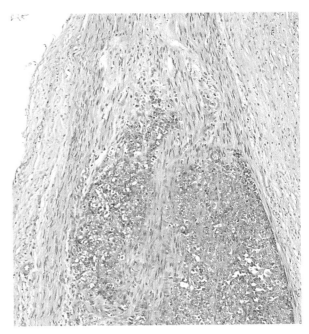

Figure 14-9

PRIMITIVE NEUROECTODERMAL TUMOR (PNET) OF SOFT TISSUE SECONDARILY INVOLVING NERVE

PNET arising in soft tissue may involve all nerve compartments by direct extension. The invasion is streak-like.

is often diffuse but nonuniform in distribution. Epineurial invasion may be seen but, unlike in carcinomatous involvement, the infiltrates often affect the subperineurial zone of the endoneurial septa or the bulk of the endoneurium (fig. 14-8). Axonal degeneration and myelin loss commonly result.

Nerve involvement by lymphoma, including angiotropic lymphoma and leukemia, typically occurs in a setting of systemic disease. In contrast, nerve involvement following CNS lymphoma has rarely been described (40). As in sciatic mononeuropathy (41), non-Hodgkin lymphomas only occasionally involve nerve in the absence of disease elsewhere (see chapter 11). So-called neurolymphomatosis (42,43), a disorder characterized by extensive, apparently selective peripheral nerve involvement, is poorly understood.

Miscellaneous Involvement

Primitive neuroectodermal tumors (PNET) of soft tissue origin may involve all nerve compartments (fig. 14-9). For the characteristics of this tumor, see chapter 12.

METASTASES TO NERVE SHEATH TUMOR

Metastasis of one tumor to another is rare and seen in only 0.1 percent of random autopsies (44). Most reported examples are encountered at autopsy. Among tumors that metastasize to others, breast and lung carcinomas do so most frequently and with nearly equal frequency (45). Most recipient tumors are benign and include longstanding lesions such as thyroid adenomas, adrenal adenomas, and meningiomas (45–47); schwannomas are also affected (fig. 14-10) (47,48). Renal cell carcinomas comprise 70 percent of malignant recipient tumors. Common to most recipient tumors is slow growth, a factor causing them to be at protracted risk of metastatic involvement. A high lipid content, as is often seen in meningioma, schwannoma, and renal cell carcinoma, is also considered a predisposing factor (49), as are such hormonal attributes as the presence of steroid hormone receptors in breast carcinoma and meningioma (50). Metastasis to schwannoma must be distinguished from the exceedingly rare occurrence of malignant transformation (MPNST ex-schwannoma), a process discussed in detail in chapter 12.

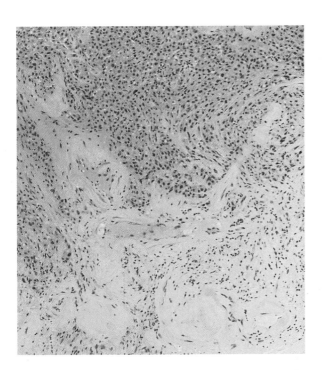 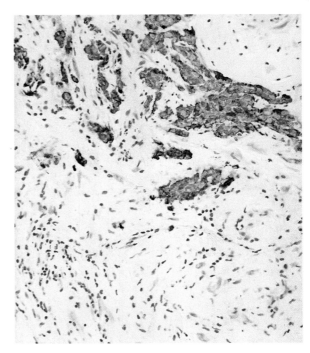

Figure 14-10

METASTASIS TO NERVE SHEATH TUMOR

Occurring in an elderly man with a lung mass, this schwannoma from the region of the elbow was the recipient of a large cell undifferentiated carcinoma (left), which stained for cytokeratin (right). (Courtesy of Dr. E. Venza, Bassano del Grappa, Italy.)

REFERENCES

1. Cruveilhier J. Maladies nes nerfs. Anatomic Pathologique du Dorps Humain, 2nd ed, Vol. 2, Part 35. Paris: J.B. Bailliere: 1829-1842.
2. Neumann E. Secondare cancroid infiltration des nervus mentalis bei einem fall von lippincroid. Arch Pathol Anat 1862;24:201.
3. Barber JR, Coventry MB, McDonald JR. The spread of soft-tissue sarcomata of the extremities along peripheral-nerve trunks. J Bone Joint Surg Am 1957;39-A:534-540.
4. Ernest P. Über das Wachstum und die Verbeitung bösartige Geschwülste insbesoderes des Krebses in den Lymphbahnen der Nerven. Beitr Pathol Anat 1907;7 (Suppl):29-51.
5. Larson DL, Rodin AE, Roberts DK, et al. Perineural lymphatics: myth or fact. Am J Surg 1966;112:488-492.
6. Rodin AE, Larson DL, Roberts DK. Nature of the perineural space invaded by prostatic carcinoma. Cancer 1967;20:1772-1779.
7. Selander D, Sjostrand J. Longitudinal spread of intraneurally injected local anesthetics. An experimental study of the initial neural distribution following intraneural injections. Acta Anaesthesiol Scand 1978;22:622-634.
8. Beggs J, Johnson PC, Olafsen A, et al. Transperineurial arterioles in human sural nerve. J Neuropathol Exp Neurol 1991;50:704-718.
9. Dodd GD, Dolan PA, Ballantyne AJ, et al. The dissemination of tumors of the head and neck via the cranial nerves. Radiol Clin North Am 1970;8:445-461.
10. Ballantyne AJ, McCarten AB, Ibanez ML. The extension of cancer of the head and neck through peripheral nerves. Am J Surg 1963;106:651-667.

11. Carter RL, Foster CS, Dinsdale EA, et al. Perineural spread by squamous carcinomas of the head and neck: a morphological study using antiaxonal and antimyelin monoclonal antibodies. J Clin Pathol 1983;36:269-275.

12. Carter RL, Pittam MR, Tanner NS. Pain and dysphagia in patients with squamous carcinomas of the head and neck: the role of perineural spread. J R Soc Med 1982;75:598-606.

13. Carter RL, Tanner NS, Clifford P, et al. Perineural spread in squamous cell carcinomas of the head and neck: a clinicopathological study. Clin Otolaryngol Allied Sci 1979;4:271-281.

14. Goepfert H, Dichtel WJ, Medina JE, et al. Perineural invasion in squamous cell skin carcinoma of the head and neck. Am J Surg 1984;148:542-547.

15. Mark GJ. Basal cell carcinoma with intraneural invasion. Cancer 1977;40:2181-2187.

16. Gonzalez-Vitale JC, Garcia-Bunuel R. Meningeal carcinomatosis. Cancer 1976;37:2906-2911.

17. Asbury AK, Johnson PC. Pathology of the peripheral nerve. Philadelphia: WB Saunders Co. 1978.

18. Johnson PC. Hematogenous metastases of carcinoma to dorsal root ganglia. Acta Neuropathol 1977;38:171-172.

19. Taylor HB, Norris HJ. Epithelial invasion of nerves in benign diseases of the breast. Cancer 1967;20:2245-2249.

20. Carstens PH. Perineural glands in normal and hyperplastic prostates. J Urol 1980;123:686-688.

21. Zimmerman KG, Johnson PC, Paplanus SH. Nerve invasion by benign proliferating ductules in vasitis nodosa. Cancer 1983;51:2066-2069.

22. Cavazza A, Asioli S, Martella EM, et al. [Neural infiltration in benign gallbladder lesions. Description of a case]. Pathologica 1998;90:42-45.

23. Costa J. Benign epithelial inclusions in pancreatic nerves. Am J Clin Pathol 1977;67:306-307.

24. Reed RJ, Leonard DD. Neurotropic melanoma. A variant of desmoplastic melanoma. Am J Surg Pathol 1979;3:301-311.

25. Mack EE, Gomez EC. Neurotropic melanoma. A case report and review of the literature. J Neurooncol 1992;13:165-171.

26. Jain S, Allen PW. Desmoplastic malignant melanoma and its variants. A study of 45 cases. Am J Surg Pathol 1989;13:358-373.

27. Jakobiec FA, Zuckerman BD, Berlin AJ, et al. Unusual melanocytic nevi of the conjunctiva. Am J Ophthalmol 1985;100:100-113.

28. Yamashiro S, Nagahiro S, Mimata C, et al. Malignant trigeminal schwannoma associated with xeroderma pigmentosum—case report. Neurol Med Chir (Tokyo) 1994;34:817-820.

29. Carlson JA, Dickersin GR, Sober AJ, et al. Desmoplastic neurotropic melanoma. A clinicopathologic analysis of 28 cases. Cancer 1995;75:478-494.

30. Smithers BM, McLeod GR, Little JH. Desmoplastic, neural transforming and neurotropic melanoma: a review of 45 cases. Aust N Z J Surg 1990;60:967-972.

31. Ackerman AB, Godomski J. Neurotropic malignant melanoma and other neurotropic neoplasms in the skin. Am J Dermatopathol 1984;6 Suppl:63-80.

32. Gibson LE, Goellner JR. Amelanotic melanoma: cases studied by Fontana stain, S-100 immunostain, and ultrastructural examination. Mayo Clin Proc 1988;63:777-782.

33. Khalil MK, Duguid WP. Neurotropic malignant melanoma of right temple with orbital metastasis: a clinicopathological case report. Br J Ophthalmol 1987;71:41-46.

34. Warner TF, Lloyd RV, Hafez GR, et al. Immunocytochemistry of neurotropic melanoma. Cancer 1984;53:254-257.

35. Warner TF, Ford CN, Hafez GR. Neurotropic melanoma of the face invading the maxillary nerve. J Cutan Pathol 1985;12:520-527.

36. David DJ, Speculand B, Vernon-Roberts B, et al. Malignant schwannoma of the inferior dental nerve. Br J Plast Surg 1978;31:323-333.

37. Scheithauer BW, Erdogan S, Rodriguez FJ, et al. Malignant peripheral nerve sheath tumors of cranial nerves and intracranial contents: a clinicopathologic study of 17 cases. Am J Surg Pathol 2009;33:325-338.

38. Burger PC, Scheithauer BW, Vogel FS. Surgical pathology of the nervous system and its coverings, 3rd ed. New York: Churchill Livingstone; 1991:359-65.

39. Russell D, Rubenstein L. Nervous system involvement by lymphomas, histiocytes and leukemias. In: Russell DS, Rubinstein LJ, eds. Pathology of the nervous system, 5th ed. Baltimore: Williams & Wilkins; 1989:608-615.

40. vanBolden V 2nd, Kline DG, Garcia CA, et al. Isolated radial nerve palsy due to metastasis from a primary malignant lymphoma of the brain. Neurosurgery 1987;21:905-909.

41. Roncaroli F, Poppi M, Riccioni L, et al. Primary non-Hodgkin's lymphoma of the sciatic nerve followed by localization in the central nervous system: case report and review of the literature. Neurosurgery 1997;40:618-621; discussion 621-612.

42. Borit A, Altrocchi PH. Recurrent polyneuropathy and neurolymphomatosis. Arch Neurol 1971;24:40-49.

43. Guberman A, Rosenbaum H, Braciale T, et al. Human neurolymphomatosis. J Neurol Sci 1978;36:1-12.

44. Barz H. [The incidence of metastatic carcinomas in meningiomas. A report of 4 cases]. Zentralbl Allg Pathol 1983;127:367-374. [German]

45. Arnold AC, Hepler RS, Badr MA, et al. Metastasis of adenocarcinoma of the lung to optic nerve sheath meningioma. Arch Ophthalmol 1995;113:346-351.

46. Bucciero A, del Basso de Caro M, Vizioli L, et al. Metastasis of breast carcinoma to intracranial meningioma. Case report and review of the literature. J Neurosurg Sci 1992;36:169-172.

47. Chambers PW, Davis RL, Blanding JD, et al. Metastases to primary intracranial meningiomas and neurilemomas. Arch Pathol Lab Med 1980;104:350-354.

48. Ni K, Dehner LP. Schwannoma with metastatic carcinoma of the breast: an unconventional form of glandular peripheral sheath tumor. Hum Pathol 1995;26:457-459.

49. Wolintz AH, Mastri A. Metastasis of carcinoma of lung to sphenoid ridge meningioma. N Y State J Med 1970;70:2592-2598.

50. di Bonito L, Bianchi C. [Metastasis of breast cancer to a meningioma]. Arch Anat Cytol Pathol 1978;26:175-176. [French]

15 NEUROFIBROMATOSIS 1 AND 2, AND SCHWANNOMATOSIS

The *neurofibromatoses* are members of the group of neurocutaneous disorders, which also include tuberous sclerosis, neurocutaneous melanosis, hypomelanosis of Ito, incontinentia pigmenti, Sturge-Weber syndrome, and von Hippel-Lindau disease. Collectively, these conditions are referred to as *phakomatoses*, a term derived from the Greek phakos, meaning a lentil or birthmark. All but Sturge-Weber syndrome, which is sporadic in occurrence, have an autosomal dominant pattern of inheritance. Only neurofibromatosis types 1 and 2, and schwannomatosis show significant involvement of the peripheral nervous system.

Neurofibromatosis is characterized by multiple lesions of diverse type affecting a variety of tissues. These processes include hyperplasias, hypoplasias, hamartomas, and both benign and malignant neoplasms. Most lesions are neuroectodermal or mesenchymal in derivation. No gender or racial predilections are seen. Although the existence of as many as eight variants of neurofibromatosis has been proposed (1), three principal genetic and clinicopathologic forms are recognized. Termed *neurofibromatosis types 1 and 2* (NF1 and NF2) as well as *schwannomatosis*, each is characterized by distinctive clinical abnormalities; overlap in manifestations is minor except in NF2 and schwannomatosis. Both NF1 and NF2 result from genetic alterations affecting tumor suppressor genes. The risk of developing a malignant neoplasm is 10-fold higher in patients with either condition. The key features of NF1 and NF2 are summarized in Table 15-1. The importance of distinguishing these conditions, conceptually as well as practically, cannot be overstressed (2). Certainly, unqualified use of the term "neurofibromatosis" lacks diagnostic precision. Thus, the variant under discussion must always be specified. Schwannomatosis is discussed separately below.

NEUROFIBROMATOSIS 1

General Features. The full expression of this frequently occurring disorder, also termed *peripheral neurofibromatosis* or *von Recklinghausen disease*, has long been recognized (fig. 15-1) (3). The responsible mutation resides in the large *NF1* gene on the long arm and near the centromere of chromosome 17 (4–7). Its precise location (17q11.2) is close to that of the nerve growth factor receptor gene (8). Spanning 350 kb of genomic DNA and consisting of 60 exons, the *NF1* gene encodes neurofibromin, a 2,818 amino acid protein. Evidence indicates that it functions as a tumor suppressor and that it also plays a role in cell proliferation and differentiation (9,10). Neurofibromin is normally expressed in many tissues.

NF1 is among the most common of mendelian disorders, sparing no races and showing a population incidence of 1 in 3,000. Since the pattern of inheritance is autosomal dominant, approximately half of affected individuals have a family history of the disorder. Its penetrance is high, but expression is variable (11). The remaining cases appear to be sporadic in occurrence given the high mutation rate of the *NF1* gene. Despite the high (100 percent) rate of penetrance, just over half of patients are only mildly affected.

Clinical Features. Although in isolation, none of the manifestations of NF1 is pathognomonic of the disorder, according to Gutmann et al. (12) a clinical diagnosis can be confirmed if a patient has two or more of the findings listed in Table 15-2. The expression of NF1 is variable, even among members of the same family. Nonetheless, concordant manifestations have been reported in affected monozygotic twins (13) and in members of the same family (14).

Among the earliest manifestations of NF1, and occasionally congenital, are smooth-contoured, pigmented cutaneous macules termed

Table 15-1

COMPARATIVE FEATURES OF NEUROFIBROMATOSIS 1 AND 2

Features	NF1[a]	NF2
Incidence	1/3000	1/40,000
Prevalence	60/100,000	0.01/100,000
Inheritance	Autosomal dominant	Autosomal dominant
Sporadic occurrence	50%	50%
Chromosome location	17q11.2	22q12
Encoded protein	Neurofibromin	Merlin (schwannomin)
Café-au-lait spots (6 or more); at least 0.5 cm (prepubertal); one or more 1.5 cm (postpubertal)	Often multiple and large At least 70% of patients About 90% of patients	Small; rarely more than 6; 40% of patients
Cutaneous neurofibromas	Most patients	Rare
Cutaneous schwannomas	Not associated	70%
Multiple Lisch nodules	Very common	Not associated
Skeletal malformations	Common	Not associated
Astrocytomas (optic, cerebellar, cerebral)	Moderate incidence	Not associated
Pheochromocytoma	Occasionally seen	Not associated
Malignant peripheral nerve sheath tumor	Approximately 5%	Not seen
Intellectual impairment	Common	Not associated
Vestibular schwannoma	Not associated	Most cases (usually bilateral)
Meningioma	Not associated	Common
Spinal cord ependymoma	Not associated	Common
Meningioangiomatosis	Not associated	Occasional
Schwannosis	Not associated	Common
Glial hamartomas	Occasional	Very common
Syringomyelia	Not associated	Associated
Posterior subcapsular cataracts	Not associated	Common (60-80%)
Ganglioneuroma	Occasional	Not associated
Gastrointestinal stromal tumor	Occasional	Not associated
Paraganglioma, including duodenal gangliocytic variant	Occasional	Not associated
Foregut carcinoid tumor, including duodenal calcifying somatostatinoma	Occasional	Not associated
Juvenile xanthogranuloma	Occasional	Not associated
Juvenile leukemia (CML)[b]	Occasional	Not associated

[a]NF1 = neurofibromatosis type 1; NF2 = neurofibromatosis type 2.
[b]CML = chronic myelogenous leukemia.

café-au-lait spots (fig. 15-2), which tend to enlarge and become more pigmented over time. Occasional macules are two-toned, with both dark and pale areas. Axillary freckling, a form of pigmentation affecting intertriginous skin, is of particular diagnostic significance (fig. 15-3). The pigmentation in café-au-lait spots and freckles is not due to an increase in melanocytes, but rather to an excess of melanin in the form of melanosome-containing phagolysosomes. Referred to as "macromelanosomes" (fig. 15-4) (15) or "melanin macroglobules" (16), they are not limited to melanocytes, but may be seen in keratinocytes, Langerhans cells, and macrophages as well. In fair-skinned people, café-au-lait spots and freckles are light tan, their color

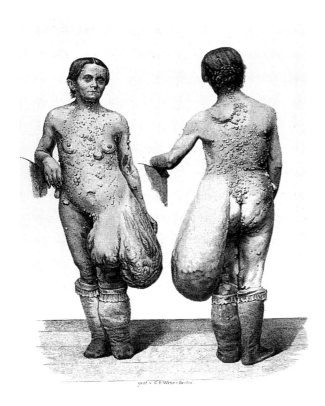

Figure 15-1

NEUROFIBROMATOSIS TYPE I (NF1) AS DEPICTED IN VIRCHOW'S "KRANKHAFTEN GESCHWUELSTE," 1856

Image from Virchow R. Die krankhaften geschwülste: dreissig vorlesungen, gehalten während des wintersemesters 1862-1863 an der Universität zu Berlin. Berlin: Verlag von August Hirschwald; 1863:II.

Table 15-2

DIAGNOSTIC CRITERIA FOR NEUROFIBROMATOSIS 1[a]

The patient should have two or more of the following:

1. Six or more café-au-lait spots
    1.5 cm or larger in postpubertal individuals
    0.5 cm or larger in prepubertal individuals

2. Two or more neurofibromas of any type or one or more plexiform neurofibromas

3. Freckling in the axilla or groin

4. Optic glioma (tumor of the optic pathway)

5. Two or more Lisch nodules (benign iris hamartomas)

6. A distinctive bony lesion
    Dysplasia of the sphenoid bone
    Dysplasia or thinning of the long bone cortex

7. A first-degree relative with NF1

[a]Table 1 from Gutmann DH, Alysworth A, Carey JC, et al. The diagnostic evaluation and multidisciplinary management of neurofibromatosis 1 and neurofibromatosis 2. JAMA 1997;278:52.

truly resembling that of coffee laced with milk; in brown or black individuals, café-au-lait spots are dark brown or black (fig. 15-3). Since café-au-lait spots are commonly found in normal persons and occur in unrelated diseases, such as the McCune-Albright syndrome (polyostotic fibrous dysplasia), their size, contour, and number must be taken into account when considering a clinical diagnosis of NF1 (Table 15-2). The presence of six macules, each measuring at least 0.5 cm, is required for a diagnosis of NF1 in prepubertal patients (12). An equal number of macules greater than 1.5 cm in diameter is required in adult patients (17). Not only the size but the number of café-au-lait spots and freckles may increase over time. At diagnosis, nearly all patients have at least one café-au-lait spot of significant size, and two thirds have six or more such spots (18).

Although occasional NF1-affected individuals have few or no café-au-lait spots, their presence can be demonstrated by examination of the skin under ultraviolet light.

The typical NF1 facies includes a broad forehead, triangular face, and dark infraorbital discoloration (figs. 15-1, 15-7, 15-20A). Pigmented iris hamartomas, termed Lisch nodules, are a common feature of NF1 (fig. 15-5) (19). Although perhaps an overestimate, they are thought to occur in 95 percent of patients over 6 years of age (20). They are readily visualized on slit lamp examination as brown, often bilateral nodules. Lisch nodules must be distinguished from other nevi of the iris.

Like café-au-lait spots, neurofibromas are hallmark lesions of NF1 (figs. 15-6–15-19). Their clinicopathologic spectrum is discussed and illustrated in detail in chapter 8. In terms of cellular makeup, they consist not only of Schwann cells, but of perineurial-like cells, fibroblasts, and cells with features intermediate between perineurial-like cells and fibroblasts. In the past, this heterogeneity prompted some to suggest that neurofibromas are polyclonal (21) and perhaps hamartomatous in nature. Recent evidence, based upon active and inactive X chromosomes in the individual tumors, suggests that neurofibromas are indeed monoclonal

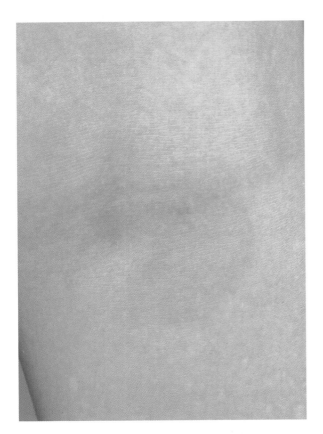 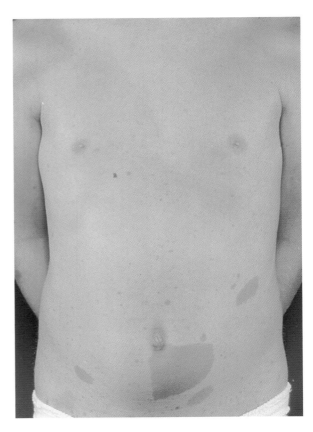

Figure 15-2

CAFÉ-AU-LAIT SPOTS IN NF1

Often oval or oblong in configuration, these hyperpigmented lesions are discrete and clearly demarcated from surrounding skin. Subtle examples could easily be missed (left) whereas others are obvious (right). Sharp demarcation of a lesion in the midline (right) suggests a dermatomal distribution. Clinical experience suggests that hyperpigmentation extending across the midline is associated with an increased risk of the development of malignant peripheral nerve sheath tumor (MPNST).

(22). As currently understood, all cells of NF1 patients harbor one nonfunctional *NF1* gene (germline mutation) (9). Neurofibromas are assumed to arise as a result of a second, somatic mutation (9). Loss or mutation of one or more tumor suppressor genes underlies transformation of neurofibroma to malignant peripheral nerve sheath tumor (MPNST) (23). As discussed in chapter 12, aberrant expression of the *p53* gene, a tumor suppressor gene on the short arm of chromosome 17, sometimes occurs in the transition of neurofibroma to MPNST (24,25).

Neurofibromas are occasionally present at birth, but most develop later in life. Usually, they first appear around puberty, with other lesions emerging later. Hyperpigmentation may overlie cutaneous and massive soft tissue

neurofibromas (see fig. 8-26), but the locations of the tumors and the pigmentations do not necessarily coincide. Both peripheral and visceral nerves are affected by neurofibromas. Small nerves of skin and subcutaneous tissue are preferentially involved. A single localized cutaneous neurofibroma is of no significance in terms of establishing a diagnosis of NF1.

Four clinically and morphologically distinct variants of neurofibroma occur in NF1 (see chapter 8): 1) cutaneous lesions of localized and diffuse type; 2) localized intraneural tumors of peripheral nerves; 3) plexiform neurofibromas typically involving major nerve trunks (26); and 4) massive soft tissue neurofibromas. Solitary neurofibromas of localized intraneural type, even sizable tumors arising in a nerve root, are

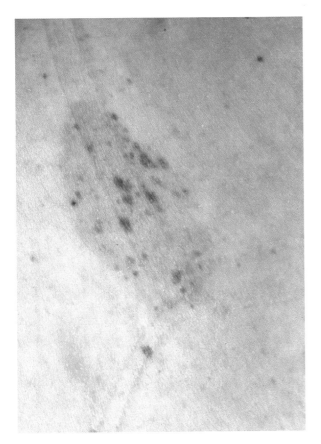
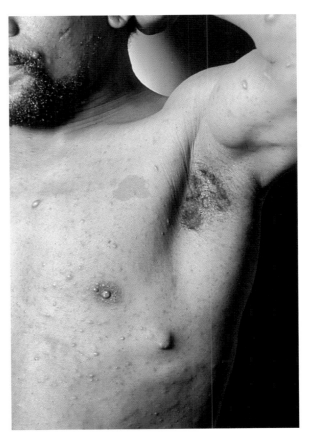

Figure 15-3

FRECKLING IN NF1

Left: Often affecting the axilla, as shown, groin, or both, these lesions may be bilateral or unilateral. In individuals not generally freckled, their presence is highly suggestive of NF1. Nonintertriginous skin is unaffected.

Right: Both café-au-lait spots and axillary freckling may be more deeply pigmented in blacks.

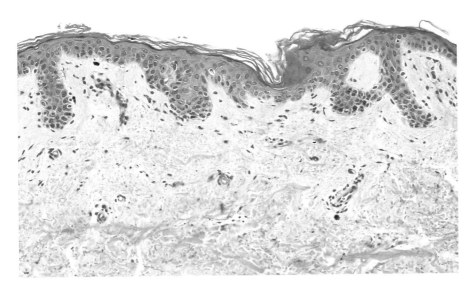

Figure 15-4

CAFÉ-AU-LAIT SPOT IN NF1

In contrast to most café-au-lait macules, here there is a slight elongation of rete ridges and a slight increase in the number of intraepidermal melanocytes.

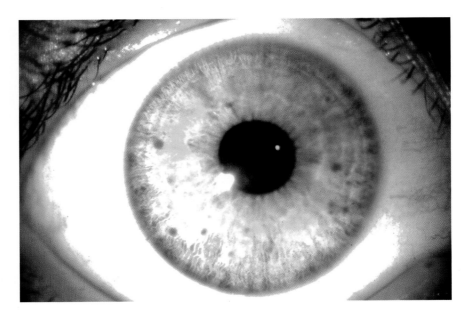

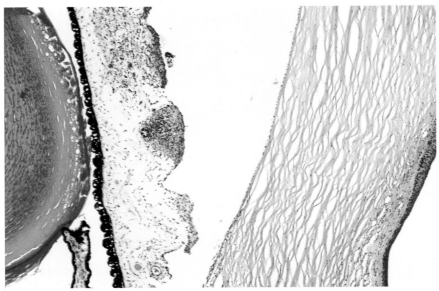

Figure 15-5

LISCH NODULES OF THE IRIS IN NF1

Top: Unlike iris freckles, these lesions are elevated above the surface of the iris. They also affect the entire area of the iris rather than the inner or outer circumference.

Bottom: A sagittal section of the eye shows that the nodules are multiple and lie on the anterior aspect of the iris.

usually sporadic in occurrence, while multiple examples are typically NF1 associated (fig. 15-7, 15-8D) (27). The same is true of large, diffuse cutaneous neurofibromas (see figs. 8-5, 8-6). Numerous localized cutaneous neurofibromas (fig. 15-7, left), plexiform examples (figs. 15-1, 15-8, 15-10), and massive soft tissue variants (fig. 15-11D; see also fig. 8-26A,B) are generally considered diagnostic of NF1.

In rare instances when a plexiform neurofibroma occurs in a patient without other manifestations of NF1 or a family history of the disorder, the tumor is likely the result of a local somatic mutation (1). This is also the mechanism underlying so-called *localized* or *segmental neurofibromatosis*, an anatomically limited form of NF1 (28). Such cases often feature cutaneous or subcutaneous neurofibromas as well as café-au-lait spots limited to one portion of the body, typically one limb or even a single dermatome (fig. 15-12). These patients do not transmit the condition to their progeny, and develop disease complications only in the distribution of the affected nerve. Other localized forms of NF1

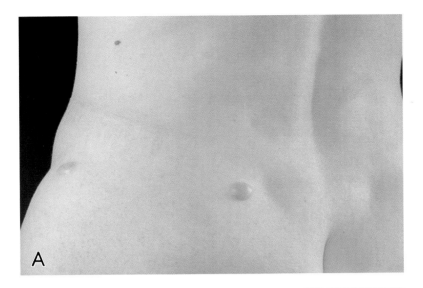

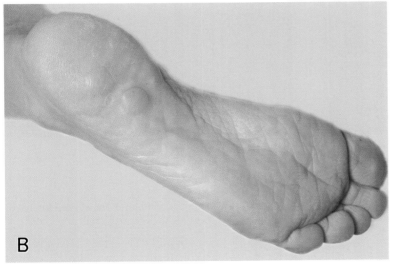

Figure 15-6

**LOCALIZED CUTANEOUS
NEUROFIBROMAS IN NF1**

A: Unlike plexiform examples, these dermal and subcutaneous neurofibromas are dome-shaped, discrete, and movable.

B: Neurofibromas affecting the palm or sole are rare outside the setting of NF1 and are thought to be associated with an increased risk of intracranial neoplasms.

C: Neurofibromas of the areola may become manifest or enlarge during pregnancy.

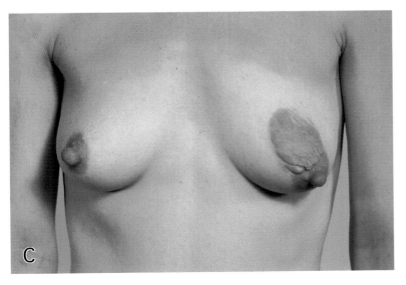

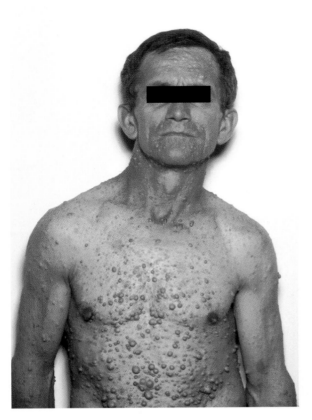
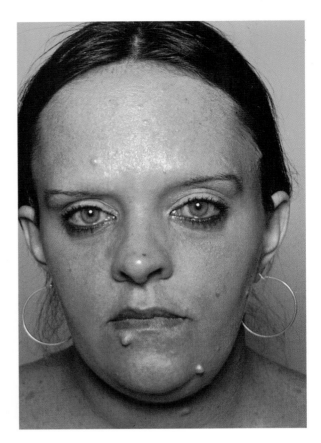

Figure 15-7

LOCALIZED CUTANEOUS NEUROFIBROMAS IN NF1

Left: Such nodular to pedunculated cutaneous examples most often affect the trunk.

Right: NF1 is occasionally associated with typical facial features, including a triangular configuration, a broad forehead, and deep-set eyes with infraorbital discoloration.

include *hemifacial hypertrophy* (fig. 15-20C,D) and *visceral neurofibromatosis* (see below). On but slim evidence, **macrodystrophia lipomatosa** (see chapter 6) has been included by some in the spectrum of localized NF1.

Visceral Neurofibromas. Neurofibromas affect viscera in a variety of ways: solitary or multiple, sporadic or NF1 associated. Visceral neurofibromatosis is a rare condition in which patients often exhibit few external manifestations of NF1. The pathobiology of visceral neurofibromatosis is unclear but it may be a result of anatomically selective *NF1* gene expression or nerve growth factor effect (29). Visceral neurofibromatosis may be the sole manifestation of NF1, or various organ systems may be affected in the generalized form of the disease (figs. 15-13–15-19). Visceral neurofibromatosis mainly

affects the gastrointestinal tract, which shows great case-to-case variation in manifestations (figs. 15-14–15-17) (29,30). The upper gastrointestinal tract (esophagus, stomach, and small bowel) is most often involved (figs. 15-14–15-16), but the colon and rectum can be affected as well (fig. 15-17, left). Hepatic neurofibromas have also been reported (fig. 15-17, right) (31,32). Urinary bladder involvement is rare but well documented (figs. 15-18, 15-19).

The spectrum of NF1-associated gastrointestinal lesions includes ganglioneuromatosis, neurofibromas of both localized and plexiform type, gastrointestinal stromal tumors, and various neuroendocrine neoplasms. Ganglioneuromatosis, whether subtle or obvious and localized or diffuse, results in a Hirschsprung-like picture in children and in pseudo-obstruction

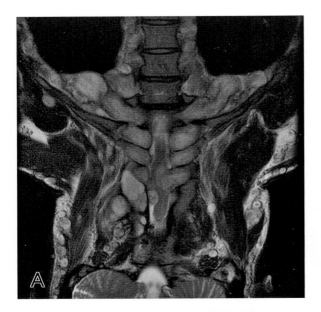

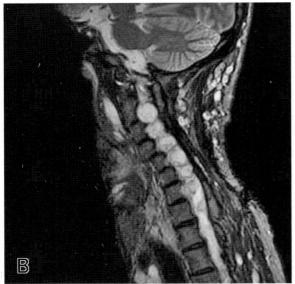

Figure 15-9

MULTIPLE BILATERAL NERVE ROOT NEUROFIBROMAS

Impressive involvement of the entire spinal axis is evident on coronal (A) and sagittal (B) magnetic resonance imaging (MRI) scans. A gross photo of the distal spinal cord demonstrates such neurofibromas; the affected nerves taper as the tumors approach the transition zone to the spinal cord (C). (C courtesy of Dr. H. Goebel, Mainz, Germany.)

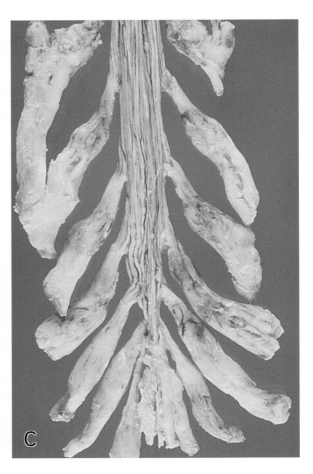

or megacolon in adults. It is characterized by an increase in ganglion cells and their processes, which affects primarily the submucosal plexus. Even "giant ganglia" featuring neurons of varying size and number may be seen. As in multiple endocrine neoplasia (MEN) 2B, the mucosa may also be involved, particularly the lower lamina propria (see fig. 5-15C).

Neurofibromas of NF1 occurring in the gastrointestinal tract are often multiple and grouped (fig. 15-15) or are large and diffuse with transmural involvement, frequently with a plexiform component (fig. 15-16). The mu-

cosa mainly features delicate neurofibromatous tissue and the presence of ganglion cells. The plexiform component varies considerably in size and extent, often involving both the submucosal and myenteric plexuses as well as the serosa. The degree to which the myenteric plexus is affected varies from markedly hypertrophic to diminished (29). In a superficial biopsy, the microscopic distinction between such lesions and the ganglioneuromatosis of MEN 2B described above may be difficult. The distinction between NF1 and MEN 2B-associated ganglioneuromatosis is discussed in chapter 5.

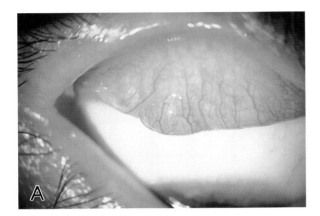

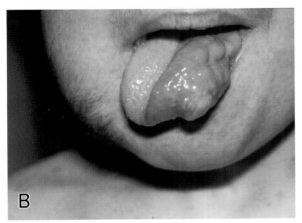

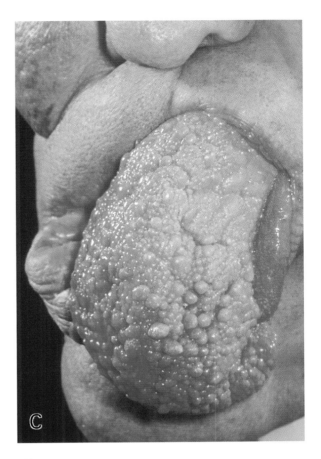

Figure 15-10

NEUROFIBROMA OF MUCOUS MEMBRANES IN NF1

A: An unbiopsied, presumably plexiform neurofibroma produced nodularity of the conjunctival mucosa and a similar tumor of the tongue.

B,C: Lesions of the tongue may be localized (B) or extensive (C), extending down through the root of the tongue into the neck. Such extensive lesions interfere with glutition and cause severe disability. The facial features of this severely affected patient are illustrated in figure 15-20C.

Much less common are visceral neurofibromas affecting the heart (33), larynx (34), or genitourinary tract (figs. 15-18, 15-19) (35). Multiple intestinal neurofibromas unassociated with NF1 have been described in association with a reciprocal translocation of chromosomes 12 and 14 (36). In addition to neurofibromas are rare purported examples of visceral MPNST (37–39) and of leiomyoma (29,30) in the setting of NF1. Patients with neurofibromatosis are also prone to develop gastrointestinal stromal tumors (see chapter 13).

NF1 and the Central Nervous System. Among central nervous system (CNS) neoplasms occurring in NF1, nearly all are neuro-ectodermal in nature. *Astrocytomas* are by far the most common. Among these, the most frequent are unilateral or bilateral *optic gliomas* of pilocytic type with leptomeningeal extension and associated arachnoid cell proliferation (fig. 15-21A,B) (20,46–51). Cerebral (52,53), brainstem, and cerebellar examples are also encountered (52,54–58). Given the presence of optic gliomas of this type in as many as 15 percent of patients with NF1, as well as their early age at presentation (80 percent are diagnosed by age 11 years), the presence of such tumors on computerized tomography (CT) scans are important to the diagnosis of NF1 (49). They may involve the intraorbital optic nerve, the

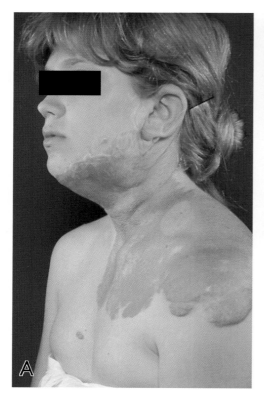

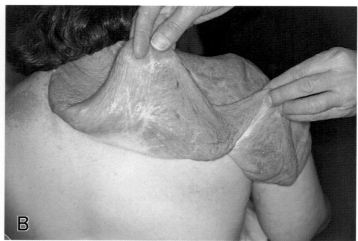

Figure 15-11

MASSIVE NEUROFIBROMAS IN NF1

These soft tissue lesions range from plaques (A) to cape-like flaps (B) and pendulous facial lesions (C). Only rarely do massive diffuse examples affect an entire limb, a lesion once referred to as "elephantiasis neuromatosa" (D). Microsections of massive soft tissue neurofibromas typically consist of both diffuse and plexiform components.

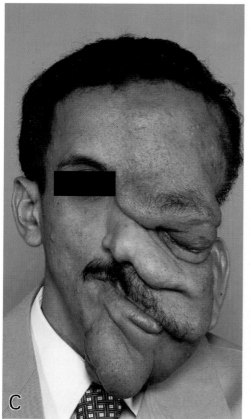

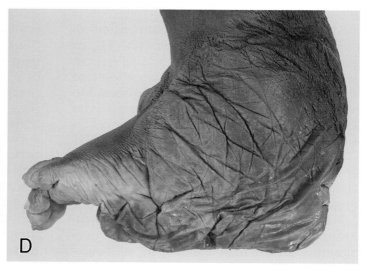

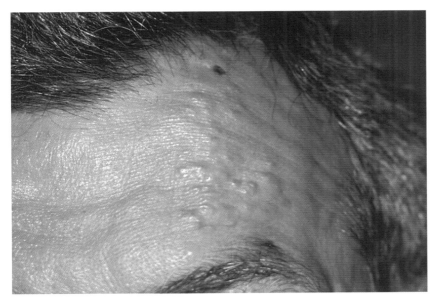

Figure 15-12

SEGMENTAL NEUROFIBROMATOSIS

Localized to one body part or even a single dermatome, this rare variant of NF1 results from a local somatic mutation. This example affects a portion of the trigeminal nerve distribution.

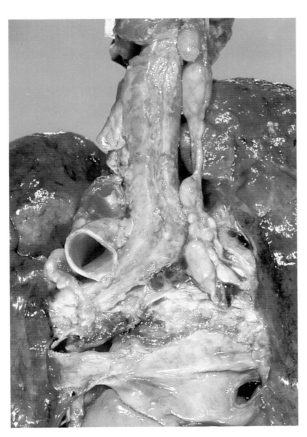

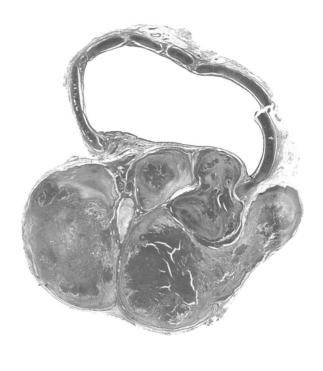

Figure 15-13

VISCERAL PLEXIFORM NEUROFIBROMAS IN NF1

Although plexiform tumors usually arise in soft tissues, where they resemble a "bag of worms," nerves in body cavities and viscera are also affected. Here an extensive plexiform neurofibroma involves the right vagus nerve and its branches (left), and another involves the posterior trachea (right).

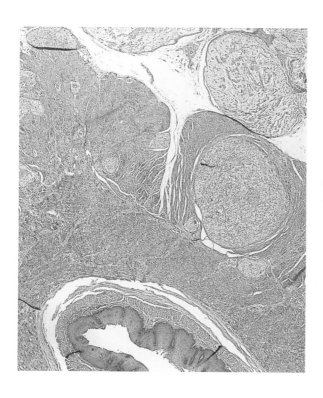

Figure 15-14

VISCERAL PLEXIFORM NEUROFIBROMAS IN NF1

A plexiform tumor affects the muscularis of the esophagus (left). Another example fills the mesentery of the small bowel (below).

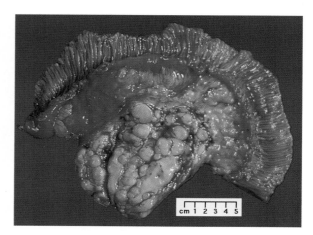

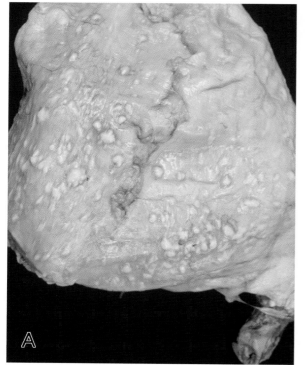

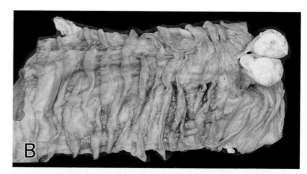

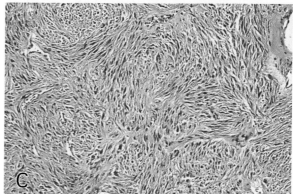

Figure 15-15

GASTROINTESTINAL NEUROFIBROMAS IN NF1

Such lesions are usually multifocal. This patient has numerous gastric mucosal lesions (A) and a jejunal submucosal lesion (B,C).

chiasm, or both. Bilateral examples are said to occur only in NF1 (59).

In addition to pilocytic astrocytomas, which are generally benign and preferentially affect the optic apparatus (fig. 15-21A,B), thalamus (fig. 15-21C), and cerebellum, ordinary diffuse or fibrillary astrocytomas also occur in the setting of NF1. Of these, half exhibit malignant behavior (52). In the Mayo Clinic experience with 100 gliomas in NF1 patients, no sex predilection was noted (52). The median age at diagnosis was 13 years. Of the tumors, 49 percent were pilocytic astrocytomas; 27 percent, diffuse infiltrative astrocytomas, of which ratio of the grades 2 to 3 to 4 was 1 to 2 to 1; and 17 percent low-grade astrocytomas of indeterminate type. Although the latter were difficult to classify, most behaved in a favorable fashion. Although tumors of the CNS are common in NF1, they differ both in type and distribution from those of NF2 (Table 15-1).

Patients with NF1 also develop *neuroglial hamartomas*, such as gliofibrillary nodules (fig. 15-21D) (53) and retinal glial hamartomas or malformations like aqueductal stenosis. Neurologic abnormalities encountered in association with NF1 include macrocephaly, learning disabilities, epilepsy, and hydrocephalus. In addition to the endocrine effects of pheochromocytoma, endocrinopathy in the setting of NF1 also includes precocious puberty, likely due to hypothalamic dysfunction.

Miscellaneous NF1-Associated Tumors and Lesions. Miscellaneous tumors associated with NF1 include bilateral pheochromocytoma, duodenal paraganglioma and carcinoid tumor (40–42), rhabdomyosarcoma (43), juvenile chronic myelogenous leukemia (fig. 15-17, right) (44,45), juvenile xanthogranuloma (44,45), and nonossifying fibroma of bone (fibrous cortical defect). Less frequently occurring manifestations of NF1 are short stature as well as skeletal and other mesodermal dysplasias. Bony lesions include "scalloping" of vertebral bodies (fig. 15-22A); kyphoscoliosis (fig. 15-22B,C), anteroposterior indentation or fusion of vertebrae; overgrowth of long bones; and dysplastic underdevelopment of long or flat bones (fig. 15-23) with tibial bowing, pseudoarthroses (fig. 15-23, right), bone cysts, and fractures. Lower thoracic acute angular scoliosis occurs almost exclusively in NF1 (60,61). Congenital pseudoarthroses, 50

to 90 percent of which occur in NF1 patients, affect primarily the tibia and fibula (62). Orbital malformations due to dysplasia or the absence of portions of the sphenoid or frontal bones (fig. 15-20A,B) result in facial asymmetry and proptosis (51). Massive osseous and soft tissue overgrowth may be particularly disfiguring (fig. 15-20C,D). Mesodermal dysplasias also affect arteries (63–66), producing a range of intimal changes including hyperplasia and fibrosis (66), the result of which is vascular stenosis (fig. 15-24) (67) or the formation of aneurysms (68). Several examples of renovascular hypertension in patients with NF1 have been attributed to intimal proliferation (69,70). Hypertrophic (obstructive) cardiomyopathy, also a hamartomatous lesion, occurs only infrequently in NF1.

NEUROFIBROMATOSIS 2

Definition and General Features. Also termed *central* or *bilateral acoustic neurofibromatosis, neurofibromatosis 2* (NF2) is inherited in an autosomal dominant manner and exhibits a penetrance of almost 100 percent at age 60 years (71). Fifty percent of cases represent new or sporadic mutations (72). These affect chromosome 22 (73) and lie near the middle of its long arm at 22q12 (74,75). The *NF2* gene has been cloned (74,75). It spans 110 kb of genomic DNA, and encodes a member of the protein 4.1 family termed merlin (schwannomin). The function of the latter may be to mediate communication between the extracellular milieu and the cytoskeleton (76).

Clinical Features. NF2 is much less common than NF1 and shows a population incidence of maximally 1 in 50,000. Most patients present in the second or third decade, but some cases are "late onset" (71). NF2 is often more clinically devastating than NF1. There are two forms of NF2: the mild *Gardner-Frazier variant* usually restricted to *vestibular schwannomas* and a severe, earlier onset type associated with *meningiomas*. The presence of intracranial meningiomas increases the relative risk of mortality 2.5-fold. A clinicopathologic comparison of NF1 and NF2 is presented in Table 15-1. Historically (12), a clinical diagnosis of NF2 was made if a patient had either bilateral 8th cranial nerve schwannomas or otherwise fulfilled the criteria listed in Table 15-3. These criteria, however, are weighted

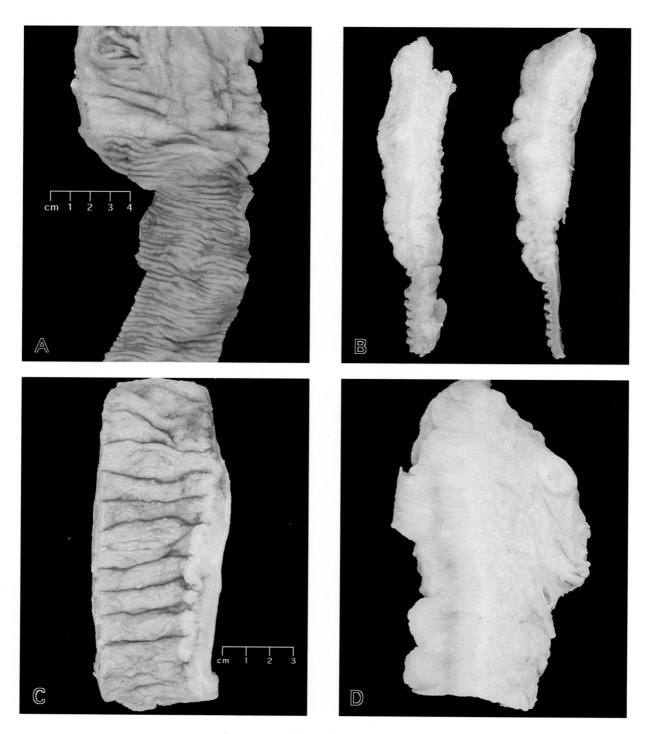

Figure 15-16

SMALL BOWEL NEUROFIBROMAS IN NF1

This 27-year-old female presented with small bowel obstruction. The transition of normal to markedly enlarged small bowel is abrupt (A,B), the mucosal folds are coarsened (C), and an obvious plexiform component is present in the serosa (D). Microsections show involvement of the mucosa by ganglioneuromatous tissue (E), diffuse and plexiform intraneural involvement of the submucosa (F), myenteric plexus over-run by tumor (G), and serosal and intramuscular plexiform neurofibroma (H). (Courtesy of Dr. W. Stahr, Cape Giradeau, MO.)

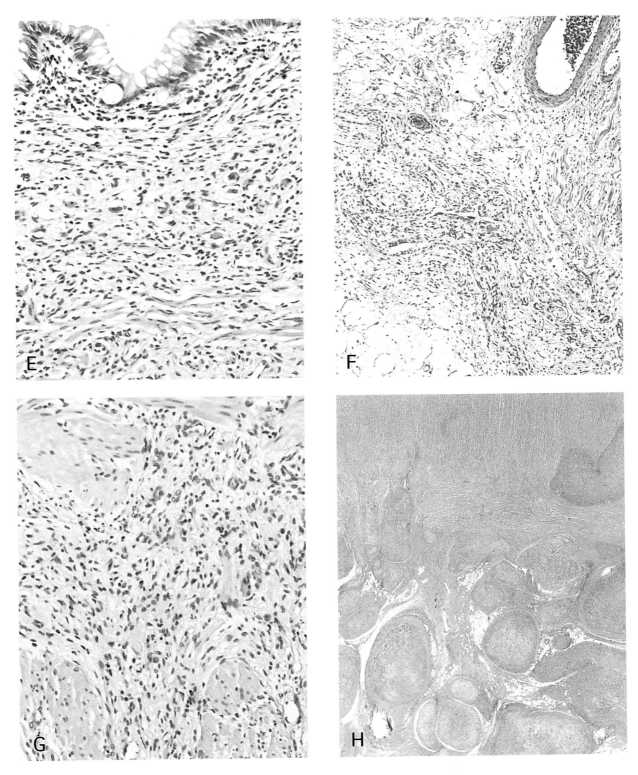

Figure 15-16, continued

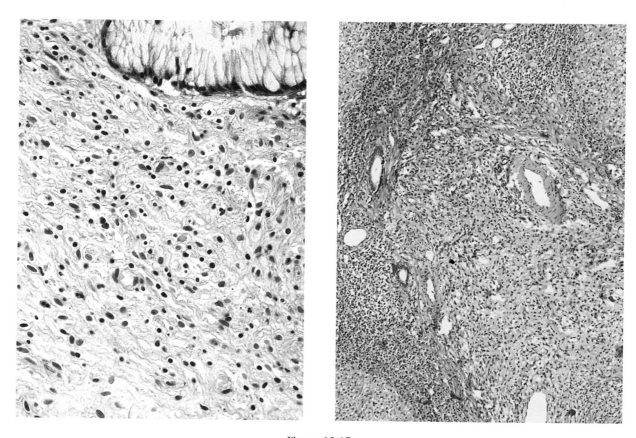

Figure 15-17

GASTROINTESTINAL TRACT NEUROFIBROMAS IN NF1

Left: Superficial biopsies, such as of the colon, may show infiltration of the lamina propria and muscularis mucosa.
Right: Hepatic involvement is rare. There is a coexisting infiltrate of juvenile chronic myelogenous leukemia. (Courtesy of Dr. J. Ludwig, Rochester, MN.)

Table 15-3

DIAGNOSTIC CRITERIA FOR NEUROFIBROMATOSIS 2

Definite	Possible
Bilateral vesicular schwannomas (VS)	Unilateral VS, age <30 years; A meningioma, glioma, other schwannoma, or JPSLO
Affected first degree relative and unilateral VS, <30 years of age or 2 of the following: menigioma, glioma, other schwannoma, or juvenile posterior subcapsular lenticular opacity (TPSLO)	Multiple menigiomas and unilateral VS or a glioma, other schwannoma or JPSLO

toward familial cases. Bilateral 8th cranial nerve schwannomas, actually vestibular rather than acoustic nerve tumors (72), may present years after the appearance of other tumors common in NF2. For this reason, Evans et al. (72) and Gutmann et al. (12) suggested the adoption of additional diagnostic criteria. Unlike in patients with NF1, café-au-lait spots, when present in NF2, are small and few in number (77). Furthermore, cutaneous neurofibromas are rare in NF2 (77). Instead, patients develop multiple schwannomas (27). No Lisch nodules are noted, but 60 to 80 percent of patients have posterior subcapsular cataracts (78,79).

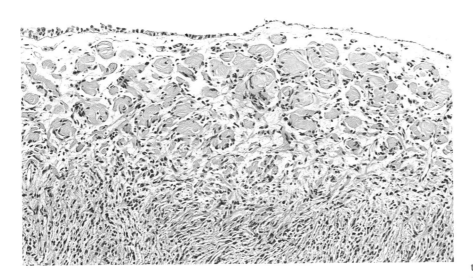

Figure 15-18

**NEUROFIBROMA OF
URINARY BLADDER IN NF1**

Top: A conspicuous feature is
the diffuse presence of pseudomeissnerian corpuscles beneath
the urothelium.

Bottom: The corpuscle-like
structures are strongly immunoreactive for S-100 protein.

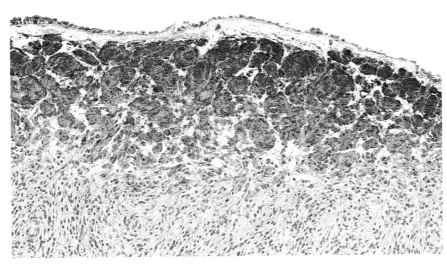

Vestibular Schwannomas. Bilateral vestibular schwannomas are the hallmark of NF2 (fig. 15-25) (80,81). Referable symptoms appear at a wide range of ages but only rarely manifest before puberty (78). As previously noted, the clinical severity of NF2 varies considerably. Genotype-phenotype correlations are reflected in the age of onset (56,82). Almost all vestibular schwannomas are benign (72). Less than 1 percent invade bone. Although bilateral in most patients, they often present metachronously, years before the appearance of symptoms of the second tumor. The demonstration of vestibular schwannomas or the exclusion of their presence requires thin-slice (3 mm) magnetic resonance imaging (MRI) examination.

Aside from vestibular examples, schwannomas in patients with NF2 affect sites similar to those of sporadic tumors, but differ in several ways. These include multifocality within a nerve (figs. 15-25, 15-26), prominent myxoid change, peritumoral nerve edema, a distinctly nodular microscopic growth pattern (83), an association with peritumoral arachnoidal cell proliferation (84), and the rare occurrence of a mixed schwannoma-meningioma phenotype (see chapter 11) (84). Cutaneous schwannomas occur in approximately 50 percent of NF2 patients, their prevalence and number varying with disease severity (77). In contrast, superficial schwannomas in schwannomatosis are subcutaneous in location. Although plexiform neurofibromas are not

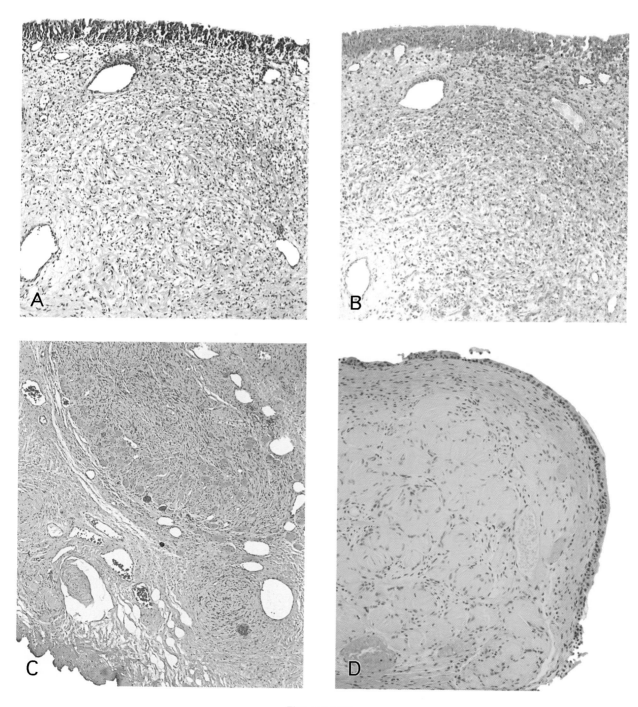

Figure 15-19

NEUROFIBROMA OF URINARY BLADDER IN NF1

A,B: The mucosa is diffusely involved (S-100 protein stain).
C: A serosal plexiform neurofibroma involves an autonomic ganglion.
D: The mucosal lesions may be polypoid rather than diffuse.

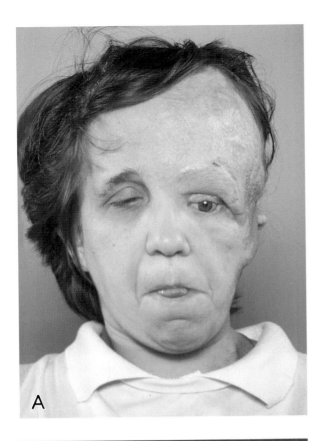

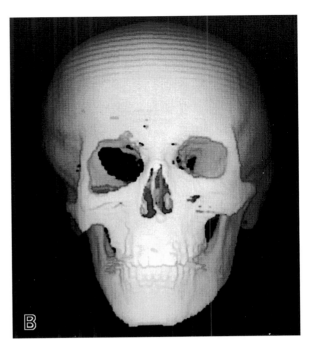

Figure 15-20

OSSEOUS DYSPLASIAS IN NF1

A,B: Dysplasia of the sphenoid with enlargement of the superior orbital fissure (B) often results in facial asymmetry and proptosis (A).

C: Massive hemifacial skeletal and soft tissue overgrowth in NF1. Such extreme examples are rare.

D: The osseous abnormalities are clearly evident on radiographs. The affected tongue of this patient is illustrated in figure 15-10C.

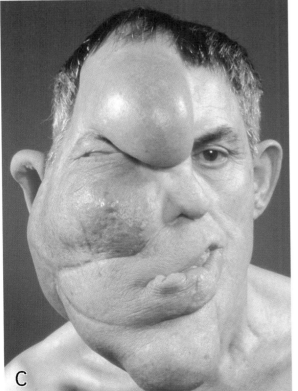

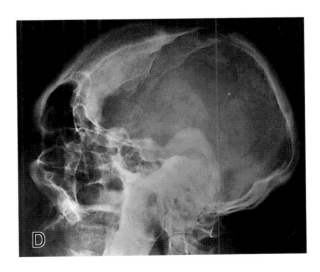

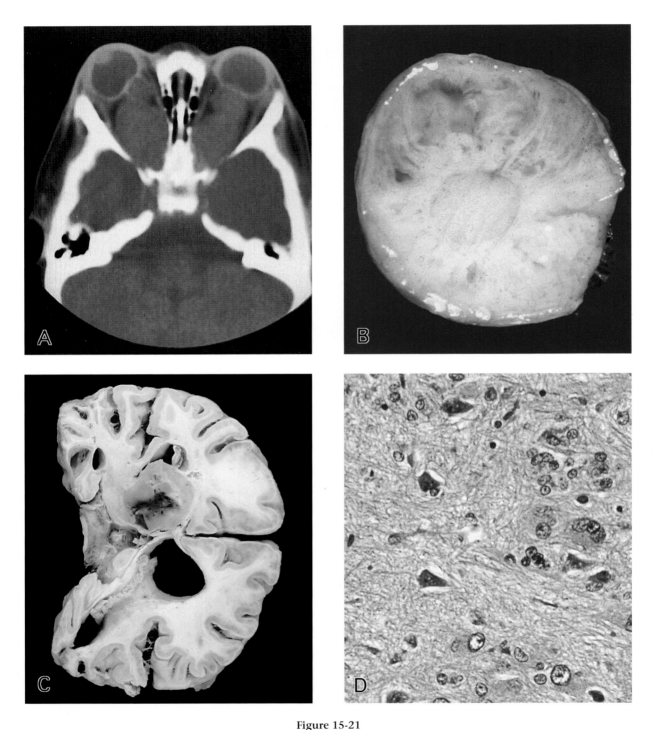

Figure 15-21

ASTROCYTOMAS IN NF1

Most common are optic nerve gliomas, nearly always low-grade tumors of pilocytic type. Such lesions may be bilateral (A) and often involve both the optic nerve and fill its surrounding leptomeningeal space (B), a pattern typical of, but not limited to, patients with NF1. Yet another favored location of pilocytic astrocytoma in NF1 is the thalamus (C). Glioneuronal hamartomas composed of dysmorphic neurons and astrocytes (D) are also seen. (A,B: Courtesy of Dr. L. Zimmerman, Washington, D.C.) (C,D: Figs. 3.495 and 3.498 from Okazaki H, Scheithauer BW. Atlas of neuropathology. New York: Gower; 1988:204-205. With permission from the Mayo Foundation.)

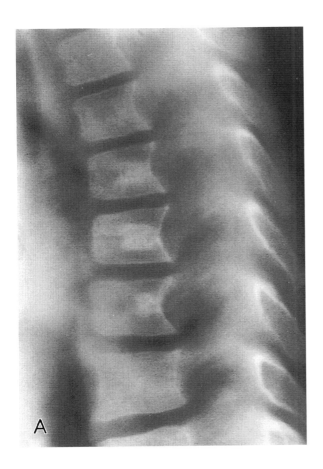

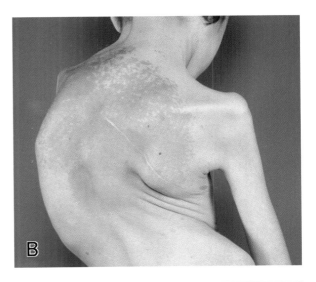

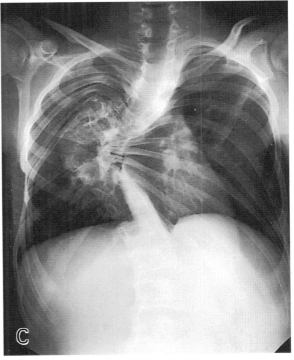

Figure 15-22

THE SPINE IN NF1

A: Abnormalities range from mild to marked. The scalloping of the vertebral bodies seen here is associated with widening of the spinal canal.

B,C: Kyphoscoliosis (B), a common manifestation of NF1, is usually related to dysplasia of vertebral bodies (C).

a component of NF2, approximately 5 percent of plexiform schwannomas occur in this setting (fig. 15-27) (85). Most sporadic schwannomas also show mutations in the *NF2* gene (86). On rare occasion, peripheral nerves show widespread nodular enlargement in the setting of a distal symmetric sensorimotor neuropathy (87,88).

Meningiomas. Meningiomas occur in the majority of patients with NF2, and multiple meningiomas may be the only feature of the

disorder (89). They arise earlier in life than sporadic examples, are often multiple or multicentric, and sometimes take the form of meningiomatosis in which diffuse or multifocal lesions involve both the cranial and spinal meninges (fig. 15-28). Multifocal meningiomas are not, however, pathognomonic of NF2. Studies of their distribution show that meningiomas occurring in NF2 are intracranial in 54 percent of cases, intracranial and intraspinal in 42 percent,

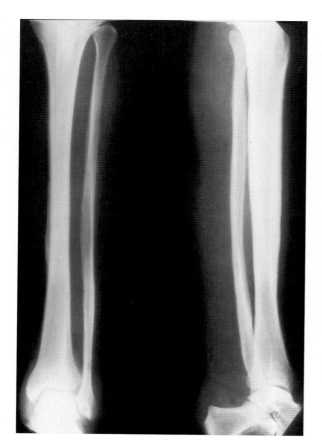
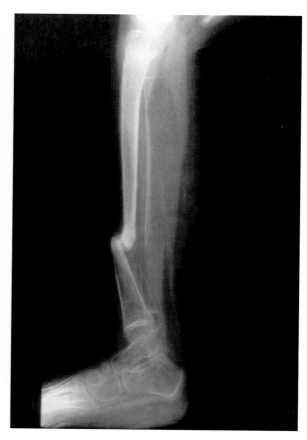

Figure 15-23

OSSEOUS ABNORMALITIES

These include dysplasia of the fibula (left) and postfracture pseudoarthroses, such as of the tibia (right).

Figure 15-24

VASCULOPATHY IN NF1

This lesion, characterized by subintimal proliferation, mild inflammation, and partial attenuation of the media, was associated with cortical infarction of the temporal lobes. (Fig. 3.505 from Okazaki H, Scheithauer BW. Atlas of neuropathology. New York: Gower; 1988:206. With permission from the Mayo Foundation.)

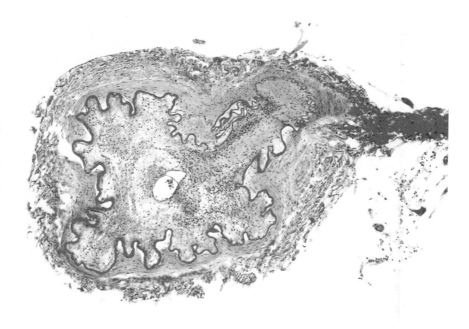

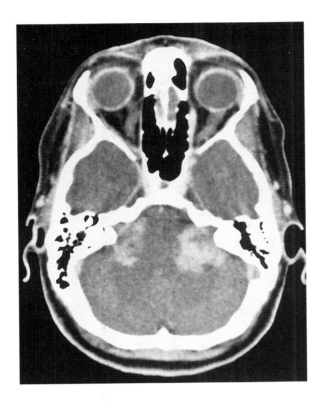

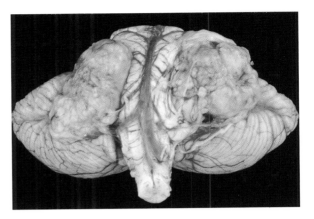

Figure 15-25

MULTIPLE SCHWANNOMAS IN NF2

Multiple schwannomas in NF2 include bilateral acoustic tumors, here shown on computerized tomography (CT) scan with contrast (left) and at autopsy (above), as well as multiple cranial or spinal nerve root schwannomas. (Left: Courtesy of Dr. P. C. Burger, Baltimore, MD; above: Fig. 3.505 from Okazaki H, Scheithauer BW. Atlas of neuropathology. New York: Gower; 1988:206. With permission from the Mayo Foundation.)

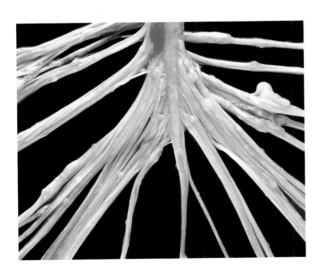

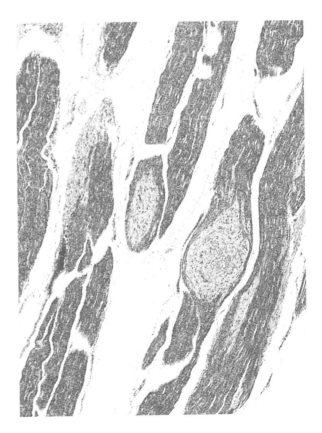

Figure 15-26

MULTIPLE SCHWANNOMAS IN NF2

Multiple cranial or spinal nerve root schwannomas arise in cauda equina nerve roots. (Right: hematoxylin and eosin [H&E]-Luxol-fast blue stain.) (Above: Fig. 3.492 from Okazaki H, Scheithauer BW. Atlas of neuropathology. New York: Gower; 1988:204. With permission from the Mayo Foundation; right: Courtesy of Dr. P.C. Burger, Baltimore, MD.)

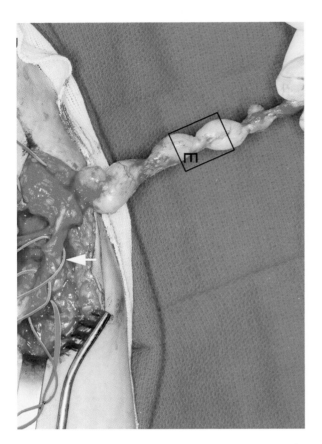 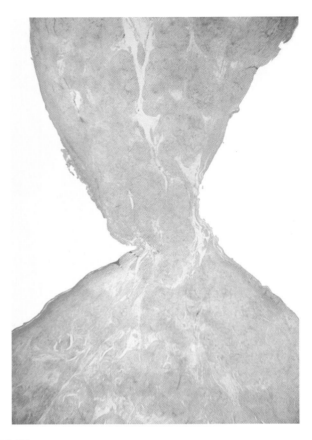

Figure 15-27

PLEXIFORM SCHWANNOMA

Left: At surgery, a multinodular lesion involves the median nerve (arrow) in a patient with NF2 presenting with neurologic impairment and a mass at the elbow. The imaging studies revealed involvement of other fascicles of the median nerve as well as of the ipsilateral radial and ulnar nerves.

Right: The microphotograph shows two joining nodules of the plexiform tumor. Continuity of the nodules is seen across the constricted portion. (Berg JC, Scheithauer BW, Spinner RJ, Allen CM, Koutlas IG. Plexiform schwannoma: a clinicopathologic overview with emphasis on the head and neck region. Hum Pathol 2008;39:633-640.)

but solely intraspinal in only 4 percent (90). The variants of meningioma occur with similar frequency in NF2-associated as compared to sporadic meningiomas, but multiple lesions (57 percent) and intraventricular tumors (13 percent) are more often observed (91).

The tumors in NF2 are not of higher grade, i.e., II or III (World Health Organization [WHO] classification 2007) than sporadic lesions, and are somewhat less often brain invasive (0 versus 7 percent). As with schwannomas, meningiomas exhibit mutations of the *NF2* gene, an occurrence highly associated with allelic loss of chromosome 22 (92,93). Other genotypic alterations are the same as those seen in sporadic meningiomas.

Meningioangiomatosis is an NF2-associated, rare lesion, in which meningothelial cells surrounding leptomeningeal and cortical vessels form single or multiple, firm, pale lesions that replace a segment of cerebral cortex (fig. 15-29A,B) (94). Some are associated with overlying coarse calcification, which often occupies a sulcus (fig. 15-29C). Similar calcifications occur in isolation, unassociated with meningioangiomatosis or NF2 (95). Meningiomas may supervene upon meningioangiomatosis (96).

Gliomas and Other CNS Lesions. In the setting of NF2, gliomas occur less commonly than either vestibular schwannomas or meningiomas. They involve the spinal cord or, less frequently, the cerebrum or cerebellum. Ependymomas account

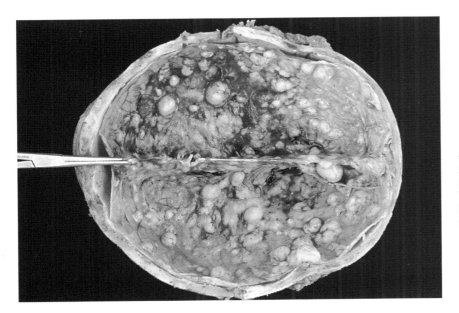

Figure 15-28

MULTIPLE MENINGIOMAS IN NF2

Such lesions sometimes cover the inner aspect of the dura. (Fig. 3.494 from Okazaki H, Scheithauer BW. Atlas of neuropathology. New York: Gower; 1988:204. With permission from the Mayo Foundation.)

for 70 percent and often present as multiple lesions (fig. 15-30) with a tendency to affect cervicothoracic levels (90). In addition, ependymomas may involve the filum terminale, a site also prone to the development of multiple schwannomas. Pilocytic or diffuse fibrillary astrocytomas of optic nerve, brainstem, cerebellum, or cerebrum are far less common in NF2 than in NF1.

Dysplastic lesions of the CNS may also be encountered but are unassociated with mental retardation. These include multiple glial microhamartomas affecting the cerebral cortex, cellular ependymal ectopias involving the spinal cord, intramedullary schwannosis, and syringomyelia (53,97,98). Of these lesions, none are preneoplastic. Other CNS lesions in NF2 include cerebral, cerebellar, periventricular, and choroid plexus calcifications (82).

Schwannoma-Meningioma Mixed Tumors. Particularly unusual are tumors composed of an intimate admixture of schwannoma and meningioma, a complex lesion most often associated with NF2 (12). Long recognized, the first example was mentioned by Cushing and Eisenhardt in their 1938 monograph entitled Meningiomas (99). To date, 10 cases have been published (84,100–103), all in the setting of NF2. The distribution of the two components varies from an admixture to very distinct zones of each tumor pattern. The pathogenesis of the lesion remains to be determined. The common cytogenesis of Schwann cells and some leptomeninges from neuroectoderm may provide an explanation. It is also tempting to consider mixed schwannoma-meningioma to be simply a collision tumor, particularly in a setting in which both lesions occur multifocally. Bona fide examples have been reported (104). Of relevance to an etiology are reports of florid meningothelial reaction in the leptomeninges surrounding optic gliomas in NF1, as well as at the periphery of 8th nerve schwannomas, both in association with NF2 (84,102) and in sporadic examples (105).

Prognosis. The majority of patients with NF2 die of CNS complications of the disorder (72), some within only 2 to 3 years of symptom onset. Most patients survive for longer periods, even into late middle age. The two distinct clinical presentations result in a different disease course. One, associated with a rapid disease course, was described by Wishart (106) and is characterized by the early onset of multiple tumors in addition to bilateral vestibular schwannomas (72,107). More protracted is the Gardner-Frazier type (108), the onset of which is late and features bilateral vestibular schwannomas alone (72,107). A 1971 study of 55 members of an NF2 kindred with bilateral acoustic schwannomas (109) found that 71 percent of the 38 patients in whom a cause of death was known died of bilateral acoustic schwannomas. The cause of death was variously attributed to brainstem compression, elevated intracranial pressure, or complications of surgery. Presently, in light of neurosurgical

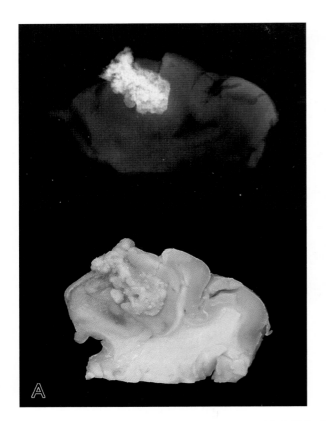

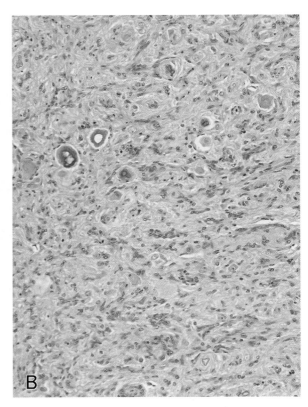

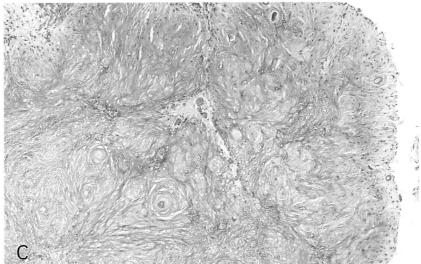

Figure 15-29

MENINGIOANGIOMATOSIS

Although this example is not NF2 associated, such lesions do show a distinct association with that disorder.

A: Fully formed, meningioangiomatosis consists of a firm pale cortical ribbon and an overlying leptomeningeal calcification. (Fig. 3.503 from Okazaki H, Scheithauer BW. Atlas of neuropathology. New York: Gower; 1988:206. With permission from the Mayo Foundation.)

B: The cortex is largely replaced by arachnoidal cells associated with an increased vasculature.

C: The often multinodular leptomeningeal calcification, which also may show osseous metaplasia, typically demonstrates peripheral hypercellularity.

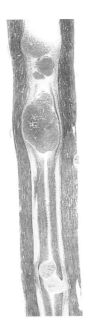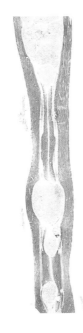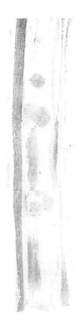

Figure 15-30

MULTIPLE SPINAL CORD EPENDYMOMAS IN NF2

This whole mount longitudinal section of the spinal cord shows numerous demarcated tumors of varying size. (Fig. 3.497 from Okazaki H, Scheithauer BW. Atlas of neuropathology. New York: Gower; 1988:205. With permission from the Mayo Foundation.)

advances, fewer patients die as a result of acoustic schwannomas. The second major cause of death, and currently the most difficult to treat, is the presence of spinal ependymomas, which are often multiple and usually occur in the cervicothoracic region. The slowly progressive growth of these tumors leads to destruction of the spinal tracts innervating the respiratory system.

SCHWANNOMATOSIS

General Features. As previously noted, NF1 and NF2 both share a predisposition to the development of nerve sheath tumors. A recent addition to the neurofibromatosis spectrum is *schwannomatosis*, an uncommon condition (estimated prevalence, 1 in 40,000) characterized by the occurrence of multiple, but not vestibular, schwannomas. Although it was long debated whether schwannomatosis is an attenuated form of NF2, it is now accepted as a separate syndrome (110).

The key feature of schwannomatosis is the occurrence of multiple schwannomas that vary in structure (fig. 15-31). Initially, schwannomas were thought to be the only neoplastic manifestation associated with this syndrome, however, recent reports suggest that schwannomatosis is also associated with meningiomas. Schwannomatosis is believed to be unassociated with non-neoplastic manifestations. Most cases are sporadic (85 percent), the remainder familial.

Clinically, pain is a key feature and may be disabling. Most patients present in the second or third decade. The distribution of schwannomas varies; in 30 percent of cases it is segmental. Peripheral, mainly spinal nerves are far more often affected (75 percent) than are subcutaneous (15 percent) or cranial (10 percent) nerves. The diagnostic criteria of schwannomatosis have been formulated by MacCollin (110) and modified by Baser (Table 15-4) (111).

All schwannomas have biallelic inactivation of the *NF2* gene, but only patients with NF2 have a germline mutation detectable in all tumors, in nontumor tissues from the same patient, and in tumors of different affected individuals in a family. *NF2* gene loss in schwannomatosis is not germline. It is detectable in tumors, but differs among various lesions in any one patient and in tumors from other affected family members. Lineage studies of schwannomatosis kindreds have placed the schwannomatosis locus centromeric to *NF2* on chromosome 22q, and mutation analysis of normal and tumor tissues in familial schwannomatosis has found germline mutations of the *SMARCB1/INI1* gene (112,113). Inactivation of this gene has been shown in malignant rhabdoid tumors to result in aneuploidy and chromosomal instability (114). Its deletion is also thought to promote chromosomal instability in Schwann cells in individuals with schwannomatosis. Although mutations of *SMARCB1/INI1* are not

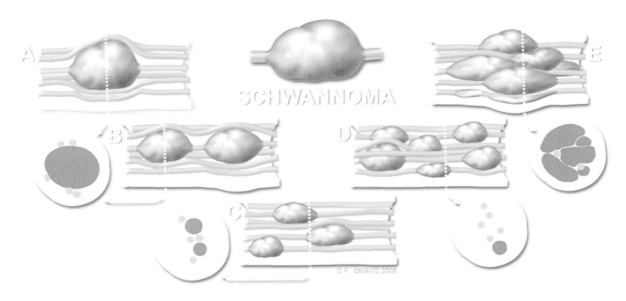

Figure 15-31

SCHWANNOMA IN SCHWANNOMATOSIS

A spectrum of gross morphologies, ranging from conventional globular lesions arising in a single fascicle (A), multiple examples affecting the same fascicle (B), and multiple tumors affecting multiple fascicles (C–E) are seen. Tumors affecting a single fascicle may be separated by normal nerve (B) or the lesions may abut one another. At surgery, complex multifascicular lesions (E) may be difficult to discern with respect the entry and exit of individual fascicles. (Copyright Mayo Foundation.)

Table 15-4

DIAGNOSTIC CRITERIA FOR SCHWANNOMATOSIS

Definite	Possible
Age >30 years	Age >30 years
2 or more nondermal schwannomas (at least 1 with histology)	2 or more nondermal schwannomas (at least 1 with histology)
No MRI evidence of a vestibular schwannoma	No vestibular schwannomas (MRI)
No known *NF2* germline mutation	No known *NF2* germline mutation
First-degree relative meeting above criteria	Age >45 years; 2 or more nondermal schwannomas (1 with histology)
One histologically proven peripheral schwannoma	No 8th nerve symptoms
	No known NF2 germline mutations

typically found in schwannomatosis (113), it has been proposed that a four-hit mechanism in which both *SMARCBI/INI1* and NF2 are inactivated (115) underlies the formation of schwannomas in this disorder (116).

Gross and Microscopic Findings. Radiographically, the schwannomas of schwannomatosis are similar to those of NF2, including the occurrence of plexiform/multinodular examples (fig. 15-32). The same is true of their gross appearance, which varies from globular lesions, sometimes multiple in a fascicle (fig. 15-33), to plexiform ones. The microscopic appearance often differs from conventional schwannoma in featuring myxoid change, often patchy, and peritumoral nerve edema in many instances

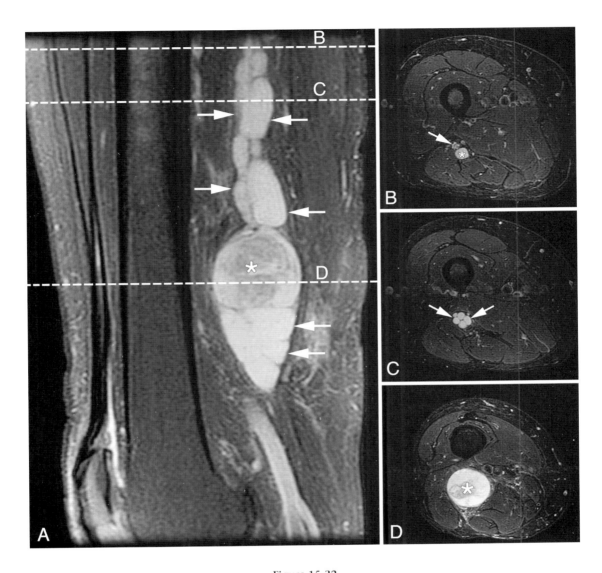

Figure 15-32

SCHWANNOMA

A: On fat suppression, the sagittal image of the right thigh reveals the longitudinal extent of the plexiform component of this sciatic nerve schwannoma. The peroneal component is more affected. Note the coexistent plexiform- (arrows) and conventional- (asterisk) appearing lesions.

B: An axial image of the upper thigh shows the enlarged fascicles (arrow) of the peroneal division of the sciatic nerve immediately adjacent to a conventional schwannoma (asterisk) arising from the tibial division.

C: An axial image of the mid thigh (inferior to B) demonstrates multiple enlarged fascicles of the peroneal division of the sciatic nerve (arrows), an appearance typical of a plexiform nerve sheath tumor.

D: The axial image of the lower third of the thigh (inferior to C) shows the typical imaging features of the more conventional schwannoma (asterisk). (Copyright Mayo Foundation.)

(figs. 15-33, 15-34). The immunophenotype of schwannomatosis-associated schwannomas is largely the same as that of conventional schwannomas (S-100 protein and collagen 4 positive).

Differential Diagnosis. The differential diagnosis includes a number of lesions, most im-

portantly neurofibroma (in particular, Schwann cell-rich neurofibroma), a tumor capable of malignant transformation. Neurofibromas also feature myxoid change and edema of peritumoral nerve. Their delicate exteriors, content of axons, occasional epithelial membrane

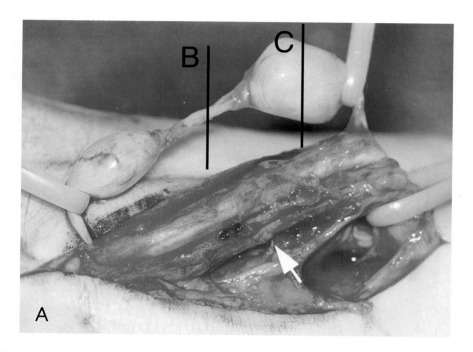

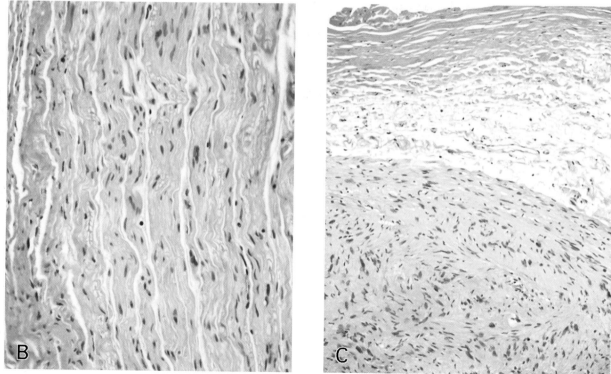

Figure 15-33

SCHWANNOMATOSIS

A: At surgery, a binodular lesion of the wrist involves a single fascicle in the median nerve (arrow) in a neurologically intact patient with schwannomatosis. There is subtle involvement of the other fascicles of the median nerve (arrow).

B: A segment of normal, unaffected myelinated nerve connects the two nodules.

C: Endoneurial edema surrounds the tumor. (Copyright Mayo Foundation.)

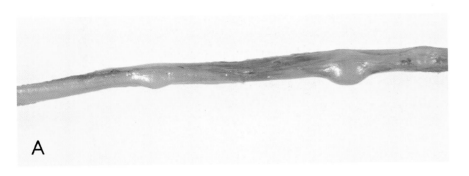

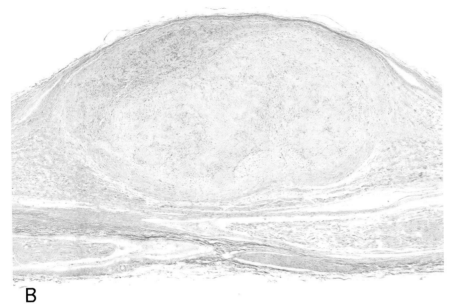

Figure 15-34

SCHWANNOMATOSIS

A: Two tumors are seen within a segment of nerve.

B: Longitudinal microsection of one schwannoma shows it to reside within a single fascicle. Three accompanying fascicles are normal (below).

C: Higher-power view of the tumor shows the endoneurium surrounding the tumor to be edematous. (Courtesy of Dr. P. Robbins, Perth, Australia.)

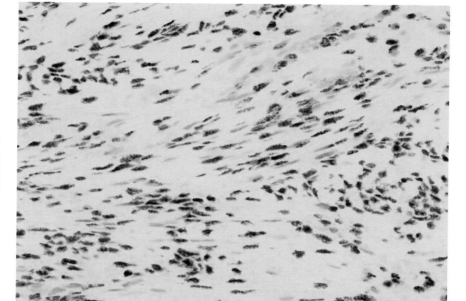

Figure 15-35

SCHWANNOMATOSIS

Loss of immunoreactivity for INI1, often partial due to mosaicism, is seen in 50% of sporadic and 90 percent of familial tumors. (Courtesy of Dr. P. Robbins, Perth, Australia.)

antigen (EMA)–positive perineurial-like cells, and frequent mast cells are of assistance in the distinction. In contrast, schwannomas of any kind only rarely become malignant.

In addition to neurofibroma, the histologic differential diagnosis includes variants of schwannoma: a cellular schwannoma that is more cellular, exhibits subcapsular chronic inflammation and histiocyte clusters, and lacks myxoid change as well as edema in peritumoral nerve; a plexiform schwannoma of the solitary type lacking myxoid change and peritumoral edema; nerve sheath myxoma; and hybrid lesions. Of the latter, those exhibiting a mixed pattern of schwannoma and perineurioma are most readily identified, given their content of S-100 protein–

positive Schwann cells as well as EMA/glut1/claudin-immunopositive perineurial cells.

Schwannomatosis lesions often show partial loss of INI-1 staining (mosaic pattern), more so in familial (93 percent) than in sporadic (50 percent) examples (fig. 15-35). NF2-associated schwannomas also often (83 percent) show a mosaic pattern of staining (112). In contrast, conventional schwannomas are only infrequently (5 percent) mosaics (113). Atypical teratoid rhabdoid tumor, a highly malignant brain tumor of childhood defined by its mutation of the *SMARCB1* gene and INI-1 immunonegativity, only rarely occurs in the setting of familial schwannomatosis (117). We have also observed an example.

REFERENCES

Neurofibromatosis

1. Riccardi VM. Neurofibromatosis: phenotype, natural history, and pathogenesis, 2nd ed. Baltimore: Johns Hopkins University Press; 1992.
2. Worster-Drought C, Carnegie-Dickson WH, McMenemey WH. Multiple meningeal and perineurial tumors of analogous changes in the glia and ependyma (neurofibroblastomatosis). With report of two cases. Brain 1937;60:85-117.
3. Riccardi VM. Von recklinghausen neurofibromatosis. N Engl J Med 1981;305:1617-1627.
4. Barker D, Wright E, Nguyen K, et al. Gene for von Recklinghausen neurofibromatosis is in the pericentromeric region of chromosome 17. Science 1987;236:1100-1102.
5. Louis DN, von Deimling A. Hereditary tumor syndromes of the nervous system: overview and rare syndromes. Brain Pathol 1995;5:145-151.
6. Viskochil D, Buchberg AM, Xu G, et al. Deletions and a translocation interrupt a cloned gene at the neurofibromatosis type 1 locus. Cell 1990;62:187-192.
7. Wallace MR, Marchuk DA, Andersen LB, et al. Type 1 neurofibromatosis gene: identification of a large transcript disrupted in three NF1 patients. Science 1990;249:181-186.
8. Seizinger BR, Rouleau GA, Ozelius LJ, et al. Genetic linkage of von Recklinghausen neurofibromatosis to the nerve growth factor receptor gene. Cell 1987;49:589-594.
9. Gutmann DH, Collins FS. Neurofibromatosis type 1. Beyond positional cloning. Arch Neurol 1993;50:1185-1193.
10. von Deimling A, Krone W, Menon AG. Neurofibromatosis type 1: pathology, clinical features and molecular genetics. Brain Pathol 1995;5:153-162.
11. Riccardi VM, Lewis RA. Penetrance of von Recklinghausen neurofibromatosis: a distinction between predecessors and descendants. Am J Hum Genet 1988;42:284-289.
12. Gutmann DH, Aylsworth A, Carey JC, et al. The diagnostic evaluation and multidisciplinary management of neurofibromatosis 1 and neurofibromatosis 2. JAMA 1997;278:51-57.
13. Akesson HO, Axelsson R, Samuelsson B. Neurofibromatosis in monozygotic twins: a case report. Acta Genet Med Gemellol 1983;32:245-249.
14. Schneider M, Obringer AC, Zackai E, Meadows AT. Childhood neurofibromatosis: risk factors for malignant disease. Cancer Genet Cytogenet 1986;21:347-354.
15. JimbJow K, Szabo G, Fitzpatrick TB. Ultrastructure of giant pigment granules (macromelanosomes) in the cutaneous pigmented macules of neurofibromatosis. J Invest Dermatol 1973;61:300-309.
16. Nevin S. Gliomatosis cerebri. Brain 1938;61:170-191.
17. Crowe FW, Schull WJ, Neel JV. A clinical, pathological, and genetic study of multiple neurofibromatosis. Springfield, IL: Thomas; 1956.
18. Tong AK, Fitzpatrick TB. The skin in neurofibromatosis. In: Rubenstein AE, Korf BR, eds. Neurofibromatosis: a handbook for patients, families, and health care professionals. New York: Thieme; 1990:88-09.
19. Lisch K. Uber Beteiligung der Augen, insbesondere das vorkommen von Irisknotchen bei der Neurofibromatose (Recklinghausen). Z Augenheilk 1937;93:137-143.
20. Lewis RA. Ocular features of neurofibromatosis. In: Rubenstein AE, Korf B, eds. Neurofibromatosis. A handbook for patients, families, and health care professionals. New York: Thieme; 1990:80-87.
21. Fialkow PJ, Sagebiel RW, Gartler SM, Rimoin DL. Multiple cell origin of hereditary neurofibromas. N Engl J Med 1971;284:298-300.
22. Skuse GR, Kosciolek BA, Rowley PT. The neurofibroma in von Recklinghausen neurofibromatosis has a unicellular origin. Am J Hum Genet 1991;49:600-607.
23. Friedman JM, Fialkow PJ, Greene CL, Weinberg MN. Probable clonal origin of neurofibrosarcoma in a patient with hereditary neurofibromatosis. J Natl Cancer Inst 1982;69:1289-1292.
24. Halling KC, Scheithauer BW, Halling AC, et al. P53 expression in neurofibroma and malignant peripheral nerve sheath tumor. An immunohistochemical study of sporadic and NF1-associated tumors. Am J Clin Pathol 1996;106:282-288.
25. Menon AG, Anderson KM, Riccardi VM, et al. Chromosome 17p deletions and p53 gene mutations associated with the formation of malignant neurofibrosarcomas in von Recklinghausen neurofibromatosis. Proc Natl Acad Sci U S A 1990;87:5435-5439.
26. Wiestler OD, Radner H. Pathology of neurofibromatosis 1 and 2. In: Huson SM, Hughes RA, eds. The neurofibromatoses: a pathogenetic and clinical overview. London: Chapman & Hall; 1994:139-155.
27. Halliday AL, Sobel RA, Martuza RL. Benign spinal nerve sheath tumors: their occurrence sporadically and in neurofibromatosis types 1 and 2. J Neurosurg 1991;74:248-253.
28. Rawlings CE 3rd, Wilkins RH, Cook WA, Burger PC. Segmental neurofibromatosis. Neurosurgery 1987;20:946-949.

29. Fuller CE, Williams GT. Gastrointestinal manifestations of type 1 neurofibromatosis (von Recklinghausen's disease). Histopathology 1991;19:1-11.

30. Hochberg FH, Dasilva AB, Galdabini J, Richardson EP Jr. Gastrointestinal involvement in von Recklinghausen's neurofibromatosis. Neurology 1974;24:1144-1151.

31. Ludwig J, Wester S, Elston AC. Evidence of neurofibromatosis and chronic myelogenous leukemia in a liver biopsy specimen. J Clin Gastroenterol 1993;16:265-267.

32. Partin JS, Lane BP, Partin JC, Edelstein LR, Priebe CJ Jr. Plexiform neurofibromatosis of the liver and mesentery in a child. Hepatology 1990;12:559-564.

33. Pung S, Hirsch EF. Plexiform neurofibromatosis of the heart and neck. AMA Arch Pathol 1955;59:341-346.

34. Pleasure J, Geller SA. Neurofibromatosis in infancy presenting with congenital stridor. Am J Dis Child 1967;113:390-393.

35. Cheng L, Scheithauer BW, Leibovich BC, Ramnani DM, Cheville JC, Bostwick DG. Neurofibroma of the urinary bladder. Cancer 1999;86:505-513.

36. Verhest A, Heimann R, Verschraegen J, Vamos E, Hecht F. Hereditary intestinal neurofibromatosis. Ii. Translocation between chromosomes 12 and 14. Neurofibromatosis 1988;1:33-36.

37. Gennatas CS, Exarhakos G, Kondi-Pafiti A, Kannas D, Athanassas G, Politi HD. Malignant schwannoma of the stomach in a patient with neurofibromatosis. Eur J Surg Oncol 1988;14:261-264.

38. Ghrist TD. Gastrointestinal involvement in neurofibromatosis. Arch Intern Med 1963;112:357-362.

39. Levy D, Khatib R. Intestinal neurofibromatosis with malignant degeneration: report of a case. Dis Colon Rectum 1960;3:140-144.

40. Dayal Y, Tallberg KA, Nunnemacher G, DeLellis RA, Wolfe HJ. Duodenal carcinoids in patients with and without neurofibromatosis. A comparative study. Am J Surg Pathol 1986;10:348-357.

41. Scheithauer BW, Nora FE, LeChago J, et al. Duodenal gangliocytic paraganglioma. Clinicopathologic and immunocytochemical study of 11 cases. Am J Clin Pathol 1986;86:559-565.

42. Stephens M, Williams GT, Jasani B, Williams ED. Synchronous duodenal neuroendocrine tumours in von recklinghausen's disease—a case report of co-existing gangliocytic paraganglioma and somatostatin-rich glandular carcinoid. Histopathology 1987;11:1331-1340.

43. Huson SM, Harper PS, Compston DA. Von recklinghausen neurofibromatosis. A clinical and population study in south-east Wales. Brain 1988;111(Pt 6):1355-1381.

44. Morier P, Merot Y, Paccaud D, Beck D, Frenk E. Juvenile chronic granulocytic leukemia, juvenile xanthogranulomas, and neurofibromatosis. Case report and review of the literature. J Am Acad Dermatol 1990;22:962-965.

45. Zvulunov A, Barak Y, Metzker A. Juvenile xanthogranuloma, neurofibromatosis, and juvenile chronic myelogenous leukemia. World statistical analysis. Arch Dermatol 1995;131:904-908.

46. Blatt J, Jaffe R, Deutsch M, Adkins JC. Neurofibromatosis and childhood tumors. Cancer 1986;57:1225-1229.

47. Borit A, Richardson EP Jr. The biological and clinical behaviour of pilocytic astrocytomas of the optic pathways. Brain 1982;105:161-187.

48. Davis FA. Primary tumors of the optic nerve (a phenomenon of Recklinghausen's disease). A clinical and pathologic study with a report of five cases and review of the literature. Arch Ophthalmol 1940;23:735-821.

49. Lewis RA, Gerson LP, Axelson KA, Riccardi VM, Whitford RP. Von Recklinghausen neurofibromatosis. II. Incidence of optic gliomata. Ophthalmology 1984;91:929-935.

50. Lund AM, Skovby F. Optic gliomas in children with neurofibromatosis type 1. Eur J Pediatr 1991;150:835-838.

51. van der Meulen J. Orbital neurofibromatosis. Clin Plast Surg 1987;14:123-135.

52. Ilgren EB, Kinnier-Wilson LM, Stiller CA. Gliomas in neurofibromatosis: a series of 89 cases with evidence for enhanced malignancy in associated cerebellar astrocytomas. Pathol Annu 1985;20(Pt 1):331-358.

53. Rubinstein LJ. The malformative central nervous system lesions in the central and peripheral forms of neurofibromatosis. A neuropathological study of 22 cases. Ann N Y Acad Sci 1986;486:14-29.

54. De Ajuriaguerra J, David M, Hagueneau F. Glios meningocerebelleuse et malidie de recklinghausen. Rev Neurol (Paris) 1955;93:645-655.

55. Manuelidis EE, Solitare GB. Glioblastoma multiforme. In: Minckler J, ed. Pathology of the nervous system. New York: McGraw-Hill; 1971:2026-2071.

56. Parry DM, MacCollin MM, Kaiser-Kupfer MI, et al. Germ-line mutations in the neurofibromatosis 2 gene: correlations with disease severity and retinal abnormalities. Am J Hum Gen 1996;59:529-539.

57. Russell, DS, Rubinstein LJ. Pathology of tumours of the nervous system, 5th ed. Baltimore: Williams & Wilkins; 1989:769-784.

58. Walker AE. Astrocytosis arachnoideae cerebelli. A rare manifestation of von Recklinghausen's neurofibromatosis. Arch Neurol Psychiatry 1941;45:520-532.

59. Chutorian A. Panel on diagnosis and natural history of optic nerve glioma. Optic gliomas in neurofibromatosis. Conference series. New York: The National Neurofibromatosis Foundation, Inc.; 1989:55-62.

60. Hunt JC, Pugh DG. Skeletal lesions in neurofibromatosis. Radiology 1961;76:1-20.

61. MacEwen GD. Orthopedic aspects of neurofibromatosis. In: Rubenstein AE, Korf BR, eds. Neurofibromatosis. A handbook for patients, families, and health care professionals. New York: Thieme; 1990:125-141.

62. Fairbank J. Orthopaedic manifestations of neurofibromatosis. In: Huson SM, Hughes RA, eds. The neurofibromatosis: a pathogenetic and clinical overview. London: Chapman & Hall; 1994:275-304.

63. Feyrter F. Uber die vasculare neurofibromatose, nach untersuchungen am menschlichen magendarmschlauch. Virchow Arch A 1949;317:221-265.

64. Greene JF Jr, Fitzwater JE, Burgess J. Arterial lesions associated with neurofibromatosis. Am J Clin Pathol 1974;62:481-487.

65. Reubi F. Les vaisseaux et les glandes endocrines dans la neurofibromatose: Le syndrome sympathi cotonique dans la maladie de Recklinghausen. Schweiz Z Pathol Bakteriol 1944;7:168-236.

66. Salyer WR, Salyer DC. The vascular lesions of neurofibromatosis. Angiology 1974;25:510-519.

67. Finley JL, Dabbs DJ. Renal vascular smooth muscle proliferation in neurofibromatosis. Hum Pathol 1988;19:107-110.

68. Malecha MJ, Rubin R. Aneurysms of the carotid arteries associated with von Recklinghausen's neurofibromatosis. Pathol Res Pract 1992;188:145-147.

69. Elias DL, Ricketts RR, Smith RB 3rd. Renovascular hypertension complicating neurofibromatosis. Am Surg 1985;51:97-106.

70. Halpern M, Currarino G. Vascular lesions causing hypertension in neurofibromatosis. N Engl J Med 1965;273:248-252.

71. Evans DG, Bourn D, Wallace A, Ramsden RT, Mitchell JD, Strachan T. Diagnostic issues in a family with late onset type 2 neurofibromatosis. J Med Gen 1995;32:470-474.

72. Evans DG, Huson SM, Donnai D, et al. A clinical study of type 2 neurofibromatosis. Q J Med 1992;84:603-618.

73. Rouleau GA, Wertelecki W, Haines JL, et al. Genetic linkage of bilateral acoustic neurofibromatosis to a DNA marker on chromosome 22. Nature 1987;329:246-248.

74. Rouleau GA, Merel P, Lutchman M, et al. Alteration in a new gene encoding a putative membrane-organizing protein causes neuro-fibromatosis type 2. Nature 1993;363:515-521.

75. Thomas PK, King RH, Chiang TR, Scaravilli F, Sharma AK, Downie AW. Neurofibromatous neuropathy. Muscle Nerve 1990;13:93-101.

76. Louis DN, Ramesh V, Gusella JF. Neuropathology and molecular genetics of neurofibromatosis 2 and related tumors. Brain Pathol 1995;5:163-172.

77. Mautner VF, Lindenau M, Baser ME, Kluwe L, Gottschalk J. Skin abnormalities in neurofibromatosis 2. Arch Dermatol 1997;133:1539-1543.

78. Eldridge R. Neurofibromatosis type 2. In: Rubinstein AE, Korf BR, eds. Neurofibromatosis: A handbook for patients, families, and health-care professionals. New York: Thieme; 1990:29-39.

79. Ragge NK, Baser ME, Klein J, et al. Ocular abnormalities in neurofibromatosis 2. Am J Ophthalmol 1995;120:634-641.

80. Eldridge R. Central neurofibromatosis with bilateral acoustic neuroma. Adv Neurol 1981;29:57-65.

81. Kanter WR, Eldridge R, Fabricant R, Allen JC, Koerber T. Central neurofibromatosis with bilateral acoustic neuroma: genetic, clinical and biochemical distinctions from peripheral neurofibromatosis. Neurology 1980;30:851-859.

82. Ruttledge MH, Andermann AA, Phelan CM, et al. Type of mutation in the neurofibromatosis type 2 gene (NF2) frequently determines severity of disease. Am J Hum Genet 1996;59:331-342.

83. Short PM, Martuza RL, Huson SM. Neurofibromatosis 2: Clinical features, genetic counselling and management issues. In: Huson SM, Hughes RA, eds. The neurofibromatoses: A pathogenetic and clinical overview. London: Chapman & Hall Medical; 1994:414-444.

84. Geddes JF, Sutcliffe JC, King TT. Mixed cranial nerve tumors in neurofibromatosis type 2. Clin Neuropathol 1995;14:310-313.

85. Berg JC, Scheithauer BW, Spinner RJ, Allen CM, Koutlas IG. Plexiform schwannoma: a clinicopathologic overview with emphasis on the head and neck region. Hum Pathol 2008;39:633-640.

86. Jacoby LB, MacCollin M, Louis DN, et al. Exon scanning for mutation of the NF2 gene in schwannomas. Hum Mol Genet 1994;3:413-419.

87. Onishi A, Nada O. Ultrastructure of the onion bulb-like lamellated structure observed in the sural nerve in a case of von Recklinghausen's disease. Acta Neuropathol 1972;20:258-263.

88. Sobel RA. Vestibular (acoustic) schwannomas: histologic features in neurofibromatosis 2 and in unilateral cases. J Neuropathol Exp Neurol 1993;52:106-113.

89. Battersby RD, Ironside JW, Maltby EL. Inherited multiple meningiomas: a clinical, pathological and cytogenetic study of an affected family. J Neurol Neurosurg Psychiatry 1986;49:362-368.

90. Rodriguez HA, Berthrong M. Multiple primary intracranial tumors in von Recklinghausen's neurofibromatosis. Arch Neurol 1966;14:467-475.

91. Perry A, Giannini C, Raghavan R, et al. Aggressive phenotypic and genotypic features in pediatric and nf2-associated meningiomas: a clinicopathologic study of 53 cases. J Neuropathol Exp Neurol 2001;60:994-1003.

92. Lekanne Deprez RH, Bianchi AB, et al. Frequent NF2 gene transcript mutations in sporadic meningiomas and vestibular schwannomas. Am J Hum Genet 1994;54:1022-1029.

93. Trofatter JA, MacCollin MM, Rutter JL, et al. A novel moesin-, ezrin-, radixin-like gene is a candidate for the neurofibromatosis 2 tumor suppressor. Cell 1993;72:791-800.

94. Halper J, Scheithauer BW, Okazaki H, Laws ER Jr. Meningio-angiomatosis: a report of six cases with special reference to the occurrence of neurofibrillary tangles. J Neuropathol Exp Neurol 1986;45:426-446.

95. Bertoni F, Unni KK, Dahlin DC, Beabout JW, Onofrio BM. Calcifying pseudoneoplasms of the neural axis. J Neurosurg 1990;72:42-48.

96. Perry A, Kurtkaya-Yapicier O, Scheithauer BW, et al. Insights into meningioangiomatosis with and without meningioma: a clinicopathologic and genetic series of 24 cases with review of the literature. Brain Pathol 2005;15:55-65.

97. Poser CM. The relationship between syringomyelia and neoplasm. Springfield, IL: Thomas; 1956.

98. Wiestler OD, von Siebenthal K, Schmitt HP, Feiden W, Kleihues P. Distribution and immunoreactivity of cerebral micro-hamartomas in bilateral acoustic neurofibromatosis (neurofibromatosis 2). Acta Neuropathol 1989;79:137-143.

99. Cushing H, Eisenhardt L. Meningiomas, their classification, regional behaviour, life history, and surgical end results. Springfield, IL: Thomas; 1938.

100. Davidoff LM, Martin J. Hereditary combined neurinomas and meningiomas. J Neurosurg 1955;12:375-384.

101. Elizabeth J, Menon G, Nair S, Radhakrishnan VV. Mixed tumour of schwannoma and meningioma in a patient with neurofibromatosis-2: a case report. Neurol India 2001;49:398-400.

102. Gelal F, Rezanko T, Uyaroglu MA, Tunakan M, Bezircioglu H. Islets of meningioma in an acoustic schwannoma in a patient with neurofibromatosis-2: pathology and magnetic resonance imaging findings. Acta Radiol 2005;46:519-522.

103. Kim DG, Paek SH, Chi JG, Chun YK, Han DH. Mixed tumour of schwannoma and meningioma components in a patient with nf-2. Acta Neurochir (Wien) 1997;139:1061-1064; discussion 1064-1065.

104. Muzumdar DP, Goel A. Acoustic schwannoma and petroclival meningioma occurring as collision tumours: a case report. J Clin Neurosci 2004;11:207-210.

105. Ludemann W, Stan AC, Tatagiba M, Samii M. Sporadic unilateral vestibular schwannoma with islets of meningioma: case report. Neurosurgery 2000;47:451-452; discussion 452-454.

106. Wishart JH. Case of tumours in the skull, dura mater, and brain. Edinburgh Med Surg J 1882;18:393-397.

107. Eldridge R, Parry DM, Kaiser-Kupfer MI. Neurofibromatosis 2 (NF2): clinical heterogeneity and natural history based on 39 individuals in 9 families and 16 sporadic cases. Proceedings of the Eighth International Congress on Human Genetics. Am J Hum Gen 1991;49:133.

108. Gardner WJ, Frazier CH. Bilateral acoustic neurofibromas. A clinical study and field survey of a family of five generations with bilateral deafness in 38 members. Arch Neurol Psychiatry 1930;23:266-302.

109. Young DF, Eldridge R, Nager GT, Deland FH, McNew J. Hereditary bilateral acoustic neuroma (central neurofibromatosis). Birth Defects Orig Artic Ser 1971;07:73-86.

Schwannomatosis

110. MacCollin M, Chiocca EA, Evans DG, et al. Diagnostic criteria for schwannomatosis. Neurology 2005;64:1838-1845.

111. Baser ME, Friedman JM, Evans DG. Increasing the specificity of diagnostic criteria for schwannomatosis. Neurology 2006;66:730-732.

112. Hulsebos TJ, Kenter SB, Jakobs ME, Baas F, Chong B, Delatycki MB. SMARCB1/INI1 maternal germ line mosaicism in schwannomatosis. Clin Genet 2010;77:86-91.

113. Rousseau G, Noguchi T, Bourdon V, Sobol H, Olschwang S. SMARCB1/INI1 germline mutations contribute to 10% of sporadic schwannomatosis. BMC Neurol 2011;11:9.

114. Vries RG, Bezrookove V, Zuijderduijn LM, et al. Cancer-associated mutations in chromatin remodeler hSNF5 promote chromosomal instability by compromising the mitotic checkpoint. Genes Dev 2005;19:665-670.

115. Sestini R, Bacci C, Sestini R, Genuardi M, Papi L. Evidence of a four-hit mechanism involving SMARCB1 and NF2 in schwannomatosis-associated schwannomas. Hum Mutat 2008;29:227-231.

116. Carroll SL. Molecular mechanisms promoting the pathogenesis of Schwann cell neoplasms. Acta Neuropathol 2012;123:321-348.

117. Swensen JJ, Keyser J, Coffin CM, Biegel JA, Viskochil DH, Williams MS. Familial occurrence of schwannomas and malignant rhabdoid tumour associated with a duplication in smarcb1. J Med Genet 2009;46:68-72.

Index*

A

Adipose lesions, 111
    classification, 111
Adrenal adenoma, 366
Alveolar soft part sarcoma, differentiation from malignant granular cell tumor, 463
Amputation neuroma, *see* Traumatic neuroma
Amyloidoma, 373
Anatomy, normal nerve, 11
    ganglia, 21
    interstitial cell of Cajal, 25
    nerve endings, 26
    peripheral nerves, 14
Ancient schwannoma, 156
Angioleiomyoma, differentiation from palisaded encapsulated neuroma, 87
Angioma, 350
Angiosarcoma, **369**, 434
    and MPNST, 434
Appendiceal neuroma, 95
Arteriovenous malformation, 350
Astrocytoma and NF1, 517
Atypical cellular perineurioma, 278
Autonomic ganglia, 22

B

Benign granular cell tumor, *see* Granular cell tumor, benign
Benign triton tumor, 122
Bilateral acoustic neurofibromatosis, *see* Neurofibromatosis 2

C

Carcinoma metastatic to nerve, 503
Carney complex, and melanotic schwannoma, 188
Cellular schwannoma, 131, **165**, 407, 540
    clinical features, 166
    differentiation from conventional schwannoma, 160; from MPNST, 162, 177, 407; from neurofibroma, 177; from leiomyosarcoma, 177; from fibrosarcoma, 177; from meningioma, 178; from schwannomatosis, 540
    DNA flow cytometry, 176

    general features, 166
    gross and microscopic findings, 166
    immunohistochemical findings, 170
    treatment and prognosis, 178
    ultrastructural findings, 176
Central acoustic neurofibromatosis, *see* Neurofibromatosis 2
Congenital and childhood plexiform cellular schwannoma, 184
Conventional schwannoma, 40, 87, 93, **129**, 253, 289, 382, 423
    ancient schwannoma, 156
    cellular schwannoma, 131, *see also* Cellular schwannoma
    clinical features, 131
    differentiation from traumatic neuroma, 40; from inflammatory pseudotumor or nerve, 71; from palisaded encapsulated neuroma, 87; from mucosal neuroma, 93; from cellular schwannoma, 131; from malignant peripheral nerve sheath tumor, 131; from neurofibroma, 131, 160, 253; from perineurioma, 131; from nerve sheath myxoma, 162, 305; from leiomyoma, 162; from ganglioneuroma, 164, 337; from gastrointestinal stromal tumor, 164, 486; from palisaded myofibroblastoma, 164; from meningioma, 165, 364; from melanotic schwannoma, 199
    epithelioid schwannoma, 152
    general features, 129
    genetics, 130
    gross findings, 139
    immunohistochemical findings, 156
    intracranial schwannoma, 137
    intraspinal schwannoma, 138
    microcystic/reticular schwannoma, 152
    microscopic findings, 141
    plexiform schwannoma, 131
    predisposing factors, 131
    pseudoglands, 155
    radiation-induced schwannoma, 131
    radiographic features, 132
    schwannomatosis, 131
    treatment and prognosis, 165

*In a series of numbers, those in boldface indicate the main discussion of the entity.

ultrastructural findings, 159
variants, 131
visceral schwannoma, 139
with epithelioid malignancy, 423
Cowden syndrome, and ganglioneuromatosis, 101
Cranial nerve lipoma, 347
Cutaneous meningioma, 366
Cutaneous myxoma, differentiation from nerve
  sheath myxoma, 303

D

Dendritic cell neurofibroma with pseudorosettes, 253
Dermatofibrosarcoma protuberans, differentiation
  from neurofibroma, 253
Development, normal nerve, 11
Diffuse cutaneous neurofibroma, 215
Dorsal root ganglia, 21
Dysplastic gangliocytoma of cerebellum, and
  mucosal ganglioneuromatosis, 101

E

Endometriosis of sciatic nerve, 57
Endoneurium, normal, 15
Epineurium, normal, 13
Epithelial differentiation, 438
Epithelial sheath neuroma, **52**
  differentiation from metastatic carcinoma, 52
Epithelioid malignant change, 423, 425
Epithelioid malignant peripheral nerve sheath
  tumor, 416
  conventional schwannoma with epithelioid
    malignancy, 423
  deep epithelioid MPNST, 416
  neurofibroma with malignant epithelioid cell
    differentiation, 427
  superficial epithelioid MPNST, 423
Epithelioid malignant peripheral nerve sheath
  tumor ex-schwannoma, 423
Epithelioid schwannoma, 152

F

Fibrolipomatosis, 111
Fibrolipomatous hamartoma, 111
Fibrosarcoma, 177, 409
  differentiation from cellular schwannoma, 177;
    from MPNST, 407

G

Ganglia,
  autonomic, 22, *see also* Autonomic ganglia
  sensory, 20, *see also* Sensory ganglia
Ganglion cells, 21
Ganglion cyst of nerve, 53
  clinical features, 54
  definition and general features, 53
  differential diagnosis, 57
  gross findings, 54
  microscopic findings, 56
  radiologic features, 54
  treatment and prognosis, 57
Ganglioneuroblastoma, 338, 450
  and MPNST, 450
  differentiation from ganglioneuroma, 338
Ganglioneuroma, 95, 164, 255, **319,** 450
  and MPNST, 450
  association with ectomesenchymoma and
    gangliorhabdomyosarcoma, 338
  association with NF1 and MEN 2B, 319
  clinical features, 320
  differentiation from conventional schwannoma,
    164, 337; from neurofibroma, 253, 337;
    from immature ganglioneuroma, 338;
    from ganglioneuroblastoma, 338
  endocrine effects, 322
  general features, 319
  gross findings, 322
  immunohistochemical findings, 332
  microscopic findings, 325
  mucosal ganglioneuroma, 98
  radiologic features, 322
  solitary polypoid intestinal ganglioneuroma, 98
  treatment and prognosis, 338
  ultrastructural findings, 334
Ganglioneuromatosis, 87, **100**
  association with Cowden syndrome, 101
  association with juvenile polyposis, colonic
    adenoma, and adenocarcinoma, 101
  association with GIST, 101
Ganglioneuromatosis polyposis, 101
Gardner-Frazier neurofibromatosis 2, 521
Gastrointestinal autonomic nerve tumor, 475
Gastrointestinal stromal tumor (GIST), 101, 139, **475**
  and interstitial cells of Cajal, 475, 476
  associated syndromes, 475
  association with ganglioneuromatosis, 101

cytologic findings, 478
differentiation from conventional schwannoma, 164, 486
familial GIST, 476, 477
general features, 475
gross and microscopic findings, 476
immunohistochemical findings, 482
molecular findings, 483
NF1 association, 476
prognosis, 487
treatment, 486
ultrastructural findings, 483
Glandular differentiation, 438
Glioma, optic, and NF1, 517
Glomangioma, 356
Glomus tumors, 351
Gorlin-Koutlas syndrome, and conventional schwannoma, 131
Granular cell tumor, benign, 305
clinical features, 305
differentiation from mammary adenocarcinoma, 317; from other granular cell tumors, 317
general features, 305
gross and microscopic findings, 307
hybrid granular cell-perineurial cell tumors, 312
immunohistochemical findings, 308
ultrastructural findings, 312
treatment and prognosis, 319
Granular cell tumor, malignant, 458
differentiation from leiomyosarcoma, 463; from alveolar soft part sarcoma, 463
Granular cell/perineurial cell tumor, 312

H

Hemangioblastoma, 356
Hemangioma, 350
Hemangiopericytoma, 369
Heterotopic ossification of nerve, 60
Histologic techniques, normal nerve, 25
Hybrid granular cell-perineurial cell tumors, 312
Hybrid peripheral nerve sheath tumors, **289**, 312
differential diagnosis, 292
Hybrid reticular (retiform) schwannoma/perineurioma, 289
Hybrid schwannoma/neurofibroma, 240
Hybrid schwannoma/perineurioma, 289
differential diagnosis, 292

Hyperplastic lesions, 81, *see also under individual entities*
localized hypertrophic neuropathy, 101
MEN 2B-associated lesions, 87
MEN 2B-unassociated lesions, 95
palisaded encapsulated neuroma, 81

I

Immature ganglioneuroma, differentiation from ganglioneuroma, 338, 339
Immunohistochemistry, normal nerve, 28
Infectious simulators of nerve tumor, 67, *see also under individual entities*
leprous neuropathy, 75
mycobacterial pseudotumor, 73
sarcoidosis, 71
Inflammatory lesions simulating nerve tumors, 67
Inflammatory myofibroblastic tumor, *see* Inflammatory pseudotumor of nerve
Inflammatory pseudotumor of nerve, 67
differentiation from schwannoma, 71; from infection, 71
Inflammatory simulators of nerve tumors, 67
Interstitial cells of Cajal (ICC), 2, **25**, 475, 476
and GIST, 475
Intestinal ganglioneuromatosis, 87
Intestinal neuroma, 95
Intestinal perineurioma, 286
differential diagnosis, 286
Intracranial schwannoma, 137
Intraneural ganglion, *see* Ganglion cyst of nerve
Intraneural injury neuroma, 50
Intraneural perineurioma, 102, **266**
differentiation from localized hypertrophic neuropathy, 104; from hypertrophic neuropathies, 274
Intraspinal schwannoma, 138

L

Leiomyoma, 162
differentiation from conventional schwannoma, 162; from plexiform schwannoma, 183
Leiomyosarcoma, 177, 407, 433, 463
differentiation from cellular schwannoma, 177; from MPNST, 407; from malignant triton tumor, 433; from malignant granular cell tumor, 463
Lepromatous leprosy, 76
Leprosy, 75

Leprous neuropathy, 75
  clinical features, 75
  differential diagnosis, 78
  general features, 75
  gross and microscopic findings, 75
  lepromatous leprosy, 76
  treatment and prognosis, 78
  tuberculoid leprosy, 75
Leukemia metastatic to nerve, 491
Lipochoristoma, 347
Lipofibroma, 111
Lipofibromatous hamartoma, 111
Lipoma, 347
  cranial nerve lipoma, 347
  of nerve sheath, 347
  spinal epidural lipomatosis, 347
Lipomatosis of nerve, 111
  differentiation from other adipose lesions, 116
Localized cutaneous neurofibroma, 213
Localized hypertrophic neuropathy, 95, **101**
  differentiation from intraneural perineurioma, 104
Localized interdigital neuritis, 35, **41**
  differentiation from traumatic neuroma, 35, 42
Localized intraneural neurofibroma, 218
Lymphoid hyperplasia, *see* Inflammatory pseudo-
    tumor of nerve
Lymphoma metastatic to nerve, 491

M

Macrodystrophia lipomatosa, 111
Malignant granular cell tumor, *see* Granular cell
    tumor, malignant
Malignant peripheral nerve sheath tumors (MPNSTs),
    122, 131, 162, 172, 177, 211, 366, **381**, 450, 499
  arising in peripheral neuroblastic tumors, 450
    in ganglioneuroma/ganglioneuroblastoma, 450
    in pheochromocytoma, 455
  association with chemicals, 384
  association with ionizing radiation, 383
  association with NF1, 382; with NF2, 383
  association with xeroderma pigmentosum, 383
  childhood MPNST, 384
  clinical features, 385
  clinical settings, 382
  cranial nerve MPNST, 385
  cytologic findings, 401
  differential diagnosis, 407; differentiation from
    neuromuscular choristoma, 122; from conven-
    tional schwannoma, 136, 162; from cellular

schwannoma, 136, 177, 407; from neurofi-
    broma, 253, 407, 408; from synovial sarcoma,
    369, 408; from perineurioma, 408; from
    leiomyosarcoma, 409; from fibrosarcoma, 409;
    from melanoma, 409; differentiation from
    neurotropic melanoma, 499
  epithelioid MPNST, 416, *see also* Epithelioid
    malignant peripheral nerve sheath tumor
  frozen section diagnosis, 410
  general features, 382
  grading, 406
  gross findings, 387
  histologic criteria, 402
  immunohistochemical findings, 403
  microscopic findings, 391
  molecular findings, 406
  nerve localization, 385
  perineurial cell MPNST, 414
  prognosis, 413
  radiologic features, 386
  recurrence and metastasis, 412
  Schwann cell-derived MPNST, 416, *see also*
    Schwann cell-derived malignant peripheral
    nerve sheath tumor
  treatment, 413
  ultrastructural findings, 403
  visceral MPNST, 386
  with divergent epithelial differentiation, 438
    with glandular differentiation, 438
    with primitive neuroepithelial tumor, 441
  with divergent mesenchymal differentiation, 431
    with angiosarcoma, 433
    with rhabdomyosarcoma, 431
Malignant peripheral nerve sheath tumor with
    angiosarcoma, 433
Malignant peripheral nerve sheath tumor with
    glandular differentiation, 438
Malignant peripheral nerve sheath tumor with
    neuroepithelial tumor, 441
Malignant peripheral nerve sheath tumor with
    rhabdomyosarcoma, 431
  differentiation from rhabdomyosarcoma, 433;
    from leiomyosarcoma, 433
Malignant triton tumor, 431, *see* Malignant
    peripheral nerve sheath tumor with
    rhabdomyosarcoma
Massive soft tissue neurofibroma, 223
Masson, Pierre, 4
Meissner corpuscles, 27

Melanocytoma, differentiation from melanotic schwannoma, 201

Melanoma, metastatic, 199, 410, 491
  differentiation from melanotic schwannoma, 201; from MPNST, 409
  neurotropic melanoma, 495

Melanotic schwannoma, 187
  association with Carney complex, 188
  clinical features, 188
  cytopathologic findings, 199
  differentiation from conventional schwannoma, 199; from pigmented neurofibroma, 201; from melanocytoma, 201; from metastatic melanoma, 202
  general features, 187
  gross findings, 190
  immunohistochemical and ultrastructural findings, 199
  malignancy, 191
  microscopic findings, 190
  psammomatous melanotic schwannoma, 190, 199
  treatment and prognosis, 202

Meningeal carcinomatosis, 491

Meningioma, 162, 165, 178, **361**, 529, 533
  and NF2, 529
  and schwannoma, 533
  cutaneous meningioma, 366
  differentiation from conventional schwannoma, 165, 364; from cellular schwannoma, 178; from perineurioma, 364

Meningiomatosis, 529

Metastases to nerve, *see* Secondary tumors

Microcystic schwannoma, 152

Microschwannoma, 240

Morton neuroma, *see* Localized interdigital neuritis

Morton node, *see* Localized interdigital neuritis

Morton toe, *see* Localized interdigital neuritis

Mucinous ganglion cyst, *see* Ganglion cyst of nerve

Mucosal ganglioneuroma, *see* Ganglioneuroma

Mucosal ganglioneuromatosis, *see* Ganglioneuromatosis

Mucosal neurogenic appendicopathy, 95

Mucosal neuroma, 35, **87**
  differentiation from traumatic neuroma, 35, 93; from palisaded encapsulated neuroma, 87

Mucosal neuromatosis, 87

Multiple endocrine neoplasia (MEN), 87

Multiple endocrine neoplasia-associated nerve tumors, **87**, 319

clinical features, 88
  differentiation from traumatic neuroma, 93; from palisaded encapsulated neuroma, 93; from schwannoma, 93
  general features, 87
  ganglioneuroma, 319
  intestinal ganglioneuromatosis, 87
  microscopic findings, 90
  mucosal neuroma, 87
  mucosal neuromatosis, 87

Multiple endocrine neoplasia (MEN)-unassociated nerve tumors, 95, *see also under individual entities*
  mucosal ganglioneuroma/ganglioneuromatosis, 95
  neuroma, 95

Muscle spindles, 28

Mycobacterial pseudotumor, 73

Myelin, 18

Myelin-associated glycoprotein, 20

Myofibroblastoma, differentiation from conventional schwannoma, 162

Myxoma, cutaneous, *see* Cutaneous myxoma

Myxopapillary ependymoma, differentiation from paraganglioma, 350

N

Nerve endings, 26
  Meissner corpuscles, 27
  muscle spindles, 28
  Pacinian corpuscles, 27

Nerve ganglion, *see* Ganglion cyst of nerve

Nerve sheath myxoma, 162, 297
  differentiation from conventional schwannoma, 162; from neurofibroma, 253; from neurothekeoma, 297, 301; from cutaneous myxoma, 303; from conventional schwannoma, 305

Neurilemoma, 129

Neurinoma, 129

Neuritis ossificans, 59

Neuroblastoma, differentiation from PNET, 457

Neurofibroma, 40, 86, 122, 129, 160, 177, 183, 201, **211**, 253, 257, 337, 403, 427, 510, 540
  association with neurofibromatosis 1, 211, 509
    neurofibroma types in NF1, 510
  dendritic cell neurofibroma with pseudorosettes, 253
  differentiation from traumatic neuroma, 40; from palisaded encapsulated neuroma, 87; from neuromuscular choristoma, 122; from schwannoma, 129, 162, 177, 183, 201, 253;

from MPNST, 255, 402, 407; from ganglioneuroma, 255, 337; from dermatofibrosarcoma protuberans, 255; from nerve sheath
myxoma, 255; from spindle cell lipoma, 255;
from congenital and neuronevi, 255;
from plexiform histiocytic tumor, 257;
from schwannomatosis, 537
  diffuse cutaneous neurofibroma, 215
  DNA flow cytometry, 245
  general features, 211
  genetics, 212
  immunohistochemical findings, 244
  localized cutaneous neurofibroma, 213
  localized intraneural neurofibroma, 218
  malignant changes, 245
  massive soft tissue neurofibroma, 223
  microscopic findings, 228, 233
  plexiform neurofibroma, 220
  Schwann cell composition, 211
  treatment and prognosis, 259
  ultrastructural findings, 244
  variants, 212
  visceral neurofibromas, 514
  with intratumoral schwannoma, 240
  with malignant epithelioid cell differentiation, 427
Neurofibromatosis 1 (NF1), 211, 382, 476, **507**
  and GIST, 476
  and MPNST, 382
  and neurofibroma, 211, 509
  central nervous system involvement, 517
    astrocytoma, 517
    neuroglial hamartoma, 521
    optic glioma, 517
  clinical features, 507
  comparison with NF2, 508
  diagnostic criteria, 509
  general features, 507
  localized/segmental, 512
  neurofibroma types, 510
  visceral neurofibromas, 514
Neurofibromatosis 2 (NF2), 130, 383, 508, **521**
  and conventional schwannoma, 130
  and ganglioneuroma, 320
  and MPNST, 383
  central nervous system involvement, 533
  comparison with NF1, 508
  diagnostic criteria, 524
  Gardner-Frazier NF2, 521
  general and clinical features, 521

  meningiomas, 521, **529**
  meningioangiomatosis, 532
  prognosis, 533
  schwannoma-meningioma, 533
  schwannomatosis, 535, *see also* Schwannomatosis
  vestibular schwannomas, 521
Neuroma, 33, 42, 50, 87, 95
  appendiceal neuroma, 95
  epithelial sheath neuroma, 52
  intestinal neuroma, 95
  intraneural injury neuroma, 50
  MEN 2B-unassociated neuroma, 95
  mucosal neuroma, 38, 87
  pacinian neuroma, 42
  traumatic neuroma, 33
Neuroglial hamartoma and NF1, 521
Neuromuscular choristoma, 117
  association with fibromatosis, 122
  clinical features, 117
  differentiation from malignant peripheral nerve
    sheath tumor with myogenic differentiation,
    122; from neurofibroma, 122; from rhabdo-
    myoma and leiomyoma, 122
  general features, 117
  gross and microscopic findings, 118
  treatment and prognosis, 123
Neuromuscular hamartoma, *see* Neuromuscular
  choristoma
Neurothekeoma, differentiation from nerve sheath
  myxoma, 297, 301
Neurotropic melanoma, 495
  differentiation from conventional MPNST, 499
Non-Hodgkin lymphoma, 369
Non-neurogenic tumors, 347, *see also under*
  individual entities
  adrenal adenoma, 366
  amyloidoma, 373
  angioma, 350
  angiosarcoma, 372
  cutaneous meningioma, 366
  glomus tumor, 351
  hemangioblastoma, 356
  hemangiopericytoma, 372
  lipoma, 347
  meningioma, 361
  non-Hodgkin lymphoma, 372
  paraganglioma, 347
  synovial sarcoma, 366

O

Optic glioma and NF1, 517
Oral pseudoperineurioma, 49

P

Pacinian corpuscles, **27**, 42
    differentiation from Pacinian neuroma, 48
Pacinian corpuscle hyperplasia, *see* Pacinian neuroma
Pacinian corpuscle neuroma, *see* Pacinian neuroma
Pacinian neuroma, 42
    differentiation from Pacinian corpuscle, 47
Pacinioma, *see* Pacinian neuroma
Palisaded encapsulated neuroma, 35, **81**
    clinical features, 81
    differentiation from traumatic neuroma, 35, 86; from schwannoma, 87, 183; from neurofibroma, 87; from mucosal neuroma, 87, 93; from angioleiomyoma, 87
    general features, 81
    immunohistochemical and ultrastructural findings, 86
    microscopic findings, 82
    treatment and prognosis, 87
Paraganglioma, 347
    differentiation from myxopapillary ependymoma, 350
Parasympathetic ganglia, 22
Perineurial cell tumors, **265**, 312
    hybrid granular cell-perineurial cell tumors, 312
    perineurioma, 265, *see also* Perineurioma
Perineurial MPNST, 414
Perineurioma, 129, **265**, 364, 407, *see also under individual entities*
    differentiation from schwannoma, 129, 282; from meningioma, 364; from MPNST, 407
    hybrid schwannoma/perineurioma, 289
    intestinal perineurioma, 286
    intraneural perineurioma, 266
    soft tissue perineurioma, 274
Perineurium, normal, 13
Peripheral neurofibromatosis, *see* Neurofibromatosis 1
Peripheral nerve tumors, 1
    anatomy, 1
    classification, 1
    histology, 1
    historical background, 2

specimen handling, 6, *see also* Specimen handling
Peripheral nerves, **14**, 25
    special stains, 25
Peripheral nervous system, normal, 11
    development, 11
    gross anatomy, **11**, 15
    immunohistochemistry, 28
    microanatomy, 14
    ultrastructure, 30
    vascular supply, 17
Phakomatoses, 507
Pheochromocytoma, and MPNST, 455
Pigmented neurofibroma, differentiation from melanotic schwannoma, 199
Plantar neuroma, *see* Localized interdigital neuritis
Plasma cell granuloma, *see* Inflammatory pseudotumor of nerve
Plexiform fibrohistiocytic tumor, differentiation from plexiform neurofibroma, 257
Plexiform neurofibroma, 183, **220**, 257
    differentiation from plexiform schwannoma, 183, 257; from plexiform fibrohistiocytic tumor, 257
Plexiform schwannoma, **178**, 187, 257
    congenital and childhood plexiform cellular schwannoma, 184
    differentiation from palisaded encapsulated neuroma, 183; from traumatic neuroma, 183; from plexiform neurofibroma, 183, 257; from leiomyoma, 183
Plexosarcoma, 475
Primitive neuroectodermal tumor (PNET), 441, **457**, 503
    and MPNST, 441
    differentiation from soft tissue PNET, 458; from neuroblastoma, 458
    general features, 457
    gross and microscopic findings, 458
    immunohistochemical and ultrastructural findings, 458
    soft tissue PNET metastatic to nerve, 503
Psammomatous melanotic schwannoma, 188, 190
Pseudocyst of nerve, *see* Ganglion cyst of nerve

R

Ramon y Cajal, Santiago, 5
Reactive lesions, 33, *see also under individual entities*
    endometriosis of sciatic nerve, 57
    epithelial sheath neuroma, 52

ganglion cyst of nerve, 53
heterotopic ossification of nerve, 59
intraneural injury neuroma, 50
localized interdigital neuritis, 35, 41
oral pseudoperineurioma, 49
Pacinian neuroma, 42
traumatic neuroma, 33
Reactive perineurial proliferations, 50
Reticular schwannoma, 148
Reticular schwannoma/perineuroma, 289
Rhabdomyosarcoma, 431, 433
and MPNST, 431
differentiation from malignant triton tumor, 433

S

Sarcoidosis of peripheral nerve, 71
Sarcoma metastatic to nerve, 494
Schwann, Theodor, 2
Schwann cell, 1, **17**
Schwann cell-derived MPNST, **416**, 429
divergent epithelial differentiation, 429
divergent mesenchymal differentiation, 431
Schwannoglioma, 129
Schwannoma, 40, 71, 87, 93, **129**, 289, 444, 533
cellular schwannoma, 165, *see also* Cellular schwannoma
conventional schwannoma, 129, *see also* Conventional schwannoma
hybrid tumors, 289
melanotic schwannoma, 187, *see also* Melanotic schwannoma
mixed schwannoma-meningioma, 533
plexiform schwannoma, 178, *see also* Plexiform schwannoma
schwannoma and MPNST, 441
schwannomatosis, 535, *see also* Schwannomatosis
Schwannoma, cellular, *see* Cellular schwannoma
Schwannoma, conventional, *see* Conventional schwannoma
Schwannoma, melanotic, *see* Melanotic schwannoma
Schwannoma, plexiform, *see* Plexiform schwannoma
Schwannoma/meningioma, 533
Schwannoma/perineuroma, 289
Schwannomatosis, 131, **535**
clinical features, 535
diagnostic criteria, 536
differentiation from neurofibroma, 537;

from cellular schwannoma, 540
gross and microscopic findings, 536
Secondary tumors, 491
carcinoma, 491
lymphoma/leukemia, 502
neurotropic melanoma, 495
PNET of soft tissue, 503
sarcoma, 494
Sensory ganglia, 20
ganglion cells, 21
Soft tissue perineurioma, 274
atypical cellular perineurioma, 278
clinical features, 275
conventional type, 274
differential diagnosis, 283
general features, 274
gross and microscopic findings, 275
immunohistochemical and ultrastructural findings, 283
molecular findings, 283
reticular type, 274
sclerosing type, 274
treatment and prognosis, 285
Solitary circumscribed neuroma, *see* Palisaded encapsulated neuroma
Solitary polypoid intestinal ganglioneuroma, 98
Specimen handling, peripheral nerve tumors, 6
diagnostic pitfalls, 6
gross features, 7
specimen types, 6
Spinal epidural lipomatosis, 347
Spindle cell lipoma, differentiation from neurofibroma, 255
Stains, peripheral nerves, 25
Stout, Arthur Purdy, 4
Synovial sarcoma, **366**, 407, 439
differentiation from MPNST, 366, 407

T

Traumatic neuroma, **33**, 86, 93, 183
differentiation from localized interdigital neuritis, 35; from palisaded encapsulated neuroma, 38, 87; from mucosal neuroma, 38, 93; from neurofibroma, 35; from schwannoma, 38, 40, 183
True neuroma, 33
Tuberculoid leprosy, 75

U

Ultrastructure, normal nerve, 30

V

Vater-Pacini corpuscles, 27
Venous angioma, 350
Verocay, Jose, 3

Vestibular schwannoma and NF2, 521, **525**
Virchow, Rudolf, 2
Visceral malignant peripheral nerve sheath tumor, 386
Visceral neurofibromas and NF1, 514
Visceral schwannoma, 139
Von Recklinghausen, Frederick, 3
Von Recklinghausen disease, *see* Neurofibromatosis